INTENSIVE REVIEW FOR THE EMERGENCY MEDICINE QUALIFYING EXAMINATION

Sassan Naderi, MD, MS

Assistant Professor of Emergency Medicine
Director of International Emergency Medicine Fellowship
North Shore-Long Island Jewish Health Systems Manhasset, New York

Richard Park, MD

Assistant Professor of Emergency Medicine
Nassau University Medical Center
East Meadow, New York

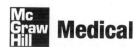

Medical

New York   Chicago   San Francisco   Lisbon   London   Madrid
Mexico City   Milan   New Delhi   San Juan   Seoul
Singapore   Sydney   Toronto

Intensive Review for the Emergency Medicine Qualifying Examination

1 2 3 4 5 6 7 8 9 0   QWD/QWD   12 11 10 9

Set ISBN   978-0-07-150280-1; MHID 0-07-150280-7
Book ISBN 978-0-07-150281-8; MHID 0-07-150281-5
CD ISBN   978-0-07-150282-5; MHID 0-07-150282-3

This book was set in Times by International Typesetting and Composition.
The editor was Catherine Johnson.
The production manager was Phil Galea.
Project managment was provided by Preeti Longia Sinha, International Typesetting and Composition.
The cover designer was Aimee Davis.
The indexer was Robert Swanson.
Quebecor World Dubuque was printer and binder.

This book is printed on acid-free paper.

NOTICE

Library of Congress Cataloging-in-Publication Data

Intensive review for the emergency medicine qualifying examination/[edited by] Sassan Naderi, Richard Park.
     p. ; cm.
    Includes bibliographical references and index.
    ISBN-13: 978-0-07-150280-1 (pbk. : alk. paper)
    ISBN-10: 0-07-150280-7 (pbk. : alk. paper)
     1. Emergency medicine—Outlines, syllabi, etc.   2. Emergency medicine—Examinations—Study guides.
    I. Naderi, Sassan.   II. Park, Richard.
    [DNLM: 1. Emergencies—Examination Questions.   2. Emergency
    Treatment—methods—Examination Questions.   WB 18.2 I6115 2009]
    RC86.92.I58 2009
    616.02′5—dc22
                                                                                    2009015303

CONTENTS

Color Insert appears between pages 150 and 151
Practice Examination

CONTRIBUTORS

Barbara Barnett, MD, FAAEM, FACEP
Assistant Professor of Clinical Emergency
Medicine and Internal Medicine
Program Director
Combined Emergency Medicine/Internal
Medicine Residency Program
Albert Einstein College of Medicine
Bronx, New York
Chapter 17, Dermatologic Emergencies

Brian Cameron, MD
Resident
Department of Emergency Medicine
Long Island Jewish Medical Center
New Hyde Park, New York
Chapter 2, Orthopedic Emergencies
Chapter 25, Questions/Answers for CD

Michael Cassara, DO, FACEP
Assistant Professor
Department of Emergency Medicine
New York University School of Medicine
New York, New York
Assistant Program Director
Emergency Medicine Residency Program
North Shore University Hospital
Manhasset, New York
Chapter 19, Hematology and Oncology
Chapter 24, Visual Stimulation

Gar Chan, MD
Assistant Professor of Clinical Emergency
Medicine
Attending Physician
Department of Emergency Medicine
New York University School of Medicine
New York, New York
Chapter 14, Gastrointestinal Emergencies

William Chiang, MD
Associate Professor of Emergency Medicine
New York University School of Medicine
Chief of Service
Department of Emergency Medicine
Bellevue Hospital Center
New York, New York
Chapter 9, Urologic and Renal Emergencies

Aaron Dora-Laskey, MD
Physician Management Group
Dayton, Ohio
Chapter 24, Visual Stimulation

Moira Davenport, MD
Assistant Professor of Emergency Medicine
Associate Fellowship Director, Primary Care
Sports Medicine
Allegheny General Hospital
Drexel University College of Medicine
Team Physician, Pittsburgh Pirates
Baseball Club
Pittsburgh, Pennsylvania
Chapter 2, Orthopedic Emergencies

Mikhail Elfond, DO
Attending Physician
Department of Emergency Medicine
Nassau University Medical Center
East Meadow, New York
Chapter 25, Questions/Answers for CD

Ugo A. Ezenkwele, MD, MPH
Assistant Professor of Clinical Emergency
Medicine
Attending Physician
Department of Emergency Medicine
New York University School of Medicine
New York, New York
Chapter 10, Ophthalmologic Emergencies

Gino Farina, MD
Associate Professor of Clinical Emergency
Medicine
Residency Director
Department of Emergency Medicine
Long Island Jewish Medical Center
Albert Einstein College of Medicine
New Hyde Park, New York
Chapter 6, Pulmonary and Critical Care
Chapter 16, Emergency Procedures

Jacob Goertz, MD, RDMS, FACEP
Assistant Professor of Emergency Medicine
Department of Emergency Medicine
Albert Einstein College of Medicine
Attending Physician and Director of Emergency
Ultrasound
Department of Emergency Medicine
Long Island Jewish Medical Center
New Hyde Park, New York
Chapter 22, Emergency Ultrasound

Dario Gonzalez, MD
Assistant Professor of Clinical Emergency
Medicine
Department of Emergency Medicine
Albert Einstein College of Medicine
Division Medical Director, NYC Fire
Department
New York, New York
Chapter 21, Prehospital Care

Howard A. Greller, MD, FACEP
Assistant Professor of Emergency Medicine
New York University School of Medicine
Attending Physician
Department of Emergency Medicine
North Shore University Hospital
Manhasset, New York
Chapter 15, Infectious Emergencies
Chapter 20, Psychiatric Emergencies

Robert Hessler, MD
Associate Professor of Emergency Medicine
and Medicine (clinical pharmacology)
Department of Emergency Medicine
New York University School of Medicine
New York, New York
Chapter 5, Cardiac Emergencies

Robert S. Hoffman, MD
Associate Professor of Emergency Medicine
and Medicine (clinical pharmacology)
Department of Emergency Medicine
New York University School of Medicine Director
New York City Poison Control Center
New York, New York
Chapter 4, Toxicologic Emergencies

Behdad Jamshahi, MD
Assistant Professor of Emergency Medicine
Department of Emergency Medicine
New York University School of Medicine
New York, New York
Chapter 11, Dental, Ear, Nose, and Throat
Emergencies

Tushar Kapoor, MD
Attending Physician
Department of Emergency Medicine
Nassau University Medical Center
East Meadow, New York
Chapter 18, Immunology and Rheumatology

Brad J. Kaufman, MD, MPH
Assistant Professor of Emergency Medicine
Albert Einstein College of Medicine
Bronx, New York
Division Medical Director, NYC Fire
Department
New York, New York
Chapter 18, Immunology and Rheumatology

Benjamin Kavinoky, DO
Chief Resident
Department of Emergency Medicine
Long Island Jewish Medical Center
New Hyde Park, New York
Chapter 10, Ophthalmology

Nicole Kriss, MD
Chief Resident
Department of Emergency Medicine
Long Island Jewish Medical Center
New Hyde Park, New York
Chapter 13, Endocrine and Metabolic
Emergencies

Eric Legome, MD
Associate Professor of Emergency Medicine
New York Medical College
Valhalla, New York
Chairman
Department of Emergency Medicine
St. Vincent's Hospital, Manhattan
New York, New York
Chapter 3, Trauma

Corey Long, MD
Department of Emergency Medicine
New York University/Bellevue Hospital Center
New York, New York
Chapter 24, Visual Stimulation

Gary Mazer, MD
Attending Physician
Department of Emergency Medicine
Long Island Jewish Medical Center
New Hyde Park, New York
Chapter 13, Endocrine and Metabolic
Emergencies

Christopher McStay, MD
Assistant Professor and Assistant Director of
Emergency Services
Bellevue Hospital Center
Department of Emergency Medicine
New York University School of Medicine
New York, New York
Chapter 8, Gynecologic and Obstetric
Emergencies

Carl A. Mealie, MD, FAAEM, FACEP
Assistant Professor of Clinical Emergency
Medicine
Albert Einstein College of Medicine
Bronx, New York
Chief of Emergency Management
Long Island Jewish Medical Center
New Hyde Park, New York
Chapter 12, Neurologic Emergencies

Francesco Mule, MD
Attending Physician
Department of Emergency Medicine
Long Island Jewish Medical Center
New Hyde Park, New York
Chapter 1, Intensive Review of Pediatric
Emergencies

Kevin Munjal, MD
EMS/Disaster Preparedness Fellow
New York City Fire Department
New York, New York
Attending Physician
Department of Emergency Medicine
Long Island Jewish Medical Center
New Hyde Park, New York
Chapter 19, Hematology and Oncology

Dimitrios Papanagnou, MD, MPH
Resident of Emergency Medicine
Department of Emergency Medicine
New York University School of Medicine
New York, New York
Chapter 7, Environmental Emergencies

Mohamed A. Peera, MD
Chief Resident
Department of Emergency Medicine
Long Island Jewish Medical Center
New Hyde Park, New York
Chapter 12 Neurologic Emergencies

Leo Pritsiolas, MD
Attending Physician Emergency Medical
Associates
Department of Emergency Medicine
Clara Maass Medical Center
Belleville, New Jersey
Chapter 13, Endocrine and Metabolic
Emergencies

Wayne Ramcharitar, MD
Chief Resident
Department of Emergency Medicine
Long Island Jewish Medical Center
New Hyde Park, New York
Chapter 14, Gastrointestinal Emergencies

Mityanand Ramnarine, MD
Resident
Department of Emergency Medicine/Internal
Medicine
Long Island Jewish Medical Center
New Hyde Park, New York
Chapter 6, Pulmonary and Critical Care

Joshua A. Rocker, MD
Assistant Professor of Pediatrics and Emergency Medicine
Albert Einstein College of Medicine
Attending Physician
Department of Pediatric Emergency Medicine
Schneider Children's Hospital at Long Island Jewish Medical Center
New Hyde Park, New York
Chapter 1, Intensive Review of Pediatric Emergencies

Adam J. Rosh, MD
Assistant Professor
Department of Emergency Medicine
Wayne State University School of Medicine
Assistant Resident Director
Detroit Receiving Hospital
Detroit, Michigan
Chapter 24, Visual Stimulation

Jasper Schmidt, MD
Attending Physician Emergency Medicine
Emergency Medical Associates
Richmond University County Medical Center
Staten Islan, New York
Chapter 9, Urologic and Renal Emergencies

David T. Schwartz, MD
Associate Professor of Emergency Medicine
New York University School of Medicine
Attending Physician
Department of Emergency Medicine
Bellevue Hospital and New York University School of Medicine
New York, New York
Chapter 24, Visual Stimulation

Kinjal Sethuraman, MD, MPH
Assistant Professor
Department of Emergency Medicine
North Shore-Long Island Jewish Health System
Manhasset, New York
Chapter 21, Prehospital Care

Anand Swaminathan, MD, MPH
Chief Resident
New York University/Bellevue Hospital Center
Department of Emergency Medicine
New York, New York
Chapter 11, Dental, Ear, Nose, and Throat Emergencies

Taku Taira, MD
Department of Emergency Medicine
State University of New York-Stony Brook
Stony Brook, New York
Chapter 5, Cardiac Emergencies

Kevin Tao, MD
New York University/Bellevue Hospital Center
Department of Emergency Medicine
New York, New York
Chapter 8, Gynecologic and Obstetric Emergencies

Paul Testa, MD, JD, MPH
Instructor
Department of Emergency Medicine
New York University School of Medicine
New York, New York
Chapter 3, Intensive Review of Trauma

Listy Thomas, MD
Attending Physician
Department of Emergency Medicine
St. Vincent's Medical Center
Bridgeport, Connecticut
Chapter 17, Dermatologic Emergencies

Deven Unadkat, DO, MPA
Attending Physician
Department of Emergency Medicine
Long Island Jewish Medical Center
New Hyde Park, New York
Chapter 23, High Yield Word Association

Kyle Vanstone, MD
Department of Emergency Medicine
Long Island Jewish Medical Center
New Hyde Park, New York
Chapter 16, Emergency Procedures

Maria Vasilyadis, MD
Chief Resident in Emergency Medicine
Department of Emergency Medicine
New York University School of Medicine
New York, New York
Chapter 2, Orthopedic Emergenices

Susi Vassallo, MD
Assistant Professor of Emergency Medicine
Attending Physician
Department of Emergency Medicine
New York University School of Medicine
New York, New York
Chapter 7, Environmental Emergencies

Diana Tran Vo, MD
Resident
New York University/Bellevue Hospital Center
Department of Emergency Medicine
New York, New York
Chapter 1, Intensive Review of Pediatric
Emergencies

Andrew Webber, DO
Attending Physician
Department of Emergency Medicine
Danbury Hospital
Danbury, Connecticut
Chapter 23, High Yield Word Association

Ethan S. Wiener, MD, FAAP
Assistant Professor of Emergency Medicine
Mt. Sinai School of Medicine
Associate Director, Pediatric Emergency
Medicine
Goryeb Children's Hospital
Morristown Memorial Hospital
Morristown, New Jersey
Chapter 1, Intensive Review of Pediatric
Emergencies

Chapter 1
INTENSIVE REVIEW OF PEDIATRIC EMERGENCIES

Ethan S. Wiener, Joshua A. Rocker, Diana Tran Vo, and Francesco Mule

I. Pediatric Infectious Disease

A. Fever: core temp >38.0°C (100.4°F)
  1. Neonates <28 days old
    a. Etiology
      i. Common Infections (in order of frequency)
        a) Urinary tract infection (UTI) ~10%
        b) Bacteremia ~3%
        c) Bacterial meningitis ~1% to 2%
        d) Cellulitis
        e) Septic arthritis
        f) Bacterial gastroenteritis
        g) Pneumonia
    b. Pathogens: unique flora from maternal genital tract
      i. Group B beta streptococcus (GBBS) most common organism
      ii. Gram-negative rods (*E. coli*)
      iii. Listeria—treat with ampicillin
      iv. *S. pneumoniae, H. influenzae,* and *N. meningitidis* in slightly older neonates
        a) 12% chance of serious bacterial infection (SBI)
      v. Viruses such as herpes simplex and varicella may also cause serious illness
    c. Risk Factors
      i. Premature rupture of membranes
      ii. Maternal fever
      iii. Maternal infection-chorioamnionitis
      iv. Maternal GBBS colonization
    d. Diagnosis
      i. Full sepsis workup and admission for antibiotics regardless of appearance
        a) Urinalysis (UA) and culture
          i) Obtain by transurethral or suprapubic route
        b) Complete blood count (CBC)
        c) Blood culture
        d) Lumbar puncture for cerebrospinal fluid (CSF)
          i) Cell count, protein, glucose, and culture
          ii) Herpes simplex virus (HSV) for polymerase chain reaction testing (PCR) in select neonates
            (a) Ill-appearing
            (b) Signs of meningitis
            (c) Maternal history of herpes
            (d) Mucocutaneous vesicles
        e) Chest x-ray (CXR)—only if respiratory symptoms
        f) Stool—only if diarrhea (think *Salmonella*)
    e. Management
      i. Treat empirically with antibiotics
        a) Ampicillin (100–200 mg/kg/day divided every 6 hours) PLUS gentamicin (2.5 mg/kg/dose every 8 hours) or
        b) Ampicillin plus cefotaxime provide important synergy for GBBS (can be resistant to ampicillin alone)
      ii. Add acyclovir if suspicious for HSV
      iii. Admit all patients <28 days with fever
      iv. Aspirin not used as antipyretic in children (Reye syndrome)
        a) Reye syndrome
          i) Etiology
            (a) Unknown mechanism
            (b) Noninflammatory condition associated with aspirin use in children during a febrile illness (especially of viral etiology)
            (c) Results in fatty liver and encephalopathy
          ii) Symptoms and signs
            (a) Vomiting or lethargy

(b) Delirium

(c) Seizures and loss of consciousness

iii) Diagnosis

(a) Fatty liver with 3-fold increase in hepatic transaminases or ammonia level

(b) CSF with <8 mm^3 white blood cells

(c) Cerebral biopsy with cerebral edema and no inflammation

iv) Prevention

(a) Centers for Disease Control and Prevention (CDC) recommends avoiding aspirin in patients <19 years

v) Management

(a) Supportive

2. Children 29 days to 3 years

a. Epidemiology

i. Viral infections are the most common cause of fever

ii. UTI is most common SBI

b. Etiology

i. Viral

a) Respiratory syncytial virus (RSV)—bronchiolitis

b) Roseola—rash with defervesence

c) Parvovirus B19—Fifth disease

d) Coxsackie A—Hand-foot-mouth disease

ii. Bacterial

a) UTI ~2%–19% (see Genito-urinary and Renal section below)

i) *E. Coli* usual pathogen

ii) Must rule out urine infection in

(a) Febrile females <2 years

(b) Males <1 year, or uncircumcised older males

(c) Viral infection, otitis, etc. do **not** change the risk of UTI

b) Bacteremia ~1%–3%

i) *S. pneumonia*, GBBS

ii) Occult bacteremia less common due to conjugated pneumococcal vaccine

c) Bacterial gastroenteritis ~2%

i) *Salmonella*

d) Meningitis ~1%

i) *S. pneumoniae, N. meningitides,* GBBS

e) Cellulitis ~1%

i) *S. aureus,* group A streptococcus

f) Pneumonia

i) *H. influenzae* and *S. pneumonia* rates decreasing as a result of Hib and pneumococcal vaccines

c. Symptoms and signs

i. Signs of serious illness include

a) Hypothermia (especially in infants and neonates)

b) Lethargy, vomiting, poor feeding, tachypnea, jaundice

d. Diagnosis

i. Low risk for SBI: rarely requires full sepsis workup

a) Well-appearing, previously healthy

b) Immunized

c) SBI risk decreases with

i) WBC between 5000 and 15,000 without bandemia

ii) Normal urinalysis

iii) Normal CXR and stool if performed

ii. High-risk children

a) Nonimmunized

b) Ill-appearing

c) Full sepsis workup (blood, urine, CSF, +/– CXR, and stool) necessary

e. Management

i. Low-risk, well-appearing child

a) Treat infection source

b) May be discharged with reliable follow-up within 24 hours

c) If no fever source

i) Antibiotics not indicated in well appearing child

ii. High-risk, ill-appearing child

a) Admission

b) Empiric antibiotics

i) Third-generation cephalosporin

(a) Ceftriaxone: 50 mg/kg/dose, or 100 mg/kg/24 hours for meningitis

(b) Cefotaxime can be given instead of ceftriaxone in hyperbilirubinemic infants

B. Common infections

1. Conjunctivitis in neonates (<28 days)

a. Chemical conjunctivitis (earlier onset than *Chlamydia trachomatis*)

i. Reaction to silver nitrate, erythromycin, or tetracycline drops given empirically at birth to protect from chlamydia and gonorrhea conjunctivitis

ii. Symptoms and signs

a) Conjunctival hyperemia and eye discharge

iii. Management

a) Resolves spontaneously within 2 to 4 days

b. *Neisseria gonorrhea*

i. Symptoms and signs

a) Onset 2 to 4 days

b) Bilateral copious purulent discharge

c) Potentially life threatening

ii. Diagnosis

a) Gram stain reveals intracellular diplococci

b) Initiate full sepsis workup because of high-risk systemic disease

c) Septic arthritis most common manifestation of disseminated disease

iii. Management

a) **Admit** for IV antibiotics (cefotaxime or ceftriaxone)

b) Copious and frequent saline irrigation

c) Treat mother, partners, and screen for other sexually transmitted diseases

c. *Chlamydia trachomatis*

i. Etiology

a) Exposure during vaginal delivery

b) Silver nitrate and erythromycin less effective for *Chlamydia* than for *N. gonorrhea*

ii. Symptoms and signs

a) Onset 5 to 14 days

i) Later onset than *N. gonococcal* conjunctivitis

b) Not as systemically ill in comparison with *N. gonococcal* conjunctivitis

c) Hyperemia, edema, watery or purulent discharge

d) Often unilateral

iii. Diagnosis

a) Cell scraping (palpebral conjunctiva)

iv. Management

a) Systemic macrolide (erythromycin 50 mg/kg/day × 14 days)

b) Cultures of blood and CSF are **not** required unless febrile or toxic-appearing

c) Treat mother and partners, and evaluate for other sexually transmitted diseases

d) Patients are usually **discharged**

v. Trachoma caused by chronic infection and scarring is a frequent cause of blindness worldwide (see Chapter 10 Ophthalmology)

d. Herpes simplex

i. Onset 2 to 14 days after birth (colonization occurs during birth)

ii. Diagnosis

a) Epithelial dendrites on slit lamp

iii. Management

a) Ophthalmology consult is required

b) Initiate full sepsis workup

i) CSF involvement common

ii) Check liver function tests (LFTs) as early sign of systemic involvement

c) IV acyclovir

2. Lymphadenitis

a. Definition: infection and/or enlargement of lymph node

b. Etiology: most often from benign viral or reactive causes

i. Anterior cervical lymphadenitis (mostly bacterial)

a) *S. aureus* and group A streptococcus account for great majority of cases

b) Occasional causes include *Mycobacterium, Tularemia, Yersinia pestis, Brucellosis*

ii. Posterior cervical lymphadenitis

a) Rubella

b) Infectious mononucleosis

c) Examine scalp for tinea capitis

c. Management

i. Do **not** attempt incision and drainage

a) Can cause persistent draining sinus

b) Computed tomography (CT) scan if abscess is suspected

ii. Ear, nose, throat (ENT) consult for

a) Airway compromise

b) Deep neck infection is source

c) Abscess is identified

iii. Antibiotics

a) Amoxicillin/clavulanic acid best coverage

b) Erythromycin or clindamycin in penicillin (PCN)-allergic patients

c) Use trimethoprim/sulfamethoxizole if cat scratch is a concern

3. Sinusitis

a. Definition: inflammation of paranasal sinuses

i. Usually precipitated by viral upper respiratory infection (URI)

a) Can distinguish from URI because symptoms last >7 days and may worsen

b. Anatomy

i. Sinus formation

a) Maxillary and ethmoid sinuses: aerate soon after birth

b) Frontal sinuses aerate ~5 to 7 years
c) Sphenoid sinuses aerate ~9 years
c. Symptoms and signs
   i. Persistent cough from postnasal drip (may be only symptom)
   ii. Purulent rhinorrhea
   iii. Fever
   iv. Headache
   v. Facial pain
d. Management
   i. Hastens resolution and avoids orbital and intracranial complications
   ii. 14-day course initially—treat until resolution
   iii. Use amoxicillin, cefuroxime, or amoxicillin-clavulanic acid
e. Complications
   i. Pott's puffy tumor (osteomyelitis of skull, usually frontal sinus)
   ii. Periorbital or orbital cellulitis
   iii. Cavernous sinus thrombosis
   iv. Epidural abscess
   v. Meningitis

II. Gastrointestinal Emergencies

A. Duodenal atresia
   1. Definition: middle portion of duodenum fails to open
   2. Epidemiology
      a. Associated with Down syndrome
   3. Symptoms and signs
      a. Bilious vomiting in the first few days of life
      b. Antenatal with polyhydramnios
      c. Early postnatal with feeding intolerance and emesis of all contents
   4. Diagnosis
      a. X-ray (Figure 1–1)
         i. "Double bubble" sign of distended stomach and proximal duodenum
         ii. Absence of bowel gas distally (obstruction pattern)
   5. Management
      a. Nasogastric tube to suction
      b. NPO
      c. IV fluids
      d. Surgical correction

B. Tracheoesophageal fistula
   1. Definition: congenital or acquired communication between trachea and esophagus
      a. 85% are proximal esophageal atresia with distal anastomosis

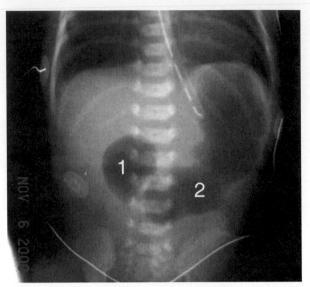

FIGURE 1–1. Duodenal atresia. "Double bubble" of stomach and proximal duodenum with absence of bowel gas. (Reproduced, with permission from Brunicardi FC, Andersen DK, Billiar TR, Dunn DL, Hunter JG, Matthews JB, Pollock RE, Schwartz SI: *Schwartz's Principles of Surgery,* 8th ed. Copyright © 2005, New York: McGraw-Hill.)

   2. Symptoms and signs
      a. Presents in the early neonatal period
         i. Copious frothy secretions
         ii. Feeding intolerance (choking and cyanosis)
   3. Diagnosis
      a. X-ray with paucity of intestinal bowel gas and coiling of nasogastric tube in proximal esophagus
   4. Management: surgical correction

C. Hirschsprung disease (congenital aganglionic megacolon)
   1. Definition: lack of ganglion cells in colon
      a. Leads to increase in muscle tone and contractility of aganglionic segment
      b. 75% occur in rectosigmoid area
   2. Symptoms and signs
      a. Neonatal presentation
      b. Delayed passage of meconium (>48 hours)
      c. Diminished stool frequency
      d. Abdominal distention
      e. Bilious emesis
      f. Less severe disease may present later with chronic constipation or failure to thrive
   3. Complications
      a. Enterocolitis
      b. Toxic megacolon

  i. Definition: massive dilation of colon proximal to aganglionic segment
  ii. Symptoms and signs: bloody stool, fever
  iii. Complications: high risk for perforation
4. Diagnosis
  a. X-ray
  b. Barium enema reveals a cone-shaped transitional zone
  c. Rectal manometry: lack of anal sphincter relaxation, rectal examination can alter results
  d. Rectal biopsy is the gold standard
5. Management
  a. Gastric decompression, rectal tube, IV fluids and antibiotics
  b. Surgical resection of segment

D. Necrotizing enterocolitis (NEC)
1. Definition
  a. Bowel necrosis of unknown etiology typically affect premature infants
2. Symptoms and signs
  a. Usually occurs in premature infants within the first 3 weeks of life
  b. Abdominal distention, pain, vomiting, poor feeding, bloody stool
  c. Systemic illness including lethargy, apnea, fever, and shock
3. Diagnosis
  a. X-ray findings are diagnostic (Figure 1–2)
    i. Pneumatosis intestinalis (intramural air) is pathognomonic for NEC
    ii. Free air (subdiaphragmatic or intraportal) is an ominous finding and a true surgical emergency
4. Management
  a. Decompression
  b. NPO
  c. Antibiotics
  d. Prolonged bowel rest
  e. Often requires surgical resection of necrotic bowel

E. Pyloric stenosis
1. Definition
  a. Idiopathic hypertrophy and elongation of pylorus causing gastric outlet obstruction
2. Risk factors
  a. Male
  b. Firstborn at highest risk
  c. Exposure to erythromycin
3. Symptoms and signs
  a. Occurs in the first 3 to 6 weeks of life
  b. Projectile **nonbilious** emesis

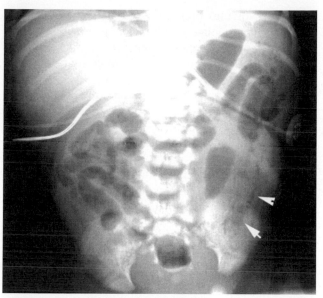

FIGURE 1–2. Necrotizing enterocolitis. Arrows point to areas of pneumatosis intestinalis. (Reproduced, with permission from Brunicardi FC, Andersen DK, Billiar TR, Dunn DL, Hunter JG, Matthews JB, Pollock RE, Schwartz SI: *Schwartz's Principles of Surgery,* 8th ed. Copyright © 2005, New York: McGraw-Hill.)

  c. Patient is hungry
  d. Olive in right upper quadrant (RUQ) —rarely palpable outside of anesthesia
4. Diagnosis
  a. Ultrasound is best
  b. Upper gastrointestinal (GI) series (string of pearls sign)
  c. Laboratory findings: **hypochloremic metabolic alkalosis** (late sign)
5. Management
  a. Surgical correction (pyloromyotomy)
  b. IV fluids

F. Malrotation and midgut volvulus
1. Etiology
  a. Incomplete rotation of intestine around superior mesenteric artery (SMA)
  b. Abnormal attachment of mesentery to the abdominal wall and ligament of Trietz
  c. Causes obstructive symptoms or volvulus (when small bowel twists around SMA causing midgut ischemia)
2. Symptoms and signs
  a. Most present with symptoms within the first year
  b. Up to 25% present >1 year, even into adulthood
  c. Malrotation may present with nonspecific signs and symptoms of incomplete obstruction (indigestion, bloating)

d. Volvulus presents with signs and symptoms of complete small bowel obstruction (**Bilious** vomiting, pain, distension)

e. Blood in stool (late finding suggesting gut ischemia)

f. Sepsis and shock with necrotic bowel

g. Chronic pain may exist with intermittent twisting and untwisting of bowel

3. Diagnosis
   a. X-ray
      i. A normal study does **not** rule out malrotation
      ii. May show partial or complete duodenal obstruction or gasless abdomen
      iii. Classic sign is double bubble sign (distended stomach and duodenum)
         a) Sign also seen in duodenal atresia
   b. Upper GI series—diagnostic study
      i. Misplaced duodenum (ligament of Treitz on the right)
      ii. With volvulus: "corkscrew" appearance of contrast

4. Management
   a. IV fluid resuscitation
   b. Nasogastric tube decompression
   c. Surgical consultation
   d. Antibiotics

G. Colic
   1. Definition
      a. Syndrome of inconsolable paroxysms of crying without an identifiable cause
      b. Typically occurs in the evening
      c. Infant typically stiffens, flexes hip, and passes flatus during episodes
   2. Etiology
      a. Unknown
      b. Occurs equally in breast-fed or formula fed infants
   3. Differential diagnosis (the inconsolable infant)
      a. Corneal abrasion
      b. Hair tourniquet
      c. Open diaper pin
      d. Nonaccidental trauma (abuse) with fracture
      e. Intracranial injury
      f. Testicular torsion
   4. Diagnosis
      a. Clinical diagnosis of exclusion
      b. Rule of 3s (Wessel criteria)
         i. Crying for >3 hours per day
         ii. >3 days per week
         iii. Lasting >3 weeks in otherwise healthy and well-fed infant
         iv. Usually within first 3 months

5. Management
   a. Self-limited and benign

H. Intussusception
   1. Definition
      a. Invagination of one portion of bowel into adjacent segment (telescoping)
      b. Predominantly in iliocecal region
         i. Ileoileal intussusception more common in patient with Henoch-Schönlein purpura
   2. Epidemiology
      a. Most common cause of intestinal obstruction in children 3 months to 5 years
      b. Average age is 7 to 8 months
      c. Male >female (3:1)
   3. Etiology
      a. Mesenteric lymphadenopathy
      b. Cystic fibrosis
      c. Meckel diverticulum
      d. Polyps
      e. Lymphoma
      f. Henoch-Schönlein purpura
      g. Idiopathic
   4. Symptoms and signs
      a. Classic triad—colicky pain, vomiting, and bloody ("currant jelly") stools
         i. All 3 signs seen in <20%
      b. Paroxysms of pain
      c. May appear completely well in between episodes
      d. Lethargy or altered mental status in between episodes
      e. Palpable vertical mass in RUQ
      f. Fever or shock with necrotic bowel
   5. Diagnosis
      a. Suggestive x-ray—target/crescent sign
      b. Ultrasound
      c. Enema (air or barium) can be both diagnostic and therapeutic
         i. Contraindicated if evidence of peritonitis or perforation
   6. Management
      a. Surgical consultation is recommended because of risk of perforation
      b. Air/barium enema
         i. Diagnostic and therapeutic
      c. Surgical reduction if enema is unsuccessful
      d. Recurrence is seen in 10% of patients (greatest in the first 48 hours)

I. Jaundice in the newborn
   1. Definitions
      a. Jaundice is the discoloration of skin and sclera caused by the accumulation of unconjugated (indirect) or conjugated (direct) bilirubin

    b. Kernicterus—neurotoxic hyperbilirubinemia

    c. Conjugated hyperbilirubinemia is always pathologic

2. Etiology (Table 1–1)

    a. Jaundice on first day of life

       i. Blood group system (ABO) or Rh incompatibility

       ii. Sepsis

       iii. Cephalohematoma

    b. Jaundice on days 2 to 3 of life

       i. Physiologic jaundice

         a) Etiology

           i) Increased breakdown of fetal reticulocytes

           ii) Decreased conjugation ability of the liver because of low uridine diphosphoglucuronyltransferase (UDPGT) activity

    c. Jaundice on days 4 to 7 of life

       i. Breast milk jaundice (BMJ)

         a) Etiology

           i) Diagnosis of exclusion

           ii) Multifactorial but poorly understood

           iii) Substance in breast milk interferes with UDPGT activity

           iv) Exclusive breast milk feeding delays establishment of gut flora and results in increased enterohepatic reabsorption of bilirubin

         b) Second peak in 2 weeks

       ii. Breast-feeding jaundice (BFJ)

         a) Etiology

           i) Distinct entity from BMJ

           ii) "Starvation jaundice"—inadequate breast milk volume leads to decreased bowel movements and decreased bilirubin excretion

    d. Jaundice >2 to 3 weeks of life

       i. Hypothyroidism

       ii. Galactosemia and other inborn errors of metabolism

3. Symptoms and signs

    a. Jaundice begins on top and progresses downward (cephalocaudal progression) as bilirubin levels increase

       i. Traditionally taught that jaundice in the face appears at bilirubin levels of 5 mg/dL and ~15 mg/dL if appreciated on the feet

       ii. Jaundice disappears in the opposite direction

    b. High-pitched "neuro" cry, seizures, and drowsiness represent severe jaundice and requires immediate attention

    c. Symptoms of pathologic jaundice (nonphysiologic, non-BMJ)

       i. Pale stool or dark urine with obstructive jaundice

       ii. Fever or evidence of focal infection

       iii. Evidence of hypothyroidism

       iv. Hepatosplenomegaly or petechiae should raise suspicion for hemolysis

4. Management

    a. Rule out and/or treat dangerous etiologies of jaundice

       i. Sepsis

         a) Treat underlying infection including meningitis

         b) Sepsis workup in the newborn

       ii. Suspected hemolysis

         a) Blood type to evaluate for ABO and Rh incompatibility

         b) Coombs testing, peripheral smear to assess erythrocyte morphology, reticulocyte count, CBC

       iii. Obstructive jaundice (conjugated hyperbilirubinemia)

         a) Fractionated bilirubin levels

         b) Ultrasound

       iv. Thyroid function testing and metabolic screening for galactosemia

    b. Treatment

       i. Treat underlying etiology

       ii. Fluids

       iii. Phototherapy indicated for levels >20 mg/dL in full-term infants and earlier for premature infants

TABLE 1–1. Causes of Neonatal Jaundice

<24 hours	**ABO, Rh incompatibility**
	Sepsis
	Congenital infections (eg, rubella, toxoplasmosis, cytomegalovirus)
	Excessive bruising from birth trauma (cephalahematoma or intramuscular hematoma)
2 to 3 days	**Physiologic**
3 days to 1 week	**Sepsis**
	Syphilis, toxoplasmosis, cytomegalovirus
>1 week	Septicemia, congenital atresia of bile ducts, serum hepatitis
	Congenital hemolytic anemias (sickle cell anemia, spherocytosis)
	Hemolytic anemia caused by drugs (G6PD deficiency)
	Rubella, herpetic hepatitis
	Hypothyroidism
	Breast milk jaundice

Source: Tintinalli JE, Kelen GD, Stapczynski JS: *Tintinalli's Emergency Medicine: A Comprehensive Study Guide,* 6th ed.

iv. Intravenous immune globulin for Rh or ABO isoimmunization

v. Exchange transfusions for severe cases (rarely performed)

vi. BMJ

   a) Increase frequency of feeds

   b) Rarely results in severe elevations requiring phototherapy

J. Bloody stool

1. Henoch-Schönlein purpura (see Rheumatologic Emergencies section below)

2. Infectious (see Pediatric GI section)

3. Intussusception

4. Milk protein allergies

5. Anal fissure

   a. Most common cause of rectal bleeding in infants up to 2 years

   b. Risk factors: constipation

   c. Management: stool softeners

6. Swallowed maternal blood

   a. Infants feeding from a cracked nipple

   b. Apt test can be used to distinguish fetal from maternal blood

      i. Maternal hemoglobin is subject to alkali denaturation, so supernatant changes from pink to brown in presence NaOH

      ii. Sample of fetal blood alone stays pink

7. Meckel diverticula

   a. Definition

      i. True diverticula of all 3 layers of the small intestines caused by incomplete obliteration of the vitelline duct

   b. Rule of 2s

      i. 2 years old

      ii. 2 feet from ileocecal valve

      iii. 2 inches long

      iv. 2% of the population

   c. Symptoms and signs

      i. Usually asymptomatic

      ii. Inflammation and bleeding (Meckel diverticulitis)—often contain heterotopic gastric tissue that can ulcerate adjacent bowel tissue

      iii. Obstruction—may become focus of volvulus, intussusception, or internal hernia

      iv. Sepsis with wall perforation

      v. Shock with severe bleeding

   d. Diagnosis

      i. Nuclear medicine scan (Meckel scan) utilizes radioactive tracer taken up by ectopic areas of gastric mucosal tissue

   e. Management

      i. Resuscitation if severe bleeding

      ii. Surgical resection

8. Hemolytic uremic syndrome (HUS)

   a. Definition

      i. Triad of microangiopathic hemolytic anemia (MAHA), thrombocytopenia, and progressive renal failure primarily in children 6 months to 4 years

      ii. Shares clinical features with thrombotic thrombocytopenic purpura (TTP)

   b. Epidemiology

      i. Most common cause of acute renal failure in children

      ii. Primarily in children 6 months to 4 years but may occur in adults

   c. Etiology

      i. Most cases associated with *E. coli* H7:0157 and production of Shiga-like toxin (verotoxin)

      ii. Less commonly a familial disease (3%)

      iii. Idiopathic

   d. Symptoms and signs

      i. Bloody diarrhea in 50% with Shiga-like toxin

      ii. Seizures and lethargy

      iii. Fever

      iv. Hypertension, edema with renal failure

      v. Petechiae

   e. Diagnosis

      i. Difficult to differentiate from TTP

         a) Renal dysfunction more pronounced with HUS

         b) Neurologic symptoms more pronounced with TTP

      ii. Urinalysis

         a) RBC casts

         b) Proteinuria

      iii. Laboratory

         a) Thrombocytopenia

         b) Anemia

         c) Evidence of renal dysfunction

      iv. Evidence of microangiopathic hemolytic anemia (nonimmune-mediated)

         a) Schistocytes on peripheral smear (RBC fragmentation)

         b) Elevated LDH

         c) Decreased haptoglobin

         d) Negative Coombs testing

   f. Management

      i. Supportive

      ii. Dialysis

      iii. Antibiotics not indicated

      iv. Plasmapharesis and intravenous immunoglobulin if unable to differentiate from TTP

K. GI foreign bodies (FBs)
1. Symptoms and signs
a. Drooling or feeding intolerance
2. Diagnosis
a. Anteroposterior (A-P) x-ray
i. Esophageal FBs seen in coronal plane "en face" (Figure 1–3)
ii. Tracheal FBs seen in sagittal plane on edge
b. Contrast CT or endoscopy may be needed to visualize radiolucent FBs
c. Obstruction occurs in areas of anatomic narrowing
i. C6—proximal third of esophagus under cricopharyngeal muscle
ii. T4—cardioesophageal junction at impingement of aortic arch
iii. Gastroesophageal junction
iv. If past pylorus: appendix, ileocecal valve, and Meckel diverticulum
3. Management
a. Swallowed objects often pass spontaneously
i. Serial x-rays to confirm passage may be needed
b. FBs likely to require removal
i. Objects >5 cm long or >2.5 cm wide (will not pass pylorus)
ii. Sharp objects
iii. Objects in esophagus >24 hours
iv. Objects that cause respiratory distress
v. Button batteries
a) Remove immediately if in esophagus
b) Observation if in stomach

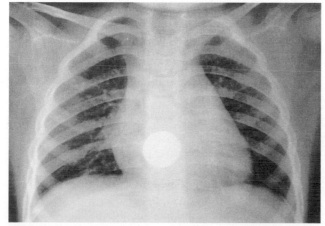

FIGURE 1–3. Coin in esophagus in coronal plane ("en face"). (Reproduced, with permission, from Stone CK, Humphries RL: *Current Diagnosis & Treatment: Emergency Medicine,* 6th ed.)

i) Requires serial x-rays to confirm passage
ii) May lodge in appendix or Meckel diverticula
c. Remove via endoscopy or interventional radiology

III. Dermatologic Emergencies (Table 1–2)

IV. Rheumatologic Emergencies

A. Henoch-Schönlein purpura (anaphylactoid purpura)
1. Definition
a. Small vessel vasculitis that occurs mainly in children presenting with triad of purpura, arthritis, and abdominal pain
2. Etiology
a. Preceded by URI in 50%
b. Drugs
i. Vancomycin, cefuroxime, and ACE inhibitors
3. Symptoms and signs
a. Purpura
i. Palpable purpura of lower extremities and buttocks
b. Colicky abdominal pain
i. May be a lead point for development of intussusception
ii. Bloody stool very common (30%)
c. Arthritis
i. Usually of wrists, elbows, and knees
ii. No permanent disability
d. Scrotal edema may mimic testicular torsion
e. Gross hematuria possible but uncommon
f. Hypertension with renal involvement
4. Diagnosis
a. Renal impairment in 40%
i. Elevated creatinine
ii. Proteinuria, hematuria, hypertension
iii. Progression to end stage renal disease (ESRD) in 1%
b. Normal or high platelets
i. In comparison with petechiae/purpura of idiopathic thrombocytopenic purpura (ITP) and TTP
c. Nonspecific elevation in erythrocyte sedimentation rate (ESR), C-reactive protein (CRP), and IgA
d. Unremitting abdominal pain may require ultrasound or barium enema to rule out intussusception
i. Ileoileal telescoping rather than more common ileocecal involvement
5. Management
a. Supportive care

TABLE 1–2.   Pediatric Rashes

DISEASE	CAUSE	RASH	TREATMENT	COMPLICATIONS
Impetigo	*S. aureus* or Group A streptococcus (GAS)	Honey crusted lesions, bullae	Mupirocin cream, oral (cephalexin)	Ecthyma (invasion dermis), poststrep-glomerulonephritis, rheumatic fever
Rubeola (measles)	Paramyxovirus	Erythematous, maculopapular (head towards feet) after cough, coryza, Koplik spots	Supportive/vaccination	Otitis media, pneumonia, laryngotracheitis
Rubella (German measles)	Rubella virus	Maculopapular, Forscheimer spots lymphadenopathy	Supportive/vaccination	Arthritis, encephalitis Congenital anomalies
Roseola (exanthem subitum)	HHV 6	Faint, blanching pink maculopapular rash (when high fever breaks)	Supportive	Febrile seizures
Fifth disease (erythema infectiosum)	Parvovirus B19	"Slapped cheek," maculopapular on trunks/extremities	Supportive	Aplastic anemia in sicklers Congenital anomalies
Scarlet fever	Group A streptococcus	"Sandpaper" rash on trunk and perineum Pastia lines on skin creases Perioral pallor	Penicillin	Rheumatic fever, glomerulonephritis (may occur despite antibiotics)
Varicella (chicken pox)	Varicella-Zoster virus	"Dew on petal" vesicles in multiple stages	Supportive/ vaccination	Bacterial superinfection, pneumonia, encephalitis, zoster Congenital abnormalities
Hand-foot-mouth disease	Coxsackie A virus	Oral ulcers, maculopapular vesicular on hands/feet	Supportive	None
Pityriasis rosea	Unknown but likely viral	"Herald Patch" Macules along cleavage lines "Christmas tree" pattern on back	Antihistamines, ultraviolet light	None

b. Most patients have spontaneous resolution of symptoms in 4 to 5 weeks

c. NSAIDs alleviate joint pain but careful with renal insufficiency

d. Steroids

   i. Indicated for severe abdominal and joint pain

   ii. Do not decrease incidence of renal involvement but lessens its severity

e. Admission

   i. Severe arthritis

   ii. Unrelenting abdominal pain

   iii. Renal involvement

     a) Elevated creatinine, hypertension, nephrotic syndrome

     b) Immunosuppressive agents or plasma-pheresis may be indicated

B. Kawasaki syndrome

1. Definition

   a. Poorly understood vasculitis most often affecting children <5 years

2. Epidemiology

   a. Leading cause of acquired heart disease in modern countries surpassing that of rheumatic heart disease

   b. More common in children of upper middle and upper class families

   c. More common in Japanese and Japanese Americans

   d. Slight male predominance

   e. Peak age 18 to 24 months

   f. Late winter and spring

   g. Epidemics of 3-year intervals

3. Symptoms and signs

   a. High fever relatively unresponsive to antipyretics

   b. Unilateral cervical lymphadenopathy >1.5 cm (least common sign)

   c. Mucous membrane involvement (strawberry tongue, lip fissures)

   d. Extremity changes (edema, erythema, and pain early on with desquamation ~10 to 14 days into course of disease)

e. Bilateral nonexudative conjunctivitis with/out iritis
f. Rash (nonvesicular)
4. Diagnosis
   a. Clinical
      i. At least 4 of the 5 signs mentioned above in addition to fever >5 days
      ii. With fever >5 days and <4 of the above signs, diagnosis also made with evidence of coronary artery disease on echocardiography
   b. Imaging
      i. Echocardiography
         a) Coronary artery aneurysms detected in 25% of untreated and 5% to 10% of those adequately treated
         b) Valvular incompetence
         c) Abnormal wall motion
         d) Pericardial effusion
      ii. Abdominal ultrasound may reveal hydrops (enlargement) of the gallbladder
   c. Laboratory
      i. Thrombocytosis (late sign when signs and symptoms begin to improve)
      ii. Sterile pyuria
      iii. Severe leukocytosis with left shift
      iv. Mild to moderate anemia
      v. Increased inflammation markers including CRP, ESR, and alpha$_1$ antitrypsin
      vi. Liver function tests may be elevated
      vii. Aseptic meningitis pattern on CSF if lumbar puncture performed
   d. ECG
      i. May reveal arrhythmias and evidence of myocarditis or even myocardial infarction
5. Management
   a. Maintain high clinical suspicion and consider treating even if all criteria are not met as most do not present classically
   b. Admit patient with cardiology consultation
   c. High-dose aspirin
   d. Intravenous gamma globulin (most important therapy)
   e. Use of steroids controversial and not currently standard practice
   f. Long-term anticoagulation often instituted after hospitalization
   g. Myocardial infarction is managed medically or with bypass surgery as cardiac catherization and stenting is not recommended
6. Complications
   a. Myocardial infarction from coronary artery aneurysms
   b. Congestive heart failure (CHF)

C. Rheumatic fever (see Chapter 18 Immunology/Rheumatology)
   1. Post group A beta-hemolytic streptococcus infection
   2. Rare in children <3 years

V. Airway Emergencies (see Chapter 11 HENT) (Table 1–3)

A. Airway Foreign Body
   1. Symptoms and signs
      a. Coughing, gagging, choking, or cyanosis
      b. Easy to miss—many present initially with postobstructive pneumonia
         i. Consider in all toddlers with respiratory symptoms
      c. Stridor, wheezing, unequal breath sounds
   2. Diagnosis
      a. CXR may be normal (usually not radiopaque)
         i. Decubitus or forced expiratory films to detect air trapping
         ii. Hyperinflated lung on affected side
         iii. ENT consult for laryngoscopy and pulmonary consult for bronchoscopy should be done based on clinical suspicion (history, history, history)
   3. Management
      a. In infants <1 year
         i. No mouth sweep
         ii. 5 back blows holding patient's abdomen on forearm and head lower than feet
         iii. 5 chest thrusts—remove object if seen in mouth
         iv. Repeat steps 2 and 3 until obstruction relieved
         v. If patient becomes unconscious, initiate CPR
            a) 2 small breaths (over nose and mouth)
            b) 30 chest wall compressions at rate of 100 compressions per minute
            c) Repeat this cycle
      b. 1 through 8 years
         i. Heimlich maneuver, mouth sweep to relieve obstruction
         ii. CPR if unconscious/apneic
            a) Sitting or straddling child
            b) 30 compressions per 2 breaths at rate of 100 compressions per minute

B. Epiglottitis
   1. Etiology
      a. *S. Aureus*, group A streptococcus, and anaerobes
      b. Classically, *H. influenza* now seen in nonimmunized children

TABLE 1–3. Airway Emergencies

	AGE	PRESENTATION	ETIOLOGY	DIAGNOSIS	TREATMENT
Peritonsillar abscess	>5 years or adolescent	Dysphagia, fever, "hot potato" voice following pharyngitis	GABHS S. aureus S. pneumoniae H. influenzae	Unilateral swelling, Uvular deviation	Drainage (needle vs. I&D) Antibiotics, steroids
Retropharyngeal abscess	<5 years	Febrile, toxic, drooling with limited neck extension	S. aureus GABHS anaerobes	Neck XR: widened retropharyngeal space, CT confirmation	Antibiotics Possible surgical debridement
Epiglottitis	Preschool-aged child (unimmunized)	Abrupt onset fever, dysphagia, dysphonia, and stridor; child in tripod/sniffing position	H. influenzae (rare post-H. influenzae vaccine) S. aureus, GABHS	Clinical, Soft tissue neck x-ray ("thumbprint" of enlarged epiglottis)	Respiratory support: Emergent/OR intubation Antibiotics in OR
Bacterial tracheitis	Infants	Symptoms similar to both croup and epiglottitis, stridor, cough fever, NO drooling	S. aureus, strep, mixed	Clinical (Laryngotracheo-bronchoscopy reveals adherant purulent membranes)	Respiratory support: Emergent/OR intubation, Antibiotics

2. Symptoms and signs
   a. Rapid onset fever, dysphagia, dysphonia, stridor
   b. Rare condition in post-*H. influenza* vaccine era
   c. Tripod positioning
3. Diagnosis
   a. Clinical, do **not** send to radiology for x-rays
   b. Lateral soft tissue of neck reveals "thumbprint" sign
4. Management
   a. Keep child comfortable
   b. Airway management by ENT and/or anesthesia in operating room
   c. Intravenous antibiotics **after** securing airway so as not to agitate child (ceftriaxone, cefotaxime)

C. Bacterial tracheitis
   1. Etiology
      a. *S. aureus, streptococcus, Moraxella catarrhalis, H. influenzae* type B (uncommon in vaccinated), *Klebsiella, pseudomonas,* anaerobes
   2. Symptoms and signs
      a. May be preceded by croup-like syndrome
      b. Toxic-appearing infant with stridor
      c. Productive cough
   3. Diagnosis
      a. Clinical suspicion should trigger emergent management
      b. Laryngotracheobronchoscopy reveals adherent purulent tracheal membranes

4. Management
   a. Similar to epiglottitis (intubation in operating room and antibiotics)

D. Peritonsillar abscess
   1. Epidemiology
      a. Uncommon in children <6 years
   2. Etiology
      a. GABHS, staphylococcus species, *S. pneumoniae, H. influenzae*
   3. Symptoms and signs
      a. Dysphagia, fever, asymmetric throat fullness, headache, "hot potato" voice following pharyngitis or tonsillitis
   4. Diagnosis
      a. Pharyngeal erythema
      b. Uvula displaced away from abscess
   5. Management
      a. Drainage—needle aspiration, I & D, or tonsillectomy
      b. Antibiotics
      c. Steroids may reduce symptoms and days of hospitalization

E. Retropharyngeal abscess
   1. Epidemiology
      a. Historically a disease of young children <6 years
      b. Increasing in frequency in adults
   2. Etiology
      a. *S. aureus,* group A streptococcus, and anaerobes
      b. Foreign body ingestion (chicken or fish bone)

3. Symptoms and signs
   a. Limited neck extension is hallmark
   b. Child febrile, toxic, and drooling
   c. Stridor
4. Diagnosis
   a. Soft tissue neck x-ray
      i. Widened retropharyngeal space that is >50% of vertebral body in width (C1 through C3)
      ii. Should be filmed with child's neck in slight extension
      iii. Neck flexion can give false-positive results
   b. CXR to rule out mediastinitis
   c. CT to determine extent of disease (cellulitis versus abscess)
5. Management
   a. Intravenous antibiotics
   b. ENT consultation for possible surgical drainage

VI. Respiratory Infections

A. Croup: (laryngotracheobronchitis)
   1. Epidemiology
      a. Children 6 to 36 months
      b. Fall and winter
   2. Etiology
      a. Parainfluenza type I
   3. Symptoms and signs
      a. URI symptoms with characteristic seal-like cough, stridor, respiratory distress, retractions
      b. Symptoms typically worse at night
      c. Hypoxia is uncommon
   4. Diagnosis
      a. CXR may show "steeple sign" caused by subglottic edema and narrowing
   5. Management
      a. Cool humidified oxygen
      b. Racemic epinephrine for severe symptoms
         i. Observe for 4 hours after treatment because of "rebound effect"
      c. Corticosteroids—dexamethasone 0.6 mg/kg PO or IM (equivalent efficacy)
      d. Heliox
         i. Decreases work of breathing by improving laminar flow
         ii. Reserved for severe croup
   6. Admit for
      a. Continued stridor after initial racemic epinephrine
      b. Hypoxemia
      c. Child is unable to eat or drink
      d. Concern about home situation or ability to return

B. Bronchiolitis
   1. Epidemiology
      a. Children <2 years
      b. Mostly seen in winter months (October through March)
      c. Ex-premature infants at greatest risk for severe disease
   2. Etiology
      a. RSV
   3. Symptoms and signs
      a. Cough, wheezing, respiratory distress/retractions
      b. Copious nasal secretions
      c. Difficulty feeding
      d. Low-grade fever
      e. May progress to respiratory failure requiring intubation
   4. Diagnosis
      a. PCR of nasotracheal aspirate for RSV
         i. Isolation of RSV-positive patients to prevent transmission
      b. CXR
         i. Hyperinflation
         ii. Increased peribronchial markings
         iii. Interstitial infiltrates
         iv. Segmental atelectasis
   5. Management
      a. Humidified oxygen and hydration
      b. Bronchodilators effective in minority of patients ($1/3$ helps, $1/3$ no change, $1/3$ worsens)
      c. Steroids not routinely recommended
   6. Admit patients who are
      a. Hypoxic
      b. Dehydrated
      c. Tachypneic (unable to feed)
      d. Most patients <1 month or premature birth
      e. Significant comorbid illnesses

C. Pneumonia (Table 1–4)
   1. Chlamydial pneumonia—seen in infants of 2 weeks to 3 months
      a. Symptoms and signs
         i. Gradually progressive **staccato** cough
         ii. Usually afebrile
         iii. Often with eye findings (erythema and discharge)
      b. Diagnosis
         i. Gold standard is positive culture from nasopharynx or conjunctiva
         ii. CXR demonstrates hyperinflation with bibasilar infiltrates, or nothing at all—can be a difficult diagnosis
      c. Management
         i. Erythromycin (50 mg/kg/day PO) based on clinical and CXR findings

TABLE 1–4. Pediatric Pneumonias

AGE	ETIOLOGY	MANAGEMENT
<28 days	Group B streptococcus, *E.coli,* *Klebsiella,* *S. aureus, streptococcus,* *Listeria, M. tuberculosis,* *Chlamydia* (see below), Viral (HSV, RSV), fungal (candida)	Ampicillin and gentamicin Vancomycin and gentamicin if suspicious of penicillin-resistant *S. aureus* Acyclovir if HSV suspected Erythromycin for chlamydia Admission, sepsis workup
1 to 3 months	Most commonly viral *S. pneumoniae,* GBBS, *H. influenzae* *Chlamydia* and *B. pertussis*	Third-generation cephalosporin, Add macrolide if chlamydia or pertussis suspected Admission
3 months to 5 years	Bacterial: Mostly by *S. pneumoniae,* also see *H. influenzae, Moraxella* *catarrhalis, S. aureus,* *S. pyogenes*	Supportive care if viral, amoxicillin is first line. Amoxicillin/clavulanate or third-generation cephalosporin for nonresponders Admit for hypoxemia, dehydration, respiratory distress, toxic appearance, underlying conditions, or concern for social situation
≥5 years	Same as above (usually *S. pneumoniae*) plus atypicals (*Mycoplasma, Chlamydia, Legionella*) Consider TB	Macrolide unless resistant *S. pneumoniae* (High-dose amoxicillin or third-generation cephalosporin)

ii. PO erythromycin also used to treat conjunctivitis alone: more effective, must assume subclinical airway involvement
iii. Treat mother and evaluate for sexually transmitted diseases

2. Pertussis ("whooping cough")
   a. Etiology-
      i. *Bordetella pertussis*
      ii. Immunity begins to wane 3 to 5 years after vaccination and essentially nonexistent after 12 years
   b. Symptoms and signs
      i. 3 stages
         a) Catarrhal phase: 1 to 2 weeks with "cold" symptoms:
            i) Rhinorrhea, mild cough, and low-grade fever
            ii) Infectious during this stage
         b) Paroxysmal phase
            i) 2 to 6 weeks of sudden paroxysmal attacks of coughing fits
            ii) Characteristic "whooping" cough
            iii) Associated with posttussive emesis, gagging, cyanosis, apnea, seizures, subconjunctival hemorrhages
         c) Convalescent phase: cough can last months, even with treatment
   c. Diagnosis

      i. Nasopharyngeal aspirate is most sensitive test—direct fluorescent antibody (DFA) and PCR
      ii. Impressive lymphocytosis (≥20 K) correlates with disease severity
      iii. Classic CXR has "shaggy right heart border"
   d. Treatment:
      i. Macrolide antibiotic
      ii. Consider admission
         a) <3 months
         b) 3 to 6 months with severe coughing paroxysms
         c) Significant comorbid illnesses
   e. Complications
      i. Pneumothorax
      ii. Encephalopathy, seizure
      iii. Young or premature infants are at risk for apnea in stage II of disease

VII. Medical Legal

A. Consent
   1. No parental consent required for[1]
      a. Life- and limb-threatening emergencies
      b. Emancipated minors (exact definition varies by state)
         i. Married
         ii. Member of armed forces
         iii. Living independently and self-supporting
         iv. Patient is a parent

          a) Pregnancy itself does **not** constitute emancipation

   c. Rights that are state dependent
     i. Child abuse
     ii. Pregnancy
     iii. Sexually transmitted disease treatment
     iv. Substance abuse

B. Child abuse and/or neglect
  1. Increased suspicion if
   a. Child lacks primary care
   b. Poor weight gain (failure to thrive)
   c. Poor hygiene
   d. Improperly dressed for climate
   e. Injuries consistent with corporal punishment
   f. Injuries in different stages of healing
   g. Injuries inconsistent with explained mechanism
  2. Munchausen syndrome by proxy
   a. Definition: type of abuse in which the caretaker feigns or induces illness in a person under their care in order to attain some type of emotional benefit
     i. Increased suspicion if a child is exposed to a harmful agent (toxin) or action (blunt trauma or smothering) by the guardian
  3. Fractures associated with abuse
   a. Very suspicious
     i. Metaphyseal fractures
       a) Also known as "bucket handle" or corner fractures (Figure 1–4)
       b) Pathognomonic for abuse
     ii. Posterior rib
     iii. Spinal process
     iv. Scapular
     v. Sternal
   b. Moderately suspicious
     i. Multiple fractures
     ii. Multiple fractures in different stages of healing
     iii. Vertebral body fractures
     iv. Complex skull fracture
     v. Fracture of digit
   c. Low suspicion
     i. Linear skull fractures
     ii. Clavicle
     iii. Long bone shaft

VIII. Apparent Life-threatening Event and Sudden Infant Death Syndrome

A. Apparent life-threatening event (ALTE)
  1. Definition[2]
   a. An episode that is frightening for the observer characterized by a combination of apnea, color change, and/or change in muscle tone

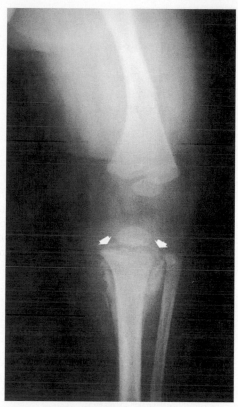

FIGURE 1–4. Bucket handle fractures suspicious for child abuse. (Reproduced, with permission from Knoop KJ, Stack LB, Storrow AB: *Atlas of Emergency Medicine,* 2nd ed.)

   b. ALTE is not a diagnosis, but rather a description of an event
  2. Etiology
   a. Idiopathic (majority)
   b. Gastroesophageal reflux disease (GERD) seen with arching of back, occurs postprandially
   c. Seizures
   d. Central apnea
   e. Infectious
     i. Meningitis, encephalitis, sepsis, pertussis, RSV
   f. Cardiac
     i. Congenital abnormality or arrhythmia
   g. Metabolic
   h. Child abuse/nonaccidental trauma
  3. Diagnosis
   a. History, vitals, and appearance of child in ED are paramount
   b. Based on history and appearance
     i. Workup may include D-stick, electrolytes, CBC, toxicology screen, urinalysis, urine/blood culture, CSF, ECG, CXR, and head CT
   c. Healthy infants may have respiratory pauses up to 20 seconds (known as "periodic breathing")

4. Management
   a. Treat underlying cause
   b. Admission with apnea monitor if
      i. Concerning history
      ii. History of cyanosis
      iii. Concerning labs

B. Sudden infant death syndrome (SIDS)[3]
   1. Definition
      a. Sudden death of any infant or young child that is unexpected by history and unexplained after a postmortem examination
         i. Examination includes an autopsy, investigation of the scene of death, and review of medical history
   2. Epidemiology
      a. Most common cause of death between 1 month and 1 year of age
      b. 1 in 750 newborns
      c. Peak incidence 2 to 4 months
      d. Rare <1 month and >6 months
   3. Risk factors
      a. Maternal smoking
      b. Maternal drug use
      c. Prone sleeping position
      d. Family history of SIDS
      e. Loose bedding
      f. Soft sleeping surfaces
      g. Male
      h. Prematurity
   4. Protective factors
      a. Breast-feeding
      b. Pacifiers
      c. "Back to Sleep" program
         i. Encourages sleeping in supine position
         ii. 50% reduction of SIDS rate

IX. Pediatric Advanced Life Support (PALS)

A. ABCs (airway, breathing, circulation)
   1. Airway
      a. Head tilt, chin lift for all ages
      b. Jaw thrust when considering cervical spine injury
      c. Intubation specifics
         i. ET tube size: age divided by 4 + 4
         ii. Traditionally, uncuffed ET tube <8 years
            a) New recommendations suggest usage of cuffed tubes >1 year (use one full size smaller than uncuffed tube)
         iii. Insertion distance = 3 × ET tube size
         iv. Cricothyroidotomy relatively contraindicated <8 years

2. Breathing
   a. Newborn: 30 to 60 breaths per minute
   b. Infant and child: 20 breaths per minute
3. Circulation
   a. Systolic blood pressure (BP) by age
      i. Birth to 1 month: >60 mm Hg
      ii. 1 month to 1 year: >70 mm Hg
      iii. 1 to 10 years: ≥70 + 2 × (age in years)
         a) Formula represents lowest fifth percentile for BP
      iv. >10 years: ≥90 mm Hg
   b. Heart rate by age
      i. <3 months: 85–205, mean 140
      ii. 3 months to 2 years: 100–190, mean 130
      iii. 2 to 10 years: 60–140, mean 80
      iv. >10 years: 60–100, mean 75
   c. Pulse check location
      i. Child: carotid
      ii. Infant: brachial or femoral
      iii. Newborn: umbilical
   d. Compressions
      i. Landmarks
         a) Child: lower half of sternum
         b) Infant and newborn: 1-finger width below intermammary line
      ii. Rate
         a) Newborn: 120 per minute
         b) Infant: >100 per minute
         c) Child: 100 per minute
      iii. Compression-ventilation ratio
         a) Two resuscitators 15:2
         b) Single resuscitator 30:2
   e. Vascular access
      i. Intraosseous
         a) Anterior tibia is the primary site
         b) 1 to 2 cm below tibial tuberosity on medial aspect of tibial plateau
         c) Safe for all medications
         d) Confirmation of insertion
            i) A decrease in resistance once the needle is advanced
            ii) The needle remains upright
            iii) Marrow can sometimes be aspirated through the needle
            iv) Fluid flows without subcutaneous infiltration
         e) Complications <1%
            i) Fracture
            ii) Compartment syndrome
            iii) Osteomyelitis
            iv) Severe extravasation
         f) Alternative sites
            i) Distal tibia on medial malleolus
            ii) Distal femur

      iii) Iliac crest
      iv) Sternum
   g) Contraindications
      i) Fracture proximal on ipsilateral extremity
      ii) Previous failed attempt at site
      iii) Overlying infection
  ii. Umbilical
    a) **2 arteries and 1 vein**
    b) Umbilical vein remains patent for 1 week
    c) Insert 5 French catheters 2 to 4 cm into the umbilical vein until flashback achieved

B. Pulseless ventricular tachycardia or fibrillation (Figure 1–5)

C. Pulseless electrical activity (PEA)/asystole
  1. Etiology (6 Hs, 5 Ts)
   a. **H**ypoxemia
   b. **H**ypoglycemia
   c. **H**ypovolemia
   d. **H**ypothermia
   e. **H**ypokalemia/hyperkalemia
   f. **H**ydrogen (acidosis)
   g. **T**amponade
   h. **T**ension pneumothorax
   i. **T**oxins
   j. **T**hromboembolism
   k. **T**rauma
  2. Management
   a. Treat underlying cause
   b. Oxygen and secure airway
   c. Epinephrine (q 3–5 minutes)

d. IV fluids
e. Atropine not found to be useful in pediatric asystole or PEA

D. Bradycardia
  1. Management of stable patient
   a. Support ABCs
   b. Evaluate cause (5 Hs, 1 T)
    i. Hypoxemia is most common cause
    ii. Hypothermia
    iii. Head injury
    iv. Heart block
    v. Heart transplant
    vi. Toxins
     a) β-blockers
     b) Calcium channel blockers
     c) Organophosphates
     d) Clonidine
  2. Management of unstable patient
   a. CPR
   b. **Epinephrine first line**
   c. Atropine second line
   d. Pace

X. Cardiology

A. Normal fetal circulation
  1. 2 parallel circuits
   a. Oxygenated blood leaves placenta by umbilical vein, bypassing liver through ductus venosus. Blood returns to right atrium (RA) via inferior vena cava and shunted across foramen ovale to left atrium (LA) → left ventricle (LV) → **ascending** aorta

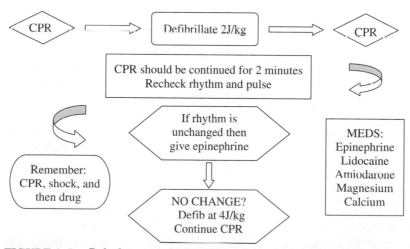

FIGURE 1–5. Pulseless ventricular tachycardia or fibrillation algorithm.

i. Results in relatively high oxygen-saturated blood → cerebral and coronary arteries, upper body and extremities

b. Desaturated blood from superior vena cava (returning from cerebral/cardiac circulation) → RA primarily directed into RV → pulmonary artery (PA). Since no alveolar oxygen, pulmonary vascular resistance (PVR) is high with majority of PA flowing via ductus arteriosus to the descending aorta → lower body and extremities → umbilical arteries → placenta

2. Circulatory changes with birth (2 circuits in series)
   a. Redirection of blood for oxygenation from placenta to lungs
   b. Fluid expelled from lungs, aeration of lungs → dilation of pulmonary vasculature, decreased peripheral vascular resistance
   c. Within minutes of improved oxygenation, umbilical arteries and vein, ductus arteriosus and ductus venosus contract
   d. Increased systemic resistance (2° no placenta >↑LA pressure) and decreased PA resistance >↓RA pressure changes flow and pressure gradient across foramen ovale causing flap of septum primum to press against septum secundum

B. Congenital heart disease
   1. Divided according to cyanotic or acyanotic presentation
      a. Cyanotic congenital heart disease (right to left shunt) (5 Ts with 1–5 mnemonic)
         i. Truncus arteriosus (vessels join to make **1**)
         ii. Transposition (**2** major vessels switched)
         iii. Tricuspid atresia (**3**)
         iv. Tetralogy of Fallot (**4** defects)
         v. TAPVR total anomalous pulmonary vascular return (**5** letters)
      b. Acyanotic (left to right shunt)
         i. ASD (atrial septal defect)
         ii. VSD (ventricular septal defect)
         iii. PDA (patent ductus arteriosus)
         iv. CoA (coarctation of aorta)
   2. Ductus arteriosus dependent—oxygenation improved with open ductus arteriosus
      a. Administration of prostaglandin E_1 keeps or reopens ductus arteriosus
      b. Ductal-dependent congenital heart disease
         i. Tetralogy of Fallot
         ii. Transposition of great arteries
         iii. Tricuspid atresia
         iv. Interrupted aortic arch
         v. Coarctation of the aorta
         vi. Hypoplastic left heart syndrome

C. Selected congenital heart diseases
   1. Transposition of great vessels (TGA)
      a. Definition
         i. Aorta rises from right ventricle and pulmonary artery arises from left ventricle
         ii. 2 sides of heart in parallel, not in series
         iii. Defect is incompatible with life unless coexisting ASD/VSD/PDA for L→R shunt
      b. Epidemiology
         i. Most common cause of cyanosis in first week of life
         ii. Male >female
         iii. More common in children of diabetic mothers
      c. Symptoms and signs
         i. Cyanotic within hours of birth
         ii. Onset of symptoms dependent on presence of PDA/VSD
            a) If only PDA, cyanosis within few days
            b) With large VSD, cyanosis days to weeks later
         iii. Signs of CHF (poor feeding, tachypnea, tachycardia)
         iv. VSD murmur
      d. Diagnosis
         i. Echocardiography
         ii. CXR may reveal "egg on a string" appearance in 30%
      e. Management
         i. Prostaglandin E_1 to promote pulmonary blood flow
         ii. Cardiac catherization may temporarily improve oxygenation by manipulating atrial septum opening
         iii. Surgery is the mainstay of treatment
   2. Truncus arteriosus
      a. Definition
         i. Single large arterial trunk from both ventricles gives rise to both aortic and pulmonary arteries
         ii. VSD of variable size
         iii. Variable right and left ventricular hypertrophy
      b. Symptoms and signs
         i. Cyanosis within first few weeks of life
         ii. Signs of CHF (poor feeding, tachypnea, tachycardia)
         iii. VSD murmur
         iv. Associated with DiGeorge syndrome—absence of thymus and hypoparathyroidism
            a) Symptoms and signs of hypocalcemia
      c. Diagnosis
         i. Echocardiography
      d. Management

i. Some subtypes benefit from prost-aglandin E_1

ii. Surgery is the mainstay of treatment

iii. 1-year mortality without surgery approaches 100%

3. Tetralogy of Fallot

  a. Definition

    i. Pulmonic stenosis

    ii. Hypertrophic right ventricle

    iii. Ventricular septal defect (VSD)

    iv. Overriding aorta

  b. Epidemiology

    i. Most common cyanotic heart defect

    ii. May present up to 3 to 4 months

    iii. Associated with DiGeorge syndrome

  c. Etiology

    i. Frequently associated with fetal alcohol syndrome, fetal carbamazepine syndrome and maternal phenylketonuria (PKU)

  d. Symptoms and signs

    i. Cyanosis

    ii. Poor feeding

    iii. Hemoptysis

    iv. Squatting to relieve symptoms

    v. Single S_2 (pulmonic valve does not audibly close)

    vi. Scoliosis common

    vii. "Tet spells"(tetralogy of Fallot)

      a) Acute respiratory distress because of increase in right ventricular outflow tract obstruction

      b) Pulmonary stenosis murmur becomes weaker because of increased shunting through VSD

  e. Diagnosis

    i. Echocardiography

    ii. ECG may reveal right atrial/ventricular hypertrophy or right axis

    iii. CXR

      a) May reveal "boot-shaped heart" or "coeur en sabot" because of right ventricular hypertrophy

      b) Decreased pulmonary vasculature

  f. Management

    i. Goal is to decrease pulmonary resistance and increase systemic resistance

      a) Calm the child

      b) Place knees to chest

      c) Oxygen

      d) Morphine

      e) IV bolus of NS at 20 cc/kg

      f) Phenylephrine

    ii. Surgery is mainstay of long-term treatment

4. Patent ductus arteriosus (PDA)

  a. Definition

    i. Persistent communication between left pulmonary artery and descending aorta >10 days after birth

    ii. Associated and required with other congenital heart diseases (see ductus arteriosus dependent lesions above)

  b. Symptoms and signs

    i. CHF may occur with a large PDA as pulmonary artery is flooded

      a) Poor feeding may be the only evidence of CHF in an infant

    ii. Wide pulse pressure

    iii. **Machine-like** murmur

    iv. Clubbing

    v. Susceptible to bacterial endocarditis

  c. Diagnosis

    i. Echocardiography

    ii. CXR—may reveal signs of CHF

    iii. ECG—notching of R waves in inferior leads II, III, and AVF known as "crochetage"

  d. Management

    i. Indomethacin

    ii. Pediatric surgery consultation

5. Coarctation of aorta (CoA)

  a. Definition

    i. Segmental narrowing of the aorta found most commonly distal to the left subclavian artery

  b. Symptoms and signs

    i. CHF symptoms (poor feeding, tachypnea, tachycardia) predominate early on

    ii. Hypertension

      a) Upper extremity >lower extremity pulse/BP

    iii. Systolic murmur

    iv. Headache and obtundation if subarachnoid hemorrhage (higher incidence in patient with CoA)

    v. Associated with Turner syndrome

      a) Webbed neck

      b) Short stature

  c. Diagnosis

    i. Echocardiography

    ii. Cardiac catherization

    iii. CXR

      a) Cardiomegaly

      b) Pulmonary congestion

      c) Rib notching

  d. Management

    i. Treat CHF with diuretics and inotropes

    ii. Treat hypertension

    iii. Prostaglandin E_1 to open ductus arteriosus

    iv. Surgical consultation
    v. Cardiac catherization/stenting

XI. Genitourinary and Renal

A. Sexual development (Table 1–5)

B. Urinary tract infection (UTI)[4]
   1. Epidemiology
    a. Present in 5% of febrile infants <12 months
    b. More common in males in the first few months of life
    c. Circumcised boys have much lower rates of UTI
   2. Symptoms and signs
    a. Fever
    b. Dysuria, frequency, and urgency
    c. Flank pain
    d. Very young may have little or no signs and symptoms
   3. Diagnosis
    a. Clinical diagnosis
    b. Urinalysis
      i. Leukocyte esterase sensitivity of 70% to 85% and specificity of 60%
      ii. Nitrate has sensitivity of 10% to 43% and specificity of 95%
    c. Culture
      i. Positive if >3000 colony-forming units (CFU) with suprapubic aspiration sample
      ii. Positive if >10,000 CFU with catherization sample
      iii. Positive if >100,000 CFU with clean catch sample
   4. Management
    a. Antibiotics—cephalosporins and penicillins
    b. Imaging for high-risk patients

      i. Indications are controversial
        a) Failure or slow response to antibiotics
        b) Abdominal mass
        c) Urinary dribbling
        d) Infection with organisms other than *E. coli*
        e) UTI in circumcised boys <1 year
        f) >2 UTI in uncircumcised boys <1 year
        g) >2 UTI episodes in school-aged girls
      ii. Imaging modality
        a) Ultrasound has supplanted intravenous pyelography
        b) Voiding cystourethrography (VCUG) or nuclear cystography to assess anatomy and presence of vesicoureteral reflux (VUR)
    c. Hospitalization
      i. Ill- or septic-appearing
      ii. Signs of urinary obstruction or underlying mass
      iii. <3 months old

XII. Hematology/Oncology

A. Leukemia (see Chapter 19 Hematology/Oncology)

B. Neuroblastoma
   1. Definition
    a. Most common extra cranial solid tumor in childhood
    b. Involves the adrenal gland (65%) and less commonly the extra adrenal sympathetic chain in the chest (20%), neck, and retroperitoneum
   2. Symptoms and signs
    a. Initial symptoms are nonspecific including fever, loss of appetite, and malaise
    b. Subsequent symptoms depend on site of tumor and sites of metastases

TABLE 1–5.   Sexual Development

TANNER STAGE	GIRLS	MEAN AGE	BOYS	MEAN AGE
1	No pubic hair, prepubital breast	–	No pubic hair, testicles <4 mL	–
2	Straight and long pubic hair, breast bud	11 years	Straight and long pubic hair, testicles >4 mL, scrotal ruggae	11.5 years
3	Darker curly pubic hair, larger breast, no secondary mound	12 years	Darker curly pubic hair, penile lengthening begins	12 years
4	Labia and mons covered, areola forms, secondary mound, menarche	13 years	Most of pubic area covered, penile lengthening begins	13 years
5	Areola is part of breast, nipples project	14 years	Pubic hair spreads to thighs and lower abdomen, adult genitals	14 years

   c. 50% with metastatic disease at time of diagnosis
   d. Classic finding of bilateral ecchymosis representing periorbital metastases uncommon
   e. Can present with opsomyoclonus; ("dancing eyes and dancing feet") nystagmus and ataxia
 3. Diagnosis
   a. CT scan
   b. Elevated urine catecholamine metabolites (vanillylmandelic acid and homovanillic acid) in 90%
   c. Biopsy is definitive
 4. Management
   a. Surgical resection
   b. Chemotherapy
   c. Radiation therapy

C. Wilms tumor (nephroblastoma)
 1. Definition
   a. Most common abdominal tumor in children involving the kidney
 2. Symptoms and signs
   a. Asymptomatic abdominal mass
   b. May present with hypertension, fever from tumor necrosis, hematuria, and anemia
   c. Associated with aniridia and genitourinary deformities
 3. Diagnosis
   a. Abdominal CT scan
   b. Renal ultrasound
   c. Biopsy is definitive
 4. Management
   a. Surgery and chemotherapy depending on the stage
   b. Prognosis is based on tumor size, stage, and histology

D. Ewing sarcoma
 1. Definition
   a. Rare malignant bone tumor most commonly affecting the long bones in children 5 to15 years
 2. Symptoms and signs
   a. Bone pain typically in the pelvis, femur, tibia, and humerus
   b. Metastases in 30% to 40% at time of diagnosis
 3. Diagnosis
   a. X-ray reveals lytic lesions with "onion skin" periosteal reaction
   b. CT scan
   c. Biopsy is definitive
 4. Management
   a. Surgical excision
   b. Chemotherapy
   c. Radiation therapy

XIII. Neurology

A. Febrile seizure[5]
 1. Definition
   a. Seizures associated with fever in children 3 months to 5 years
   b. Diagnosis of exclusion
 2. Epidemiology
   a. 3% to 4% of population
   b. Genetic predisposition
   c. Peak occurrence 14 to 18 months
   d. Associated with *Roseola*
 3. Symptoms and signs
   a. Simple febrile seizures (85%)
     i. Generalized tonic-clonic seizure
     ii. Occurs in children 3 months to 5 years
     iii. <15-minutes duration
     iv. Nonfocal neurologic examination
     v. No recurrence of seizure within 24 hours
   b. Complex febrile seizures (15%)
     i. Any event not meeting criteria above for simple febrile seizures
     ii. Should raise suspicion for serious disease such as meningitis, encephalitis, intracranial bleeding, or mass
 4. Management
   a. Primary management involves ruling out more serious disease
   b. Uncover and treat underlying infection
   c. Antipyretics have NOT been shown to decrease frequency or prevent recurrence
   d. CT scan and lumbar puncture with complex febrile seizures
   e. Strongly consider lumbar puncture <12 months[6]
   f. Educate parents
 5. Prognosis
   a. 30% chance of having another febrile seizure
     i. Risk factors for recurrence
       a) <1 year
       b) Seizure occurs with low fever
       c) Complex seizure
   b. Risk of epilepsy is 2% to 10% (vs. 1% for general population)

B. Neurocutaneous disorders—neurologic syndromes with skin manifestations
 1. Neurofibromatosis type I (autosomal dominant)
   a. Dermatologic manifestations
     i. Neurofibromas—soft, nonpainful, flesh-colored tumors
     ii. Café au lait, skin fold freckling , iris harmartomas (Lisch nodules)
   b. Neurologic manifestations
     i. Seizures

       ii. Increased risk for central nervous system (CNS) tumors (benign and malignant) such as optic gliomas, astrocytomas, meningiomas

       iii. Hydrocephalus

    c. Miscellaneous associations

       i. Lisch nodules—tiny noncancerous tumor on iris confirm diagnosis

       ii. Growth hormone deficiency and short stature

       iii. Precocious puberty

       iv. Pheochromocytoma

       v. Wilms tumor

  2. Tuberous Sclerosis (autosomal dominant)

    a. Dermatologic manifestations

       i. Ashleaf spot

         a) Earliest appearing symptom

         b) Hypopigmented macules accentuated with Wood lamp

       ii. Shagreen patch (diagnostic of disease)

         a) Flesh-colored plaque with orange peel appearance

         b) Typically located on trunk or lower back

       iii. Adenoma sebaceum

         a) Red maculopapular lesions on face in butterfly pattern consisting of blood vessels

    b. Neurologic manifestations

       i. Tubercle growths

         a) Potato-like growths in the brain that calcify and become sclerotic with time

       ii. Seizures

       iii. Mental retardation

    c. Miscellaneous manifestations

       i. Renal hamartomas

       ii. Rhabdomyomas of the heart

       iii. Multiple lung cysts

  3. Sturge-Weber syndrome

    a. Dermatologic manifestations

       i. Port wine stain usually involving the trigeminal nerve

    b. Neurologic manifestations

       i. Developmental delay

       ii. Seizures

       iii. Hemiplegia

       iv. Homonymous hemianopsia

    c. Miscellaneous manifestations

       i. Glaucoma

C. Select seizure syndromes

  1. Benign Rolandic (benign partial epilepsy)

    a. Definition

       i. Benign seizure of childhood characterized by facial twitching and aphasia

    b. Epidemiology

       i. Most common epilepsy syndrome of childhood

       ii. 2 to 16 years

    c. Symptoms and signs

       i. Seizures occurring mostly at night or upon awakening

       ii. Hemifacial motor and/or sensory seizure

       iii. Speech arrest and drooling

       iv. Consciousness intact unless seizure becomes generalized

         a) May generalize to tonic clonic seizures

       v. Normal neurologic examination in between episodes

       vi. Normal development in majority

    d. Diagnosis

       i. EEG with characteristic high voltage slow wave forms

       ii. CT or MRI with atypical symptoms to rule out more serious pathology

    e. Management

       i. Seizures usually resolve by adolescence even without treatment

       ii. Refractory or frequent seizures may benefit from carbamazepine

  2. Infantile spasms (West syndrome)

    a. Definition

       i. Triad of

         a) Clusters of myoclonic seizures on awakening

         b) Hypsarrhythmia pattern on EEG

         c) Mental retardation

    b. Symptoms and signs

       i. Usually begin 4 to 8 months

       ii. Brief contractions of neck, trunk, and extremities lasting 5 to 10 seconds, each occurring in clusters

         a) May be accompanied by a cry

       iii. Often accompanied by developmental delay

    c. Diagnosis

       i. Brain imaging with CT or MRI often abnormal

       ii. Characteristic EEG finding termed hypsarrhythmia

       iii. Consider lumbar puncture to rule out meningitis/encephalitis

    d. Management

       i. Treatment with adrenocorticotropic hormone (ACTH), prednisone, and antiseizure medications

       ii. Ketogenic diet advocated by some

D. Miscellaneous

  1. Night terrors

a. Definition
  i. Parasomnia sleep disorder characterized by
    a) Inability to be fully awakened during episode of extreme fearfulness
    b) Occurrence during nonrapid eye movement sleep
      i) Stages 3 to 4 of sleep
    c) Return to sleep without fully awakening
    d) Lack of ability to recall the event
b. Epidemiology
  i. Boys >Girls
  ii. Peaks 5 to 7 years
2. Breath-Holding Spells
a. Screaming fit that ends in breath holding and possible loss of consciousness
b. Begins 6 to 18 months
c. 90% disappear by 6 years

XIV. Pediatric Trauma[7]

A. Epidemiology
1. Pediatric trauma is the leading cause of death and morbidity in children > 1 year
2. Child abuse must always be ruled out

B. Pathophysiology
1. Children have smaller mass than adults, so any external force is dissipated over a smaller area, causing more injury
2. Children have greater surface area relative to volume than adults
  a. Prone to hypothermia during resuscitation

C. Airway (see PALS, Breathing above)
1. Anatomy
  a. A child's larynx is higher and more anterior than in the adult
  b. Shorter trachea prone to right mainstem intubation
  c. Relatively larger tongue requires chin lift or jaw thrust to maximize airway
  d. Larger head causes relative flexion and airway obstruction when lying supine
2. Management
  a. Infants are obligate nose breathers so do not forget suctioning or if not contraindicated, consider a nasal-pharyngeal airway
  b. Position the patient in the sniffing position
  c. Oral airways should not be rotated 180 degrees but placed with a tongue depressor

D. Shock
1. Recognition
  a. A 25% loss of circulating blood volume is required to manifest minimal signs of shock

b. The first sign is tachycardia
c. Hypotension represents uncompensated shock and indicates a 45% loss of circulating blood volume
2. Management
  a. A child's blood volume is calculated as 80 mL/kg, so a 20 cc/kg bolus will replenish 25% of volume
  b. Consider blood transfusion after the third fluid bolus. This is the 3:1 rule
  c. Early intraosseous access if venous access failed

E. CNS Injuries
1. Head injury
  a. Proportionately larger head in comparison with adults' head
  b. Injuries often produce diffuse edema rather than focal injury
    i. Initial head CT may not be as impressive as symptoms suggest
  c. May have nonfocal examination despite significant injury
    i. Pliable skull and sutures allow for significant bleeding to occur before signs of increased intracranial pressure become apparent
  d. CNS hemorrhage in an infant can lead to hypotension
2. Spinal cord injury
  a. Cervical
    i. <8 years: C1 through C3 more likely to be injured
    ii. >8 years: injury pattern similar to adults
    iii. Normal predental space in child may be up to 5 mm in comparison with 3 mm in adults
    iv. Pseudosubluxation—anterior displacement of C2 on C3
      a) 40% of children <7 years
      b) 20% of children up to 16 years
      c) Line of Swischuk
        i) Line is drawn from anterior aspect of C1 to C3. The anterior aspect of C2 should be within 2 mm of this line.
  b. Lumbar
    i. Chance fractures
      a) Transverse fracture through vertebrae
      b) Associated with hyperflexion injury with an automobile lap belt
  c. Spinal cord injury without radiographic abnormality (SCIWORA)

   i. Epidemiology
     a) 20 % of pediatric spinal cord injuries fall under SCIWORA
     b) Up to 60% of cervical injuries in children <8 years
   ii. Definition
     a) Acute or latent traumatic myelopathy despite normal plain radiographs and CT scans
   iii. Etiology
     a) Underdeveloped spinal cord blood supply susceptible to injury
     b) Ligamentous laxity and relatively large head
     c) Fracture of the cartilaginous end plates not visualized by radiographs
     d) Spontaneous reduction of displaced vertebral bodies
   iv. Symptoms and signs
     a) The younger the patient, the more severe the symptoms
     b) Delayed presentation can occur hours to days after injury
     c) Varying degrees of motor weakness and sensory loss depending on severity of lesion
   v. Diagnosis
     a) Clinical examination
     b) MRI abnormal in majority
   vi. Management
     a) Controversial
     b) Prognosis and management correlate with MRI findings and presenting symptoms
     c) Hard cervical collar for 3 to 4 months
     d) Limited physical activity

F. Thoracic trauma
  1. Anatomy
    a. Pliable rib cage
    b. Relatively mobile mediastinum
  2. Epidemiology
    a. Bronchial and diaphragmatic injuries more common than in adults
    b. Great vessel injury less common than in adults
  3. Symptoms and signs
    a. Significant intrathoracic injury may exist with minimal external signs of trauma
    b. Pneumothorax and pulmonary contusions may occur without evidence of rib fracture
  4. Traumatic asphyxiation
    a. Definition: abrupt transthoracic compression resulting in retrograde superior vena cava pressures

    b. Symptoms and signs: cervical and facial petechiae and subconjunctival hemorrhage
    c. Good prognosis
  5. Commotio cordis
    a. Epidemiology: highest incidence 5 to 15 years
    b. Definition: sudden death secondary to blunt trauma to the chest by a missile (baseball, hockey puck)
    c. Etiology: arrhythmia, commonly ventricular fibrillation

G. Abdominal/Pelvic injuries
  1. Epidemiology
    a. Blunt trauma is the most common mechanism
    b. Splenic injuries are most common in pediatric abdominal trauma
    c. Pelvic injuries are less common
     i. Pelvic fractures in children rarely leads to life-threatening hemorrhage
  2. Anatomy: abdomen begins at level of nipple in young children
    a. Pliable cartilaginous rib cage increases the risk of compression of abdominal organs
     i. Significant abdominal injuries can exist with few external signs
    b. Children have larger solid organs, less protective muscle, and less subcutaneous fat
  3. Mechanism
    a. Lap belt injury consists of small bowel injury (duodenal hematoma) in 5% to 10% of restrained children in a motor vehicle accident (MVA)
    b. Handle bar/bicycle-induced duodenal hematoma may not present until 24 hours after episode

REFERENCES

1. American Academy of Pediatrics, Committee on Pediatric Emergency Medicine: Consent for emergency medical services for children and adolescents. *Pediatrics.* 2003;111:703.
2. Dewolfe CC: Apparent life-threatening event: a review. *Pediatr Clin North Am.* 2005 Aug;52(4):1127.
3. Mitchell EA, Thach BT, Thompson JM, et al: Changing infants' sleep position increases risk of sudden infant death syndrome. New Zealand Cot Death Study. *Arch Pediatr Adolesc Med.* 1999 Nov;153(11):1136.
4. American Academy of Pediatrics, Committee on Quality Improvement Practice parameter: The diagnosis, treatment, and evaluation of the initial urinary tract infection in febrile infants and young children. *Pediatrics.* 1999;103:843.
5. American Academy of Pediatrics, Committee on Quality Improvement, Subcommittee on Febrile Seizures Practice

parameter: Long-term treatment of the child with simple febrile seizures. *Pediatrics.* 1999;103:1307.

6. Provisional Committee on Quality Improvement, Subcommittee on Febrile Seizures. Practice Parameter: The neurodiagnostic evaluation of the child with a first simple febrile seizure. *Pediatrics.* 1996;97(5):769.

7. Kapklein MJ, Mahadeo R: Pediatric trauma. *Mt Sinai J Med.* 1997;Sep-Oct; 64(4-5):302.

BIBLIOGRAPHY

Kadish HA, Loveridge B, Tobey J, et al: Applying outpatient protocols in febrile infants 1–28 days of age: can the threshold be lowered?. *Clin Pediatr.* 2000;39:81.

Ferrera PC, Bartfield JM, Snyder HS: Neonatal fever: utility of the Rochester criteria in determining low risk for serious bacterial infections. *Am J Emerg Med.* 1997;15:299.

Hammerschlag MR, Cummings C, Roblin PM, et al: Efficacy of neonatal ocular prophylaxis for the prevention of chlamydial and gonococcal conjunctivitis. *N Engl J Med.* 1989;320:769.

Baskin MN, O'Rourke EJ, Fleisher GR: Outpatient treatment of febrile infants 28 to 89 days of age with intramuscular administration of ceftriaxone. *J Pediatr.* 1992;120:22.

Baker MD, Bell LM, Avner JR: The efficacy of routine outpatient management without antibiotics of fever in selected infants. *Pediatrics.* 1999;103:627.

Lieu TA, Schwartz JS, Jaffe DM, et al: Strategies for diagnosis and treatment of children at risk for occult bacteremia: clinical effectiveness and cost-effectiveness. *J Pediatr.* 1991; 118:21.

Chen JY: Prophylaxis of ophthalmia neonatorum: comparison of silver nitrate, tetracycline, erythromycin and no prophylaxis. *Pediatr Infect Dis J.* 1992;11:1026.

Bell TA, Sandstrom KI, Gravett MG, et al: Comparison of ophthalmic silver nitrate solution and erythromycin ointment for prevention of natally acquired Chlamydia trachomatis. *Sex Transm Dis.* 1987;14:195.

Mahon BE, Rosenman MB, Kleiman MB: Maternal and infant use of erythromycin and other macrolide antibiotics as risk factors for infantile hypertrophic pyloric stenosis. *J Pediatr.* 2001;139:380.

Cooper WO, Griffen MR, Arbogast P, et al: Very early exposure to erythromycin and infantile hypertrophic pyloric stenosis. *Arch Pediatr Adolesc Med.* 2002;156:647.

Isenberg SJ, Apt L, Wood M: A controlled trial of povidone-iodine as prophylaxis against ophthalmia neonatorum. *N Engl J Med.* 1995;332:562.

American Academy of Pediatrics. Chlamydial trachomatis. In: Pickering LK, ed. *Red Book: 2006 Report of the Committee on Infectious Diseases,* 27th ed. Elk Grove Village, IL: American Academy of Pediatrics; 2006:252.

Kohen DP: Neonatal gonococcal arthritis: three cases and review of the literature. *Pediatrics.* 1974;53:436.

Babl FE, Ram S, Barnett ED, Rhein L, et al: Neonatal gonococcal arthritis after negative prenatal screening and despite conjunctival prophylaxis. *Pediatr Infect Dis J.* 2000;19:346.

Rothrock SG, Pagane J: Acute appendicitis in children: emergency department diagnosis and management. *Ann Emerg Med.* 2000;36:39.

Slutsker L, Ries AA, Greene KD, et al: Escherichia coli O157:H7 diarrhea in the United States: clinical and epidemiologic features. *Ann Intern Med.* 1997;126:505.

Talan D, Moran GJ, Newdow M, et al: Etiology of bloody diarrhea among patients presenting to United States emergency departments: prevalence of Escherichia coli O157:H7 and other enteropathogens. *Clin Infect Dis.* 2001;32:573.

Ozbek C, Aygenc E, Tuna EU, et al: Use of steroids in the treatment of peritonsillar abscess. *J Laryngol Otol.* 2004 Jun;118(6):439.

Herzon FS, Martin AD: Medical and surgical treatment of peritonsillar, retropharyngeal, and parapharyngeal abscesses. *Curr Infect Dis Rep.* May 2006;8(3):196.

Marx JA: *Rosen's Emergency Medicine: Concepts and Clinical Practice.* 6th ed. St. Louis, MO: Mosby; 2006.

Mahadevan G: *An Introduction to Clinical Emergency Medicine.* New York, NY: Cambridge University Press; 2005.

Barone MA, ed: *The Harriet Lane Handbook: A Manual for Pediatric House Officers.* 17th ed. St. Louis, MO: Elsevier; 2005.

Chapter 2
ORTHOPEDIC EMERGENCIES

Moira Davenport, Brian Cameron, and Maria Vasilyadis

I. Principles of Orthopedic Care

A. Definitions
  1. Fractures
     a. Fractures are described by the relationship of the distal segment to the proximal segment
     b. Comminuted: fracture with more than 2 fragments
     c. Impaction: fracture with ends compressed together
     d. Displacement: amount by which the fracture segments are maligned
     e. Angulation: angle between imaginary line drawn parallel to normal axis of bone and fracture fragment
     f. Rotation: spin around an imaginary line drawn through the center of the long axis of a bone
     g. Fractures are associated with more blood loss than apparent on external examination
        i. Radius and ulna: 200 mL
        ii. Humerus: 250 mL
        iii. Pelvis: 1500 to 3000 mL
        iv. Femur: 1000 mL
        v. Tibia and fibula: 500 mL
     h. Fracture line direction
        i. Transverse: fracture perpendicular to long axis of bone
        ii. Spiral: fracture line associated with twisting or torsion stress
        iii. Oblique: transverse-like fracture at an angle without torsion appearance
     i. Simple (closed) versus compound (open)
        i. Simple: overlying skin intact
        ii. Compound: overlying skin broken
  2. Sprains versus strains
     a. Sprains: injury to ligaments (bone to bone attachment)
     b. Strains: injury to tendons (bone to muscle attachment) or muscles

B. Management axioms
  1. Rotational deformity should be corrected prior to angulation
     a. Angulation may correct itself over time as natural tension lines straighten while rotational deformities do not correct on their own
  2. Application of circumferential casts should be accompanied by good education regarding ischemia secondary to swelling within an overly tight casting
  3. Tendon ruptures should be repaired as soon as possible

II. Upper Extremity Injuries

A. Acromioclavicular (AC) separations (Figure 2–1)
  1. Mechanism
     a. Fall directly onto adducted shoulder
     b. Fall onto outstretched arm
  2. Symptoms and signs
     a. Pain and deformity over the AC joint
  3. Classification
     a. Type I injury
        i. Partial tear of the AC ligament
        ii. Coracoclavicular ligament (CC) remains intact
        iii. AC joint maintains normal alignment
        iv. Normal x-ray
     b. Type II injury
        i. Full tear of the AC ligament
        ii. Intact CC ligament
     c. Type III injury
        i. Full tear of the AC ligament
        ii. Full tear of the CC ligaments
        iii. An obvious deformity is present
     d. Type IV injury—Type III with posterior displacement of the distal clavicle
     e. Type V injury—Type III with superior displacement of clavicle
     f. Type VI injury—Type III with inferior displacement of the clavicle

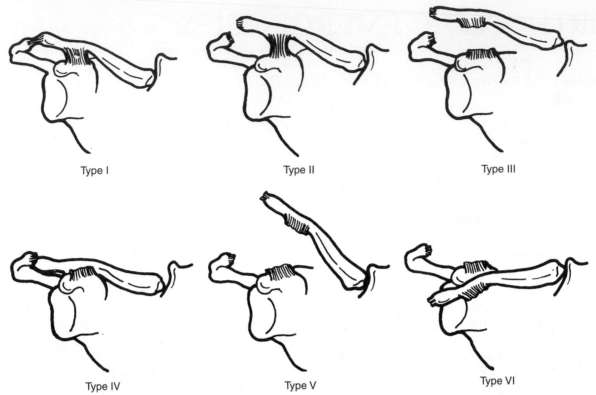

FIGURE 2–1. Types of acromioclavicular (AC) injuries. (Reproduced with permission from Perry CR, Elstrom JA, Pankovich AM. *Handbook of Fractures.* Copyright © 2005, New York: McGraw-Hill.)

4. Diagnosis
   a. Anteroposterior (A-P) and lateral x-ray
   b. Consider x-ray of contralateral side for comparison
   c. Stress views no longer recommended in the ED
5. Management
   a. Types I and II managed with sling and analgesia
   b. Type III surgical therapy only if conservative therapy fails
   c. Types IV through VI generally managed surgically

B. Sternoclavicular (SC) dislocations
   1. Symptoms and signs
      a. Joint pain
      b. Pain with motion of the affected extremity
      c. Anterior dislocation much more common than posterior
      d. Posterior dislocation
         i. Up to 25% associated with mediastinal injury
         ii. May present with dyspnea secondary to tracheal compression

      iii. Rule out pneumothorax
      iv. Rule out great vessel injury
   2. Classification
      a. First-degree injury involves incomplete tears of SC and costoclavicular ligaments
      b. Second-degree injury involves subluxation of clavicle from manubrium
      c. Third-degree injury, involves complete dislocation, tear of SC, and costoclavicular ligaments
   3. Diagnosis
      a. Physical examination
         i. Pain
         ii. Slight decrease in range of motion (ROM)
      b. X-ray
         i. Plain chest x-ray (A-P and lateral views)
         ii. Sternal views
         iii. Computed tomography (CT) scan if plain radiographs negative but clinical suspicion high
            a) Additional benefit of evaluating mediastinum
   4. Management
      a. Posterior dislocations
         i. A medical emergency

    ii. Immediate reduction necessary
      a) Abduct and apply traction to arm
      b) Grasp clavicle with towel clip and pull back
      c) May require surgical intervention
  b. Anterior dislocations
    i. Sling and analgesia for first- and second-degree injury
    ii. Third-degree dislocations require reduction
      a) Apply traction with 90 degrees abduction and 15 degrees extension
      b) May require posterior and inferior pressure on medial clavicle

C. Shoulder dislocation
  1. Epidemiology
    a. Most mobile joint and therefore most frequently dislocated
    b. Anterior dislocations account for >95% followed by posterior dislocations (<5%) and inferior dislocations (luxatio erecta <1%)
    c. Bimodal incidence
      i. Age 20 to 30 years: men >women (9:1 ratio)
      ii. Age 60 to 80 years: women >men (3:1 ratio)
    d. Recurrence rate
      i. 80% to 90% if first dislocation <20 years
      ii. 10% to 15% if first dislocation >40 years
  2. Anterior dislocation
    a. Mechanism
      i. Abduction, extension, and external rotation as demonstrated when a baseball is pitched in full extension
      ii. Fall on abducted and externally rotated hand
    b. Symptoms and signs
      i. Pain and decreased ROM
      ii Held in slight abduction and external rotation
      iii. "Squaring-off" of shoulder with deltoid indentation
    c. Diagnosis
      i. Clinical examination
      ii. A-P and scapular Y views on x-ray (Figures 2–2A, 2B, and 2C)
    d. Management
      i. Stimson
        a) Lay patient prone with affected arm hanging off bed
        b) Apply 10-lb weight to wrist of affected shoulder
        c) Passive reduction with minimal manipulation by practitioner

      ii. Scapular rotation
        a) Perform Stimson technique as above plus
        b) Apply medially directed force to inferior tip of scapular and lateral force to superior portion of scapula
      iii. Traction-countertraction
        a) Traction applied using bed sheet tied to the flexed elbow
        b) Axial countertraction applied to chest using bed sheet
        c) Gentle internal/external rotation to engage humeral head
      iv. External rotation
        a) Gentle external rotation applied to adducted and flexed elbow
        b) Often performed without procedural sedation
      v. Kocher method
        a) Flex adducted elbow (arm to side of torso)
        b) External rotate arm until resistance felt
        c) Lift anteriorly in sagittal plane as far as possible
        d) Internally rotate until reduction occurs
      vi. Milch method
        a) Abduct and externally rotate elbow
      vii. Hippocrates technique
        a) Apply traction to arm with foot placed in ipsilateral axilla
        b) This technique is prone to axillary nerve injury and is **no longer recommended**
  3. Posterior dislocation
    a. Etiology
      i. Severe internal rotation and adduction
        a) Seizures and electrical injuries, less commonly caused by direct posterior force
        b) Internal rotators are stronger than external rotators, therefore posterior dislocations are rare
    b. Symptoms and signs
      i. Pain and decreased ROM
      ii. Adducted and internally rotated shoulder
      iii. Difficult to diagnose clinically and is often a missed injury
    c. Diagnosis
      i. "Light bulb" sign results from internal rotation and loss of greater and lesser tuberosity contour on A-P view x-ray (Figure 2–2D)
      ii. Posterior displacement of humeral head on scapular Y view or swimmer's view (Figure 2–2E and 2–2F)

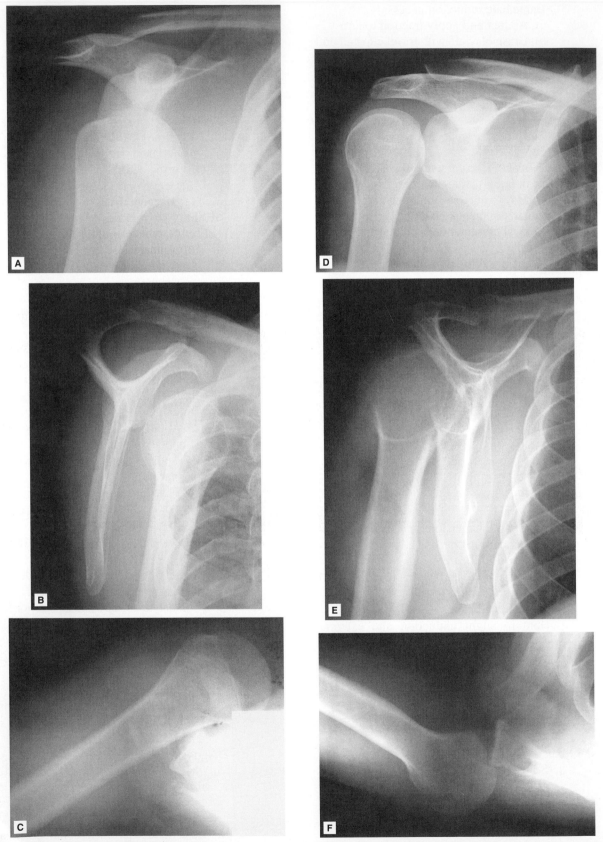

FIGURE 2–2. Shoulder dislocation. Anterior: *A.* AP view. *B.* Y view. *C.* Axillary view. Posterior. *D.* AP view. *E.* Y view. *F.* Axillary view. (Reproduced with permission from Schwartz DT: *Emergency Radiology: Case Studies.* Copyright © 2008, New York: McGraw-Hill.)

    d. Management
        i. Apply firm and steady axial traction to humerus
        ii. Anteriorly directed force from behind with gentle external rotation of humerus

4. Inferior dislocation (Luxatio erecta)
    a. Mechanism
        i. Axial load to outstretched arm
        ii. Hyperabduction
    b. Symptoms and signs
        i. Patient's shoulder is completely abducted with elbow flexed behind head (as if going to sleep using the forearm as a pillow)
    c. Diagnosis
        i. Clinical presentation is unique and unmistakable
        ii. X-ray reveals humeral head inferior to glenoid
    d. Management
        i. Overhead traction-countertraction

5. Complications of shoulder dislocations
    a. Rotator cuff injury is the most common complication
    b. Fractures occur in 30%
        i. Perform pre- and postreduction films
        ii. Hill-Sachs deformity
            a) Compression fracture of posterolateral humeral head
            b) Associated with anterior dislocation
        iii. Reverse Hill-Sachs deformity
            a) Associated with posterior dislocation
            b) Compression fracture of anterolateral humeral head
        iv. Bankart fracture
            a) Anterior rim fracture of glenoid
        v. Greater tuberosity avulsion fracture
    c. Nerve injury
        i. Perform pre- and postreduction neurovascular checks
        ii. Axillary nerve—loss of sensation over deltoid and weakness of external rotation and abduction of arm
        iii. Musculocutaneous nerve—loss of sensation over dorsum of forearm
    d. Vascular injury
        i. Axillary artery rupture
            a) Inferior dislocations have highest association (3%)
            b) Axillary hematoma
            c) Cool and pulseless extremity

D. Rotator cuff injuries
1. Mechanism
    a. Spectrum of injury from reversible tendonitis to full-thickness tears
    b. Acute injury and trauma
        i. Overhead shoulder use
        ii. Heavy lifting
        iii. Direct trauma
    c. Chronic tendonitis
        i. Age-related degeneration
            a) Repetitive trauma and stress
            b) Ischemia
        ii. Outlet impingement
            a) High-riding humerus compresses tendons against the coracoacromial arch

2. Clinical anatomy
    a. Injury to shoulder stabilizers (use the mnemonic **SItS**)
        i. **S**upraspinatus—most commonly injured
        ii. **I**nfraspinatus
        iii. **T**eres minor (lower case "t" in mnemonic intentional)
        iv. **S**ubscapularis
    b. Stabilizes much larger humeral head on glenoid fossa
        i. Glenohumeral joint likened to a golf ball sitting atop a golf tee
    c. Rotator cuff tendons originate from scapula and insert on humeral head
        i. Subscapularis inserts into lesser tuberosity to stabilize internal shoulder rotation
        ii. Remaining tendons insert into greater tuberosity to stabilize external rotation

3. Symptoms and signs
    a. Less common in patients <40 years
    b. Overhead laborers such as painters
    c. Pain
        i. Typically located on anterolateral shoulder
        ii. Worse at night especially when lying on affected shoulder
        iii. Acute pain with trauma
        iv. Insidious onset with chronic tendonitis
        v. Followed by weakness with significant tears
        vi. Exacerbated by overhead use
    d. Clicking, catching, or crepitus
    e. Palpation of greater tuberosity often elicits pain

4. Diagnosis
    a. Difficult to differentiate clinically from shoulder bursitis
    b. Provocative testing
        i. Supraspinatus—most commonly injured
            a) Neer impingement test
               i) Pain with forceful internal rotation with arm in full overhead forward flexion constitutes positive test
            b) Hawkins-Kennedy test
               i) Forward flex shoulder and elbow at 90 degrees

        ii) Pain with internal rotation constitutes positive test
    ii. Infraspinatus
      a) External rotation lag sign
        i) With patient's elbow flexed to 90 degrees and shoulder abducted to 20 degrees, attempts are made to hold maximal external rotation of arm
        ii) Inablity to hold in external rotation (lag) constitutes positive test
    iii. Subscapularis
      a) Lift-off test
        i) Internally rotate arm and place dorsum of hand on lower back
        ii) Pain with lifting off against resistance to palmar surface of hand constitutes positive test
  c. Imaging
    i. Plain radiography
      a) Generally not required in the ED unless fracture suspected
      b) May detect abnormal acromion anatomy or bone spurs
    ii. Outpatient
      a) Magnetic resonance imaging (MRI)
      b) Ultrasonography
 5. Management
  a. Conservative initially
    i. Rest, ice, compression, elevation
    ii. NSAIDs
    iii. Sling for no more than 2 days
    iv. Physical therapy and exercise
    v. Steroid injection into bursa if no response to above
  b. Orthopedic follow-up for elective surgery if conservative therapy fails

E. Scapular fractures
 1. Mechanism
  a. Uncommon injury (<1% of all fractures)
  b. Associated with high-velocity trauma (blunt trauma)
 2. Clinical anatomy
  a. Body and spine (50% of scapular fractures)
  b. Glenoid neck (medial to the glenoid fossa) (25%)
  c. Glenoid cavity (10%)
  d. Acromion (8%)
  e. Coracoid (7%)
 3. Symptoms and signs
  a. Pain with shoulder abduction (rotates scapula)
  b. Coracoid fractures painful with forced adduction and elbow flexion

 4. Diagnosis
  a. Plain radiographs including A-P, lateral, and axillary views of shoulder and scapula diagnose majority of fractures
  b. CT scan displaced scapular fracture in preparation for possible surgery
 5. Management
  a. Nonoperative in majority of scapular fractures
  b. Displaced acromion fractures may require surgery
  c. Scapulothoracic dislocation
    i. Scapular fracture with AC separation, clavicle fracture or SC dislocation that results in a free-floating shoulder
    ii. Considered a closed amputation and a surgical emergency
 6. Complications
  a. Rule out concomitant injury
    i. **Pulmonary injury** (15% to 50%)
    ii. Skull fracture (25%)
    iii. Vascular injury (11%)
    iv. Splenic injury (8%)
    v. Central nervous system (CNS) injury (5%)
  b. **Brachial plexus** injury especially with acromion and coracoid fractures

F. Proximal humeral fractures
 1. Mechanism
  a. Trip and fall onto outstretched arm (indirect trauma)
  b. Less commonly, direct trauma onto shoulder
 2. Symptoms and signs
  a. Pain, edema, ecchymosis
  b. Decreased ROM
 3. Clinical anatomy
  a. Proximal humerus divided into 4 parts using Neer classification
    i. Anatomic neck (old epiphyseal plate)
    ii. Surgical neck (weakened area below the tuberosity and humeral head, 2 cm below the anatomic neck)
    iii. Greater tuberosity
    iv. Lesser tuberosity
 4. Classification
  a. Class I: any fracture without significant displacement (>1 cm) or angulation (>45 degrees)
    i. >80% of proximal humeral fractures Class I
  b. Class II: any fracture part with significant displacement and angulation
  c. Class III: displaced surgical neck with either greater **or** lesser tuberosity involvement
  d. Class IV: displaced surgical neck with both greater **and** lesser tuberosity involvement

5. Diagnosis
   a. Plain x-ray including A-P, Y, and axillary views
6. Management
   a. Most proximal humeral fractures managed with sling and analgesia
   b. Classes III and IV fractures typically require surgery
7. Complications
   a. Axillary nerve injury
      i. Wraps around surgical neck
      ii. Most common nerve injury with proximal humerus fractures
      iii. Loss of sensation on deltoid
      iv. Impaired shoulder abduction caused by weak deltoid
   b. Axillary artery injury (rare)
   c. Brachial plexus injury (rare)
   d. Rotator cuff injury

G. Humeral shaft fractures
   1. Mechanism
      a. Direct trauma or fall on outstretched arm (transverse or oblique fractures)
      b. Torsion or twisting forces produce spiral fractures
   2. Symptoms and signs
      a. Pain, swelling, deformity
   3. Diagnosis
      a. Plain radiography
   4. Management
      a. With good closed reduction, most fractures managed without surgery
         i. <20 degrees of angulation
         ii. <2 cm overriding/shortening (bayonet position)
         iii. Spiral fractures have greater fracture surface area and heal better
      b. Coaptation splint (sugar-tong-like splint with closed end on elbow and open ends on humerus/shoulder)
   5. Complications
      a. Radial nerve injury most commonly injured nerve (15%)
         i. Particularly susceptible with mid to distal third fractures
         ii. Wrist drop
         iii. Sensation loss over radial aspect on the dorsum of the hand
      b. Brachial plexus injury

H. Elbow fractures (proximal ulna, radial head, olecranon/supracondylar fracture)
   1. Mechanism

   a. Most commonly, fall on outstretched hand (>90%)
   b. Direct trauma
2. Fracture type by age
   a. Pediatrics (<10 years)
      i. Supracondylar fractures—60% of elbow fractures in children
      ii. Radial neck fractures
      iii. Olecranon fractures rare
   b. Adults
      i. Intercondylar and condylar fractures
      ii. Radial head fractures
      iii. Olecranon fractures common
3. Symptoms and signs
   a. Pain, ecchymosis, edema, deformity
   b. Pain with pronation and supination with radial head fracture
   c. Pain with flexion and extension with olecranon fracture
4. Diagnosis
   a. Plain radiography (A-P and lateral)
      i. Fractures not always apparent
      ii. Radial head should point to capitellum in all views
      iii. Anterior humeral line should intersect the middle third of capitellum
      iv. Fat pad signs
         a) Anterior fat pad sign may be normal
         b) Posterior fat pad sign is always pathologic
5. Management
   a. Supracondylar fractures
      i. Splint with outpatient follow-up if only minimally displaced
      ii. Do not apply circumferential cast
      iii. Admit for neurovascular monitoring
      iv. Surgical management in majority of patients
   b. Radial head fractures
      i. Minimally displaced fractures are managed with sling, analgesia, and early ROM exercises to avoid stiffness
      ii. Surgery indicated if >3 mm displacement, >30% of articular surface involvement, or >30% angulation exists (rule of 3s)
   c. Olecranon fractures
      i. Managed nonoperatively in majority
      ii. Operative management if
         a) >2 mm displacement
         b) Comminuted fracture
         c) Triceps tendon rupture
6. Complications
   a. Volkmann ischemic contracture
      i. Compartment syndrome associated with supracondylar fractures

    ii. Permanent flexion contracture of the hand that results in a "claw-like" deformity

    iii. Unwilling to open hand, forearm tenderness, and pain with passive extension of fingers

  b. Cubitus varus deformity—gunstock deformity

    i. Occurs with poorly managed supracondylar fractures in children

  c. Brachial artery injury

    i. Associated with supracondylar fractures

    ii. Cool extremity

    iii. Weak or absent pulse

  d. Median nerve injury most commonly injured with supracondylar fractures

    i. Unable to oppose and flex thumb

    ii. Loss of sensation on the palmar side of the thumb, index, middle, and radial half of ring finger

    iii. Unable to make OK sign with thumb and index finger caused by anterior intraosseous nerve injury (branch of median nerve)

      a) Difficulty flexing interphalangeal joint of thumb and distal interphalangeal (DIP) joint of index and middle finger

  e. Ulnar nerve injury associated with condylar and olecranon fractures

    i. Loss of finger abduction (spread) and adduction (intraosseous muscles)

    ii. Sensory loss and change of pinky and ulnar aspect of ring finger

I. Elbow dislocation

  1. Mechanism

    a. Fall onto outstretched arm leads to posterior elbow dislocation (majority)

    b. Direct trauma to olecranon may result in anterior dislocation

  2. Symptoms and signs

    a. Pain, swelling, deformity

    b. Posterior dislocation—elbow in flexion at 45 degrees

    c. Anterior dislocation—upper arm appears shortened and held in supination and full extension

  3. Diagnosis

    a. Plain radiographs

      i. Review—fractures and dislocations described by the distal segment relative to proximal

      ii. Posterior dislocation would appear with humerus anterior to olecranon

  4. Management

    a. Early reduction with analgesia and muscle relaxant

    b. Gentle traction with elbow at ~30 degrees flexion

    c. May use modified Stimson technique (shoulder relocation technique) with patient lying prone and weight attached to flexed elbow at 30 degrees

  5. Complications

    a. Anterior dislocations have higher incidence of complications

    b. Ulnar nerve injury in 8% to 21%

    c. Median nerve injury less common

    d. Brachial artery injury

    e. Complete avulsion of triceps with anterior dislocation

J. Radial and ulnar fractures

  1. Mechanism: direct trauma

  2. Symptoms and signs: pain, swelling, deformity

  3. Diagnosis: plain radiographs

    a. Radial head should point toward capitellum in all views

    b. Pay attention to distal radial-ulnar junction (DRUJ)

      i. Distal radius and ulnar should not overlap

      ii. DRUJ should not be >2 mm apart

  4. Management

    a. Reduction, splinting, and emergent orthopedic follow-up

    b. Radial fractures

      i. Displaced fractures and **distal** third fractures are typically surgically managed in a semi-elective manner

    c. Ulnar fractures

      i. Displaced fractures and **proximal** third fractures are typically surgically managed

  5. Complications

    a. Compartment syndrome

    b. Posterior intraosseous nerve injury (deep branch of radial nerve)

      i. Associated with mid-distal ulnar fracture

      ii. Inability to extend fingers against resistance

    c. Radius and ulna are a parallel paired structure such that an injury to one frequently results in an injury to the other

      i. Monteggia (MUgr)

        a) Fractures of the proximal mid ulna with proximal radial head dislocation (Figures 2–3A and 2–3B)

        b) Patient requires open reduction and internal fixation (ORIF)

      ii. Galeazzi (muGR)

        a) Much more common than Monteggia fractures (3:1 ratio)

  b) Distal radial fractures with distal radioul-
     nar joint disruption (Figure 2–3C)
  c) Suspect if
     i) >5 mm radius shortening
     ii) >2 mm DRUJ widening
     iii) Subluxation of DRUJ
     iv) Ulnar styloid fracture
  d) Patient requires open reduction with
     external fixation (ORIF)

K. Distal radius fractures
  1. Colles fracture
     a. Mechanism
        i. Hyperextension as in "fall onto out-
           stretched hand" (FOOSH)
           a) Hand is pronated
     b. Symptoms and signs
        i. "Dinner-fork" deformity
        ii. Decreased sensation of median nerve
            distribution

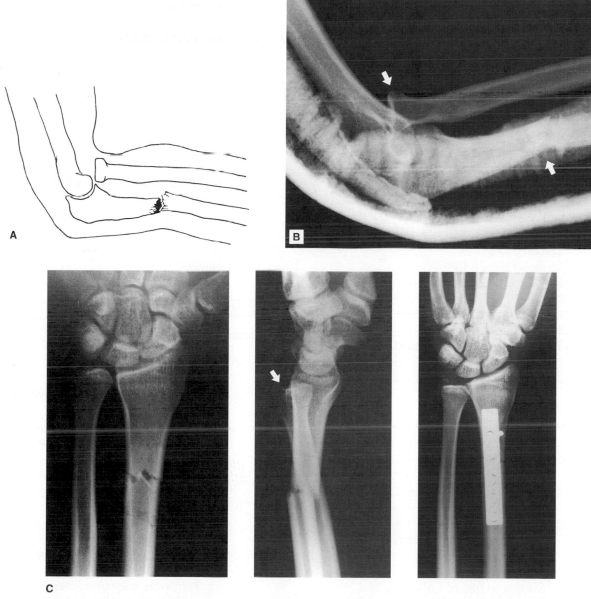

FIGURE 2–3. Forearm fractures. *A.* and *B.* Monteggia fracture. Fracture of the proximal ulnar shaft and volnar dislocation of the radial head *(arrows)*. *C.* Galeazzi fracture. Displaced fracture through the distal third of the radial shaft. (Reproduced with permission from Schwartz DT, Reisdorff EJ: *Emergency Radiology.* Copyright © 2000, New York: McGraw-Hill.)

c. Diagnosis
  i. X-ray (Figure 2–4A)
    a) Dorsally displaced and angulated fracture of distal radius
d. Management
  i. Early reduction and splint/casting decreases complications
  ii. Sugar-tong splint
  iii. Consider positioning in slight flexion, pronation, and ulnar deviation to maintain radial length (controversial)
  iv. Urgent orthopedic referral
e. Complications
  a) Median nerve injury most common followed by ulnar neuropathy
  b) Associated ulnar styloid fracture in 50%

2. Smith fracture
  a. Mechanism
    i. Fall onto outstretched supinated hand
    ii. Backward fall onto the palm of pronated hand
  b. Symptoms and signs
    i. "Garden-spade" deformity
    ii. Median or ulnar neuropathy
  c. Diagnosis (Figure 2–4B)
    i. X-ray reveals volarly displaced and angulated distal radius
  d. Management
    i. Early reduction
    ii. Sugar-tong splint
  e. Complications similar to those of Colles fracture

3. Barton fracture
  a. Mechanism
    i. Volar Barton mechanism similar to Smith fracture
    ii. Dorsal Barton mechanism similar to Colles fracture
  b. Diagnosis
    i. Intra-articular distal radius fracture with radiocarpal dislocation
    ii. Volar or dorsal displacement and angulation possible
      a) Volar injury more common than dorsal
  c. Management
    i. Most require surgical intervention despite reduction and splinting
  d. Complications
    i. Similar to that of Colles fracture

4. Hutchinson or Chauffeur fracture
  a. Etiology
    i. Scaphoid impaction into radius with wrist in dorsiflexion and ulnar deviation
    a) Name derived from era when cars were cranked and "backfired" leading to this pattern of wrist injury
  b. Diagnosis
    i. A-P films best demonstrate this injury
  c. Management includes immobilization in volar splint and orthopedic referral for likely percutaneous fixation

L. Carpal bone fractures
  1. Scaphoid fractures
    a. Epidemiology: most common carpal fracture
    b. Mechanism: FOOSH
    c. Symptoms and signs
      i. Pain with radial deviation
      ii. Axial loading of thumb elicits pain
      iii. Anatomical snuffbox tenderness
        a) Base defined by distal radius
        b) Radial border—abductor pollicis longus
        c) Ulnar border—extensor pollicis longus
    d. Diagnosis
      i. Plain radiographs (Figure 2–5)
        a) A-P and lateral wrist x-ray
        b) Scaphoid view—A-P of wrist in ulnar deviation
        c) Fracture may not be apparent for 1 to 2 weeks
      ii. CT scan advocated by some
      iii. MRI if diagnosis unclear
    e. Management
      i. When in doubt, treat as if fracture present
        a) Thumb spica splint
        b) Early orthopedic follow-up
      ii. Treat fractures with cast immobilization for 8 to 12 weeks
    f. Complications
      i. Avascular necrosis and nonunion
        a) Vascular supply to scaphoid occurs distal to proximal
        b) Proximal fractures more likely to result in nonunion and avascular necrosis
  2. Triquetral fractures
    a. Epidemiology: second most common carpal fracture
    b. Mechanism
      i. Extreme dorsiflexion with ulnar deviation
      ii. Direct blow to dorsum of hand
    c. Symptoms and signs
      i. Pain over triquetrum best isolated with radial deviation
    d. Diagnosis
      i. Dorsal chip fractures associated with hyper-dorsiflexion, seen on lateral x-ray

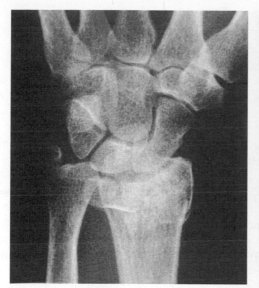
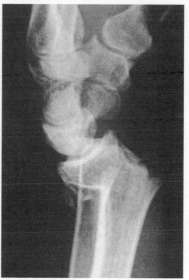

A

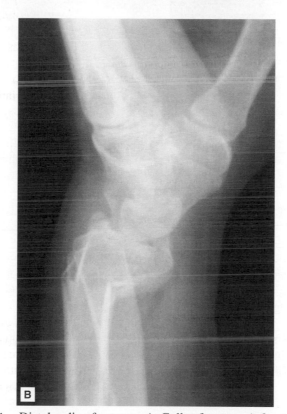

B

FIGURE 2–4.   Distal radius fractures. *A.* Colles fracture. A fracture through the metaphysic of the distal radius with dorsal displacement. *B.* Smith fracture. A volarly displaced fracture of the distal radius. (Reproduced, with permission from Schwartz DT, Reisdorff EJ: *Emergency Radiology.* Copyright © 2000, New York: McGraw-Hill.)

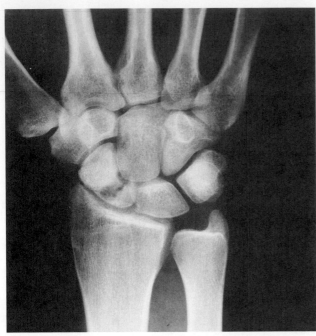

FIGURE 2–5. Scaphoid fracture. Displaced fracture through the proximal third of the scaphoid. (Reproduced, with permission from Schwartz DT, Reisdorff EJ: *Emergency Radiology.* Copyright © 2000, New York: McGraw-Hill.)

      ii. Transverse fractures secondary to direct blow, seen on A-P view
  e. Management
      i. Volar splint
  f. Complications
      i. Deep branch of ulnar nerve palsy
  3. Lunate fractures
    a. Mechanism
      i. Third most common carpal fracture
      ii. Hyperextension injury as in FOOSH
    b. Symptoms and signs
      i. Pain with axial loading of third metacarpal
      ii. Lunate tenderness
        a) Located in depression just distal and ulnar to Lister tubercle
        b) Flexion of wrist brings lunate bone to surface
    c. Diagnosis
      i. X-ray
        a) Multiple coned views may be necessary
    d. Management
      i. Based on clinical or radiographic evidence of fracture
      ii. Thumb spica splint if tender, even if x-rays appear normal
    e. Complications
      i. Avascular necrosis (Kienböck disease)

M. Carpal instability
  1. Scapholunate ligament rupture
    a. Mechanism
      i. Hyperextension injury as in FOOSH
    b. Symptoms and signs
      i. Pain and swelling at scapholunate junction
      ii. Clicking of wrist
      iii. May present with weak grip strength
    c. Diagnosis
      i. A-P x-ray of wrist shows widening of space (>3 mm) between scaphoid and lunate (Terry Thomas or David Letterman sign)
      ii. Signet ring sign—rotary subluxation results in shadowing of distal scaphoid onto body of scaphoid
    d. Management
      i. Thumb spica and orthopedic referral
      ii. Surgery usually indicated
    e. Complications
      i. Carpal bone instability
      ii. Arthritis
  2. Lunate and perilunate dislocations
    a. Mechanism
      i. High-energy injury as in fall from height
      ii. Hyperextension and ulnar deviation injury as in FOOSH
      iii. Spectrum of injury beginning with scapholunate dissociation to perilunate dislocation to lunate dislocation
        a) The capitate is dislocated dorsally (perilunate dislocation) and with higher energy injuries, rebounds to knock lunate in volar direction (lunate dislocation)
    b. Symptoms and signs
      i. Pain and swelling
      ii. Decreased ROM
      iii. Palpable fullness of volar wrist with lunate dislocations
      iv. Palpable fullness of dorsal wrist with perilunate dislocations
      v. Decreased sensation in median nerve distribution
    c. Diagnosis (Figure 2–6)
      i. A-P x-ray
        a) Increased spacing between carpal bones
        b) "Pizza-pie" sign with lunate dislocation
          i) Lunate-shaped like pizza slice (normally rectangular)
      ii. Lateral x-ray
        a) Single most important view
        b) Normally the distal radius, lunate, and capitate line up in a vertical row

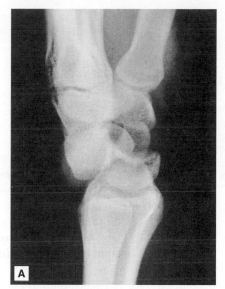

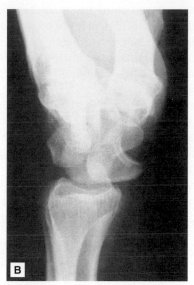

FIGURE 2–6. Perilunate and lunate dislocations. *A.* Perilunate. *B.* Lunate. (Reproduced, with permission from Schwartz DT, Reisdorff EJ: *Emergency Radiology.* Copyright © 2000, New York: McGraw-Hill.)

c) Capitate dorsally dislocated with perilunate dislocations
d) Lunate tilted and displaced volarly with lunate dislocation ("spilled teacup" sign)

d. Management
 i. Immediate orthopedic consultation in ED
 ii. Closed reduction may be attempted but rarely successful
 iii. Both injuries typically require open reduction and fixation

e. Complications
 i. Median nerve injury
 ii. Arthritis

N Selected metacarpal injuries
 1. Metacarpal neck fractures
  a. Definition
   i. Fracture of fifth metacarpal neck is known as a "boxer fracture"
  b. Mechanism
   i. Punch with clenched fist
  c. Symptoms and signs
   i. Tenderness and swelling
   ii. Rotational deformity of affected finger
  d. Diagnosis
   i. A-P and lateral x-rays (Figure 2–7)
  e. Management
   i. As in all fractures, address rotational deformity prior to angulation

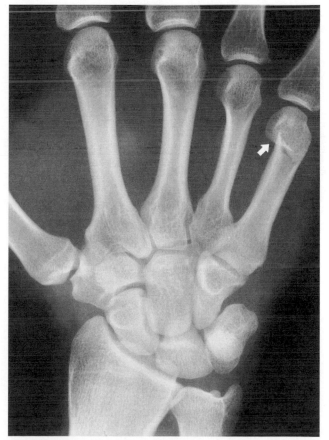

FIGURE 2–7. Boxer fracture. Fracture of the neck of the little finger metacarpal. (Reproduced, with permission from Schwartz DT, Reisdorff EJ: *Emergency Radiology.* Copyright © 2000, New York: McGraw-Hill.)

    ii. The second and third metacarpal necks can tolerate up to 15 degrees of angulation without functional impairment

    iii. The fourth and fifth necks are more mobile and can tolerate up to 30 to 40 degrees of angulation

    iv. Reduce angulation

    v. Volar splint with wrist in 30 degrees extension and metacarpophalangeal (MCP) joint flexed at 90 degrees

  f. Complications

    i. Missed "fight bites"

      a) Open wounds over MCP joint may indicate contamination with oral organisms

      b) Cover for Gram-positives, *Eikenella corrodans,* and oral anaerobes

      c) Examine extensor tendon through the full ROM with emphasis on the closed-fist position

      d) Strongly consider intravenous antibiotics and admission

      e) Never suture closed

    ii. Missed foreign body

      a) Consider x-ray to rule out tooth fragments

2. First metacarpal fractures

  a. Bennett fracture

    i. Definition

      a) Intra-articular fracture dislocation of base of first carpometacarpal joint

    ii. Mechanism

      a) Axial loading of partially flexed metacarpal

      b) Most common thumb fracture

    iii. Management

      a) Reduction and thumb spica

      b) Requires percutaneous pinning or ORIF

  b. Rolando fracture

    i. Definition

      a) Comminuted intra-articular fracture of thumb base

    ii. Mechanism

      a) Severe axial loading

    iii. Management

      a) Thumb spica and orthopedic referral

      b) Most ultimately require ORIF or percutaneous fixation

      c) Less common but worse outcome than Bennett fractures

O. Infections of the hand

  1. Paronychia and eponychia

  a. Definition: soft tissue infection of the lateral and proximal nail folds respectively

  b. Etiology

    i. Typically involve *Staphylococcus aureus* or *Streptococcus*

    ii. Fungal infection less common

  c. Symptoms and signs

    i. Cellulitis can progress to frank pus and extension into eponychium or with severe cases, into the pulp of fingertip (felon)

  d. Management

    i. Warm soaks and antibiotics for mild cases

    ii. Drainage of pus with elevation of lateral nail skin folds with blunt instrument or blunt edge of blade

    iii. Extensive pus collection may require incision and drainage after ring block

2. Felon

  a. Definition: infection of fingertip pulp

  b. Etiology: most commonly *S. aureus*

  c. Symptoms and signs

    i. Swelling and erythema pad of fingertip

  d. Management

    i. Incision and drainage

    ii. Antibiotics if concurrent cellulitis

  e. Complications

    i. Inadequate drainage from failure to relieve septated pus

    ii. Osteomyelitis

    iii. Flexor tenosynovitis

    iv. Sensation loss

3. Herpetic whitlow

  a. Etiology

    i. Herpes simplex virus

    ii. Auto-inoculation from genital or oral herpes

  b. Risk factors

    i. Health-care workers

    ii. Nail salon workers

  c. Symptoms and signs

    i. Prodrome of fever or malaise

    ii. Grouped vesicles on erythematous base

    iii. Lymphangitic streaking

  d. Management

    i. Self-limiting illness

    ii. Do **not** I&D

    iii. Topical acyclovir may decrease length of illness

    iv. Oral acyclovir may decrease recurrence

4. Infectious flexor tenosynovitis

  a. Etiology

    i. Penetrating trauma

    ii. *S. aureus* is most common organism

    iii. Human or animal bites

a) Cover for *Eikinella corrodens* if human bite

b) Early infection <24 hours after cat bite suspicious for *Pasteurella multocida*

iv. Consider disseminated gonorrhea in sexually active young adults

b. Symptoms and signs

  i. Pain, redness, and fever

  ii. Kanaval 4 cardinal signs

    a) Finger held in slight flexion

    b) Symmetric finger swelling

    c) Tenderness along flexor tendon

    d) Pain with passive extension

c. Management

  i. Very early infection may be managed conservatively with admission for intravenous antibiotics

  ii. Most patients will require surgery and open irrigation and debridement

P. Soft tissue injuries of the hand

1. De Quervain tenosynovitis

  a. Etiology

    i. Idiopathic inflammation of abductor pollicis longus and extensor pollicis brevis

    ii. May occur from repetitive stress injury, direct trauma, or in pregnancy

    iii. Thyroid disease

  b. Symptoms and signs

    i. Pain and thickening of dorsal compartment along radial styloid

    ii. Pain with thumb and wrist motion

  c. Diagnosis

    i. Finkelstein test

      a) Ulnar deviation of wrist with thumb in fist reproduces symptoms

  d. Management

    i. Thumb spica immobilization

    ii. Steroid injection in first dorsal compartment effective in 50% to 85% of patients

    iii. Surgical release if injections fail

2. Gamekeeper thumb (ulnar collateral ligament disruption)

  a. Mechanism

    i. Extreme radial extension of thumb

    ii. Most common cause today is hyperextension on skiing pole, but historically acquired by gamekeepers while twisting the neck of rabbits

  b. Symptoms and signs

    i. Pain along ulnar aspect of MCP joint of the thumb

    ii. Weak pinching grasp

c. Diagnosis

  i. X-ray to rule out avulsion fracture

  ii. Laxity of ulnar collateral ligament

    a) Place thumb in 30 degrees of flexion and apply valgus stress. >30 degrees laxity or >15 degrees difference from unaffected thumb constitutes a positive test

      i) Contraindicated if fracture present

  iii. Stener lesion

    a) Palpable lump at thumb MCP representing distal end of torn ligament

d. Management

  i. Thumb spica splint

  ii. Operative repair may be required based on the extent of ligamentous disruption

3. Mallet finger

  a. Definition

    i. Disruption of extensor tendon mechanism to the DIP joint

    ii. Results in flexion attitude of DIP joint

  b. Mechanism

    i. Forced flexion of the distal phalanx

      a) Classically from "jammed" finger playing volleyball or basketball

    ii. Disruption of extensor tendon at base of distal phalanx

  c. Diagnosis

    i. Clinical diagnosis

    ii. X-ray useful in diagnose of avulsion fragments (Figure 2–8)

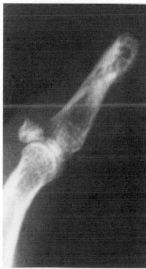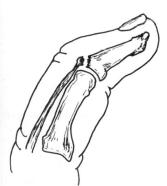

FIGURE 2–8. Mallet finger. Forced flexion of the DIP joint causes avulsion of the extensor tendon from the base of the distal phalanx. (Reproduced, with permission from Schwartz DT, Reisdorff EJ: *Emergency Radiology.* Copyright © 2000, New York: McGraw-Hill.)

d. Management
  i. Splint finger in full extension
    a) 6 to 8 weeks if ligamentous injury
    b) 4 to 6 weeks if avulsion fracture
  ii. Surgery rarely indicated
e. Complications
  i. Cosmetic deformity but rarely of functional consequence
  ii. Swan neck deformity may result (uncommon)
4. Swan neck deformity
  a. Definition
    i. DIP flexion and proximal interphalangeal (PIP) hyperextension
  b. Etiology
    i. Chronic inflammation or disease of PIP volar plate
      a) Rheumatoid arthritis
      b) Cerebral palsy, Parkinson disease, stroke
      c) Trauma (mallet finger)
    ii. Disease of DIP joint
  c. Management
    i. Nonsurgical if PIP joint relatively disease free and not stiff
    ii. Surgical management for severe deformity
    iii. Physical therapy
5. Boutonniere deformity
  a. Definition
    i. Reverse swan neck deformity with hyperextension of DIP joint and flexion of PIP joint
  b. Etiology
    i. Deformity and defect of central slip causing volar migration of lateral bands
      a) Trauma and lacerations
      b) Chronic inflammation as in rheumatoid arthritis
  c. Management
    i. Finger splinting in extension for mild disease
    ii. Surgery for severe deformity but risk worse disability
    iii. Physical therapy

III. Pelvic and Hip Injuries

A. Pelvic fractures
  1. Mechanism
    a. Tile-Young classification by mechanism
      i. A-P fracture: crush injury (Figure 2–9A)
        a) External iliac rotation
        b) Potential open book injuries
        c) Highest mortality and blood loss
      ii. Vertical shear: fall from height (Figure 2–9B)
        a) Anterior pubic ramus fractures
        b) Sacrum fractures or sacroiliac diastasis
        c) Iliac wing fractures
      iii. Lateral compression: pedestrian struck (Figure 2–9C)
        a) Internal iliac rotation
        b) Lowest mortality and blood loss caused by inherent compression
  2. Symptoms and signs
    a. Hypotension, tachycardia, and shock with significant blood loss

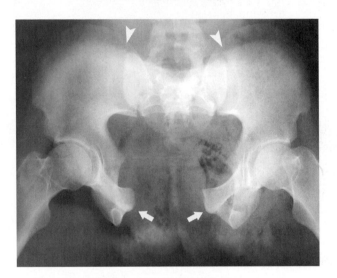

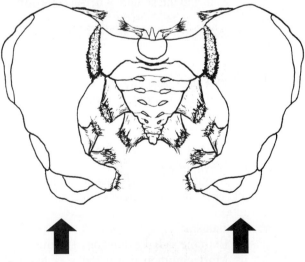

A

FIGURE 2–9. Pelvic fracture classification. *A.* A-P crush injury. *B.* Vertical shear injury. *C.* Lateral compression injuries. (Reproduced, with permission from Schwartz DT, Reisdorff EJ: *Emergency Radiology.* Copyright © 2000, New York: McGraw-Hill and Schwartz DT, *Emergency Radiology: Case Studies.* Copyright © 2008, New York: McGraw-Hill.)

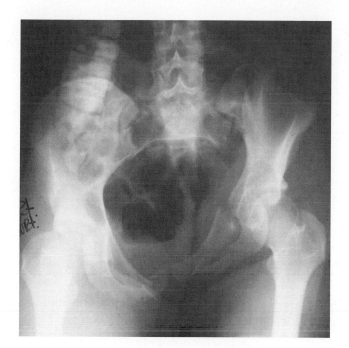

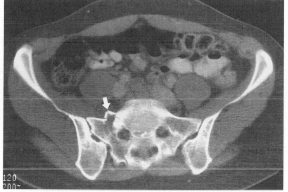

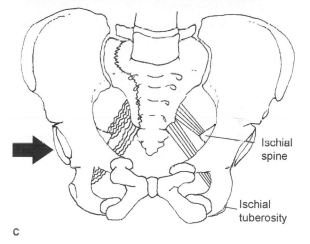

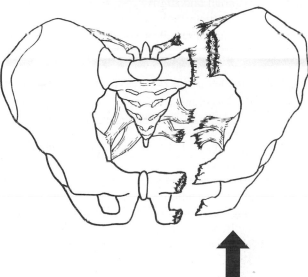

Ischial
spine

Ischial
tuberosity

B

C

FIGURE 2–9.   (*Continued*)

i. Up to 6 L of blood can collect into retroperitoneal space
   a) A-P crush injury—average 15 units blood loss
   b) Vertical shear—average 9 units blood loss
   c) Lateral compression mechanism—3.5 units blood loss
b. Pelvic instability

c. Fracture line may be palpable on bimanual examination
d. Secondary signs of pelvic fracture
   i. Destot sign—hematoma above inguinal ligament
   ii. Earle sign—tender fracture line or hematoma felt on rectal examination
e. Secondary genitourinary injury common
   i. Tenderness on rectal examination
   ii. High-riding prostate

        iii. Scrotal hematoma

        iv. Gross hematuria

        v. Blood at urethral meatus

        vi. Inability to urinate

3. Diagnosis
   a. X-rays
      i. A-P and lateral views
         a) Symphysis pubis normally <1 cm in width
            i) If >2.5 cm, assume posterior diastasis
         b) Sacroiliac joint normally <5 mm in width
      ii. Inlet views evaluate anterior and posterior displacement of hemipelvis
      iii. Outlet views evaluate vertical shear displacement
   b. CT scans
      i. Better at evaluating acetabulum
      ii. Better at evaluation of posterior pelvic elements
      iii. Helps rule out concomitant genitourinary, abdominal, and thoracic injuries

4. Management
   a. Follow standard advanced trauma life support (ATLS) protocol
   b. Pelvis stabilization and tamponade of blood
      i. External binder (commercially available splinting device)
      ii. Sheets tied around patient's pelvis at the level of **greater trochanter**
      iii. External fixators
      iv. Pneumatic antishock garment (PASG)
   c. Management of hypotensive patient with potential abdominal trauma
      i. Distracting injury makes abdominal examination unreliable
      ii. Laparotomy versus angiography
         a) Hypotensive with a positive FAST (Focused Assessment with Sonography for Trauma) examination, intra-abdominal fluid on CT scan, or positive peritoneal lavage—proceed to laparotomy
         b) Negative evaluation for intra-abdominal fluid should prompt angiographic evaluation in the hypotensive patient
         c) Perform peritoneal lavage via **supraumbilical** approach
   d. Ultimate management may involve
      i. Operative fixation
      ii. Embolization for arterial bleeding, although venous plexus injuries are most common

5. Complications
   a. Urethral injury and bladder rupture are the most common concomitant visceral injury (see Trauma chapter)
      i. Urethral injuries more common in men
      ii. Urethral injury highest with straddle injury
   b. Pulmonary embolus
   c. Fat emboli
   d. Rectal injuries with ischial fractures—administer antibiotics
   e. Thoracic aortic rupture associated with the high-energy trauma
   f. Overall mortality 10% in adults
   g. 50% mortality if hypotensive on arrival

B. Hip dislocations
   1. Mechanism
      a. Motor vehicle collision (MVC) and fall most common causes
         i. Dashboard injury to flexed hip in MVC
      b. Football and rugby
         i. Athlete lands with hip flexed, adducted, and internally rotated
      c. Native hip dislocation associated with high-energy trauma
      d. Prosthetic hips prone to dislocation with minimal trauma
      e. Children with congenital hip abnormalities prone to dislocation
      f. Patients with Down syndrome prone to hip dislocations
   2. Symptoms and signs
      a. Ability to ambulate does not rule out fracture
      b. Internally rotated and shortened extremity with posterior dislocations (posterior more common than anterior dislocations)
      c. Externally rotated and shortened with anterior dislocation
      d. Vascular injury may lead to loss of distal pulses
      e. Nerve injury may lead to motor weakness and sensory disturbance
   3. Diagnosis
      a. A-P and lateral hip and pelvis x-ray (Figure 2–10)
      b. CT scan patients with negative x-rays with high clinical suspicion
   4. Management
      a. Native hip dislocations are true orthopedic emergencies
         i. >6-hour delay in reduction increases likelihood of avascular necrosis of femoral head
      b. Neurovascular injury necessitates immediate reduction

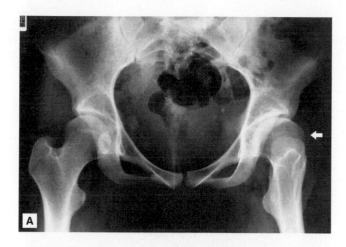

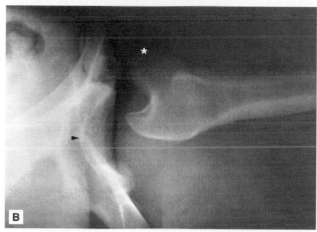

FIGURE 2–10. Anterior hip dislocation. *A.* AP view. *B.* Cross-table lateral view. (Reproduced, with permission from Schwartz DT, Reisdorff EJ: *Emergency Radiology.* Copyright © 2000, New York: McGraw-Hill.)

  c. Adequate conscious sedation
  d. Distract inferiorly in an attempt to disengage femoral head from the acetabulum and once cleared, the femoral head is able to relocate into the bony pelvis; slight internal and external rotation may facilitate this process
 5. Complications
  a. Posterior dislocations
   i. Sciatic nerve injury
    a) Pain along lateral thigh and calf
    b) Lower leg weakness
  b. Anterior dislocations
   i. Femoral nerve injury
    a) Weak quadriceps
    b) Medial thigh paresthesias
   ii. Femoral artery injury
   iii. Femoral vein thrombosis and pulmonary embolism
  c. Avascular necrosis of femoral head

C. Hip fractures
 1. Definition
  a. 4 subtypes of proximal femur fractures colloquially referred to as "hip fractures"
   i. Femoral head
    a) Usually high-energy trauma (typical hip fractures associated with low-energy trauma such as minor falls)
    b) Associated with dislocations
   ii. Femoral neck
    a) Between the head and greater trochanter
    b) Often interrupts blood supply to femur
    c) Highest risk of avascular necrosis without arthroplasty
   iii. Intertrochanteric
    a) Fracture line between greater and lesser trochanter
    b) Most common hip fracture
    c) Good prognosis for healing with conservative therapy
   iv. Subtronchanteric
    a) Fracture below intertrochanteric line
 2. Risk factors
  a. Elderly, female, white, osteoporosis, malignancy
 3. Symptoms and signs
  a. Externally rotated and shortened lower extremity
  b. Hypotension and tachycardia with blood loss (up to 1500 mL)
 4. Diagnosis
  a. X-ray
   i. Pelvis and hip
   ii. Cross-table lateral
   iii. Frog-leg lateral views **not** recommended in trauma patients
  b. CT and MRI with high clinical suspicion for fracture with negative plain films
 5. Management
  a. ATLS
  b. Orthopedic consult
 6. Complications
  a. 30% to 50% 1-year mortality
  b. Avascular necrosis and nonunion

IV. Lower Extremity Injuries

A. Knee injuries
 1. Tibial plateau fractures—most commonly proximal tibial fracture
  a. Definition: fractures involving the medial and/or lateral tibial condyles

b. Mechanism
  i. Axial load with valgus or varus rotation (fall from height)
  ii. Laterally directed force (as in pedestrian struck by car)
c. Symptoms and signs: knee effusion, point tenderness
d. Diagnosis: A-P and lateral x-rays plus tibial plateau views
  i. Most plateau fractures involve the lateral condyle
e. Management
  i. Nondisplaced fracture—immobilize and non-weight-bearing
  ii. >3 mm depressed fracture—orthopedic referral for ORIF

2. Dislocations and relocations
  a. True orthopedic and vascular emergency
  b. Mechanism
    i. Anterior dislocations
      a) Hyperextension injury as in running and stepping into a hole
    ii. Posterior dislocation
      a) Knee to dashboard injury
    iii. Medial dislocation
      a) Lateral to medial force on tibia
    iv. Lateral and rotary
  c. Symptoms and signs
    i. Often present after relocation
    ii. May appear deceptively normal
    iii. Popliteal artery injury may present with cool or pulseless leg
    iv. Peroneal nerve injury may present with sensation loss between first webspace and foot drop
      a) Seen commonly with posterior and medial dislocations
  d. Diagnosis
    i. Maintain high clinical suspicion
      a) An unstable knee is a reduced dislocation until proven otherwise
      b) Popliteal artery injury possible even with normal examination
    ii. X-ray—A-P and lateral views
      a) Anterior and posterior dislocations most common
    iii. Suspicion of popliteal artery injury warrants angiogram
      a) Historically, knee dislocations were evaluated with angiograms
      b) Recent literature supports the role of the ankle brachial index (ABI) as a screening tool but this remains controversial

e. Management
  i. Orthopedic and vascular consultation
  ii. Reduction and immobilization
  iii. Assessment of neurovascular injuries
    a) Vascular injuries require emergent repair
    b) Nerve injury results in poor outcome without surgery
f. Complications
  i. Popliteal artery injury is the most-feared complication (30%)
    a) Seen commonly with anterior dislocations
    b) Uncommon with posterior and medial dislocations
    c) Failure to operate and repair within 6 to 8 hours may lead to irreversible ischemia and limb amputation
  ii. Peroneal nerve injury (30%)
  iii. Compartment syndrome (see below)
  iv. Joint instability caused by concomitant ligamentous injury

3. Soft tissue injuries to the knee
  a. Meniscus injury
    i. Mechanism
      a) Rotary stress in varying degrees of flexion or extension
      b) Repeated squatting and standing
      c) Medial >lateral meniscus injured
    ii. Symptoms and signs
      a) Joint line pain and edema (late effusion)
      b) Locking of knee
      c) Feeling of knee "giving out"
      d) Joint line tenderness
    iii. Diagnosis
      a) MRI
      b) Apley test
        i) Differentiates meniscus versus ligamentous injury
        ii) Patient prone with knee flexed at 90 degrees
        iii) Pain with distraction of calf away from joint with internal and external rotation indicative of ligamentous injury
        iv) Pain with compressive "grinding" of knee with internal and external rotation indicative of meniscus injury
      c) McMurray test
        i) Patient supine with hip flexed at 90 degrees
        ii) Fully flex knee

iii) Pain and click with extension of knee with valgus stress and external rotation indicative of medial meniscus injury

iv) Pain with varus stress and internal rotation indicative of lateral meniscus injury

d) Payr test

    i) Sit patient with legs crossed

    ii) Pain with downward pressure on medial aspect of knee suggestive of medial meniscus injury

iv. Management

a) Acute locked knee

    i) Sit patient on edge of table with knee hanging

    ii) Gently apply traction with rotation

    iii) Manipulation may cause further injury so only a few gentle reduction attempts should be performed

    iv) Orthopedic consultation advised

    v) Failure to manually reduce a locked knee is an indication for arthroscopy (within 24 hours)

b) Apply splint and keep non-weight-bearing

c) Orthopedic follow-up

b. Anterior cruciate ligament (ACL) injury

i. Mechanism

a) ACL injury

b) Hyperextension/pivot combination ("I planted my foot, twisted, and heard a pop")

ii. Risk factors

a) Women >men

b) Sports requiring landing from jump, cutting, or rapid changes in direction

iii. Symptom and signs

a) Immediate swelling and pain (in contrast to late effusion associated with meniscal tears)

iv. Diagnosis

a) MRI

b) X-ray

    i) Usually normal

    ii) Segond fracture (associated with ACL tear)—avulsion fracture of lateral proximal tibia below articular surface

c) Pivot shift test

    i) Keep patient supine and flex hip to 45 degrees

    ii) Apply valgus stress and internally rotate fully extended knee

iii) An audible/palpable click representing reduction of an anteriorly subluxed tibia indicates a positive test

iv) Maneuver may be uncomfortable for patient

d) Lachman maneuver

    i) Test knee in 20 degrees of flexion

    ii) Pull tibia anteriorly while stabilizing femur

    iii) Excessive anterior movement relative to unaffected knee constitutes a positive test

e) Anterior drawer test

    i) Least reliable provocative maneuver

    ii) Patient seated with hip in 45 degrees flexion and 90 degrees knee flexion

    iii) Pull on tibia while stabilizing femur and foot

    iv) Increased anterior laxity compared to unaffected knee constitutes a positive test (>6 mm)

v. Management

a) Elastic bandage and crutches to help bear weight

b) Outpatient orthopedic consultation

c. Posterior cruciate ligament

i. Mechanism

a) Posteriorly directed force to proximal tibia on flexed knee

b) Typically high-energy mechanism as in knee-to-dashboard injuries with MVC

ii. Symptoms and signs

a) Immediate swelling

b) Pain and limping

iii. Diagnosis

a) MRI

b) Posterior drawer test

    i) Very sensitive and specific

    ii) Patient sitting with hip in 45 degrees flexion and 90 degrees knee flexion

    iii) Apply posteriorly directed force on tibia

    iv) >5-mm posterior translation constitutes positive test

c) Reverse pivot shift test

    i) Valgus stress applied to externally rotated knee in 90 degrees of flexion

    ii) Audible or palpable click with extension of knee represents reduction of a posteriorly subluxed tibia and a positive test

iv. Management
  a) As in suspected ACL injuries
d. Medial collateral ligament (MCL) injury
  i. Mechanism
    a) Valgus stress as in football tackle and blow to lateral knee of a planted foot
  ii. Symptoms and signs
    a) Medial knee pain and swelling
    b) Knee "feels loose"
  iii. Diagnosis
    a) MRI
      i) May also help diagnose associated medial meniscus and ACL tear (the unhappy triad)
    b) Valgus stress testing at 20 degrees of flexion isolates MCL from ACL
      i) Increased laxity (typically >10 mm) in comparison with unaffected knee constitutes positive test
  iv. Management
    a) Elastic bandage and crutches to help bear weight
    b) Orthopedic referral
e. Lateral collateral ligament injury
  i. Mechanism
    a) Least common soft tissue knee injury
    b) Varus stress to partially flexed knee
      i) Running into a hole on the street
      ii) Wrestlers
  ii. Symptoms and signs
    a) Lateral knee pain and swelling
    b) Peroneal nerve injury possible
  iii. Diagnosis
    a) MRI
    b) Varus stress testing reveals increased laxity
  iv. Management
    a) As in suspected MCL injuries

B. Extensor mechanism injuries
  1. Clinical anatomy
    a. The rectus femoris, vastus lateralis, intermedius, and medialis condense to form the quadriceps tendon and inserts into the superior pole of the patella
    b. The patellar tendon originates on the inferior pole of the patella and inserts onto the tibial tuberosity
    c. Injury to any of the above structures can interrupt proper knee extension
  2. Epidemiology
    a. Quadriceps tendon rupture occurs more commonly in the elderly
    b. Patella tendon ruptures are rare but occur in the young
    c. Tibial tuberosity injuries occur in active adolescents
  3. Quadriceps rupture
    a. Mechanism
      i. Sudden forced extension
      ii. Direct trauma
    b. Symptoms and signs
      i. Suprapatellar pain and swelling
      ii. Inferior displacement of patella
      iii. Palpable defect above patella
      iv. Unable to extend knee
    c. Management
      i. Surgery
  4. Patellar fracture (Figure 2–11)
    a. Mechanism
      i. Direct trauma to patella
      ii. Forceful quadriceps contraction
    b. Symptoms and signs
      i. Tenderness and small effusion
      ii. May look deceptively benign
      iii. Severe injury may disrupt extensor mechanism
        a) Always check to see if patient able to extend knee

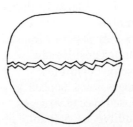 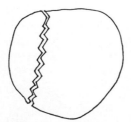 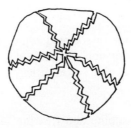 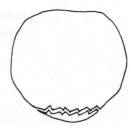

| Horizontal (Transverse) | Vertical | Stellate | Marginal |

FIGURE 2–11. Types of patellar fractures. (Reproduced, with permission from Schwartz DT, Reisdorff EJ: *Emergency Radiology.* Copyright © 2000, New York: McGraw-Hill.)

c. Diagnosis
   i. A-P, lateral, and sunrise views on x-ray
d. Management
   i. Splint in full extension with weight-bearing as tolerated
   ii. Operative management if loss of extensor mechanism or >3 mm displacement of fracture fragments

5. Patellar dislocation
   a. Mechanism: tibial rotation against flexed knee during quadriceps contraction
   b. Symptoms and signs: hip and knee are typically flexed to 90 degrees with the patella dislocated laterally (more common than medial dislocation)
   c. Diagnosis: x-ray also rules out fractures
   d. Management
      i. Reduction of lateral dislocation
         a) Apply valgus force to patella while extending knee
      ii. Knee immobilizer
      iii. Orthopedic follow-up

6. Chondromalacia patellae (patellar malalignment syndrome/runner knee)
   a. Mechanism—various theories
      i. Anterior knee pain caused by erosion of cartilage beneath patella as it tracks up and down
      ii. Patellar tendon laxity leading to excessive patellar mobility
      iii. Affects females significantly more than males
      iv. Wide Q-angle (angle measured between lines drawn patella and shaft of femur)
   b. Symptoms and signs
      i. Pain walking down stairs and rising after extended time sitting
      ii. Slightly more motion is expected laterally than medially
      iii. Pain occurring after exercise
   c. Diagnosis
      i. Patellar grind
         a) Downward pressure on patella during quadriceps contraction elicits pain and constitutes a positive test
      ii. Apprehension test
         a) Pain or apprehension with lateral force applied to patella constitutes a positive test
   d. Management
      i. RICE therapy (rest, ice, compression, elevation)
      ii. Quadriceps-strengthening exercises
      iii. Splinting contraindicated

7. Patellar tendonitis and rupture (jumper knee)
   a. Mechanism
      i. Repetitive stress injury in sports requiring frequent jumping and extension at the knee
   b. Diagnosis
      i. Tenderness at the inferior pole of patella
      ii. No fractures on x-ray
      iii. With rupture of tendon
         a) High-riding patella
         b) Palpable defect beneath patella
         c) Inability to extend knee
   c. Management
      i. RICE therapy and NSAIDs
      ii. Physical therapy
      iii. Surgical repair

8. Tibial tuberosity avulsion fractures
   a. Mechanism
      i. Avulsion injury that occurs in adolescence caused by powerful contraction of knee extensors, as in jumping
      ii. Direct trauma uncommon
   b. Symptoms and signs
      i. Adolescents may have had history of bilateral tuberosity pain with history of Osgood-Schlatter (see Pediatric Orthopedics below)
      ii. Pain and swelling at tibial tuberosity
      iii. High-riding patella
      iv. Inability to extend knee
   c. Diagnosis
      i. A-P and lateral x-ray
   d. Management
      i. Most patients require surgical intervention

9. Iliotibial band syndrome
   a. Definition: common cause of lateral knee pain in athletes
   b. Clinical anatomy
      i. Originates from iliac crest and inserts into lateral portion of proximal tibia to help abduct and flex the hip
   c. Symptoms and signs
      i. Frequent flexion and extension, as in running or cycling
      ii. Pain with climbing steps or walking down incline
   d. Management
      i. RICE therapy and NSAIDs
      ii. Steroid injection may benefit refractory pain

C. Ankle injuries
   1. Anatomy
      a. Ankle is made up of 2 joints
         i. The true joint
            a) Consists of distal tibia, distal fibula, and the talus

b) Responsible for allowing dorsiflexion and plantar flexion

ii. The subtalar joint

    a) Consists of talus and calcaneus

    b) Responsible for inversion and eversion of ankle

b. Lateral ligaments (in order of injury occurrence)

    i. Anterior talofibular ligament (ATFL)

    ii. Calcaneofibular ligament

    iii. Posterior talofibular ligament

c. Deltoid ligaments (medial aspect of ankle)

    i. Medial ligamentous complex

    ii. Particularly strong

d. Syndesmotic ligaments (posterior aspect of ankle)

    i. Anterior tibiofibular ligament

    ii. Posterior tibiofibular ligament

    iii. Inferior transverse ligament

    iv. Intraosseous membrane

2. Ankle sprains

  a. Mechanism

    i. Inversion: injuries to lateral ligaments, most commonly the ATFL

    ii. Eversion: injuries to deltoid ligaments

    iii. Forceful external rotation: injury to syndesmotic ligaments

  b. Symptoms and signs

    i. History of prior ankle sprains

    ii. Hearing a "pop"

    iii. Pain and swelling

    iv. Syndesmotic injuries

      a) Compression of calf with 2 hands causes ankle pain

      b) May present with deceptively minimal swelling

      c) May present with weak heel lift and toe walking

  c. Diagnosis

    i. X-rays to rule out fracture

      a) Indications as per Ottawa ankle rules (Table 2–1)

TABLE 2–1. Ottawa Foot and Ankle Rules

X-rays are not necessary if
- The patient can walk 4 steps at the time of injury and in the ED
- There is no tenderness over the distal 6 cm of the tibia/fibula
- There is no tenderness over the medial or lateral malleolus
- There is no tenderness over the fifth metatarsal
- There is no tenderness over the navicular

b) >4 mm diastasis between medial malleolus and talus suspicious for unstable deltoid ligament

c) >4 mm diastasis between tibia and fibula suspicious for unstable syndesmosis

d. Management

    i. Stable ankle sprains treated with RICE therapy

    ii. Deltoid and syndesmotic injuries may require casting, non-weight-bearing, and surgical intervention

3. Peroneal tendon subluxation

  a. Definition

    i. Subluxation of peroneal brevis tendon anterior to lateral malleolus

    ii. An uncommon injury requiring surgical intervention

    iii. Commonly misdiagnosed as a lateral ankle sprain

  b. Mechanism

    i. Forced hyperdorsiflexion and eversion of the ankle

  c. Diagnosis

    i. Suspected only after "ankle sprain" not improving as expected

    ii. MRI

  d. Management

    i. Most require surgery

4. Ankle fractures

  a. Definition

    i. Single malleolar: fracture involving either distal fibula or tibia

    ii. Bimalleolar: fracture involving both distal fibula and tibia

    iii. Trimalleolar: bimalleolar fracture and posterior tibial involvement

  b. Eponyms

    i. Pilon fracture

      a) Axial load mechanism such as fall from height

      b) Distal tibial fracture with disruption of talar dome

      c) Associated with lumbar fractures

    ii. Tillaux fracture

      a) Severe lateral rotation injury

      b) Type III Salter-Harris injury of lateral tibia

    iii. Maisonneuve fracture

      a) Severe eversion and external rotation injury

      b) Medial malleolar fracture (or deltoid ligament rupture) associated with concomitant proximal fibular fracture

c. Symptoms and signs
   i. Pain, swelling, and obvious deformity
   ii. Pallor and coolness if vascular injury exists
d. Diagnosis
   i. A-P, lateral, and mortise view x-rays
   ii. Consider knee x-ray
       a) "Ring axiom"—a fracture in one part of the ring is associated with another injury
   iii. Ottawa ankle rules as above
e. Management
   i. Most single malleolar fractures involve the distal fibula
       a) Medical management if fracture is below level of mortise
   ii. Bimalleolar and trimalleolar fractures are unstable, require ORIF
   iii. Vascular injuries require reduction and surgery consultation

5. Achilles tendon rupture
   a. Mechanism
      i. Sudden dorsiflexion
          a) Jumping
          b) Running and stepping into a hole
   b. Risk factors
      i. Steroids (oral or injection)
      ii. Fluoroquinolone use
      iii. Rheumatoid arthritis
   c. Symptoms and signs
      i. May report hearing a loud "pop"
      ii. A palpable defect is often in the midsubstance of the tendon
   d. Diagnosis
      i. Ultrasound
      ii. Thompson test
          a) Absent plantar flexion with calf squeezed
          b) Partial tears may not have positive Thompson test
   e. Management
      i. Splint foot in 20 degrees of plantar flexion (equinas)
      ii. Definitive management (surgical versus serial splinting)

D. Foot injuries
   1. Calcaneal fractures
      a. Mechanism
         i. High-energy axial load as in fall from height
         ii. Osteoporotic patients can have fractures with trivial trauma
      b. Symptoms and signs
         i. Heel pain and swelling
         ii. Back pain with concomitant lumbar/thoracic spine fractures

c. Diagnosis
   i. X-ray
       a) Suspect fracture if Bohler angle <25 degrees
       b) CT scan with high suspicion
d. Management
   i. Intra-articular fractures involving subtalar joint requires surgery
   ii. RICE for nondisplaced and minor extraarticular fractures

2. Jones versus Pseudo-Jones fractures
   a. Pseudo-Jones fracture (Figures 2–12A and 2–12B)
      i. Avulsion fracture at the base of the fifth metatarsal
      ii. Treated with a bulky dressing or hard-sole shoe for 6 weeks
      iii. The prognosis for full fracture healing is excellent
   b. Jones fracture is a fracture of the fifth metatarsal diaphysis
      i. Injury is prone to nonunion
      ii. Cast within 48 to 72 hours of injury
      iii. Patient should be non-weight-bearing
      iv. Surgical pinning may be indicated (Figure 2–13)

3. Lisfranc fracture
   a. Definition
      i. Midfoot dislocation and fracture injury involving the second metatarsal
   b. Mechanism
      i. Direct injury and crush
      ii. Axial load applied to a plantar flexed foot
      iii. Driver involved in MVC (MVC occurs while slamming on the brakes)
   c. Symptoms and signs
      i. Pain out of proportion to external deformity
      ii. Unable to bear weight, given main stabilizer of foot is affected
      iii. Injury at the base of the second metatarsal
   d. Diagnosis (Figure 2–14)
      i. A-P, lateral, and oblique x-ray views, and stress (weight-bearing) views
          a) >2 mm diastasis between first and second metatarsals
      ii. CT scan
   e. Management
      i. Immediate orthopedic and podiatry consultation
      ii. Analgesics
      iii. Splinting
      iv. Operative repair ideally within 24 hours

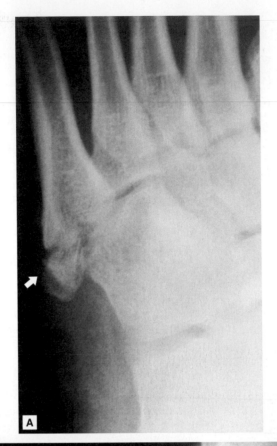

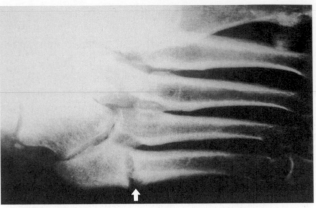

FIGURE 2–13. Jones fracture. A transverse fracture through the proximal fifth metatarsal that involves the articular surface between the bases of the fourth and fifth metatarsals. (Reproduced, with permission from Schwartz DT, Reisdorff EJ: *Emergency Radiology.* Copyright © 2000, New York: McGraw-Hill.)

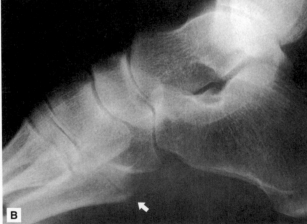

FIGURE 2–12. "Pseudo-Jones" fracture. An avulsion fracture of the fifth metatarsal tuberosity. (Reproduced, with permission from Schwartz DT, Reisdorff EJ: *Emergency Radiology.* Copyright © 2000, New York: McGraw-Hill.)

V. Compartment Syndrome

A. Definition
   1. Ischemia resulting from increasing pressure within a closed space

B. Mechanism
   1. Trauma

    a. Crush
    b. Burns
    c. Long bone fractures (tibial fractures are the most common cause)
   2. Nontraumatic
    a. Anticoagulation
    b. Rhabdomyolysis
    c. Carbon monoxide poisoning
    d. Snake envenomation

C. Symptoms and signs
   1. The **5-Ps** (**P**ain out of proportion to examination, **P**aresthesia, **P**allor, **P**ulselessness, **P**oikilothermia)
   2. Pain with passive extension of limb or joint
   3. Tense limb
   4. Paresthesias and paralysis

D. Diagnosis
   1. Labs
    a. Creatine kinase (CK) levels to rule out rhabdomyolysis
    b. Check for hyperkalemia and abnormal renal function
    c. Urinalysis may be dip positive for blood but no RBCs on microscopic, indicating the presence of myoglobin
    d. Consider international normalized ratio (INR) and carbon monoxide levels in appropriate setting
   2. Measure compartment pressures
    a. Measure as close to the fracture site as possible
    b. Measure twice to avoid false-negative readings

E. Management
   1. Compartment pressures should be <10 mm Hg
    a. Admit and observe if pressures between 10 and 30 mm Hg

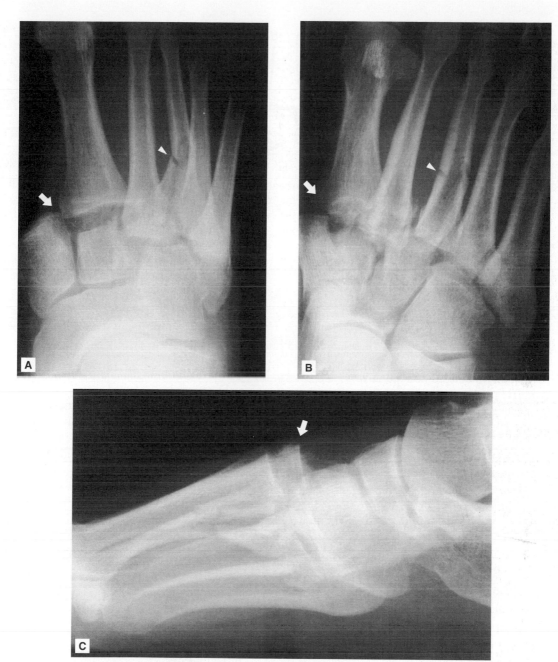

FIGURE 2–14. Lisfranc fracture/dislocation, homolateral type. *A.* A-P view. *B.* Internal oblique view. *C.* Lateral view. (Reproduced, with permission from Schwartz DT, Reisdorff EJ: *Emergency Radiology.* Copyright © 2000, New York: McGraw-Hill.)

b. Emergent fasciotomy with pressures >30 mm Hg

c. Interpretation

VI. Pediatric Orthopedics

A. Definitions
1. Greenstick: pediatric incomplete fracture pattern (bending) along one cortex

2. Torus or buckle: pediatric incomplete fracture pattern (buckling)

B. Growth plate (epiphyseal) injuries
1. Epiphyseal injuries more common than ligamentous injuries
2. Salter-Harris classification (Figure 2–15)
   a. Type I: transverse fracture through physis (widening of epiphyseal plate)
   b. Type II: physis and metaphysis

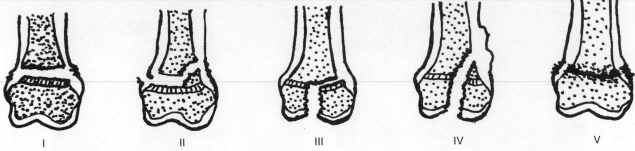

FIGURE 2–15. Salter-Harris classification of fractures through the epiphyseal growth plate. (Reproduced, with permission from Schwartz DT, Reisdorff EJ: *Emergency Radiology.* Copyright © 2000, New York: McGraw-Hill.)

    c. Type III: physis and epiphysis
    d. Type IV: metaphysis, epiphysis, and physis
    e. Type V: crush fracture of epiphyseal plate
  3. Management
    a. Types I and II
      i. Type II most common Salter-Harris fracture
      ii. Excellent prognosis
      iii. Usually managed nonoperatively
    b. Type III
      i. Management based on size and displacement of fracture
      ii. Often unstable
    c. Types IV and V
      i. Require surgical intervention
      ii. Prone to limb length discrepancies despite treatment
      iii. Type V injury difficult to appreciate on x-ray
      iv. Type V fracture often diagnosed after growth delay occurs

C. Supracondylar humeral fractures (see elbow fracture section above)

D. Nursemaid elbow
  1. Mechanism
    a. Hyperextension and pulling injury
    b. Swinging injury pattern
    c. Small radial head subluxed under loose annular ligament
    d. Incidence decreases as radial head size increases (aged 5 years)
  2. Symptoms and signs
    a. Presents with the elbow flexed and pronated
    b. The child is reluctant to use extremity but otherwise comfortable
  3. Diagnosis
    a. Clinical diagnosis
    b. X-ray if fracture suspected

  4. Management (2 methods)
    a. Flex and supinate elbow or hyperpronate and extend forearm
    b. Patient will begin using arm in 5 to 10 minutes

E. Congenital hip dislocation (<1 year)
  1. Epidemiology
    a. Firstborn females
    b. Uncommon in Asians and African Americans
  2. Diagnosis
    a. Ortolani and Barlow maneuvers
      i. Ortolani—abduct hips while patient lies supine with knees flexed
        a) A palpable clunk constitutes positive testing
      ii. Barlow—adduct hips with a second clunk (as the femoral head relocates) constitutes a positive test
  3. Management
    a. Refer to pediatric orthopedist for ultrasound and Pavlick bracing

F. Legg-Calves-Perthes (2 to 13 years)
  1. Epidemiology
    a. Males >females (4:1)
    b. Median age 7 years
  2. Definition
    a. Idiopathic avascular necrosis of the femoral head
  3. Risk factors
    a. Sickle cell disease
    b. Steroid use
  4. Symptoms and signs
    a. Hip pain that refers to knee or groin
    b. Limp
    c. Short stature (generalized delayed bone age)
    d. Leg length discrepancy
  5. Diagnosis
    a. A-P, lateral, and frog-leg views x-rays
      i. Joint space widening or sclerotic changes of femoral head

6. Management
   a. Orthopedic referral
   b. Bed rest and abduction exercises

G. Slipped capital femoral epiphysis (adolescence)
   1. Epidemiology
      a. African American adolescents
      b. Mild obesity
      c. Male >female
      d. Left >right hip affected
   2. Definition
      a. Slippage at the proximal femur epiphysis
   3. Symptoms and signs
      a. Limp/ hip or groin pain
      b. Hip externally rotated and adducted
   4. Diagnosis
      a. A-P and lateral pelvis and bilateral hips (Figure 2-16)
         i. Abnormal Klein line
            a) A straight line drawn along lateral aspect of the femoral neck should normally intersect part of the femoral head
         ii. Loss of Shenton line
            a) Curved line from the femoral neck to the obturator foramen
         iii. The slipped epiphysis resembles "ice cream falling off the cone"
      b. MRI for equivocal cases
   5. Management
      a. Orthopedic consultation for pinning
      b. Non-weight-bearing

H. Septic hip versus transient synovitis
   1. Septic hip
      a. Etiology
         i. *S. aureus* most common followed by *Streptococcus* species and *Pseudomonas*
         ii. Prior to vaccination, *H. influenzae* type B was most common
         iii. In children <3 years, consider *Kingella kingae*
         iv. Most cases from hematogenous seeding
      b. Symptoms and signs
         i. Children <6 years
         ii. Ill-appearing with fever
         iii. Refusal to walk
         iv. Hip held in flexion and external rotation (caused by capsule distention)
      c. Diagnosis
         i. Labs
            a) Complete blood count (CBC), erythrocyte sedimentation rate (ESR), C-reactive protein (CRP) blood cultures, basic electrolytes

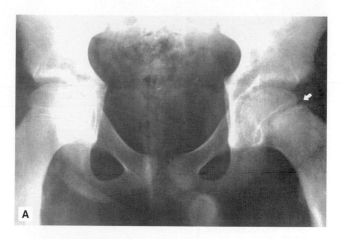

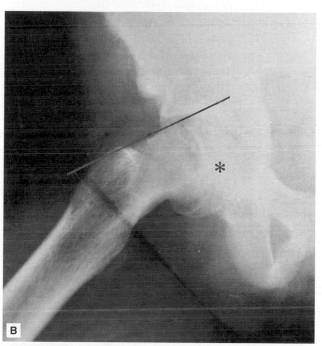

FIGURE 2–16. Two examples of subtle slipped capital femoral epiphysis (SCFE). *A.* A-P view. *B.* Frog-leg view. (Reproduced, with permission from Schwartz DT, Reisdorff EJ: *Emergency Radiology.* Copyright © 2000, New York: McGraw-Hill.)

            b) Normal CBC, ESR, or CRP does not definitively rule out
         ii. X-rays of the hip may reveal widened joint capsule
         iii. Ultrasound may confirm presence of joint effusion
         iv. CT to rule out psoas abscess, a clinically indistinguishable mimic
         v. MRI has no role
         vi. Fluoroscopically or ultrasound guided aspirate is definitive

    d. Management
      i. Orthopedic consultation
      ii. Joint aspiration
      iii. Antibiotics, preferably after blood and aspirate cultures

2. Transient synovitis
    a. Etiology
      i. Recent infection in 50% of patients
      ii. Unknown etiology
    b. Risk factors
      i. Boys >girls (2:1)
      ii. Usually <10 years
      iii. Association with Legg-Calves-Perthes disease
    c. Symptoms and signs
      i. Sometimes clinically indistinguishable from septic arthritis
      ii. May have mild fever
      iii. Non-toxic-appearing
      iv. Present with hip, groin and thigh, or knee pain
      v. Hip held in flexion, abduction, and external rotation
      vi. Responds well to NSAIDs

    d. Diagnosis
      i. Basic laboratory studies are usually normal, but ESR, CBC, and CRP may be slightly elevated
      ii. Diagnosis of exclusion
      iii. May require joint aspiration to rule out septic hip if not improving
    e. Treatment
      i. NSAIDs and rest

I. Osgood Schlatter disease
  1. Definition
    a. Inflammation over insertion point of patellar tendon on tibial tuberosity
  2. Etiology
    a. Repetitive traction injury
    b. Rapid growth
  3. Risk factors
    a. Boys >girls
    b. Sports involving repetitive jumping
  4. Symptoms and signs
    a. Tibial tuberosity tenderness, edema
    b. Pain increases with repetitive activity
  5. Treatment
    a. RICE therapy
    b. NSAIDs

Chapter 3

INTENSIVE REVIEW OF TRAUMA

Eric Legome and Paul Testa

I. Initial Approach to Trauma

A. Primary survey
   1. Airway
   2. Breathing
      a. Takes precedence over airway in penetrating chest trauma with tension pneumothorax
   3. Circulation
      a. Hemorrhage control-pressure is usually sufficient for external trauma
      b. Standard answer is use 2 L normal saline (NS) or lactated ringers (LR) followed by blood products
   4. Deficits
      a. Glasgow coma scale (GCS) and gross motor examination
      b. AVPU (**a**lert, responds to **v**oice, **p**ain, **u**nresponsive)
   5. Exposure
      a. Critical action to completely expose (then cover to keep warm)

B. Resuscitation
   1. Hemorrhage control
   2. Neurovascular compromise
   3. Permissive hypotensive resuscitation practiced but remains controversial

C. Secondary survey
   1. Determine what really happened
   2. System-based injury evaluation
   3. AMPLE history (**a**llergies, **m**edication, **p**ast medical history, **l**ast meal, **e**vents leading up to/**e**nvironmental)

D. Specific injuries of importance
   1. Traumatic arrest
      a. Penetrating chest trauma
      b. Vitals on arrival, then lost

   c. If both a and b are present, strongest indication for ED thoracotomy
   2. Traumatic head injury (severe)
      a. Intubate for hypoxia/airway protection
      b. C-spine precautions
      c. Identify neurosurgical candidates

II. Hemorrhagic Shock

A. Classification
   1. Class I hemorrhage: blood loss 0% to 15% (0–750 cc)
      a. Heart rate (HR) <100
      b. Treat with crystalloids, no blood products necessary
      c. Asymptomatic as typical blood donations involve 8% to 10% loss
   2. Class II hemorrhage: blood loss 15% to 30% (750–1500 cc)
      a. Tachypnea, **tachycardia >100**, narrow pulse pressure, cool skin. Initial treatment with crystalloids, may then use blood products
   3. Class III hemorrhage: blood loss 30% to 40% (1500–2000 cc)
      a. Tachypnea, tachycardia (HR >120), **<systolic blood presure** (BP), anxiety
      b. Blood products and crystalloids, typed blood if possible
   4. Class IV hemorrhage: blood loss >40% (>2 L)
      a. Tachycardia >140, < systolic BP, **confusion**, lethargy

B. Symptoms and signs
   1. Earliest signs are tachycardia and vasoconstriction (decreased pulse pressure)
   2. Tachycardia (class II), hypotension and anxiety (class III), mental status change and hypotension (class IV)

C. Management
  1. Initial treatment is volume resuscitation using warmed crystalloids
  2. Use blood warmers, 2 L crystalloid
  3. Type O Rh **negative** for women, Rh negative or positive for men

D. Massive transfusion
  1. Definition
    a. No strict definition but commonly referred to as the replacement of entire body blood volume within 24 hours, or >10 units of packed red blood cells (PRBC) transfusions within a few hours
  2. Complications
    a. Metabolic alkalosis and hypocalcemia secondary to citrated blood
    b. Hyperkalemia or **hypo**kalemia
    c. Hypothermia
    d. Dilutional coagulopathy
    e. Thrombocytopenia
    f. Acute respiratory distress syndrome (ARDS)
  3. Management
    a. Administer via blood warmer (not microwave)
    b. Factor replacement as necessary based on coagulation studies (no definitive guidelines or formulas)
    c. Calcium gluconate only if electrocardiogram (ECG) changes or tetany

III. Head Trauma

A. Classification by GCS (Table 3–1)
  1. Minor head trauma
    a. Definition: variably described as GCS 13 to 15
    b. Concussion
      i. Confusion and amnesia (retro- or anterograde)
      ii. Functional disturbance without evidence of structural injury
  2. Severe head trauma
    a. Definition: GCS <8
    b. Intubate a patient with GCS <8

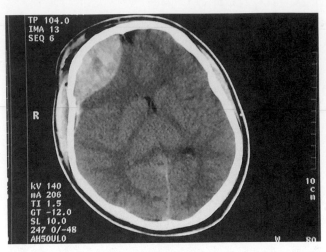

FIGURE 3–1. Epidural hematoma. (Reproduced, with permission from Stone CK, Humphries RL: *Current Diagnosis and Treatment: Emergency Medicine*, 6th ed. Copyright © 2008, New York: McGraw-Hill.)

B. Classification by injury type (see Neurology chapter)
  1. Epidural hematoma (Figure 3–1)
    a. Definition: blood collection between dura and the skull vault
    b. Etiology: laceration of middle meningeal artery from temporal bone fracture classically described
      i. Symptoms and signs: classic loss of consciousness followed by a lucid interval and rapid decompensation present in only 30%
    c. Diagnosis
      i. **Lenticular** shape on computed tomography (CT)
      ii. Crosses midline, but **not** suture lines
    d. Management
      i. Immediate hematoma evacuation
  2. Subdural hematoma (Figure 3–2)
    a. Definition: blood between the dura and arachnoid mater
    b. Etiology: disruption of bridging veins most common
    c. Symptoms and signs: headache and mental status change

TABLE 3–1. Glasgow Coma Scale

BEST EYE RESPONSE (4)	BEST VERBAL RESPONSE (5)	BEST MOTOR RESPONSE (6)
+ 1 No eye opening	+ 1 No verbal response	+ 1 No motor response
+ 2 Opening to pain	+ 2 Incomprehensible sounds	+ 2 Extension to pain
+ 3 Opening to verbal command	+ 3 Inappropriate words	+ 3 Flexion to pain
+ 4 Eyes open spontaneously	+ 4 Confused	+ 4 Withdrawal from pain
	+ 5 Orientated	+ 5 Localizing pain
		+ 6 Obeys commands

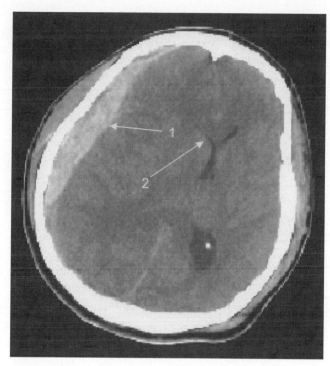

FIGURE 3–2. Subdural hematoma. (Reproduced, with permission from Tintinalli JE, Kelen GD, Stapczynski JS: *Tintinalli's Emergency Medicine: A Comprehensive Study Guide*, 6th ed. Copyright © 2004, New York: McGraw-Hill.)

   d. Diagnosis
     i. CT appearance of blood is crescent-shaped
     ii. Does **not** cross midline but crosses suture lines
   e. Management
     i. Depends on size of collection
     ii. Indications for surgery include >5 mm midline shift and neurologic deterioration

3. **Traumatic** subarachnoid hemorrhage (SAH)
   a. Definition
     i. Blood between the arachnoid and pia mater secondary to trauma
     ii. Entity distinct from spontaneous SAH caused by ruptured aneurysms (see Neurology chapter)
   b. Etiology
     i. Traumatic tears of subarachnoid vessels lead to bleeding
   c. Diagnosis
     i. Noncontrast head CT may reveal focal/ diffuse blood in cortical sulci in a pattern distinct from aneurismal bleeding into suprasellar cistern and ventricles
   d. Management
     i. Supportive

     ii. Prevent ischemia caused by increased intracranial pressure (ICP), cerebral vasospasm, and hydrocephalus
       a) Increased ICP (see management of herniation syndromes below)
       b) Vasospasm—oral nimodipine (may or may not prevent vasospasm, but is associated with better prognosis)
       c) Hydrocephalus—occurs more commonly with spontaneous SAH and may require shunt placement
       d) Triple H therapy—intentional **h**emodilution, **h**ypertension, and **h**ypervolemia

4. Intracerebral hematoma
   a. Definition
     i. Parenchymal contusions with direct injury to the brain
   b. Etiology
     i. Sudden acceleration and deceleration particularly along bony inner skull structures
     ii. Contracoup injury can occur opposite site of impact
   c. Diagnosis: head CT
   d. Management: supportive

5. Diffuse axonal injury (shear injury)
   a. Definition
     i. Diffuse axonal injury causing severe depressed level of consciousness out of proportion to radiographic findings
   b. Etiology
     i. White and grey matter have different densities and therefore tears one from another with sudden acceleration and deceleration or rotation motor vehicle accident (MVA), shaken baby syndrome
   c. Symptoms and signs
     i. Spectrum of illness related to degree of injury and mechanism ranging from brief loss of consciousness to persistent vegetative state
     ii. Complex ongoing biochemical cascade may cause delayed injury and worsening symptoms and signs
   d. Diagnosis
     i. Clinical and unfortunately, often a histologic diagnosis
     ii. MRI is superior to CT, but both modalities may be nondiagnostic
   e. Management: supportive

6. Skull fractures
   a. Definition
     i. Linear
       a) Rarely clinically significant in and of itself

b) Concern is for underlying brain injury, vascular bleeding, thrombosis, or suture diastasis
  ii. Comminuted
    a) In many fragments
  iii. Depressed
    a) A comminuted fracture with inward displacement
    b) If depression is greater than the thickness of adjacent inner table, may require surgical elevation
  iv. Basilar skull fracture
    a) Linear fractures running through the base of the skull, often through the petrous portion of temporal bone
    b) Usually high-energy injury
b. Symptoms and signs
  i. Linear fractures may present with pain and hematoma
  ii. Depressed fractures may present with skull crepitus
  iii. Basilar skull fracture
    a) Battle sign—ecchymosis behind the ear
    b) "Raccoon eyes"—periorbital ecchymosis with anterior cranial fossa bone injuries
    c) Cerebrospinal fluid (CSF) otorrhea/rhinorrhea
    d) Hemotympanum
    e) Cranial nerve injuries particularly CN VII and CN VIII
      i) Facial palsy, nystagmus, vertigo, hearing change
c. Diagnosis
  i. Palpation
  ii. Plain radiographs or CT scan
    a) Linear fractures may be missed on axial CT scans
    b) Basilar skull fractures may be missed on CT scans
  iii. CSF leaks with basilar skull fractures
    a) "Halo" or "ring" sign—bloodstain encircled by a clear or yellow ring
    b) CSF otorrhea and rhinorrhea can also be tested for high glucose and tau-transferrin
d. Management
  i. Open skull fractures (overlying skin broken) require antibiotics
  ii. Linear fractures rarely require repair and may be discharged if otherwise asymptomatic
  iii. Depressed skull fractures may require surgical elevation if depression greater than adjacent inner skull table thickness

  iv. Basilar skull fracture
    a) No consensus if patients with CSF leak should receive prophylactic antibiotics
    b) Steroids may aid recover of facial nerve palsy
C. Herniation syndromes
  1. Anatomy (Figure 3–3)
    a. The falx cerebri separates the left and right hemispheres
    b. The tentorium cerebelli divides the hemispheres (supratentorial) from the cerebellum and brainstem (infratentorial)
    c. Both structures are rigid and relatively sharp causing injury as tissue slides under/over and against them
    d. Each consist of a central opening that permits herniation to compensate for unequal pressures
  2. Classification
    a. Subfalcine
      i. Most common brain herniation syndrome
      ii. CT shows midline shift of frontal lobe under falx
      iii. May simultaneously put downward pressure on brainstem
    b. Central (transtentorial)—temporal lobes herniated through tentorium
      i. May injure basilar artery
    c. Uncal herniation—uncus of a temporal lobe herniates through tentorium and into brainstem
      i. May cause an ipsilateral CN III palsy (blown pupil that is "down and out")

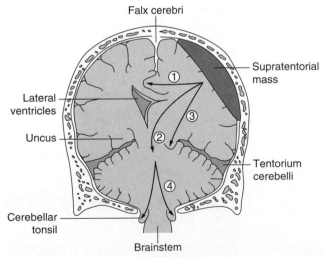

FIGURE 3–3. Herniation syndromes. (Reproduced, with permission from McPhee SJ, Ganong WF: *Pathophysiology of Disease: An Introduction to Clinical Medicine*, 5th ed. Copyright © 2006, New York: McGraw-Hill.)

ii. Therefore, when CT scan unavailable, place emergent burr hole **ipsilateral** to affected eye

d. Upward or cerebellar—posterior fossa mass causes upward herniation of cerebellum through tentorium

e. Tonsillar—downward cerebellar herniation through foramen magnum

  i. May exhibit brainstem dysfunction

D. Supportive care in traumatic brain injury

1. Hypotension

  a. Hypotension (systolic BP <90 mm Hg) and hypoxia (PaO_2 <60 mm Hg) associated with poor outcome

  b. Cerebral perfusion pressure (CPP) is mean arterial pressure (MAP) minus intracranial pressure (normal ICP 0–15)

  c. CPP should be maintained at >70 mm Hg

  d. Maintain ICP <20 mm Hg

   i. Mild hyperventilation (PCO_2 ~30: short-lived effect)

   ii. Mannitol if evidence of impending transtentorial herniation; CSF drainage preferable to mannitol

   iii. Elevate the head of the stretcher from 20 to 30 degrees if not contraindicated

  e. MAP should be kept at >90 mm Hg throughout the resuscitation of severe traumatic brain injury patients

2. Hypertension

  a. Management of hypertension based on incomplete evidence

  b. Recommend MAP at ~110 for intracerebral hemorrhage

3. Controversial

  a. Short-term phenytoin to prevent secondary seizures generally administered despite lack of supporting evidence

  b. Steroids historically administered to decrease brain edema, but the largest study to date by Ghajar et al (CRASH) in 2006 showed **increased** mortality

  c. Role of hypothermia in traumatic brain injury unclear at this time

   i. Mixed results

   ii. Appears to increase risk for pneumonia

IV. Facial Trauma

A. Orbital "blowout" fracture

1. Etiology

  a. Direct trauma resulting in orbital floor fracture

2. Symptoms and signs

  a. Diplopia

   i. Most obvious with **upward gaze** limitation

   ii. Inferior rectus caught between bony fragments of orbital floor

  b. Paresthesia

   i. Infraorbital nerve palsy and neuropraxia or transsection common

    a) Upper lip paresthesia

    b) Maxillary teeth paresthesia

    c) Cheek paresthesia (less likely)

3. Diagnosis

  a. Perform thorough ophthalmologic examination, including visual acuity, slit lamp, and fluorescein staining

  b. Plain x-rays may be helpful

   i. Teardrop sign: radiographic visualization of periorbital fat and inferior rectus muscle protruding into maxillary sinus

  c. CT scan

   i. Opacification of maxillary sinus with blood

   ii. Helpful to plan operative repair

4. Management

  a. Analgesics

  b. Tetanus prophylaxis as indicated

  c. Prophylactic antibiotics if sinuses disrupted

  d. Follow-up needed with ophthalmologist

B. Le Fort fractures

1. Definition: maxillary fractures from high-energy blunt trauma

2. Classification: advent of CT has blurred the classification lines (Figure 3–4)

  a. Le Fort I fracture: maxilla separated from pterygoid and nasal septum by transverse fracture

   i. Upper alveolar bone mobile

  b. Le Fort II fracture: maxilla (central) and palate fractured

   i. Area between upper teeth and infraorbital region is mobile

  c. Le Fort III fracture: fracture crosses the orbits, the zygomatic sutures, and the nose (craniofacial dissociation)

   i. Area between upper teeth and supraorbital region to zygomatic arch is mobile

3. Diagnosis

  a. CT scan is gold standard

   i. Reveals the Le Fort classification to be an oversimplification as most fractures are mixed

  b. Physical examination

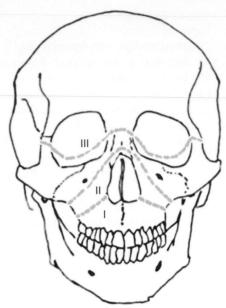

FIGURE 3–4. Le Fort fractures. (Reproduced, with permission from Brunicardi FC, Andersen DK, Billiar TR, et al: *Schwartz's Principles of Surgery*, 8th ed. Copyright © 2005, New York: McGraw-Hill.)

4. Management
   a. Aggressive airway management
   b. Rule out concomitant injuries (eg, cervical spine, central nervous system [CNS], eye)
      i. Increasing risk with greater Le Fort injuries
   c. Involve specialty consults early

C. Mandible fractures
   1. Epidemiology
      a. Second most commonly fractured facial bone (nasal fractures most common)
   2. Symptoms and signs
      a. Trismus
      b. Tooth misalignment
         i. Tongue blade test—detects subtle fractures
            a) Patient bites blade while examiner attempts to break it; inability to stabilize blade is an indication for imaging
      c. Intraoral lacerations
      d. Missing teeth
   3. Diagnosis
      a. Plain mandibular x-rays is a screening test only
      b. Panoramic radiograph is a better screening test
      c. CT scan of the facial bones is the gold diagnostic standard (a dedicated mandibular scan)
      d. Fracture location is (in decreasing order) body, angle, condyle

4. Management
   a. Open fractures require IV antibiotics and admission.
      i. Penicillin or clindamycin
   b. Closed fractures may be discharged with dental follow-up
      i. Adequate anesthesia
      ii. Instruct to avoid chewing on the affected side
   c. Many fractures require open reduction with internal fixation

V. Neck Trauma

A. Anatomy
   1. Multiple organ systems compressed into small space
      a. Airway (trachea), gastrointestinal (pharynx, esophagus), vascular (carotid arteries), endocrine (thyroid), neurologic (stellate ganglia)
   2. Multiple organ systems in close proximity to the neck
      a. CNS (spinal cord, brain, brachial plexus, CN IX through CN XII, laryngeal nerve)
      b. Respiratory (lungs)
      c. Cardiac (heart)

B. Penetrating trauma
   1. Etiology: gunshot wounds, knife attacks, impalement injury
   2. Classification of injury by zone (Figure 3–5)
      a. Zone I: clavicle to cricoid cartilage

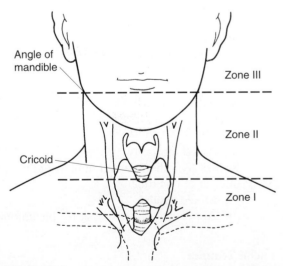

FIGURE 3–5. Penetrating trauma: zones of the neck. (Reproduced, with permission from Doherty GM, Way LW: *Current Surgical Diagnosis and Treatment*, 12th ed. Copyright © 2006, New York: McGraw-Hill.)

       i. Structures at risk overlap in each zone but include the trachea, esophagus, thoracic duct, carotid and vertebral arteries, thymus

      ii. Highest morbidity/mortality

  b. Zone II: cricoid cartilage (inferior margin) to mandible

      i. Larynx, esophagus, recurrent laryngeal nerve, thyroid

      ii. Most common neck injury

    iii. Best prognosis as anatomy is most accessible

  c. Zone III: mandible (angle of the mandible) to skull base

      i. Carotid and vertebral arteries

3. Symptoms and signs

  a. Symptoms are myriad depending on injured organ

      i. Dyspnea may result from tracheobronchial tree disruption, expanding carotid hematoma, pneumothorax, etc.

      ii. Stroke-like symptoms may result from carotid injury, spinal cord transaction, or even cortical injury from zone III penetration

  b. Vascular injury

      i. Hard signs of injury necessitate surgical exploration with or without angiography (expanding hematoma, diminished pulse, paralysis, rapid bleeding, stroke)

      ii. Soft signs (paresthesias, small hematoma)

4. Diagnosis

  a. Platysma integrity should be assessed

      i. If intact, local exploration is sufficient

      ii. Do **not** explore neck wounds that penetrate the platysma

  b. Zone-dependent (see Management below)

5. Management

  a. General rules

      i. Aggressive intervention and diagnostic testing is the rule as a wait-and-see approach can lead to disaster

      ii. External inspection may appear deceptively benign

    iii. Probing a wound may dislodge a clot and cause catastrophic bleeding

    iv. Do not remove impaled object, knives, etc. in the ED

  b. Airway management

      i. Sit patient up

      ii. C-collar if blunt injury or neurologic findings exist

    iii. Watch for hematoma formation

    iv. Consider transection of larynx

      a) Advance endotracheal tube gently to avoid extending a partial tear into a complete tracheal disruption

  c. **Unstable** patients should go to operating room (certain centers with rapid dedicated angiography suites may elect to perform angiography with zone I and III injuries despite instability)

  d. Stable patient should be evaluated based on the zone

      i. Zone I: angiography and CT angiogram and esophagram, +/– bronchoscopy

      a) Chest x-ray (CXR) to rule out pneumothorax

      b) Echo or ultrasound to rule out cardiac injury

      ii. Zone II: angiography and CT angiogram and esophagram +/– bronchoscopy +/– Doppler ultrasound **and/or** operative exploration

      a) In comparison with zone I and III injuries, it is easier to explore and identify zone II injuries; therefore lower threshold to surgically and visually inspect

    iii. Zone III: angiography and CT angiogram

  e. Zone assessment does not apply to gunshot-wound management

      i. Trajectory of bullet difficult to predict and may traverse all zones and even violate the skull or abdomen

C. Blunt trauma

  1. Etiology

    a. Seatbelt injury

    b. "Padded dash syndrome"—anterior neck strikes steering wheel

    c. Chiropractic manipulation

    d. Assault (especially strangulation)

    e. Suicide attempt

    f. Snowmobile and motorcycle ('clothesline injury')

  2. Symptoms and signs

    a. Laryngotracheal injury

      i. Vague symptoms; delayed presentation common

      ii. Hoarse voice, dysphagia, dyspnea, crepitus, and stridor

    b. Vascular injury

      i. Bruits and thrills, expanding hematoma, stroke

    c. Tracheobronchial injuries may present with dyspnea and subcutaneous crepitus

    d. Subconjunctival hemorrhage and petechiae may accompany strangulation and hanging

3. Diagnosis
   a. C-spine evaluation
      i. Plain radiography or CT
   b. Laryngeal fractures
      i. CT scan
      ii. Direct laryngoscopy
   c. Tracheobronchial injury evaluation
      i. CXR or chest CT may reveal subcutaneous emphysema
      ii. Bronchoscopy
   d. Vascular injuries
      i. Angiography is the preferred study
      ii. Computed tomographic angiography (CTA)
      iii. Doppler ultrasound
4. Management
   a. Airway management
   b. ENT and vascular surgery evaluation as indicated

VI. Injuries of the Spine

A. Cervical spine fractures and dislocations
   1. Stable
      a. Clay shoveler
         i. Avulsion fracture of spinous process of C6 and C7
         ii. Abrupt flexion of the neck with contraction of lower neck muscles or direct trauma
      b. Type I odontoid
      c. Unilateral facet dislocation
   2. Unstable (mnemonic: Jefferson bit off a hangman's thumb)
      a. **J**efferson burst fracture (C1) (Figure 3–6)
         i. Axial load (eg, diving)
         ii. Forces transmit to atlas with bilateral lateral mass fracture
      b. **B**ilateral facet dislocation
      c. **O**dontoid fractures (C2) (Figure 3–7)
         i. Type I: tip fracture (stable)
         ii. Type II: fracture at the base (most unstable)
         iii. Type III: fracture into the base (unstable)
      d. **A**ny fracture dislocation
      e. **H**angman fracture (C2)
         i. Extreme hyperextension
         ii. Fracture of posterior processes with protrusion into canal
      f. **T**eardrop fracture (Figure 3–8)
         i. Displaced anteroinferior aspect, typically of C2
         ii. Hyperextension of the anterior longitudinal ligament causes a true avulsion fracture

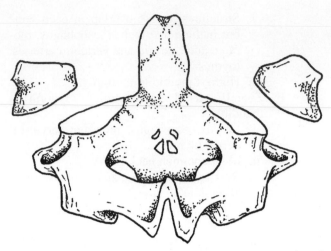

FIGURE 3–6. Jefferson burst fracture of C1. (Reproduced, with permission from Tintinalli JE, Kelen GD, Stapczynski JS: *Tintinalli's Emergency Medicine: A Comprehensive Study Guide*, 6th ed. Copyright © 2004, New York: McGraw-Hill.)

         iii. Flexion mechanism causes fragment to form caused by compression of anterior vertebra
         iv. Both are unstable
      g. Atlanto-occipital dislocation
         i. Severe flexion or extension leads to complete disruption of ligaments between occiput and atlas
         ii. Pressure on brainstem leads to respiratory failure and death

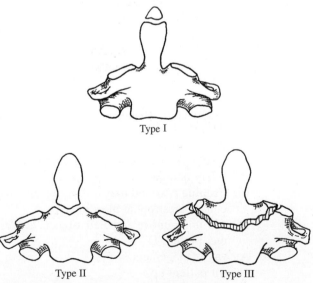

Type I

Type II   Type III

FIGURE 3–7. Odontoid fractures. (Reproduced, with permission from Tintinalli JE, Kelen GD, Stapczynski JS: *Tintinalli's Emergency Medicine: A Comprehensive Study Guide*, 6th ed. Copyright © 2004, New York: McGraw-Hill.)

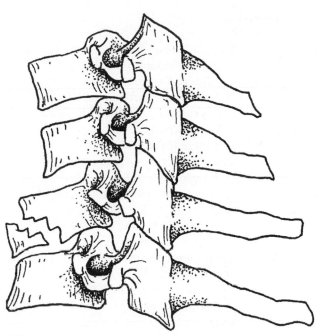

FIGURE 3–8. Teardrop fractures. (Reproduced, with permission from Tintinalli JE, Kelen GD, Stapczynski JS: *Tintinalli's Emergency Medicine: A Comprehensive Study Guide*, 6th ed. Copyright © 2004, New York: McGraw-Hill.)

3. Diagnosis
   a. NEXUS criteria used to clinically clear and remove cervical spine immobilization if patients meet certain criteria
      i. No focal neurologic deficits
      ii. Normal level of alertness
      iii. No evidence of intoxication
      iv. No painful distracting injury
      v. No posterior midline cervical tenderness
   b. Canadian c-spine rules include 3 high- and 5 low-risk variables
      i. High-risk factors—mandatory imaging if any exist
         a) >65 years
         b) Paresthesias in extremities
         c) Dangerous mechanism (fall >3 ft or >5 stairs; axial load; high speed >100 km/h; rollover and ejection, collision involving a motorized recreational vehicle; bicycle collision)
      ii. Low-risk factors—clinically clear if none present and able to rotate 45 degrees right and left
         a) Simple rear-end MVA
         b) Seated position in ED
         c) Ambulatory at any time

   d) Delayed onset of neck pain
   e) No midline c-spine tenderness
   c. Imaging
      i. Plain radiography (at least 3 views)
         a) Cross-table lateral view
            i) Visualize C1 to top of T1
            ii) Check alignment of anterior and posterior longitudinal line
            iii) Check alignment of spinolamina line (spinolamina of C2 should be within 2 mm of a line drawn between C1 and C2)
            iv) Prevertebral soft tissue no wider than vertebral body at any level (alternatively, 6 mm at C2 and 22 mm at C6)
            v) Predental space <3 mm in adults, <5 mm in children
            vi) Subluxation of >25% of 1 vertebral body on another should raise suspicion for bilateral facet dislocation
         b) Odontoid (open-mouth) view
            i) Check for odontoid fracture
            ii) Interspace between lateral mass and odontoid should be symmetric bilaterally
            iii) Lateral masses of C1 should align well with the body of C2
         c) Anteroposterior view
            i) Least useful of the 3 views
            ii) Spinous processes should line up, otherwise, suspect a rotational injury
         d) Always look for the second or third fracture as any fracture is associated with more
         e) 12% to 16% of fractures missed on plain films[1,2]
      ii. Cervical spine CT scan
      iii. Indications for MRI
         a) Assessment for ligamentous injury
         b) Patients with neurologic deficits despite negative plain radiography and CT scan results
         c) Spinal cord injury without radiographic abnormality (SCIWORA) in children (see Pediatric chapter)
4. Management
   a. C-spine immobilization
   b. Traction tongs
   c. Neurosurgical evaluation
   d. Steroids for blunt spinal trauma (not limited to cervical spine)

      i. Controversially practiced by most physicians in North America

      ii. Congress of Neurologic Surgeons position regarding steroids[3]

        a) "Recommended as an option with acute spinal cord injuries that should be undertaken only with the knowledge that the evidence suggesting harmful side effects is more consistent than any suggestion of clinical benefit."

      iii. Cochrane review

        a) "Treatment with this steroid does improve movement but it must start soon after the injury . . . within eight hours. It should be continued for 24 to 48 hours."

      iv. If used, administer within first 8 hours of injury at 30 mg/kg bolus of methylprednisolone followed by 5.4 mg/kg/h for 23 hours

B. Spinal cord syndromes (see Neurology chapter)
1. Cauda equina syndrome
2. Conus medullaris syndrome
3. Central cord syndrome
4. Anterior cord syndrome
5. Brown-Sequard syndrome

VII. Thoracic Trauma

A. Traumatic aortic rupture
1. Epidemiology
   a. Accounts for up to 15% of MVA-related deaths
   b. Most patients with complete transection die on scene leaving those with partial transections to seek care
2. Etiology
   a. Sudden deceleration injury as in MVA or fall from height
   b. Severe crush injury
   c. Most tears are transverse and incomplete
   d. Most occur at aortic isthmus (area between origin of left subclavian and the fixed ligamentum arteriosum)
3. Symptoms and signs
   a. Asymmetric pulses, shortness of breath, chest pain, back pain
   b. Small partial tears may be relatively asymptomatic
   c. External evidence of chest wall trauma may not be apparent
   d. Suspect if red blood exits tube thoracostomy placed during multiorgan trauma resuscitation

4. Diagnosis
   a. CXR
      i. Relatively insensitive and nonspecific
      ii. Common findings include
         a) Widened mediastinum >8 cm at the level of the aortic arch (70%)
         b) Abnormal shadow of descending aorta (67%)
         c) Left apical cap (65%)
         d) Downward displacement of left bronchus (65%)
         e) Rightward tracheal deviation (63%)
         f) Blurring of aortic arch (55%)
         g) Abnormal contour of aortic arch (40%)
         h) Left hemothorax (35%)
   b. CT and aortography are the primary modalities but institution dependent
   c. Transesophageal echocardiography
      i. Performed at bedside or in the operating room
      ii. Some loss of sensitivity with proximal disruptions
5. Management
   a. Unstable patients need rapid transport to operating room or endovascular interventional suite (institution dependent)
      i. Consider thoractomy if vital signs are lost during resuscitation but rarely successful in context of blunt trauma
   b. Stable patients require BP and heart rate management in preparation for surgery
      i. Target heart rate 60 to 80 beats per minute with use of a β-blocker (propranolol or esmolol)
      ii. Target systolic BP <120 mm Hg with use of nitroprusside
      iii. May use labetolol as a single agent
   c. Avoid "cyclical resuscitation"
      i. Cyclical restoration of BP followed by hypotension after repeated fluid administration
      ii. May lead to frank rupture

B. Blunt cardiac injury (cardiac contusion)
1. Definition
   a. Blunt cardiac trauma resulting in "stunning" of heart muscle that can lead to arrhythmias and heart failure
2. Etiology
   a. MVA
   b. Crush injuries
3. Symptoms and signs (rare)
   a. Chest pain, shortness of breath, palpitations
   b. Evidence of external chest trauma common
   c. Fractures or steering wheel imprints

d. Arrhythmias

e. Sudden death caused by arrhythmias (commotio cordis)

4. Diagnosis

a. No gold standard

i. Positive cardiac enzymes or abnormal echocardiography have been used by some as diagnostic criteria

b. Despite "diagnosis" very low incidence of complications[4]

c. Strategy should not be to "diagnose" but to admit and monitor those at high risk for poor outcome

d. Neither abnormal echocardiography nor nuclear studies, or positive cardiac enzymes correlate with morbidity and mortality

5. Management

a. Obtain ECG and place on cardiac monitoring for fixed period of time (duration is controversial—4 to 12 hours)

b. Admit for monitoring if

i. Abnormal ECGs or dysrhythmias

ii. >50 years (controversial)

C. Penetrating cardiac injury

1. Etiology

a. High-velocity—gunshot, shotgun wounds

b. Low-velocity—stab wounds, screwdrivers, ice picks

c. Iatrogenic—pacemaker and central line placement

2. Relevant anatomy

a. Position of heart in thorax determined chamber of injury

i. Right ventricle injury (43%) >left ventricle (33%)

ii. Right atria (14%) >left atria (5%)

b. Great vessel injuries occur in ~5% to 10%

c. Coronary arteries involved in 3% to 5%

i. Left anterior descending artery >right coronary artery

3. Symptoms and signs

a. Dichotomous presentation

i. Hemorrhagic hypotension with significant injuries

ii. Pericardial tamponade with smaller injuries

b. Beck triad (hypotension, muffled heart sounds, jugular venous distension) with pericardial tamponade

c. Pulsus paradoxus

4. Diagnosis

a. Ultrasound focus assessment with sonography for trauma (FAST) examination (see Ultrasound chapter)

b. CT scan if patient stable

c. CXR of limited utility

i. 250 cc of blood required before cardiac silhouette enlarged

d. ECG may detect pulsus alternans

5. Management

a. Fluid resuscitation and blood transfusion

b. Cardiothoracic surgery

c. Mechanical ventilation prior to relief of tamponade may cause sudden refractory hypotension

d. Pericardiocentesis

i. As little as 200 cc of acute accumulation may result in hypotension

ii. As little as 50 cc of pericardial aspiration may result in clinical improvement

iii. Preferable to leave catheter in pericardial sac

e. Emergency thoracotomy

i. Indicated for patients who lose vital signs in the ED

ii. See Procedures chapter

D. Pulmonary contusion

1. Definition

a. Blunt trauma leading to edema and bleeding into lung parenchyma

2. Epidemiology

a. Occurs in up to 20% of patients admitted for trauma

b. Most common chest injury in children

3. Symptoms and signs

a. Develop over 24 hours

b. Dyspnea and chest pain

c. Tachypnea, cyanosis, tachycardia, hypotension

d. May occur with or without rib fractures

e. Crackles are a late finding

4. Diagnosis

a. CXR

i. Detect most significant contusions

ii. Initial films may underestimate degree of injury until 24 to 48 hours later

iii. May detect rib fractures and flail segments

b. CT scan is much more sensitive than CXR

i. Most small contusions diagnosed on CT are not clinically significant

5. Management

a. Supportive respiratory care

i. Position patient so that the **good lung is down** to improve oxygenation (in contrast to pulmonary hemorrhage in which bad lung is down to prevent spillage over to good lung)

ii. Central lines should be placed ipsilateral to injured lung to prevent possible pneumothorax to good lung

    b. Fluid restriction as classically taught may lead to hypotension and worsening of symptoms—target euvolemia

E. Simple rib fractures
1. Epidemiology
    a. Most common thoracic injury
    b. 10% have multiple fractures
2. Symptoms and signs
    a. Tenderness, crepitus, and ecchymosis
    b. Subcutaneous air is consistent with underlying pneumothorax
    c. Lower rib fractures (8 through 12) have higher association with intraabdominal injury (liver, spleen, kidneys)
    d. Fractures of first rib traditionally taught to be indication of severe trauma (pneumothorax, aorta, brachial plexus)
3. Diagnosis
    a. CXR: insensitive for nondisplaced fracture
      i. Assess for pneumothorax, hemothorax, pulmonary contusion
      ii. Ribs 4 through 9 most commonly fractured
      iii. Most fractures occur at posterolateral angle (weakest point)
    b. Utility of dedicated rib films unclear
      i. Rarely provides additional useful information
      ii. Rarely impacts management
4. Management
    a. Analgesia: consider intercostal nerve blocks
    b. Pulmonary toilet: discharged patients should receive an incentive spirometer for home use to prevent atelectasis
    c. Consider admitting patients with severe pain, multiple rib fractures, and the elderly

F. Flail chest
1. Definition
    a. Occurs when a section of ribs separates from the rest of the chest wall
    b. Free-floating "section of ribs"—2 fractures in each rib involving at least 2 ribs
2. Symptoms and signs
    a. Pain and dyspnea
    b. Presence of flail segment highly predictive of underlying pulmonary contusion
    c. Palpation will reveal tenderness and bony crepitus
    d. Paradoxical chest wall movement—segment moves inwards during inspiration and outwards during expiration
3. Diagnosis
    a. Physical examination is diagnostic
    b. CXR is used to visualize fracture fragments

    c. CT scan if concern for concomitant chest or abdominal injuries
4. Management
    a. Supportive care
    b. Management related to care of pulmonary contusion
    c. Mechanical ventilation for respiratory failure
      i. Consider prophylactic chest tube placement
    d. In an out-of-hospital setting, stabilize patient with injured side down
    e. Admit

G. Simple and tension pneumothorax (see Pulmonary chapter)

H. Open pneumothorax
1. Definition
    a. A pneumothorax with communication to the environment through a chest wall defect
2. Pathophysiology
    a. Because the distance (L) of the chest wall opening to the lungs is shorter than to the trachea, air preferentially enters the wall defect when its diameter approaches 75% of the trachea's
    b. Results in a one-way valve phenomenon and tension pneumothorax
3. Symptoms and signs
    a. Large chest wall defects may lead to inadequate ventilation caused by reasons explained above
4. Management
    a. Seal the opening and place a chest tube
    b. If chest tube unavailable, apply bandage to wound with only 3 sides taped down
      i. In theory acts as a flap valve preventing air entry during inspiration but allowing exit on expiration

I. Hemothorax
1. Definition
    a. Bloody fluid within the pleural cavity
2. Etiology
    a. Pulmonary contusion
    b. Rib fractures
    c. Great vessel injury
3. Symptoms and signs
    a. Chest pain, dyspnea
    b. External evidence of trauma
    c. Decreased breath sounds and dullness to percussion
    d. Decreased chest wall expansion
    e. Hypotension if severe
4. Diagnostic testing (Table 3–2)
    a. CXR

TABLE 3–2. Diagnostic Testing of Hemothorax

TEST	FINDINGS
CXR A-P upright view	Upright CXR: may reveal fluid level with meniscus on affected side. Need ~400 to 500 cc to obscure diaphragm on an A-P film. Primary diagnostic tool.
CXR A-P supine view	Supine CXR: may opacify hemithorax with lung marking visible underneath. Fluid level rarely visible unless massive as fluid lies posteriorly.
CT scan	Highly sensitive. May be useful to differentiate blood from areas of contusion or aspiration. Shows amount and location of bleeding.
FAST ultrasound	May detect hemothoraces above the diaphragm as a hypoechoic area. Ultrasound highly sensitive for hemothorax and pneumothorax but not the primary diagnostic means.

  b. CT scan
  c. FAST examination (see Ultrasound chapter)
 5. Management
  a. Chest tube drainage
   i. 32 French minimum in adults
   ii. Direct tube posteriorly
   iii. Failure to adequately drain may lead to undrainable hematoma and abscess and empyema formation
  b. Indications for surgical thoracotomy
   i. Rarely indicated as most traumatic hemothoraces result from self-limiting venous bleeding
   ii. Base decisions on clinical status and presence of ongoing hemorrhage rather than the absolute numbers following below in (iii)
   iii. Traditional indications include initial bloody output >1 L or 250 mL/h × 4 hours

VIII. Abdominal Trauma

A. Blunt abdominal trauma
 1. Anatomy
  a. Intraabdominal organs
   i. Solid organs (liver and spleen)
   ii. Hollow viscus organs (stomach, ileum, jejunum, transverse colon)
  b. Retroperitoneal organs
   i. Duodenum, pancreas, kidneys, ureters, bladder, ascending and descending colon, major vessels, and rectum
 2. Mechanism
  a. MVA, pedestrian struck, fall from height, explosions
  b. Fall from height often results in rupture of hollow viscus and retroperitoneal injury
  c. Movement of tethered organs at fixed points
   i. Ligament of Treitz
   ii. Junction of large and small bowel
  d. Handlebar to abdomen injury may result in duodenal hematoma or pancreatic injury

 3. Injured organs in descending order of frequency
  a. Spleen, liver, small intestines, large intestines
 4. Symptoms and signs
  a. Solid organ injury
   i. Symptoms and signs result from associated hemorrhage, hemoperitoneum, and hypotension
   ii. Kehr sign—referred left shoulder pain from diaphragmatic irritation
   iii. Rib fractures associated with liver and splenic injuries
  b. Hollow viscus injuries
   i. Gastric injury causes peritonitis secondary to acid irritation
   ii. Intestinal injury may lead to delayed peritonitis secondary to spillage of bacteria and fecal matter
   iii. Seat belt sign—contusion of lower abdomen suspicion for intraperitoneal injury (duodenum, pancreas)
  c. Retroperitoneal injury
   i. Hematuria may result from injury to ureter and bladder
   ii. Grey-Turner sign—flank ecchymosis indicative of retroperitoneal bleeding
   iii. Cullen sign—periumbilical ecchymosis indicative of retroperitoneal bleeding
   iv. Duodenal wall hematoma
    a) May be asymptomatic at time of injury
    b) May cause gastric outlet obstruction
 5. Diagnosis
  a. Laboratory tests
   i. CBC and type and screen
   ii. Elevated amylase or lipase neither sensitive nor specific for pancreatic or bowel injury
   iii. Gross hematuria should raise suspicion for renal injury
  b. Plain radiography
   i. May detect free air indicative of perforated hollow viscus

    ii. CXR may detect diaphragmatic injury (eg, bowel or nasogastric tube in chest cavity)

    iii. "Chance fracture"—transverse fracture of vertebral body associated with bowel injury

  c. Diagnostic peritoneal lavage (DPL) in **blunt** trauma

    i. Positive if 10 mL of gross blood

    ii. Lavage fluid >100,000 RBC/mL, >500 WBC/mL, elevated lipase

    iii. Contains gross urine, fecal or vegetable matter

    iv. See Procedures chapter

  d. FAST

    i. See Ultrasound chapter

  e. CT scanning

    i. Excellent at detecting solid organ injury

    ii. Able to detect retroperitoneal bleeding (unlike FAST and DPL)

    iii. Poor sensitivity for diaphragmatic, pancreatic, and hollow viscus injuries

6. Management

  a. ATLS resuscitation

  b. Surgical subspecialty consultation

  c. In the multitrauma patient, identification of system source of hypotension, (eg, thoracic, abdominal, pelvic) takes priority over identification of specific organ injury

  d. Laparotomy indications

    i. Hemodynamically unstable

    ii. Peritonitis

    iii. Free air on CXR

    iv. CT diagnosed injury requiring surgery (eg, duodenal rupture)

  e. Angiographic embolization for select injuries (see Management of Organ Specific Injuries below)

B. Penetrating abdominal injury

  1. Mechanism

    a. High-velocity—Gunshot most common

    b. Low-velocity—Stab wound, impalement

  2. Injured organs in descending order of frequency

    a. Liver, small bowel, diaphragm, large bowel

  3. Diagnosis

    a. Physical examination more accurate and arguably more important with penetrating than with blunt trauma

    b. Thorough physical required, especially with gunshot wounds as path of injury is unpredictable

    c. Perform thorough pelvic and rectal examination

    d. Threshold for positive DPL is lowered to >5000 to 10,000 RBCs (institution dependent)

    e. Plain radiographs may reveal metallic bullet fragments

    f. Imaging as in blunt trauma

  4. Management

    a. Indications for laparotomy

      i. Hemodynamically unstable

      ii. Progressing abdominal examination

      iii. Obvious evisceration injuries

      iv. All gunshot wounds (high-velocity)

      v. Identified injury absolutely requiring repair (eg, asymptomatic patients with ureter or pancreas transaction on CT scan)

      vi. Positive DPL

      vii. Positive local wound exploration

      viii. Suspicion for diaphragmatic injury

    b. Indications for conservative management (watchful waiting)

      i. Low-velocity **and** hemodynamically stable

        a) Unnecessary (negative) laparotomy rate ~50% to 60% in prior era where all stab injuries were explored

      ii. Requires careful serial abdominal examinations

    c. Surgical consultation

    d. Consider antibiotics and tetanus status

C. Organ-specific injuries

  1. Liver

    a. Epidemiology

      i. Second most common injured organ after blunt trauma

      ii. Most common cause of death after blunt trauma

      iii. Mortality with blunt trauma >penetrating trauma

    b. Symptoms and signs

      i. Reflect degree of hemorrhage

      ii. Bile duct injury may result in peritonitis

    c. Diagnosis

      i. CT scan, ultrasound, DPL

    d. Management

      i. Most hemodynamically stable patients are managed nonoperatively

      ii. Hypotension or suspicion for bile leak or infection are indications for intervention

        a) Laparotomy

        b) Angiographic embolization

  2. Spleen

    a. Epidemiology

      i. Most commonly injured organ in blunt trauma

    b. Symptoms and signs

      i. Reflect degree of hemorrhage

    c. Diagnosis

  i. Plain radiography
  - a) Left hemidiaphragm elevation, left lower lobe atelectasis, and left pleural effusion
  - b) Leftward displaced gastric bubble
  - c) Inferiorly displaced splenic flexure
  ii. CT scan, ultrasound, DPL
  d. Management
  i. Observe hemodynamically stable patients especially in children
  ii. Persistent bleeding or "rebleed" common
  iii. Angiographic embolization may be therapeutic and prognostic
3. Pancreatic injury
  a. Etiology
  i. Penetrating injury much more common than blunt
  ii. Relatively protected high in the retroperitoneal space
  iii. Handlebar injuries
  b. Symptoms and signs
  i. Can be relatively asymptomatic early
  ii. Cullen sign, Grey-Turner sign
  iii. Seat belt marks
  c. Diagnosis
  i. An uncommon diagnostic enigma with poor outcomes if not promptly identified
  ii. Laboratory
  - a) Amylase poorly sensitive and specific (may be elevated with bowel wall, ovarian, or salivary gland injury)
  - b) Lipase poorly sensitive and specific
  iii. CT
  - a) Sensitivity only 40% to 70%
  iv. Endoscopic retrograde cholangiopancreatography (ERCP) may detect ductal injuries
  d. Management
  i. Most patients require surgical exploration and intervention
  ii. Surgery is both diagnostic and therapeutic
  iii. Ductal injury requires drainage and total parenteral nutrition to advance healing
4. Diaphragm
  a. Etiology
  i. Blunt or penetrating trauma
  ii. Most commonly after MVA
  iii. Left posterolateral involvement most common
  - a) Right diaphragm relatively protected by liver
  iv. Intraabdominal pressure is greater than intrathoracic pressure so that diaphragmatic defects place abdominal contents at risk for strangulation in the chest

  b. Symptoms and signs
  i. Respiratory distress
  ii. Chest pain
  iii. Symptoms and signs secondary to herniation of abdominal contents
  - a) Evidence of obstruction and strangulation
  - b) Hypotension caused by cardiac and great vessel compression
  iv. Small injuries may be asymptomatic and not present until years later (especially small stab wounds)
  v. Associated with rupture of **thoracic aorta**
  c. Diagnosis
  i. CXR is most important screening tool
  - a) Elevated hemidiaphragm
  - b) Bowel or stomach in chest
  - c) Nasogastric tube curled into chest
  ii. CT
  - a) Axial CT poorly visualizes the diaphragm
  - b) Sagittal, coronal, and 3D reconstructions better
  - c) May detect abdominal contents in chest
  iii. Drainage of DPL fluid through chest tube diagnostic
  iv. MRI stable patients
  v. Laparotomy
  d. Management
  i. ED management focused on suspecting and diagnosing injury
  ii. Nasogastric tube placement may reduce herniated contents and aid diagnosis
  iii. Surgically repair as abdomen-chest pressure gradient favors enlargement of even small defects

IX. Genitourinary Trauma

A. Upper genitourinary (GU) system
  1. Definition
    a. Consists of kidneys and ureters
  2. Etiology
    a. MVA is most common cause followed by gunshot wounds
    b. Ureter injuries most commonly iatrogenic or of penetrating etiology
  3. Symptoms and signs
    a. Gross hematuria
    b. Flank pain and ecchymosis (Grey-Turner sign)
    c. Lower rib fractures
    d. Injuries to ureters may be asymptomatic early on
  4. Diagnosis
    a. Rule out lower GU system injury first
      i. Down-up evaluation

    ii. Order of evaluation begins with urethra, bladder, ureters, and ends with the kidneys so as not to miss or exacerbate existing injuries

  b. Laboratory

    i. Assess renal function and electrolytes

    ii. Hematuria absent in 5%

  c. Imaging

    i. Indications for imaging

      a) Hemodynamically unstable

      b) **Gross** hematuria

      c) Persistent microscopic hematuria

    ii. Contrast CT scan

    iii. Intravenous pyelogram

    iv. Retrograde ureterogram if ureter injury suspected

5. Management

  a. Urology consultation

  b. Need for surgery dependent on extent of injury

  c. Injury to ureter requires surgical repair

B. Lower GU system

1. Definition

  a. Consists of bladder, urethra, and external genitalia

2. Bladder rupture

  a. Etiology

    i. Blunt trauma most common

    ii. Frequently occurs with **pelvic fractures**

    iii. Consider in the alcoholic who falls on a full bladder

  b. Classification

    i. **Extraperitoneal** more common and associated with pelvic ramus fractures

    ii. **Intraperitoneal** associated with penetrating injury or rupture of distended bladder

  c. Symptoms and signs

    i. Suprapubic pain

    ii. Inability to void

    iii. Gross hematuria

  d. Diagnose

    i. Rule out urethral injury first (down-up evaluation)

    ii. Retrograde cystogram (see Procedures chapter)

  e. Treatment

    i. Bladder: catherization

    ii. Intraperitoneal: surgical repair

    iii. Extraperitoneal: nonsurgical unless failure not healing

3. Urethral injury

  a. Etiology

    i. Blunt trauma

    ii. Iatrogenic injuries

    iii. Anterior segment injury associated with straddle (bicycle) or penetrating injuries

    iv. Posterior segment injury associated with pelvic fracture

  b. Symptoms and signs

    i. Hematuria

    ii. Blood at urethral meatus

    iii. Scrotal and penile swelling

    iv. Inability to void

  c. Diagnosis

    i. Retrograde urethrogram (see Procedures chapter)

  d. Management

    i. Avoid bladder catherization with high-riding prostate or blood at meatus until urethral injury ruled out

    ii. Bladder drained with suprapubic cystostomy

    iii. Surgical repair

4. External genitalia (penis and scrotum)

  a. Penile fractures

    i. Genitourinary (GU) emergency

    ii. Etiology

      a) Buck fascia and corpus cavernosum rupture

      b) Penile trauma during erection

    iii. Symptoms and signs

      a) Angulation

      b) Acute pain, loss of erection, and swelling

    iv. Management

      a) Identify and treat concomitant urethral injury if necessary (see Management of Urethral Injury below)

      b) Functional outcome better with surgery

  b. Penile amputation

    i. Obvious emergency

    ii. Reimplantation successful if performed < 4 hours

  c. Testicular trauma

    i. Etiology: blunt trauma most common

    ii. Diagnosis: Doppler ultrasound most useful

    iii. Indications for surgical exploration

      a) Most testicular injuries benefit

      b) Penetrating testicular injuries

      c) Testicular fracture, expanding hematomas >5 cm, absence of blood flow, disruption of tunica albuginea

X. Pelvic Trauma (see Orthopedic chapter)

XI. Trauma in Pregnancy

A. Epidemiology

1. Majority of maternal deaths in pregnancy are traumatic

2. Approximately 5% to 10% experience some form of trauma
3. Most occur during in third trimester

B. Etiology
   1. MVA most common
   2. Domestic violence
   3. Accidental fall
   4. Improper seat belt use

C. Symptoms and signs
   1. Evidence of head trauma
      a. Most common cause of maternal death
   2. Vaginal bleeding
      a. Placenta abruptio is the second leading cause of fetal death (maternal shock is the leading cause)
   3. Premature rupture of membrane (see Obstetrics and Gynecology chapter)
   4. Palpate for uterine contractions and tenderness
      a. Uterus rises out of its pelvic protection at 12 weeks' gestation
   5. Absent or decreased fetal movement
   6. Abdominal pain is less pronounced because of peritoneal stretching and resulting decrease in nerve density

D. Diagnosis
   1. Laboratory
      a. Standard trauma panel
      b. Determine Rh status
      c. Kleihauer-Betke
         i. Assess degree of maternal-fetal hemorrhage
         ii. Determines need for additional RhoGAM (clears only 15 mL of fetal RBCs)
         iii. Positive testing may indicate severe trauma and guide duration of observation period
   2. Assess fetal heart rate with Doppler or ultrasound
   3. Radiation exposure in trauma
      a. Best care for fetus is caring appropriately for the mother
      b. Greatest risk during organogenesis (2 to 8 weeks' gestation)
      c. CNS teratogenesis at 10 to 17 weeks' gestation
      d. <50 to 100 mGy (5 to 10 rads) cumulative exposure during entire pregnancy is considered safe
      e. Select radiation exposures
         i. CXR (0.0007 mGy), c-spine (0.02 mGy), pelvis (0.4 mGy), head CT (0.5 mGy), chest CT (1.0 mGy), abdominal CT (25 to 30 mGy)

E. Management
   1. Obstetric consultation
   2. RhoGAM if Rh negative
   3. Left lateral decubitus to prevent supine hypotension syndrome
   4. Watch and manage for abruptio placentae
   5. Cardiotocographic monitoring if >20 weeks' gestation
      a. Minimum of 4 hours observation
      b. Major trauma as indicated by mechanism, positive Kleihauer-Betke testing, and bleeding may require longer observation

XII. Miscellaneous Trauma

A. Amputation
   1. Definitions
      a. Complete amputations lack bridging tissue and are replanted
         i. Incomplete amputation: retain tissue between the distal and proximal portions and are revascularized
   2. Management
      a. Tetanus and antibiotics
      b. Care of proximal wound
         i. Irrigate with NS for gross contamination
         ii. Any debridement should be done by a specialist
         iii. Do not clamp bleeding arteries
         iv. Cover with a saline-moistened sterile dressing and place splint
      c. Care of amputated part
         i. Preserve at 4°C but be careful not to freeze
         ii. Wrap tissue part in saline-moistened gauze, place inside plastic bag, and immerse in ice water (1:1 water and ice)
         iii. Immediate transport to a specialty center
      d. Indications for replantation
         i. Relatively clean-cut
         ii. Young age
         iii. Functional benefit
            a) Thumb involvement
            b) Multiple digit involvement
            c) Wrist or distal forearm
            d) Distal humerus
      e. Indicators of poor prognosis
         i. Severe crush injuries
         ii. Severe contamination
         iii. Amputation proximal to the proximal interphalangeal joint (PIP) (because of stiffness)
         iv. Prolonged ischemia
            a) Digit amputations can tolerate up to 24 hours of cold ischemia at 4°C (12 hours warm ischemia)

        b) Replantation of limbs tolerate less ischemia time because of higher muscle content (does not tolerates ischemia well)

B. High pressure injection
1. Definition
   a. Injection of foreign material <2000 to 10,000 pounds per square inch (psi)
2. Etiology
   a. Grease gun, paint sprayers, fuel injectors, air guns
   b. Injectants distribute along fascial planes, tendon sheaths, and neurovascular bundles
   c. Chemical irritation is the major determinant of digit ischemia
3. Symptoms and signs
   a. Depend on nature of injectant
      i. Air and clean water have a relatively benign course
      ii. Paint and grease cause severe inflammation
   b. Injuries to the **nondominant** index finger most common
   c. External examination may look deceptively innocuous
   d. Delayed pain as inflammation sets in
   e. Distended and swollen digit

    f. Vascular involvement may result in a pale ischemic digit
4. Management
   a. Surgical emergency requiring immediate debridement and exploration
   b. Severely injured digits often require amputation
   c. Tetanus prophylaxis, analgesia, and intravenous antibiotics

REFERENCES

1. Widder S, Doig C, Burrowes P, et al: Prospective evaluation of computed tomographic scanning for the spinal clearance of obtunded patients: preliminary results. *J Trauma.* 2004; 56:1179.
2. Ajani A, Cooper D, Scheinkestel C: Optimal assessment of cervical spine trauma in critically ill patients: a prospective evaluation. *J Trauma.* 1998;26:487.
3. Hadley MN, Walters BC, Grabb PA, et al: Pharmacological therapy after acute cervical spinal cord injury. *Neurosurgery.* 2002;50(3):S63.
4. Wisner DH, Reed WH, Riddick RS, et al: Suspected myocardial contusion. Triage and indications for monitoring. *Annals of Surgery.* 1990;212(1):82.

Chapter 4
TOXICOLOGIC EMERGENCIES

Robert S. Hoffman

I. General Management

A. Emesis
1. Indications
   a. In 2003, the American Academy of Pediatrics issued a policy statement recommending that syrup of ipecac no longer be used routinely as a home treatment strategy in children following ingestion of a potentially poisonous substance. The first action of a caregiver should be to contact the local poison control center
   b. By the time poisoned patients reach the ED the use of emesis is rarely if ever considered
   c. Essentially no remaining indications
2. Contraindications
   a. Nontoxic ingestions—emesis should not be used as a method of punishment.
   b. Prior significant vomiting
   c. Any patient who is comatose, seizing, hypotensive, or has lost his or her protective airway reflex
   d. The patient who is presently awake, but may be expected to rapidly deteriorate before emesis has been completed. Examples of this type of ingestion include (tricyclic antidepressant [TCA], β-blockers, camphor, and many others
   e. Caustic agents may cause additional injury during emesis
   f. Aspiration risk: ingestions of poorly absorbed hydrocarbons
   g. Sharp objects and other foreign body ingestions
   h. Late in pregnancy
   i. Hypertensive crisis or intracranial hypertension
3. Complications
   a. Intractable vomiting (rare)
   b. Diarrhea
   c. Aspiration
   d. Myocardial toxicity—associated with **extract of ipecac** (has 14 times the alkaloidal content of the syrup; production ceased in 1970) or with repeated dosing of syrup as in patients who have bulimia
   e. Neuromuscular weakness (seen with chronic abuse in bulimia or with Munchausen by proxy)
   f. Mallory-Weiss tear of the esophagus
   g. Pneumomediastinum
   h. Lethargy
   i. Threatened abortion possibly induced by ipecac

B. Gastric lavage
1. Indications
   a. Acute poisoning where gastric emptying is indicated. It is **preferred** when the ingestion occurred recently and a rapid deterioration in mental status or vital signs is expected (ie, TCAs), or for which even a small decrease in toxic exposure may be critical (ie, calcium channel blockers, colchicine, lithium)
   b. Lavage is preferred in patients who have lost their gag reflexes, who are intubated for airway protection, and in patients intubated for other reasons
   c. If the ingestion occurs >1 hour prior to presentation, the above indications must be weighed against the contraindications; >1 hour is not a contraindication
2. Contraindications
   a. Caustic ingestions
   b. Large foreign bodies or sharp objects
   c. Inability to protect the airway (or no endotracheal tube)
   d. When drug is no longer considered to be accessible in the stomach
3. Complications
   a. Aspiration pneumonia
   b. Esophageal or gastric perforation
   c. Tension pneumothorax and empyema
   d. Decreased oxygenation during the procedure

C. Activated charcoal (AC)
  1. Method
     a. AC is a fine black powder prepared by pyrolysis (burning) of carbonaceous products. Activation increases the surface area of the particle
     b. Toxins adsorb (stick) to AC, and thus the total surface area of the charcoal preparation is related to the amount of drug able to be adsorbed
     c. Some toxins are not well adsorbed to AC. Included are most small molecules (eg, iron, the alcohols, lithium, strong acids and alkalis, sodium, chloride)
  2. Dose
     a. The optimal dose of charcoal for most well-adsorbed toxins is a 10:1 charcoal to drug ratio. For unknown ingestions dosing is based on ability to tolerate the agent: adults: 60 to 90 g; children: 1 g/kg body weight

D. Multiple-dose activated charcoal (MDAC)
  1. MDAC has shown efficacy in patients with ingestions of phenobarbital, dapsone, theophylline, digitoxin, phenytoin, carbamazepine, and several other drugs. Most toxins have not been investigated
  2. In general, MDAC is given to decrease ongoing absorption of drug ingested (sustained-release [SR] preparations, drugs that form concretions in the gastrointestinal [GI] tract, etc)
  3. MDAC is also used to enhance elimination of drugs in patients who are clinically ill and have ingested drugs whose pharmacokinetics (low Vd, long $t_{1/2}$, enterohepatic or enteroenteric circulation) makes them accessible to adsorb to charcoal
  4. Contraindications
     a. Absent gut motility or perforation. When GI motility is decreased, residual charcoal can be removed from the stomach with a nasogastric tube to avoid aspiration
     b. When endoscopic visualization will be required, as in caustic ingestions
     c. Loss of protective airway reflexes
  5. Cautions
     a. Advise health-care professionals to ascertain that their AC preparation does not contain a cathartic. Repeat dosing of AC that contains a cathartic should never be administered, as significant fluid and electrolyte abnormalities can result
  6. Complications
     a. Clinically significant complications occur infrequently
        i. Fatal aspiration
        ii. Small bowel obstruction

E. Whole bowel irrigation (WBI)
  1. Indications
     a. The potentially toxic ingestion of a substance not well adsorbed to AC
     b. Substances with a prolonged absorption phase—SR preparations
     c. Rising drug levels despite gastric emptying and the use of AC (SR preparations)
     d. GI drug smuggling
  2. Contraindications
     a. Absent bowel sounds
     b. Bowel obstruction or perforation
     c. Unprotected compromised airway
     d. Hemodynamic instability
  3. Dose: polyethylene glycol
     a. Adults: 1.5-2 L/h (minimally)
     b. Children: 500 mL/h or 25 mL/kg/hour
     c. This is given orally or via a nasogastric tube (preferred)
     d. Administration is continued until **rectal effluent is clear**
     e. Administer AC before and after WBI for drugs adsorbed to AC
  4. Complications
     a. Vomiting or bloating occurs frequently
     b. Rectal irritation has also been reported
  5. Adjuncts
     a. Antiemetics (preferably metoclopramide) are often required
     b. Consider promotility agents (erythromycin, metoclopramide) in addition to WBI for patients with well-constructed drug packets

F. Cathartics
  1. Indications
     a. Not routinely recommended
     b. Not recommended in pediatric patients, or in a patient with a low risk, or trivial ingestion
     c. Use only a single dose if desired
  2. Contraindications
     a. Children <1 year
     b. Presence of diarrhea, or following exposure to a toxin expected to produce significant diarrhea
     c. Absent bowel sounds

II. Tricyclic Antidepressants

A. Mechanism
  1. Block reuptake of biogenic amines
  2. Anticholinergic (antimuscarinic) effects
  3. Sodium channel blockade
  4. TCAs block fast inward sodium channels
     a. Type IA antidysrhythmic or "quinidine-like" or "membrane-stabilizing" effects on the myocardial conduction system

b. Phase 0 depolarization is prolonged with resultant QRS widening and characteristic "wide complex dysrhythmias"

c. Negative inotropy also contributes to hypotension

5. α_1-Adrenergic receptor blockade—vasodilation, contributes to hypotension

6. Antihistamine effects—contribute to sedation

7. γ-aminobutyric acid (GABA) antagonism may contribute to seizures

B. Symptoms and signs

1. Vital signs: hypertension initially with some agents, normo- to hypotensive subsequently, tachycardia routinely

2. Anticholinergic signs: dilated pupils, tachycardia, dry, hot, and flushed skin, decreased bowel sounds, urinary retention

3. Neurologic symptoms: myoclonus or seizures. Mental status may range from lethargy to coma or may be normal if early, and rapidly deteriorate while in the ED

C. Diagnosis

1. Electrocardiogram (ECG) as screening tool (Table 4–1)

D. Right axis deviation between 130 and 270 degrees in patients poisoned with TCAs

E. Management

1. Acute toxicity

a. Intubate and hyperventilate (as clinically indicated)

b. GI decontamination

c. Syrup of ipecac is absolutely contraindicated

d. Consider orogastric lavage if ingestion is recent

e. AC 1 g/kg and occasionally followed by MDAC

2. Diazepam or lorazepam for seizures

a. Phenytoin is contraindicated

3. Sodium bicarbonate bolus for dysrhythmias

a. If QRS >100 ms, sodium bicarbonate bolus 1 to 2 mEq/kg

b. If QRS narrows, then start infusion. 3 amps NaHCO$_3$ in 1L D$_5$W and infuse at 2 to 3 times maintenance. Carefully monitor potassium levels

TABLE 4–1. ECG Finding and Corresponding Tricyclic Toxicity

QRS DURATION	CLINICAL EFFECT
QRS <100 ms	No significant toxicity
QRS >100 ms	33% of patients had seizures
QRS >160 ms	50% of patients had ventricular dysrhythmias

c. Consider hyperventilation and/or hypertonic saline if sodium bicarbonate becomes problematic. The goal is a maximum serum pH 7.55 if narrowing of QRS has not occured

4. Hypotension

a. Intravenous (IV) fluids, normal saline or lactated Ringer

b. Sodium bicarbonate bolus to enhance inotropy and increase intravascular volume

c. Pressors: norepinephrine is preferable to dopamine if fluids fail to increase the blood pressure (BP) because it is direct-acting

5. Physostigmine is contraindicated to treat anticholinergic effects

6. No role for flumazenil in benzodiazepine (BZD) or TCA OD

7. Disposition

a. Admit patient with a QRS >100 msec

b. Admit patient with a seizure, dysrhythmia, altered mental status, or complication

c. Patients who have been decontaminated, who never seize or develop abnormal ECGs (other than sinus tachycardia that should resolve) can be safely discharged after 6 hours of observation if otherwise stable

d. Although not scientifically substantiated, most patients with ECG abnormalities should be placed in the ICU on bicarbonate therapy for 12 to 24 hours

III. Other Antidepressants

A. Selective serotonin reuptake inhibitors (SSRIs)

1. Mechanism

a. SSRIs preferentially block the reuptake of serotonin into the nerve terminal. This theoretically alters the downstream regulation of central nervous system (CNS) serotonin receptors that over time lead to improved mood using unclear mechanisms

2. Toxicity profile

a. Therapeutic dose

i. GI symptoms, sexual dysfunction, jitteriness, headache, insomnia, fatigue

ii. Syndrome of inappropriate secretion of antidiuretic hormone (SIADH)—reported in elderly woman also on diuretic therapy

iii. Extrapyramidal signs (akathisia and dystonia)—more common with concomitant use of dopamine antagonist

b. Overdose (OD)

i. Nausea, vomiting, lethargy, and sedation

ii. Seizures have been reported (rarely) following OD of most SSRIs

iii. Citalopram ODs are associated with QT prolongation, which may be delayed up to 24 hours. Escitalopram (the S-enantiomer of citalopram) has also been associated with QT prolongation in OD, thus OD involving either of these SSRIs requires 24-hour ECG monitoring

c. Serotonin syndrome
   i. Etiology: drugs that inhibit serotonin breakdown (MAOI), block serotonin reuptake (cocaine, meperidine, dextromethorphan), enhance serotonin release (MDMA or ecstasy), or serve as serotonin precursors or agonists (tryptophan, lithium)
   ii. Symptoms and signs: develop within minutes to hours after exposure to the offending agent(s)
      a) Mental status changes (mild agitation, slightly pressured speech)
      b) Autonomic instability (tachycardia without fever, diarrhea, shivering, diaphoresis, mydriasis)
      c) Neuromuscular abnormalities (myoclonus, ocular clonus, inducible clonus, hyperreflexia greater in lower extremities, tremor, seizures)
      d) **Hyperthermia**
   iii. Differential diagnosis
      a) Neuroleptic malignant syndrome
         i) Definition: a combination of hyperthermia, muscle rigidity, and autonomic dysregulation associated with the use of antipsychotic medications, leading to hypothalamic D_2 antagonism
            (a) Butyrophenone or phenothiazenes
            (b) Dopamine depletion
            (c) Withdrawal of dopaminergic drugs, such as levodopa (L-dopa)
         ii) Treatment
            (a) Cooling, BZDs, physical restraints, discontinuation of neuroleptic agent, IV fluids
      b) Malignant hyperthermia
         i) Etiology: increased release of calcium from the sarcoplasmic reticulum associated with certain anesthetics (eg, halothane and halogenated volatile anesthetics), as well as succinylcholine, a neuromuscular blocking agent
         ii) Symptoms and signs: rigidity with induction

iii) Treatment: dantrolene, cooling, paralysis
   a) Block the release of calcium from the sarcoplasmic reticulum
d. Management
   i. Overdose
      a) Rule out TCA by ECG
      b) Consider AC
   ii. Serotonin syndrome
      a) BZDs, hydration, and cooling are the mainstay of therapy
      b) Cyproheptadine may be helpful

B. Monoamine oxidase inhibitors (MAOIs)
   1. Mechanism
      a. Monoamine oxidase degrades norepinephrine, epinephrine, dopamine, and serotonin
      b. MAOIs induce an increase in neuronal biogenic amine levels
   2. Toxicity
      a. Overdose
         i. Release of excess catecholamines causes the initial sympathomimetic appearance of the patient
         ii. Severe cases may progress to cardiovascular collapse causing hypotension, dysrhythmias, disseminated intravascular coagulopathy (DIC), death
         iii. Symptoms onset after isolated MAOI OD can be delayed 12 to 24 hours
      b. Food/drug interaction
         i. Hypertensive reactions
         ii. Occur because MAO in the gut normally degrades ingested tyramine that is present in many protein foods
         iii. Undegraded tyramine is an indirect-acting sympathomimetic which induces the release of presynaptic neuronal catecholamines
         iv. Identical reaction occurs when patients ingest medicinal indirect-acting sympathomimetics, like pseudoephedrine (previously ephedrine or phenylpropanolamine). Patients taking reversible MAOIs can have an unrestricted diet
         v. Serotonin syndrome
   3. Treatment
      a. Overdose
         i. Because of the delayed onset of effect, all patients with suspected MAOI OD should be admitted
         ii. Treatment is supportive with avoidance of drugs that can interact further with MAOIs

iii. Hyperthermia, agitation, myoclonus, and seizures are managed with cooling and sedation (BZDs)

iv. Initial hypertension is controlled with short-acting agents (nitroprusside, phentolamine, nitroglycerine) that can be rapidly stopped if hypotension develops. Avoid β-blockers (unopposed alpha)

v. Paralysis (with EEG monitoring) may be necessary in those with severe hyperthermia or rigidity

vi. Hypotension is treated with fluids

    a) Direct-acting pressor, such as norepinephrine, may be needed

    b) Indirect-acting pressors, such as dopamine, have unpredictable effects and should be avoided

b. Food/drug interactions—hypertensive reaction

i. Oral terazosin (α-blocker) should be effective if patient has normal baseline BP

ii. Oral nifedipine (immediate release) often effective if patient has normal baseline BP

    a) Use caution in patients with hypertensive medical history to avoid reduction of perfusion to critical organs

iii. Phentolamine, a parenteral α-blocking agent, an be used at doses of 3 to 5 mg IV in adults

iv. BZDs for anxiolysis and sedation may be helpful

IV. Acetaminophen (APAP)

A. Clinical presentation following acute OD

1. 0.5 to 24 hours

a. The patient may present with nausea, vomiting, anorexia, and an unremarkable physical examination.

b. If vital sign abnormalities or significant symptoms are present **think of a potential co-ingestant**

2. 24 to 48 hours

a. Initial symptoms resolve

b. The patient develops right upper quadrant (RUQ) abdominal pain/tenderness and an elevation of hepatic enzymes, prothrombin time, international normalized ratio (INR) and bilirubin

3. 48 to 96 hours

a. Marked hepatic dysfunction occurs and includes coagulopathy, peak hepatic enzymes elevation, acidosis, hypoglycemia, spontaneous bleeding, jaundice, anuria, cerebral edema, and coma

b. Death occurs in this stage, often caused by cerebral edema

4. 4 to 14 days—hepatic dysfunction resolves

B. Evaluation

1. Predicting the risk of toxicity

a. History

i. A reliable time of ingestion and amount ingested must be obtained

ii. 150 mg/kg is a potentially toxic dose

2. Serum APAP level

a. Obtain this level at 4 hours after ingestion or as soon as possible thereafter

b. It should be sent in all cases of suicidal ingestion. 1 of 500 patients without a history of APAP ingestion will have a potentially toxic level

c. The APAP treatment nomogram may be used to interpret levels in acute ingestions. The nomogram cannot be applied to levels obtained <4 hours

C. Treatment

1. N-acetylcysteine (NAC)

a. Dosing

b. Oral dosing

i. The loading dose is 140 mg/kg

ii. Maintenance doses are 70 mg/kg every 4 hours × 17 total doses

iii. The total dose delivered is 1330 mg/kg over 72 hours

c. Intravenous dosing is now available in the United States

i. A 20-hour protocol is administered IV for adults

ii. The loading dose is 150 mg/kg over 15 minutes

iii. The loading dose is followed by 50 mg/kg over 4 hours

iv. This is followed by 100 mg/kg over 16 hours

v. The total dose delivered is 300 mg/kg over ~21 hours

vi. After the 21-hour protocol, recheck both LFTs and an APAP level. If APAP is measureable or the LFTs elevated, restart IV NAC at the second maintenance dose (100 mg/kg in 1 L of 5% dextrose over 16 hours)

V. Aspirin

A. Symptoms and signs

1. Gastrointestinal: nausea and vomiting, hemorrhagic gastritis, decreased gastric motility, pylorospasm

2. Pulmonary: hyperpnea, tachypnea, acute lung injury

3. Cardiovascular: tachycardia

4. CNS
   a. Tinnitus
   b. Vertigo, confusion, agitation, hyperactivity, delirium, hallucination, convulsions, lethargy, stupor, coma (rare)
   c. Cerebral edema
5. Diaphoresis and hyperthermia
6. Fluid and electrolytes
   a. Dehydration
      i. Secondary to vomiting, diaphoresis (caused by hyperthermia), and insensible losses (caused by increased respiratory rate)
      ii. Hypoglycemia secondary to impaired gluconeogenesis
      iii. Renal loss of sodium and bicarbonate (compensation for respiratory alkalosis)
      iv. Hypokalemia develops from potassium movement intracellularly (in response to initial alkalemia) and potassium loss in the urine

B. Diagnosis
   1. Urinalysis
      a. Ketones, pH, glucose, specific gravity
   2. Arterial or venous blood gas (ABG/VBG) with lactate concentration
   3. Serum electrolytes
      a. Increased—anion gap metabolic acidosis caused by lactic acid, ketoacids, salicylic acid, and metabolites
      b. Glucose abnormalities
      c. Hyperglycemia—glycogenolysis
      d. Hypoglycemia—depletion of easily mobilized glucose stores, impaired gluconeogenesis
      e. Relative CNS hypoglycemia
      f. Potassium
      g. Hypokalemia is an important finding since it impairs urinary alkalinization
   4. Serum salicylate level
      a. Toxicity correlates poorly with serum levels
      b. Reference levels
         i. Acute ingestions
            a) Therapeutic level 15 to 30 mg/dL
            b) Signs or symptoms commonly present at >30 mg/dL
            c) Critically poisoned requiring hemodialysis at >100 mg/dL
         ii. Chronic toxicity
            a) Serum levels have more limited role. Patient can be critically ill with level of 50 mg/dL

C. Management
   1. GI decontamination
      a. Gastric emptying in patients with an acute OD

b. Multiple doses (2 to 4 doses) of AC. Important for large ingestions
c. Potential for the formation of aspirin concretions
d. Must be aggressive to restore fluid and electrolyte balance as most patients are hypovolemic as a result of vomiting, hyperpnea, hyperthermia, and diaphoresis
e. There is no reason to give fluids beyond restoring fluid balance
   i. Forced diuresis does not substantially enhance elimination
2. Airway management
   a. Intubation may lead to the development of respiratory acidosis, thereby **increasing morbidity**
3. Urine alkalinization
   a. Indications
      i. Signs and symptoms consistent with salicylism
      ii. Serum level >40 mg/dL
   b. Technique
      i. Bolus 1 to 2 mEq/kg sodium bicarbonate IV
      ii. Then begin IV bicarbonate infusion at 2 × maintenance rate
      iii. 1 L D_5W + 3 amps sodium bicarbonate (132 mEq) + 40 mEq KCl
      iv. Goal is to achieve a urine pH of 7.5 to 9 and a blood pH of 7.45 to 7.55
      v. It is essential to maintain a normal serum potassium (>4.5)
4. Extracorporeal removal
   a. Methods
      i. Hemodialysis—method of choice because it is able to correct acid-base and electrolyte abnormalities in addition to removing drug
      ii. Exchange transfusions possible for infants
   b. Indications for hemodialysis
      i. Manifestations of salicylism in vital end organs
      ii. Pulmonary edema
      iii. Altered mental status
      iv. Coagulopathy
      v. Clinical deterioration despite adequate supportive care
      vi. Inability to alkalinize the serum because patient cannot tolerate the fluid load (pulmonary edema, renal failure)
      vii. Renal failure (unable to eliminate drug)
      viii. Absolute serum level
         a) Acute >100 mg/dL
         b) Chronic >60 mg/dL (relative indication)

VI. Iron

A. Symptoms and signs
1. History
   a. History of emesis and if so how many times—**key element of the history**
   b. Poisoning without emesis is extremely uncommon
   c. 3 to 4 episodes of emesis in a well-looking patient may be attributed to local toxicity
   d. Patients with more than 4 episodes of emesis or those who look ill probably have systemic (ie, free iron) poisoning
   e. Predicted toxicity of calculated iron load by history (Table 4–2)
2. 3 acute and 2 subacute stages
   a. Local GI irritation occurring with an onset no >6 hours post-ingestion
      i. Nausea, vomiting, diarrhea
   b. Latent stage
      i. A period of improvement in GI symptoms only. If severe poisoning is present, the patient will still have clinical or metabolic evidence of illness
   c. Metabolic and cardiovascular stage
      i. GI symptoms return as well as hypotension and shock, metabolic acidosis, lethargy, and stupor
      ii. This is stage when patients die!
      iii. May begin early (within first 6 to 8 hours) and last up to 2 days postingestion
   d. Hepatic stage
      i. Develops 2 to 5 days post-ingestion and manifests itself with elevation of transaminases
   e. Delayed GI effects
      i. 4 to 6 weeks post-ingestion, may present with early satiety or nausea secondary to pyloric outlet obstruction

B. Diagnosis
1. Abdominal radiograph
   a. Several compounds are radiopaque including iron (**CHIPES** is a helpful mnemonic)

Chloral hydrate, calcium carbonate
Heavy metals
Iron, iodine
Phenothiazines
Enteric-coated pills
Solvents, halogenated ones (carbon tetrachloride, chloroform, and SR preparations such as Lithobid)

   b. Adult preparations are often visualized
   c. Chewable and liquid preparations are rarely visualized
   d. The greater the duration since ingestion the lower the yield of an abdominal radiograph
   e. A negative x-ray does **not** imply lack of ingestion or toxicity
2. Serum iron level
   Iron levels tend to correlate grossly with clinical toxicity if obtained within 4 to 6 hours of ingestion (Table 4–3)

C. Management
1. General supportive care
   a. Limited role for emesis, lavage, or charcoal
2. Deferoxamine (DFO)
   a. DFO chelates free iron-forming ferrioxamine which is water soluble; the urine excretes the complex, which discolors the urine a classical "vin-rose" but usually brown or rusty color is seen
   b. Dosing
      i. IV—15 mg/kg/h is ideal but should start drip gradually (5 mg/kg/h) to prevent hypotension

VII. Caustics

A. Definition: a substance that causes both clinical and histologic damage on contact with tissue surfaces
1. Typically acids or alkalis
2. May include other agents that function as desiccants, vesicants, or protoplasmic poisons

B. Pathophysiology
1. Caustic agents are classified as acid or alkali

TABLE 4–2. Iron Ingestion and Corresponding Clinical Effects

DOSE (ELEMENTAL)	CLINICAL EFFECT
<20 mg/kg	Nontoxic
20 to 60 mg/kg	Mild to moderate toxicity
>60 mg/kg	Severe toxicity

TABLE 4–3. Iron Level and Corresponding Clinical Effects

SERUM LEVEL	CLINICAL EFFECT
<300 mcg/dL	Nontoxic
300 to 500 mcg/dL	Expect GI symptoms, and potential for significant metabolic toxicity
>500 mcg/dL	Severe toxicity

2. Acid: proton donator
   a. H+ ions desiccate epithelial cells: **coagulation** necrosis → cell death
3. Alkali: proton acceptor
   a. Dissociated OH⁻ ions penetrate tissue surfaces: **liquefactive** necrosis → cell death
4. Extent of injury by caustic agents is determined by
   a. Duration of tissue contact
   b. Ability of the substance to penetrate tissues
   c. Volume
   d. pH
   e. Concentration

C. Symptoms and signs
   1. GI tract: severe pain of the lips, mouth, throat, chest, abdomen; drooling; dysphagia; odynophagia; vomiting; hematemesis
   2. Respiratory tract: hoarseness, stridor, respiratory distress leading to epiglottitis, laryngeal edema and ulceration, pneumonitis, impaired gas exchange
   3. Eyes—pain, tearing, irritation, clouding of the cornea, chemosis, decreased vision
   4. Skin—drible marks on the face chest and legs, which can be first, second, or third degree burns with associated pain
   5. The presence or absence of oropharyngeal burns in children does not predict the presence of esophageal or gastric burns

D. Diagnosis
   1. Endoscopy
      a. Indicated in all patients with intentional ingestions
      b. Indicated in patients with unintentional ingestions with stridor, pain, vomiting, or drooling
      c. Should be performed within 12 hours and preferably not >24 hours post-ingestion
      d. Laparoscopy/laparotomy may be indicated when endoscopy cannot be performed
   2. Imaging
      a. X-rays of chest and abdomen—useful to detect gross signs of esophageal/gastric perforation; look for pneumomediastinum, pneumoperitoneum, pleural effusion
      b. CT of chest and abdomen—useful in detecting perforation; more sensitive than x-ray
      c. Esophagram/upper GI series—useful when endoscopy is not possible; extravasation of contrast outside of the GI tract is diagnostic for perforation

E. Management of esophageal exposures
   1. Acute management
      a. Decontamination of the patient's skin, eyes
      b. Gastric decontamination
         i. Induced emesis, lavage, AC generally not indicated
         ii. Exceptions—large ingestions of acids
      c. Airway
         i. Inspection for signs of airway edema—stridor, change in voice
         ii. Intubation if necessary following direct visualization of the cords (ie, direct laryngoscopy or fiberoptic endoscopy)
         iii. Avoid paralytics—may distort airway anatomy
         iv. IV dexamethasone (adults 10 mg; children 0.6 mg/kg to 10 mg) for airway edema
      d. Constant monitoring of heart rate, respiratory rate, BP, urine output
      e. Examination of the oropharynx for injury, drooling, vomitus
      f. Empiric hydration using central venous pressure/neck vein distension as guidelines
      g. Serial physical exams of oropharynx, neck, chest , abdomen for any new changes
      h. Dilution
         i. Should be considered only in patients with no airway compromise, vomiting, drooling, oropharyngeal/chest/abdominal pain
         ii. Liquid caustic ingestions—milk or water when administered within seconds to minutes post-ingestion may be helpful
         iii. Solid caustic ingestions (crystal lye)—delayed administration of milk or water may be helpful
      i. Neutralization should be avoided
      j. Surgical intervention
         i. Indicated with perforation, severe abdominal rigidity, persistent hypotension

VIII. Carbon Monoxide

A. Epidemiology
   1. Leading cause of poisoning morbidity and mortality in United States
      a. 50% are suicides
      b. 33% are from fires

B. Sources of CO
   1. Incomplete combustion of any carbonaceous fossil fuel (complete combustion forms CO_2)
      a. Fires, particularly coal and wood
      b. Engine exhaust, such as motor vehicles or other gas-powered engines/tools, such as boats
         i. Car exhaust contains little CO now owing to efficient catalytic converters

c. Propane-powered vehicles—Zamboni machines, power mowers, tractor exhaust
d. Non-vehicular sources—home heating, natural gas stoves, kerosene heaters, indoor hibachi use with inadequate ventilation, clothes dryers, hot water heaters, indoor gas-powered machinery

C. Risk factors for poor outcome following CO poisoning
1. Extremes of age (less than 6 months and over 60 years old)
2. Pregnant women (poor fetal outcome)
3. Preexisting coronary artery disease/respiratory disease

D. Pathophysiology
1. Carboxyhemoglobin (COHb) does not carry oxygen → decreased oxygen content of the blood
2. Shifts O_2–Hb dissociation curve to the left (impaired cooperativity and decreased 2, 3 DPG) → decreased O_2 delivery to tissues
3. Binding to myoglobin → impairs tissue oxygen delivery → myocardial and skeletal muscle hypoxia
4. Binding to cytochrome oxidase → impaired mitochondrial utilization of oxygen
5. Induces lipid peroxidation in CNS → delayed neurologic sequelae

E. Symptoms and signs
1. Acute symptoms are caused by tissue hypoxia. Heart and brain most affected
   a. CNS: most sensitive to CO poisoning
      i. Headache, dizziness, nausea, blurred vision, altered mental status, ataxia, seizures, coma
   b. Cardiovascular system
      i. Exertional dyspnea, weakness, angina, palpitations, tachycardia, tachypnea, hypotension, myocardial ischemia, dysrhythmias
   c. Respiratory: acute respiratory distress syndrome (ARDS), pulmonary edema
   d. Renal: acute renal failure (2° to rhabdomyolysis or acute tubular necrosis)
   e. Musculoskeletal: rhabdomyolysis (atraumatic)
   f. Ocular: blindness reported rarely, venous engorgement
   g. Dermal: cherry-red color (seen with severe exposure, generally after the patient dies)
2. COHb levels
   a. Nonsmokers: 1% to 2%; smokers: 5% to 10%
   b. Poor correlation of levels with symptoms, especially with chronic exposure
   c. Do not predict development of delayed neurologic or neuropsychiatric sequelae

F. Management
1. Remove from exposure and resuscitate
2. Give 100% oxygen by face mask as soon as diagnosis suspected
3. COHb level by co-oximetry (may be venous)
4. Pulse oximeter does not detect COHb; will be normal with elevated COHb
5. Assess end-organ damage:
6. ECG, cardiac monitor, measure pH (ABG/VBG)
7. Detailed neurologic examination/neuropsychiatric testing
8. Pregnancy test if appropriate
9. Hyperbaric oxygen (HBO) for those who meet indications

G. Hyperbaric oxygen
1. Indications for HBO
   a. Evidence of end-organ damage regardless of COHb level
   b. Loss of consciousness, coma, seizures
   c. Confusion, cognitive deficits, focal findings, visual symptoms
   d. Myocardial ischemia, life-threatening dysrhythmias
   e. Persistent symptoms (after treatment with 1 atm O_2—headache, ataxia, abnormal neuropsychiatric testing
   f. COHb Levels: (regardless of symptoms)
      i. COHb >25%
      ii. COHb >15% in pregnant women

IX Methemoglobin

A. Methemoglobin (MetHb) forms when hemoglobin (Hb) becomes oxidized
1. An iron atom in Hb loses one electron to an oxidant and is oxidized from the ferrous (Fe^{2+}) state to the ferric (Fe^{3+}) state

B. Pathophysiology
1. MetHb cannot bind oxygen
   a. Iron must be in the ferrous (Fe^{2+}) state in order to bind oxygen
2. MetHb impairs oxygen release from normal Hb
   a. Leftward shift of the oxyhemoglobin (oxyHb) dissociation curve

C. Etiologies
1. Medications: amyl nitrite, benzocaine, dapsone, lidocaine, nitroglycerin, nitroprusside, phenacetin, phenazopyridine, prilocaine, quinines, sulfonamide
2. Chemical agents: aniline dye derivatives, butyl nitrite, chlorobenzene, food containing nitrites, isobutyl nitrite, naphthalene, nitrophenol, nitrous gases, silver nitrate, trinitrotoluene, well water contaminated with nitrates

TABLE 4–4. Methemoglobin Level and Corresponding Findings

METHEMOGLOBIN LEVEL	SIGNS AND SYMPTOMS
0% to 3%	Normal levels. No symptoms.
10% to 20%	Mild symptoms. Cyanosis. Chocolate-brown-colored blood
20% to 50%	Dyspnea, exercise intolerance, fatigue, headache, dizziness, confusion, tachycardia, syncope
>50%	CNS hypoxia: CNS depression, seizures, coma
	Cardiac hypoxia: dysrhythmias, ischemia
	Systemic hypoxia: tachypnea, metabolic acidosis
>70%	Severe hypoxic symptoms, death

3. Fires
   a. Heat-induced Hb denaturation
   b. Inhalation of nitrogen oxide in smoke

D. Symptoms and signs (Table 4–4)
   1. Cyanosis
      a. Related to impaired oxygen delivery to the tissue
      b. Severity corresponds to an increasing percentage of MetHb
      c. Severity also corresponds to the rate of formation and elimination
      d. Primarily affects the cardiovascular system and CNS
      e. Develops when 1.5 g/dL of MetHb is present
         i. This corresponds to MetHb level of 10% in a normal person with a Hb of 15 g/dL. Other than cyanosis, these patients are often asymptomatic
         ii. This corresponds to a MetHb level of 20% in an anemic patient with a Hb of 7.5 g/dL. In addition to cyanosis, this patient will manifest signs and symptoms of MetHb poisoning
      f. Cyanosis caused by hypoxemia requires 5 g/dL of deoxyhemoglobin (deoxyHb)
         i. This represents a 33% reduction in oxygen-carrying capacity in patients with a Hb of 15 g/dL. In addition to cyanosis, these patients are always symptomatic

E. Diagnosis
   1. Exposure history is critical, but not always present or available

2. Cyanosis
   a. Is out of proportion to clinical signs and symptoms
   b. Does not improve with supplemental oxygen
   c. Is not associated with a right-left cardiac shunt
   d. Is associated with a normal PO_2 and oxygen saturation on arterial blood gas (ABG)
3. Blood that is chocolate brown in color and remains so with exposure to oxygen
4. A saturation gap is present—the difference between the O_2 saturations measured by blood gas and co-oximeter, blood gas and the pulse oximeter, or co-oximeter and pulse oximeter
5. ABG often demonstrates a normal oxygen saturation
   a. Measures the PO_2 (dissolved oxygen content of the blood) which is usually normal
   b. The O_2 saturation is calculated from the PO_2, temperature, and pH
   c. It assumes that only normal Hb is present
6. Pulse oximetry readings frequently hover around 85%; may be lower depending on oximeter
7. Co-oximeter
   a. Measures light absorbance at multiple wavelengths
   b. Uses multiple equations to calculate an accurate percentage of oxyHb, deoxyHb, MetHb, and COHb. Some newer machines have an expanded spectrum and are also able to read fetal hemoglobin and sulfhemoglobin

F. Management
   1. Supportive care
   2. Administer 100% oxygen to maximize oxygenation of normal Hb
   3. Methylene blue
      a. Dosing: 1 to 2 mg/kg (0.1–0.2 mL/kg of 1% methylene blue) IV over 5 minutes
      b. Indications for methylene blue
         i. Significant tissue hypoxia
         ii. Tachycardia or tachypnea
         iii. Metabolic acidosis
         iv. End-organ dysfunction
         v. Altered mental status, seizures
         vi. Dysrhythmias, myocardial ischemia
         vii. Levels >20%, even in asymptomatic patients

X. Cyanide

A. Sources of cyanide
   1. Ingestion of cyanide salts
   2. Smoke inhalation

3. Occupational exposures
   a. Jewelry production
   b. Fumigation for insect and woody plant control
4. Medicinal sources of cyanide
   a. Nitroprusside
5. Food sources
   a. Plants of *Prunus* species contain amygdalin in their pits
      i. Apricot, bitter almond, cherry, peach
   b. Cassava (*Manihot*), a tuber, contains 2 cyanogens, linamarin, and lotaustralin
6. Cyanogenic chemicals
   a. Acetonitrile

B. Pathophysiology
1. Cyanide inhibits cytochrome oxidase at the cytochrome a_3 portion of the electron transport chain
2. CNS injury occurs as a result of impaired oxygen utilization, oxidant stress, and enhanced release of excitatory neurotransmitters
   a. Impaired oxygen utilization
      i. Injury occurs in the most oxygen-sensitive areas (basal ganglia)
   b. Induction of cellular oxidant stress
      i. Inhibition of antioxidant enzymes such as catalase, glutathione dehydrogenase and reductase, or superoxide dismutase
   c. Enhanced release of excitatory neuro-transmitters
   d. Cyanide-induced lipid peroxidation

C. Symptoms and signs
1. Routes of exposure
   a. Inhalational: immediate onset
   b. Parenteral: rapid onset (seconds to minutes)
   c. Ingestion: onset delayed ~20 minutes
2. Acute cyanide toxicity is characterized by catastrophic symptomatology with multi-organ system failure
   a. CNS: headache, anxiety, agitation, confusion, lethargy, coma, seizures
   b. Cardiac
      i. Initially, hypotension and bradycardia
      ii. Followed by hypotension and reflex tachycardia
      iii. Terminal event is consistently bradycardia and hypotension
   c. Respiratory
      i. Early: tachypnea
      ii. Late: bradypnea; pulmonary edema (both acute lung injury and cardiogenic pulmonary edema)
   d. Gastrointestinal: abdominal pain, nausea, vomiting

   e. Metabolic: severe lactic acidosis (increased anion gap metabolic acidosis)
   f. Skin: cherry-red skin color as a result of increased venous hemoglobin oxygen saturation
      i. Cyanide does not directly cause cyanosis
      ii. The occurrence in some cases is likely secondary to shock

D. Diagnosis
1. Tentative diagnosis and treatment are based on historical circumstances and initial clinical presentation
2. Suspicious for cyanide
   a. Bitter-almond odor of HCN should not be relied upon for diagnostic purposes
   b. Fire victim with coma and acidosis (associated with a serum lactate >10 mmol/L)
   c. Unexplained coma and acidosis
3. Laboratory testing
   a. Severe metabolic acidosis with increased anion gap and elevated lactate
   b. Elevated central venous O_2 saturation caused by reduced tissue oxygen extraction
      i. Decreased arterial-venous oxygen difference
4. Cyanide levels are used to confirm diagnosis. They cannot typically be obtained rapidly and do not serve a role in acute management

E. Management
1. Supportive care
   a. Airway patency, ventilatory support, administer 100% oxygen
   b. Avoid mouth-to-mouth resuscitation
   c. IV fluid and vasopressors for hypotension
   d. Administer sodium bicarbonate; titrate according to the ABG and serum bicarbonate
   e. Decontamination (health-care workers should exercise extreme caution in order to avoid exposure)
   f. Inhalation exposure: removal from the source of exposure
   g. Oral exposure: orogastric lavage, AC
   h. Dermal exposure: remove clothing, flush with water
2. Cyanide antidote kit (formerly the Lilly kit) contains the only antidotes available in the United States
   a. Three components
      i. Amyl nitrite pearls (amyl nitrite is released when glass pearls are crushed)
         a) Should be used only until IV access is established
         b) Inhaled for 30 seconds to 1 minute. May be introduced into the ventilator
         c) Results in ~5% MetHb

    ii. Sodium Nitrite (3%)
       a) Pediatric dose: 0.33 mL/kg (maximum dose is 10 mL)
       b) Dose is decreased in anemic patients
       c) Adult dose: 10 mL (300 mg)
       d) Infuse over 2 to 4 minutes
       e) Adverse effects of nitrites include vasodilation, hypotension, and tachycardia
       f) Induces up to 7% to 14% methemogobin (MetHb)
       g) Goal is to induce 20% to 30% MetHb
    iii. Sodium thiosulfate (25%)
       a) Pediatric dose: 1.65 mL/kg (max 50 mL)
       b) Adult dose: 50 mL (12.5 g)
       c) A second dose may be necessary

3. Hydroxocobalamin (vitamin B_{12} precursor)
   a. FDA-approved in December 2006 for the treatment of known or suspected cyanide poisoning. Has been widely used since 1996 in Europe and Canada for use in the fire brigades for smoke-inhalation victims
   b. Cyanokit
    i. Vials: 2.5 g each of Hydroxocobalamin for dilution in 100 cc NS (final concentration 25 mg/mL)
    ii. Starting dose: 5 g (2 vials) for adult; 70 mg/kg for children, infused over 15 minutes
    iii. Additional doses of 5 g each (up to 15 g total) are recommended for incomplete or transient response. Second and subsequent doses should be infused over a longer period (6 to 8 hours) unless the patients is in cardiac arrest or is hemodynamically unstable
   c. Mechanism
    i. Hydroxocobalamin binds (chelates) cyanide to form cyanocobalamin (vitamin B_{12}). Cyanocobalamin is eliminated in the urine or releases the cyanide moiety at a rate sufficient to allow detoxification by rhodanese
    ii. Mild vasopressor effects are likely mediated by "NO scavenging"
   d. Complications
    i. Does not carry risks of MetHb formation associated with nitrities
    ii. Red color of hydroxocobalamin causes chromaturia (up to 5 weeks) and red skin discoloration for up to 2 weeks
    iii. Interferes with colorimetric laboratory tests which may present a diagnostic dilemma in a subset of patients. If given pre-hospital, EMS should provide pre-drawn blood tubes to the ED

    iv. Marked hypertension may occur in the first hour of administration (as a result of NO scavenging)
    v. Should not be administered via the same IV line as thiosulfate (sodium thiosulfate binds and inactivates hydroxocobalamin)
   e. Efficacy data
    i. In a Beagle model of cyanide toxicity, hydroxocobalamin administered alone (without thiosulfate) a 150 mg/kg infusion was superior to a 75 mg/kg dose, but both conferred a significant mortality benefit over saline placebo)
    ii. One retrospective study reported a 42% survival rate when prehospital hydroxocobalamin was administered to smoke inhalation victims
    iii. One prospective series reported 71% survival in 14 severe cyanide-poisoned victims whose pretreatment CN concentrations were considered lethal

XI. Organophosphates

A. Mechanism
  1. Organophosphates bind to cholinesterase preventing breakdown of acetylcholine

B. Symptoms and signs
  1. Excess acetylcholine at muscarinic and nicotinic receptors, including autonomic ganglia and skeletal muscle, induces a variety of manifestations
  2. Predominant findings vary with route of exposure, dose, lipid solubility, and affinity of agent for acetylcholinesterase
   a. Muscarinic- postganglionic parasympathetic
    i. SLUDGE = **S**alivation, **l**acrimation, **u**rination, **d**iarrhea, **G**I cramps, **e**mesis
   b. Nicotinic: autonomic ganglia
    i. Diaphoresis, mydriasis
    ii. Tachycardia, hypertension
   c. Nicotinic: neuromuscular junction (skeletal muscle)
    i. Fasciculations
    ii. Muscle weakness
    iii. Paralysis
   d. CNS effects: confusion, agitation, lethargy, coma and seizures

C. Management
  1. Decontamination
   a. Personnel should take protective measures and wear gowns and gloves to prevent contamination

b. Ocular and dermal exposures require thorough irrigation and decontamination

c. Clothing should be removed and discarded in a well-ventilated area
   i. Leather can be a reservoir for the agent and cannot be decontaminated
   ii. Shoes, belts, watchbands must be discarded

2. Stabilization
   a. ABCs
      i. Mouth-to-mouth resuscitation is a potential hazard to health-care providers and should not be performed
      ii. Early intubation
   b. Orogastric lavage or nasogastric lavage is indicated if liquid was ingestion and patient has not vomited yet (part of decontamination, but should be deferred until ABCs addressed)
      i. Remember that lavaged fluid is a potential hazard to health-care providers
   c. IV access for antidotes and fluids

3. Antidotes
   a. Atropine
      i. Works by competitive inhibition of ACh at muscarinic (M_1, M_2, M_3) receptors in CNS and periphery
      ii. No effects on neuromuscular junction/weakness (nicotinic receptors)
      iii. Titrate dose to **drying of bronchial secretions**; may need large amounts ultimately, but start with 0.5 to 1 mg initially in adults; 0.02 mg/kg in children. A doubling philosophy may be required to reach effective doses; administer double the previous dose every 2 to 3 minutes until bronchorrhea controlled or saturations normalize
      iv. A minimum dose of 0.1 mg atropine in children to avoid potential paradoxical bradycardia which occurs via a central mechanism
      v. Tachycardia should not prohibit drug dosing; most often it is the result of bronchorrhea induced hypoxia and more atropine is required
   b. Pralidoxime (2-PAM, Protopam)
      i. Mechanism: forms a complex with the organophosphate-bound acetylcholinesterase enzyme. The organophosphate-pralidoxime portion of the complex is released from the enzyme, regenerating its ability to metabolize acetylcholine. Decreases atropine requirement
      ii. Efficacy increased by early treatment; once the acetylcholinesterase-OP complex "ages", 2-PAM becomes ineffective

iii. Dose
   a) Adult: 1 to 2 g in 100 mL 0.9% NaCl IV over 15 to 30 minutes, then q 6 to 12 hours **or**
   b) Adult: 1 to 2 g in 100 mL 0.9% NaCl IV over 15 to 30 minutes then 500 mg/h continuous infusion in adults for 24 hours
   c) Pediatric: 25 mg/kg to a maximum of 1 g per dose, then q 6 to 12 hours **or**
   d) Pediatric: 20 to 40 mg/kg loading dose over 30 to 60 minutes with an infusion of 20 mg/kg/h

XII. Mushrooms (Table 4–5)

XIII. Cocaine

A. Toxic dose
   1. Any dose is potentially toxic
      a. Death is reported with first use; 20 mg reported to cause fatality
   2. Maximum intranasal cocaine dosage recommended 80 to 200 mg for medical use (1 to 2 mg/kg)
   3. 1 to 1.2 g intranasal cocaine is a typical fatal dose

B. Symptoms and signs
   1. Onset
      a. IV: onset 10 to 60 seconds; peak 3 to 5 minutes; duration 20 to 60 minutes
      b. Inhalation (smoking): onset 3 to 5 seconds; peak 1 to 3 minutes; duration 5 to 15 minutes
      c. Oral or intranasal: onset 1 to 5 minutes; peak 15 to 20 minutes; duration 60 to 90 minutes
   2. Hyperthermia (psychomotor agitation)
   3. Skin: soft tissue necrosis is possible if it infiltrates
   4. HEENT: mydriasis, rhinorrhea, and septal perforation
   5. CNS: euphoria, hyperactivity, agitation, convulsions, intracranial hemorrhage (ruptured aneurysm)
   6. Cardiovascular
      a. Tachycardia, hypertension, coronary vasoconstriction, and their sequelae (aortic dissection, myocardial ischemia [may delayed up to 24 hours])
         i. The risk of an acute myocardial infarction during the 60 minutes after use is increased 24-fold
         ii. 6% of patients with cocaine-induced chest pain will have enzyme elevation
         iii. ECG is less sensitive and less specific for MI in patients who have recently used cocaine when compared to patients with traditional atherosclerotic heart disease

TABLE 4-5. Mushroom Toxicity

GENUS/SPECIES	TOXIN	TIME OF ONSET OF SYMPTOMS	PRIMARY SITE OF TOXICITY	SYMPTOMS	MORTALITY	SPECIFIC THERAPY[a]
I. Amanita phalloides, A. tenuifolia, A. virosa Galerina autumnalis, G. marginata, G. venenata Lepiota josserandi, L. helveola	Cyclopeptides Amatoxins Phallotoxins	5 to 24 hours	Hepatic	Phase I: GI toxicity-N V D Phase II: Quiescent Phase III: Gastroenteritis, jaundice, ↑AST, ↑ALT N/V, weakness, hepatorenal failure	10% to 30%	Activated charcoal Hemoperfusion Penicillin G Silibinin
II. Gyromitra ambigua, G. esculenta, G. infula,	Gyromitrin (metabolite: monomethylhydrazine)	5 to 10 hours	CNS	Seizures, abdominal pain, N/V, weakness, hepatorenal failure	Rare	BZDs, Pyridoxine, 70 mg/kg IV
III. Clitocybe dealbata, Omphalotus olearius, Most Inocybe spp	Muscarine	0.5 to 2 hours	Autonomic nervous system	Muscarinic effects: salivation, bradycardia, lacrimation, urination, defecation, diaphoresis	Rare	Atropine: Adults: 1–2 mg Children: 0.02 mg/kg with a minimum of 0.1 mg
IV. Coprinus atramentarius	Coprine (metabolite: 1-aminocyclopropanol)	0.5 to 2 hours	Aldehyde dehydrogenase	Disulfiram-like effect with ethanol, tachycardia, N/V	Rare	—
V. Amanita gemmata, A. muscaria, A. pantherina	Ibotenic acid, muscimol	0.5 to 2 hours	CNS	GABAergic effects, rare delirium, hallucinations, dizziness, ataxia	Rare	BZDs during excitatory phase
VI. Psilocybe caerulipes, P. cubensis, Gymnopilus spectabilis, Psathyrella foenisecii	Psilocybin, psilocin	0.5 to 1 hours	CNS	Ataxia, N/V, hyperkinesis, hallucinations	Rare	BZDs
VII. Clitocybe nebularis, Chlorophyllum molybdites, C. esculentum, Lactariusspp Paxillus involutus	Various, GI irritants	0.5 to 3 hours	GI	Malaise, N/V/D	Rare	—
VIII. Cortinarius orellanus, C. speciosissimus, C. rainierensis	Orelline, orellanine	>24 hours days to weeks	Renal	Phase I: N/V, Phase II: Oliguria, renal failure	Rare	Hemodialysis for renal failure
IX. Amanita smithiana,	Allenic norleucine	0.5 to 12 hours	Renal	Phase I: N/V, Phase II: Oliguria, renal failure	None	Hemodialysis for renal failure
X. Tricholoma equestre	Unidentified myotoxin	24 to 72 hours	Muscle (skeletal and cardiac)	Fatigue, nausea, muscle weakness, myalgias (↑CPK), facial erythema, diaphoresis, myocarditis	25%	—

Key: D, diarrhea; N, nausea; V, vomiting.

[a]Supportive care (fluids, electrolyes, and antiemetics) as indicated.
Reprinted, with permission, from Flomenbaum NE, Goldfrank LR, Hoffman RS, et al. Goldfrank's Toxicologic Emergencies, 8th ed. New York: McGraw-Hill, 2006: 1566 as adapted from Lincoff G, Mitchel DH. Toxic and Hallucinogenic Mushroom Poisoning: A Handbook for Physicians and Mushroom Hunters. New York: Van Nostrand Reinhold, 1977: 246-247.

iv. Cocaine can also directly injure endothelium, increase platelet aggregation, and reduce endogenous thrombolysis

b. Virtually all types of tachydysrhythmias are reported including atrial fibrillation/flutter, torsade de pointes, and ventricular tachycardia/fibrillation. QRS prolongation occurs through sodium channel blockade. QT prolongation is possible

7. Pulmonary: pneumothorax, pneumomediastinum, and pneumopericardium (barotrauma), acute exacerbation of asthma (including fatal and near-fatal asthma), acute lung injury , diffuse alveolar hemorrhage, recurrent pulmonary infiltrates with eosinophilia , nonspecific interstitial pneumonitis, bronchiolitis obliterans with organizing pneumonia (BOOP), and acute pulmonary infiltrates associated with "crack lung": acute pulmonary infiltrates associated with a spectrum of clinical and histologic findings

8. Gastrointestinal: ischemic bowel, perforation

9. Genitourinary: renal failure from rhabdomyolysis or hypertension

10. Uterus: placental abruption in the second and third trimesters of pregnancy

C. Management

1. BZDs and cooling measures only are demonstrated to decrease mortality from cocaine intoxication in animal studies; thus external cooling and reduction in psychomotor agitation with BZDs are critical early maneuvers

2. GI decontamination: limited efficacy

XIV. Opioids

A. Symptoms and signs

1. Depression of BP, pulse, and temperature; likely mediated by CNS depression

2. Miosis

3. CNS depression

4. Hypoventilation

B. Management

1. Respiratory depression

a. Respiratory support: bag valve mask ventilation, or endotracheal intubation is lifesaving

b. Mechanical ventilation and oxygenation critical, not naloxone

c. Naloxone

i. Administered in incremental doses starting at 0.05 mg

ii. Redose based on clinical response, with observation for signs of withdrawal

iii. Continuous infusion of naloxone may be needed to maintain ventilation

iv. Typically, 66% of the effective reversal dose can be delivered hourly

XV. Anticonvulsants

A. Types

1. 5 agents in common use: phenytoin, carbamazepine, valproic acid, ethosuximide, and phenobarbital

2. 4 recently approved drugs, all structurally unrelated: felbamate, gabapentin, lamotrigine, and vigabatrin

B. Phenytoin/fosphenytoin

1. Fosphenytoin is a water-soluble precursor of phenytoin that avoids some of the problems associated with propylene glycol. It is for parenteral (IM/IV) use

2. Symptoms and signs: acute oral or parenteral toxicity

a. CNS: dizzy, nystagmus (>15 mcg/mL), ataxia (>30 mcg/mL), lethargy (>40 mcg/mL), dysarthria, vomiting, athetoid movements, hyperactive deep tendon reflexes, ophthalmoplegia

b. Seizures are unlikely but possible at high levels in patients with a seizure history

c. Cardiac dysrhythmias are distinctly uncommon with oral OD

3. Symptoms and signs acute: parenteral only

a. Rate-related, and in part related to **propylene glycol** solvent

i. **Hypotension**, cardiac arrest, bradycardia, impaired cardiac contractility

4. Management

a. AC may be given

b. Symptomatic and supportive care is the mainstay of therapy

c. Consider admitting the patient if the ataxia is too severe for patient to care for him- or herself. Admission does not require a monitored setting

C. Carbamazepine: structurally similar to TCAs

1. Symptoms and signs of toxicity

a. CNS: confusion, agitation, drowsiness, ataxia, diplopia, nystagmus, stupor, coma, **cyclical coma**, seizures, respiratory arrest, choreiform movements, dyskinesias, myoclonus, dystonia

b. Cardiac: QRS complex widening on ECG; suppresses phase 4 depolarization, tachycardia or bradycardia, AV block, ventricular arrhythmias

2. Serum concentrations
    a. Adults: levels >40 mcg/mL are associated with coma, seizures, respiratory failure, and cardiac conduction defects
    b. Children: appear more sensitive than adults; no correlation found with levels
3. Management
    a. GI Decontamination
        i. Consider orogastric lavage with large ODs
        ii. Repeat dose AC enhances clearance
    b. Sodium bicarbonate may be beneficial for a wide QRS
    c. Hemoperfusion clearance is equal to MDAC. A 4-hour run with good blood flow removes ~800 mg

D. Valproic acid
1. Symptoms and signs of toxicity
    a. GI: nausea, vomiting
    b. CNS: sedation, ataxia, coma, respiratory depression, hypertonia, tremor, cerebral edema
    c. Cardiac: arrest
    d. Other: hyperammonemia, hypernatremia, hypocalcemia, metabolic acidosis; drug interactions
    e. Overall, OD with valproic acid is usually benign with death rare. No correlation with serum concentrations exists. Liver enzymes remain normal
2. Management
    a. GI decontamination with several doses of AC decreases GI absorption
    b. Naloxone—several cases report success with naloxone. The mechanism of action is unclear
    c. Symptomatic and supportive care is generally all that is required
    d. Extracorporeal removal is rarely considered
        i. Its efficacy is based on multiple case reports, but unclear if it improves outcome
    e. L-carnitine improves hyperammonemia, but will not reverse the CNS depression seen in valporic acid (VPA) OD

XVI. Digoxin

A. Symptoms and signs of toxicity
1. Extracardiac
    a. Gastrointestinal
        i. Acute OD—nausea, vomiting almost always present and are usually the first symptoms
        ii. Chronic OD—anorexia, nausea, vomiting common

    b. Central nervous system
        i. Acute OD—lethargy, confusion, weakness
        ii. Chronic OD—headaches, delirium, confusion, disorientation, drowsiness, visual disturbances (halos, blurring, color aberrations) and seizures (rare; reported in children)
    c. Metabolic
        i. Acute: hyperkalemia is a marker for severe poisoning in acute OD (Table 4–6)
        ii. Mechanism of hyperkalemia: blockade of cardiac Na^+/K^+ ATPase increases extracellular $[K^+]$; release of K^+ from tissues (especially liver); inhibition of K^+ uptake into skeletal muscle
        iii. Hyperkalemia increases AV block exacerbating bradydysrhythmias and conduction delays
        iv. Importance of hyperkalemia in acute OD: potassium is an accurate predictor of outcome in adult patients with acute digitoxin (and probably digoxin) OD
2. Cardiac
    a. Digitalis ("dig") effect (may be seen with therapeutic levels)
        i. Scooped ST segments (Salvador Dali mustache), PR prolongation
    b. Keys to understanding digoxin toxicity
        i. Digoxin increases vagal tone → sinus bradycardia, impaired AV node conduction
        ii. Digoxin enhances automaticity → ventricular dysrhythmias
    c. Rhythm disturbances with digoxin toxicity
        i. Think digoxin whenever you see **increased automaticity with high-degree AV block**
        ii. Any dysrhythmia is possible except a rapidly conducted supraventricular rhythm, such as atrial fibrillation, with a rapid ventricular rate (unless the patient also has a congenital accessory pathway)

B. Management
1. Supportive
    a. The following measures are used in addition to digoxin-specific Fab or for patients who do not meet indications for antidotal therapy. Digoxin-specific Fab (Digibind or DigiFab) provides definitive treatment
        i. Decontamination
            a) AC: adsorbs digoxin well
            b) Orogastric lavage is not recommended unless the patient has life-threatening coingestants that warrant

TABLE 4–6. Potassium Level and Prognosis with Acute Digoxin Toxicity

POTASSIUM	OUTCOME
K^+ <5 mEq/dL	all survived
5 <K <5.5 mEq/dL	~50% survival
K^+ >5.5 mEq/dL	all died

decontamination, arrives within 1 to 2 hours, and has not already vomited

    c) Caution—lavage may increase vagal tone and worsen bradydysrhythmias

2. Management of dysrhythmias
   a. Bradydysrhythmias
      i. Atropine
         a) Internal pacemakers are contraindicated
   b. Tachydysrhythmias
      i. Potassium or magnesium replacement
         a) Often effective if serum [K^+] or [Mg^{++}] low
         b) **Never** use magnesium in bradycardia/AV block
         c) Use magnesium cautiously if patient has renal insufficiency
      ii. Phenytoin
         a) Reported success for the treatment of digoxin-related ventricular dysrhythmias
3. Management of hyperkalemia and hypokalemia
   a. **Hyper**kalemia
      i. It is usually not clinically significant except as a **marker** for digoxin toxicity in **acute** OD
      ii. Severe hyperkalemia may require treatment—insulin/glucose, sodium bicarbonate. (β-receptor agonists should be

used with caution because of their prodysrrhythmic effects
      iii. Calcium is contraindicated
   b. **Hypo**kalemia sensitizes the heart to digoxin, worsening signs and symptoms in **chronic digoxin toxicity** and thus requires repletion
      i. Replace potassium if K^+ < 4 and there are ventricular dysrhythmias
4. Definitive management: digoxin-specific antibody fragments (Digibind, DigiFab) (Table 4–7)
   a. Indications for Digibind, DigiFab
      i. Rhythm and conduction disturbances
         a) Ventricular dysrhythmias
         b) Bradydysrhythmias not responsive to atropine
      ii. Serum [K^+] >5 mEq/dL in an acute ingestion in an otherwise healthy individual
      iii. Serum digoxin level 10 to 15 ng/mL in an acute ingestion
      iv. A digoxin ingestion of >10 mg (4 mg in a child)
      v. Empirically for undiagnosed bradycardia (clinical judgment)
         a) Digibind and DigiFab are dosed the same way as is described in Table 4-7

XVII. β-Adrenergic Antagonists (β-Blockers) and Calcium Channel Blockers

A. β-Adrenergic Antagonists (β-Blockers)
   1. Symptoms and signs of toxicity
      a. Often benign, particularly in young healthy individuals (those not dependent on adrenergic tone); ~33% remain asymptomatic
      b. Comorbid conditions like congestive heart failure (CHF), sick sinus syndrome, and coingestion, especially of cardioactive toxins increase likelihood of toxicity

TABLE 4–7. Dosing of Fab in Digoxin Toxicity

SITUATION	CALCULATION
If dose ingested is known	$\text{Dose (vials)} = \dfrac{\text{amount ingested (mg)} \times 0.8}{0.5 \text{ mg (ie, amount digoxin bound/vial)}}$
If serum digoxin level is known	$\text{Dose (vials)} = \dfrac{(5 \text{ L/kg}) \times (\text{digoxin level (ng/mL)}) \times (\text{wt in kg})}{(0.5 \text{ mg}) \times (1000 \text{ mL L})}$
Simplified formula	$\text{Dose (vials)} = \dfrac{(\text{digoxin level in ng/mL}) \times (\text{wt in kg})}{100}$
Empiric dosing with unknown digoxin level	Acute OD: 10 vials (adult or child)* Chronic OD: Adult: 5 vials >Child: 2 vials

*Empiric dose is identical for acute poisoning in children

c. Cardiovascular toxicity
  i. Hypotension, bradycardia, CHF
  ii. QRS and QT prolongation on ECG
d. Respiratory depression and apnea
e. Central nervous system
  i. Delirium, coma, seizures
  ii. Occurs most often in setting of hypotension
  iii. More lipophilic β-blockers (propranolol) may cause delirium in the absence of cardiovascular effects; in the elderly this may occur even in therapeutic dosing
f. Hypoglycemia (relatively common in children after β-blocker ingestion)
g. Hyperkalemia occasionally complicates acute OD
h. Bronchospasm appears to occur only in susceptible patients
i. Toxicity generally manifests early, within 6 hours
  i. Sotalol may cause delayed and prolonged toxicity
  ii. Little known about SR preparations but reasonable to expect delayed and prolonged toxicity

B. Calcium channel blockers
1. Symptoms and signs of toxicity
  a. Symptoms and physical findings usually reflect the degree of hypoperfusion
    i. Mild or moderate toxicity: weak and dizzy, mild confusion, bradycardia
    ii. Severe: profound bradycardia and shock, cardiovascular collapse
  b. Presentation is often rapid and fulminant with immediate-release formulations; with SR preparation signs may be delayed 6 to 8 hours and delays up to 15 hours have been reported
  c. Cardiovascular: hypotension, bradycardia, dysrhythmias, cardiogenic shock
    i. CNS: dizziness, altered mental status, seizures, stroke, coma may occur in setting of cardiogenic shock
  d. Pulmonary: acute lung injury/ARDS
  e. Hyperglycemia: insulin release from pancreatic β-islet cells also calcium-mediated. In CCB OD, get decreased calcium influx leading to decreased insulin release and hyperglycemia

C. Management of β-blocker and calcium channel blocker OD
1. The primary goal is to prevent and correct the hypotension caused by the negative inotropy and peripheral vasodilation
2. ABCs, particularly aggressive fluid resuscitation
3. GI decontamination
4. Syrup of ipecac

a. Contraindicated because of the potential for rapid deterioration
5. Orogastric lavage
  a. Possibly indicated following large ingestions or in seriously ill patients
  b. SR preparations are often too large to fit up the lavage tube
  c. Theoretical concern of increasing vagal tone and worsening bradycardia (atropine prior may be useful)
6. Activated charcoal
  a. Indicated in a patient whose airway is protected regardless of the time since ingestion
  b. MDAC indicated for patients with ingestions of SR preparations
7. Whole bowel irrigation
  a. May be useful in patients with SR ingestions
  b. Begin early with 2 L/h of PEG (0.5 L/h in children) until the rectal effluent is clear
  c. Often a nasogastric tube is required
  d. Not associated with significant fluid or electrolyte shifts
8. Atropine
  a. May have limited effect because the hypotension is primarily caused by global myocardial depression and not by increased vagal tone
  b. Hold in patients who will be receiving WBI as atropine's anticholinergic properties will decrease bowel motility
9. Calcium
  a. Increases extracellular calcium creating a concentration gradient across the cell membrane promoting intracellular calcium flux (remember several types of channels exist and only 1 is blocked by CCBs)
  b. Dosing depends on the type of calcium salt used.
    i. 1 g calcium chloride contains 13.4 mEq calcium
    ii. 1 g calcium gluconate contains 4.3 mEq calcium
    iii. Calcium chloride ($CaCl_2$) provides 3 times as much calcium as calcium gluconate
  c. Initially 1 to 2 ampules of $CaCl_2$ (10–20 mL of a 10% $CaCl_2$ solution) or 3 to 6 ampules of calcium gluconate (30–60 mL of a 10% calcium gluconate solution) given by slow IV push over 3 to 5 minutes
  d. Ascertain digoxin is not the causative agent of the bradydysrhythmias before calcium administration
10. Glucagon
  a. Activates adenyl cyclase through the glucagon receptor (via G_s protein), bypassing the β-receptor

i. Likely to be unhelpful with CCB toxicity as the lesion is "downstream" from adenylate cyclase—but should still be considered with refractory hypotension 2° to CCB toxicity

b. Adult dose is initially 2 to 5 mg slowly IVP, which can be repeated in 5 to 10 minutes up to a total dose of 10 mg

c. Follow the bolus with a continuous infusion starting at a rate equal to the minimum effective dose (eg, if the patient requires 3 mg, followed by 5 mg for a response, the drip should be set at 8 mg/h). Prolonged glucagon infusion may require adequate intravenous glucose supplementation for continued clinical effect

XVIII. Clonidine

A. Mechanism of action
1. Central α_2 agonism: acts on the brain as a postsynaptic α_2-adrenergic agonist ($\downarrow$ NE release in the brain = $\downarrow$ sympathetic outflow from the brain = decreased heart rate, BP, cardiac output)
2. Peripheral α_2 agonism: acts on peripheral vessels as a postsynaptic α_2-adrenergic agonist ($\uparrow$ NE release = peripheral vasoconstriction and early transient hypertension)

B. Symptoms and signs
1. Cardiovascular: transient initial **hypertension** from peripheral vasoconstriction gives way to hypotension and bradycardia from central effects
2. CNS: lethargy
3. Respiratory: hypoventilation, hypoxia, Cheynes-Stokes respiration, periodic apnea
4. Ocular: pinpoint pupils

C. Management
1. GI decontamination: consider orogastric lavage if early and massive ingestion (rarely indicated), otherwise give AC
2. Syrup of ipecac is contraindicated as decreased mental status is a common finding
3. Naloxone: may reverse some or all of the sedation associated with clonidine (mechanism unclear)
   a. High doses of naloxone (4 to 10 mg) may be required and many patients will not respond at any dose
4. Hypotension and bradycardia
   a. Initial treatment should be IV fluids
   b. If bradycardia is symptomatic, standard doses of atropine are effective, but re-dosing may be required
   c. If hypotension is unresponsive to fluids, consider a vasoconstrictor agent

XIX. Lithium

A. Symptoms and signs of toxicity (Table 4–8)
1. Must distinguish acute versus chronic toxicity from acute on chronic OD
2. Poor correlation with serum levels; toxicity does not occur until lithium distributes into cells
3. Acute toxicity is characterized by early GI symptoms; neurologic symptoms are delayed since there is a slow distribution of lithium into the brain
4. Chronic toxicity is characterized by neurologic symptoms (resembles later stages of acute toxicity) and is caused by a high total body burden of lithium (including the brain); any additional increase in lithium results in immediate toxicity

TABLE 4–8. Clinical Manifestations of Acute versus Chronic Lithium Ingestion

	ACUTE	CHRONIC
GI	Nausea, vomiting	Minimal
Renal	Concentrating defects	Nephrogenic diabetes insipidus, interstitial nephritis, renal failure
Neurologic	Mild: Weakness, light-headedness, fine tremor	Mild: Same
	Moderate: Muscle twitching, tinnitus, drowsiness, hyperreflexia, slurred speech, apathy	Moderate: Same
	Severe: Confusion, clonus, coma, seizure, extrapyramidal symptoms	Severe: Parkinson disease, psychosis, memory deficits, idiopathic intracranial hypertension
Cardiovascular	Prolonged QT interval, ST- and T-wave changes	Myocarditis
Endocrine	Hypothyroidism	Hypothyroidism
Hematologic	Leukocytosis	Aplastic anemia
Cutaneous	None	Dermatitis, ulcers, edema

5. Acute OD: higher levels with less symptoms; chronic OD: more symptoms with lower levels
6. Acute on chronic OD: intermediate findings

B. Predisposing factors for chronic toxicity
1. Dehydration
2. Sodium depletion
3. Preeclampsia
4. Continuation of high lithium doses after control of acute mania
5. Renal dysfunction
6. Drug interactions leading to elevated lithium concentrations
   a. NSAIDs, antipsychotics, diuretics, SSRIs, ACE inhibitors, carbamazepine

C. Management
1. Consider orogastric lavage if spontaneous emesis has not already occurred
   a. May not be helpful
      i. Immediate-release preparations are rapidly absorbed
      ii. SR preparations are usually too large to pass through the tube
2. Initiate WBI if ingestion is of SR preparations
3. AC for known or potential coingestants
4. Normal saline hydration, twice maintenance if tolerated, to correct dehydration and electrolyte depletion and to maximize renal lithium clearance
5. Diuretics **not** recommended since they may worsen lithium toxicity as patients become dehydrated
6. Reassess neurologic status frequently
7. Notify nephrologist for elevated levels, significant ingestion, and/or neurologic signs
   a. Hemodialysis recommended for patients with
      i. Li^+ concentration >4 mEq/L in acute toxicity, even in the absence of symptoms
      ii. Elevated Li^+ concentration and moderate to severe toxicity, particularly neurologic (including altered mental status)
      iii. Renal failure (unable to clear lithium)
      iv. Inability to tolerate saline hydration caused by underlying medical conditions (CHF)

XX. Toxic Alcohols

A. Definition
1. General formula for an alcohol: R-OH (alcohol)
2. The term toxic alcohol is generally used to refer to
   a. Methanol
   b. Ethylene glycol
   c. Isopropanol

3. The agents are ingested for several reasons
   a. Ethanol substitutes
   b. Unintentional ingestions of household products
   c. Suicide attempts

B. Methanol (CH_3OH, MW 32)
1. Uses
   a. Gasoline antifreeze: 100% solution
   b. Windshield washer fluid: up to 30%
   c. Denaturants in paint and varnish removers
   d. Fuel (eg, Sterno): ~4%
   e. "Denatured" alcohol for the laboratory
   f. In 1979, 46 cases of methanol poisoning and 3 fatalities were reported after a mass ingestion of photocopy fluid by a group of prison inmates
2. Properties
   a. High volatility, low freezing point
3. Symptoms and signs of toxicity
   a. Ethanol coingestion may delay onset of methanol metabolism and subsequent poisoning since ADH has a higher affinity for it. This is the basis for ethanol therapy
   b. Possible inebriation (CNS sedation), often no symptoms with small, but consequential ingestions
   c. Any time from 1 hour to, typically, 12 to 24 hours post-ingestion
   d. High anion gap metabolic acidosis
   e. Absence of significant lactate or ketone concentrations to explain acidosis
   f. Visual changes ("snow field vision"), blindness. Funduscopic examination may reveal disc hyperemia or pallor and/or retinal edema
   g. Abdominal complaints

C. Ethylene glycol (CH_2OH-CH_2OH, MW 62)
1. Uses
   a. Automobile coolant and antifreeze (eg, radiator)
   b. Solvents
   c. De-icers (eg, methanol or isopropanol)
2. Properties
   a. Low volatility
   b. High boiling point
   c. Sweet tasting
3. Symptoms and signs of toxicity
   a. Possibly inebriation, often no symptoms with small, but consequential ingestions
   b. Ethanol coingestion may delay onset of ethylene glycol metabolism and subsequent poisoning since ADH has a higher affinity for it. This is the basis for ethanol therapy
   c. High anion gap metabolic acidosis (glycolic acid)
   d. Absence of significant lactate or ketone concentrations to explain acidosis

e. Oxalate formation can chelate serum calcium resulting in hypocalcemia. Calcium oxalate may precipitate out in renal tubules causing **acute renal failure** 12 to 48 hours after ingestion (if untreated)

f. Cranial nerve deficits are reported

g. Abdominal complaints

D. Evaluation of patients with methanol or ethylene glycol exposure
1. Inebriation ability based loosely on the number of carbons: methanol < ethanol < ethylene glycol < isopropanol
2. Serum toxic alcohol levels
    a. Not routinely available in a clinically relevant, rapid fashion
    b. Danger level (methanol and ethylene glycol): 25 mg/dL
3. If serum levels are unavailable, try to collect objective evidence for poisoning
    a. Osmol gap = **measured** osmolality to **calculated** osmolarity
    b. Blood gas analysis
    c. Urine for ketones and crystals
    d. Lactate

E. Management of methanol and ethylene glycol toxicity
1. ABCs, substrates (especially glucose), GI decontamination
2. Syrup of ipecac—not useful because of potential for CNS depression
3. Nasogastric lavage—useful early (within 30 minutes or in intentionally large ingestions)
4. AC—methanol and ethylene glycol adsorb well to charcoal
5. Sodium bicarbonate—keep serum pH normal; alkalinization enhances elimination of glycolate and keeps the amount of undissociated formic acid low and thereby out of the CNS. (Watch for fluid overload)
6. Consider ethanol or fomepizole therapy and nephrology consult early; consult poison center or medical toxicologist early
7. Hemodialysis indications
    a. Methanol or ethylene glycol level ≥25 mg/dL
    b. High osmol gap without other cause
    c. End-organ manifestations of toxicity
    d. Severe acid/base abnormalities
8. Adjunctive therapy
    a. Methanol: folate or folinic acid (leucovorin): dose 1 mg/kg up to 50 mg every 4 to 6 hours
    b. Ethylene glycol: thiamine (100 mg) and pyridoxine (50 mg) every 4 to 6 hours
    c. When in doubt administer all 3 vitamins (folate, thiamine, and pyridoxine)

d. Sodium bicarbonate to alkalinize the patient's urine to enhance the clearance of acid metabolite (eg, formate)

F. Isopropanol
1. Uses
    a. Rubbing alcohol
    b. Solvents
    c. De-icer
2. Symptoms and signs
    a. Early presentation compared to methanol and ethylene glycol
    b. CNS depression, coma
    c. Ketosis without acidosis
    d. Gastritis, may be severe
    e. Hypotension, may be severe and prolonged (large ingestions)
    f. Hemorrhagic tracheobronchitis (rare)
    g. Renal failure
3. Diagnosis
    a. Osmol gap elevated, no increase in anion gap
    b. Weakly to briskly positive urinary ketones caused by acetone metabolite
    c. No acidosis
4. Management
    a. GI decontamination (rarely indicated): nasogastric lavage if early and is thought to be a large ingestion
    b. No need for ethanol or fomepizole therapy
    c. Supportive care with fluid replacement
    d. Hemodialysis for hypotension refractory to fluids and pressors (rare)

XXI. Hydrocarbons

A. Aspiration results from the unique characteristics of hydrocarbons
1. Viscosity: resistance to flow
2. Surface tension or van der Wals forces: ability to creep (as up a capillary tube)
3. Volatility

B. Large volume (>30mL) ingestions are a risk for aspiration caused by regurgitation

C. Symptoms may result immediately or may be delayed for up to 6 hours
1. Coughing, choking, dyspnea, grunting, rales, hypoxia

D. Hydrocarbons in lung cause
1. Pneumonitis
    a. Mimics pneumonia clinically
2. Destruction of alveolar lipid membranes

E. Symptoms and signs
  1. Cough and bronchospasm are typical initial signs
  2. Progressive respiratory distress may follow
  3. Infiltrate on CXR, hyperthermia, and leukocytosis commonly follow
  4. Acute lung injury and respiratory failure may occur

F. Management—largely supportive
  1. Most hydrocarbon aspirations are complications of ingestions
  2. Historical information is helpful in managing patients
  3. Asymptomatic, unintentional ingestions of hydrocarbons which do not result in systemic toxicity may be observed at home
  4. Intentional ingestions, ingestions of hydrocarbons with systemic toxicity, and all symptomatic patients should be evaluated in a hospital setting

G. Hospital management
  1. Gastric decontamination is almost never indicated
  2. Gastric decontamination may be indicated for hydrocarbons with systemic toxicity, but these cases are exceedingly rare
  3. Diagnosis
    a. Assess for clinical evidence of aspiration and observe for 6 hours
    b. If still asymptomatic at 6 hours, obtain chest radiograph
    c. Patients with a normal chest radiograph at 6 hours who are asymptomatic may be discharged
  4. Bronchospasm, hypoxia, respiratory failure are treated as they otherwise would be treated
  5. Antibiotics and steroids have little if any role in the absence of a documented infection
  6. Surfactant has been used anecdotally with success

Chapter 5
CARDIAC EMERGENCIES

Robert Hessler and Taku Taira

I. Ischemic Heart Disease and Coronary Artery Disease

A. Epidemiology
1. Leading cause of death in United States in both men and women
2. Accounts for 30% of all U.S. deaths[1]
3. Projected to cost more than $258 billion in 2006[2]

B. Etiology
1. Insufficient blood supply to myocardium
   a. Fixed obstructing lesions
      i. Atherosclerosis
      ii. Etiology of stable angina
   b. Ruptured plaque
      i. Leading to exposure of thrombogenic core and thrombus formation
      ii. Etiology of acute coronary syndrome
   c. Prinzmetal angina—coronary artery vasospasm
   d. Systemic hypotension
2. Inadequate oxygen delivery
   a. Severe anemia, hypoxia, acidosis, carbon monoxide, cyanide, methemoglobinemia
3. Increased myocardial oxygen demand
   a. Tachycardia, increased contractility, increased systemic vascular resistance, aortic valve disease (rare)[3], hypertrophic cardiomyopathy (rare)[3]

C. Coronary anatomy
1. Left main coronary artery
   a. Originates in the left aortic sinus giving rise to the left anterior descending and left circumflex arteries
      i. Left anterior descending artery
         a) Feeds the anteroseptal portions of the heart
      ii. Left circumflex artery
         a) Feeds the anterolateral portions of the heart

   b) May feed posterior structures in left dominant individuals (see discussion on dominance below)
2. Right coronary artery (RCA)
   a. Feeds the right ventricle and extends to supply the inferior and posterior portions of the heart
3. Posterior descending artery (PDA)
   a. Coronary dominances determined by which artery feeds the PDA
      i. Right dominant in 80% to 90%—supplied by RCA
      ii. Left dominant in 10% to 15%—supplied by LCX
      iii. Codominant in 5% to 10%
   b. PDA supplies the atrioventricular (AV) node and posteromedial papillary muscle
      i. Ischemia involving PDA can lead to mitral regurgitation and bradycardia and heart block

D. Risk factors[6]
1. Family history, smoking, hypertension, diabetes, cholesterol, male, >55 years
2. Others: cocaine[7], antiretroviral treatment[8,9,10,11], lupus

E. Risk stratification
1. Thrombolysis in Myocardial Infarction (TIMI) scoring system
   a. Elements of score
      i. >65 years
      ii. ≥3 cardiac risk factors (see risk factors above)
      iii. Prior coronary stenosis >50%
      iv. ST-segment deviation
      v. 2 anginal events in 24 hours
      vi. Aspirin use within the week
      vii. Elevated CK or CK-MB

   b. Score and risk of death, myocardial infarction (MI), or reinfarction
      i. (0 to 1) 4.7% risk
      ii. (2) 8.3 % risk
      iii. (3) 13.2 % risk
      iv. (4) 19.9 % risk
      v. (5) 26.2 % risk
      vi. (6 to 7) 40.9% risk[12]
   c. For ED physicians, it is important to note that a TIMI risk score of 0 to 1 still has a 4.7% risk of death or MI which many would argue is too high

F. Symptoms and signs
   1. Symptoms
      a. Chest pain
      b. Atypical chest pain
         i. Women, diabetics, and elderly more likely to present atypically[4,3]
         ii. Symptoms range from fatigue, nausea, epigastric pain, palpitations, and chest wall pain
         iii. Chest pain absent in 18% of MI[5]
      c. Associated symptoms
         i. Diaphoresis
         ii. Nausea or hiccups with inferior wall ischemia
         iii. Radiation to jaw, shoulder(s), back
   2. Signs
      a. Vital signs: tachycardia or bradycardia, hypertension or hypotension
      b. Cardiac examination
         i. New S_3—sudden halting of rushing blood into the ventricle
         ii. New S_4—atrial contraction forcing blood into a noncompliant ventricle
         iii. New murmur
            a) Papillary muscle dysfunction or rupture
            b) Interventricular septal rupture
         iv. New rub—pericardial inflammation
         v. Pulmonary crackles indicating congestive heart failure (CHF)
         vi. Hypotension
         vii. Tachycardia
         viii. Bradycardia (common with RCA infarct)

G. Diagnosis
   1. ECG
      a. Initially abnormal in <50% of patients with ischemic chest pain
         i. Often normal in ACS with episodic ischemia
      b. ECG changes

      i. Hyperacute T waves
         a) Earliest ECG sign of myocardial infarction
         b) T waves are more prominent, symmetrical, and pointed
      ii. T wave flattening/inversion
         a) Differential includes, myocardial contusion, CNS disease, digoxin effect, and right ventricle (RV) or left ventricle (LV) strain
      iii. ST segment elevation
         a) Elevation >1 mm in 2 anatomically contiguous leads
         b) Differential includes
            i) Early repolarization
            ii) Pericarditis
            iii) Left bundle branch block (LBBB)
            iv) Intracranial hemorrhage
            v) Hyperkalemia
            vi) Brugada syndrome
            vii) Pulmonary embolism[13]
      iv. ST segment depression
         a) Measured from the PR segment to the ST segment
         b) Depression >1 mm in 2 or more anatomically contiguous leads indicates myocardial ischemia
      v. New bundle branch block or AV block may be secondary to a new infarction
         a) New left bundle branch block, in the setting of chest pain is considered a criteria for acute thrombolysis
         b) Associated with increased mortality[14]
      vi. Arrhythmias
         a) Bradyarrythmias secondary to dysfunction of sinoatrial (SA) or AV node
         b) Tachyarrhythmias caused by reperfusion, altered autonomic tone, or hemodynamic instability
         c) Ventricular fibrillation in the acute setting is an indication for immediate catheterization
         d) Accelerated idioventricular rhythms (AIVR) and junctional rhythms can occur in the setting of acute MI
            i) May be reperfusion rhythms after thrombolysis
            ii) May resemble VT except slower (50 to 100 bpm)
            iii) Anti-arrhythmics (eg, lidocaine) contraindicated as they suppress ventricular activity and may lead to asystole
   c. Infarction patterns

    i. Septal

       a) ST elevations in V_1 and V_2

    ii. Anterior

       a) ST elevations in V_3 and V_4

       b) Primarily from occlusion of the LAD

       c) Associated with malignant high-grade heart block

    iii. Lateral

       a) ST elevations in I, aVL, V_5, and V_6

    iv. Inferior

       a) ST elevations in II, III, and aVF

       b) Primarily RCA occlusion

       c) Arrhythmia secondary to heightened vagal tone[15] or AV node dysfunction

       d) Up to 25% of inferior wall MIs are complicated with right ventricular infarction

    v. Right ventricle

       a) Inferior wall MI should prompt repeat ECG with right-sided leads

         i) ST elevations in V_4R and V_5R diagnostic

       b) ST elevations in V_1 may be diagnostic with late presenting infarcts

    vi. Posterior

       a) Large R waves and ST depression in V_1 and V_2

         i) Should prompt posterior lead placement on patient's back

         ii) ST elevations in V_7 and V_8 are diagnostic

  d. Other

    i. Acute infarction in the setting of a preexisting LBBB is indicated by

       a) ST segment elevation >1 mm concordant with the QRS complex

       b) ST segment depression of >1 mm in V_1, V_2, V_3

       c) ST segment elevation >5 mm discordant with the direction of the QRS[16]

    ii. Wellen sign—critical stenosis of proximal LAD

       a) Deep T wave inversions or less commonly biphasic T waves in V_2 and V_3

2. Cardiac enzymes

  a. Troponin T and I

    i. Specific for cardiac injury (trop T 94%, trop I 100%)[5]

    ii. Positive in 2 to 6 hours and remain elevated for at least 1 week

    iii. Can be positive with pulmonary embolus, pericarditis, heart failure, myocarditis, shock, and renal failure[17]

    iv. Elevations in troponin and CK MB have both diagnostic and prognostic utility[18]

  b. CK MB—positive in 3 to 8 hours, less specific than troponin

    i. Calculating a CK index (CK MB and total CK) can increase the specificity of a MB elevation

    ii. May be used to diagnose recurrent infarction in the periinfarction period, caused by more rapid clearance when compared to troponin

  c. May be positive in patients without myocardial infarction

    i. Sepsis, supraventricular tachycardia (SVT), left ventricular hypertrophy (LVT), trauma, myocarditis and pericarditis, heart transplant, CHF, pulmonary embolism (PE), pulmonary disease, renal failure[17,19]

3. Echocardiogram

  a. Regional wall motion abnormality may be evident

  b. Poor correlation between the regional infarction pattern and the echo diagnosed regional wall motion abnormality[20]

4. Treadmill testing

  a. Continuous ECG monitoring while exertion on treadmill

  b. Sensitivity 65% to 70%, specificity 70% to 75%

5. Stress echo

  a. Echocardiographic evaluation of wall motion immediately following exertion with treadmill testing

  b. Sensitivity 80% to 85%, specificity 80% to 85%

6. Pharmacological stress echo

  a. For patients unable to exert themselves physically

  b. Cardiac function is evaluated in the same fashion as a stress echo after injection of dobutamine or persantine

  c. Sensitivity 80% to 85%, specificity 85% to 90%

7. Exercise and pharmacologic myocardial perfusion single photon emission computed tomography (SPECT), with quantitative analysis

  a. Injection of radioactive material (Tc 99m or thallium) allows detection of perfusion defects in the myocardium during cardiac exertion

  b. Sensitivity 80% to 90%, specificity 80% to 90%

H. Management

1. Oxygen

2. Antiplatelet agents

  a. Aspirin[21,22,23]

    i. Dosage should be between 162 and 326 mg

  ii. Nonenteric-coated aspirin should be chewed to allow more rapid absorption

  iii. Contraindications: aspirin allergy or possibility of aortic dissection

 b. Clopidogrel[24]

  i. Indicated in patients with ACS

  ii. Can be given instead of aspirin for patients with true aspirin allergies

3. Nitroglycerin

 a. Smooth muscle dilator

  i. Improves myocardial oxygen supply by dilating coronary arteries

  ii. Provides preload and afterload reduction

 b. Contraindications

  i. Sildenafil (Viagra) use within past 24 hours

  ii. Right ventricular infarction

4. Morphine

 a. Blocks catecholamine surge

 b. Reduces preload and afterload by means of its histamine effects

 c. Use with extreme caution if suspect RCA infarct or patient is hypotensive

5. β-Blockers

 a. Use in ACS controversial since COMMIT trial[26]

 b. Administration of PO β-blocker in patients with suspected MI is still considered a Centers for Medicare and Medicaid Service patient quality measurement

 c. Stable patients may have mortality benefit

  i. Decreases incidence of ventricular arrhythmias

 d. Contraindicated with cocaine chest pain

 e. Relative contraindication

  i. CHF, active asthma, hypotension, bradycardia

6. Antithrombotic agents

 a. Heparin

  i. Activates antithrombin III which inactivates thrombin, to block the coagulation cascade

  ii. Bolus of 60 to 70 U/kg (maximum of 5000 U)

  iii. Infusion of 12 to 15 U kg/h[27]

 b. Low-molecular-weight heparin has demonstrated 16% relative risk reduction in rates of infarction and death but with increased rates of bleeding[28-30]

 c. Bivalirudin

  i. A direct thrombin inhibitor

  ii. May be superior to heparin for patients going to PTCA[31]

  iii. There is limited evidence showing equivalent efficacy in treatment of ACS between bivalirudin and heparin[32]

  iv. Use in patients with heparin induced thrombocytopenia

 d. GP IIB and GP IIIA inhibitors

  i. The majority of the evidence for improved outcomes comes from studies where GP IIB and GP IIIA inhibitors were used in patients undergoing catheterization

  ii. The role of GP IIB and GP IIIA inhibitors in the medical management of ACS remains controversial[25]

7. Thrombolytics and cardiac catheterization

 a. Indications

  i. ST elevations >1 mm in 2 anatomically contiguous limb leads

  ii. ST elevations >2 mm in 2 anatomically contiguous chest leads

  iii. New LBBB

  iv. High clinical suspicion for MI with pre-existing LBBB

  v. Reciprocal ST segment depression V_1 through V_3 from a posterior wall infarction

 b. Absolute contraindications for thrombolysis

  i. Strong suspicion for dissection of the aorta

  ii. Active GI or other internal bleeding (excluding menses)

  iii. Intracranial tumor, hemorrhage, or arteriovenous malformation

  iv. Significant closed-head or facial trauma within 3 months

  v. Known allergy

 c. Relative contraindications

  i. History of chronic, severe, poorly controlled hypertension

  ii. Persistently elevated blood pressure >180/110 mm Hg

  iii. History of prior ischemic stroke >3 months

  iv. Major surgery within 3 weeks

  v. Recent (within 2 to 4 weeks) internal bleeding

  vi. Noncompressible vascular punctures

  vii. Pregnancy

  viii. Active peptic ulcer

  ix. Current use of anticoagulation[33]

 d. Percutaneous coronary intervention (PCI) is preferred if

  i. Absolute contraindication to thrombolysis

  ii. PCI available with contact to balloon time <90 minutes

  iii. Cardiogenic shock

  iv. Presentation >3 hours from onset[33]

 e. Thrombolysis is preferred if

  i. Prolonged transport to a catherization capable facility

ii. Medical contact to balloon time is anticipated to be >90 minutes

II. Congestive Heart Failure

A. Definitions
   1. Left-sided versus right-sided heart failure for etiology and symptoms and signs (Table 5–1)
   2. Systolic versus diastolic heart failure
      a. Systolic heart failure
         i. Poor ability of the left ventricle to contract
         ii. Echocardiography shows decreased ejection fraction with increased left ventricular size
            a) Higher risk for arrhythmia
      b. Diastolic heart failure
         i. Poor diastolic compliance because of hypertension, and left ventricular hypertrophy
         ii. Systolic function is preserved
         iii. Echocardiography shows signs of impaired relaxation, concentric ventricular hypertrophy and normal or increased ejection fraction
         iv. Estimated to be 20% to 50% of patients with heart failure[35]
   3. High-output versus low-output heart failure
      a. High-output
         i. Secondary to high metabolic state or shunting of blood that increases myocardial oxygen demand
            a) Hyperthyroidism, beriberi, AV fistulas, Paget disease, severe anemia, and pregnancy
      b. Low-output
         i. Most commonly caused by a depressed ejection fraction

B. Epidemiology
   1. Account for 3.4 million ED visits a year

2. 70% to 80% of patients with heart failure die within 8 years[34]

C. Pathophysiology
   1. Hemodynamic model of heart failure
      a. Left ventricular >elevated diastolic filling pressures → pulmonary congestion
   2. Neurohormonal model of heart failure
      a. Inadequate end-organ perfusion → sympathetic nervous system and renin-angiotensin–aldosterone axis activation → vasoconstriction/fluid retention → increased afterload → worsening cardiac output/ventricular dilatation

D. Symptoms and signs
   1. Symptoms
      a. Exertional dyspnea, orthopnea, paroxysmal nocturnal dyspnea (PND), nocturia
   2. Signs
      a. Diminished pulse pressure
      b. Pulsus alternans—alternating weak and strong pulse
      c. Bilateral rales
      d. Pitting edema
      e. Hepatomegaly/hepatojugular reflux
      f. Ascites
      g. Jugular venous distension
      h. S_3 gallop
      i. Loud P_2

E. New York Heart Association (NYHA) classification
   a. Class I: no limitation of physical activity
   b. Class II: slight limitation of physical activity; comfortable at rest
   c. Class III: marked limitation of physical activity; comfortable at rest
   d. Class IV: unable to carry out any physical activity; symptoms at rest

F. Diagnosis
   1. No defined gold standard
   2. Chest x-ray

TABLE 5–1. Right and Left Ventricular Failure

	RIGHT VENTRICULAR FAILURE	LEFT VENTRICULAR FAILURE
Signs and symptoms	• JVD • Dependent edema • Liver congestion	• Pulmonary edema • Orthopnea • Paroxysmal nocturnal dyspnea
Causes	• Left ventricular failure • Mitral stenosis/regurgitation • Pulmonary hypertension (COPD, sleep apnea, idiopathic, pulmonary embolism, pneumonia) • Pulmonic stenosis/regurgitation • Cardiomyopathy • Right ventricular infarction	• Mitral regurgitation • Systemic hypertension • Aortic stenosis/regurgitation • Cardiomyopathy • Left ventricular infarction • Right heart failure

a. Cardiomegaly (not sensitive or specific)
b. Cephalization
c. Kerley B lines (lymphatic vessels)
d. Pleural effusion (when unilateral, right side more common)
e. Interstitial perihilar infiltrates (bat winging)
f. X-ray may identify other potential cause of shortness of breath

3. Echo
   a. LV EF <40% is considered to be systolic dysfunction
   b. LV EF >40% with thickened myocardial wall is evidence for diastolic dysfunction
   c. Can diagnose valvulopathy as a cause or contributing factor

4. Brain type natriuretic peptide (BNP)
   a. Secreted by the ventricles in response to stretch
   b. Elevated by any process that increases ventricular afterload
      i. Values <50 pg/mL has a negative predictive value of 98%
      ii. Values >100 pg/mL has a 83% accuracy[36]
      iii. Cardiac causes of elevated BNP
         a) Heart failure
         b) Diastolic dysfunction
         c) Acute coronary syndrome
         d) Hypertension with LVH
         e) Valvular heart disease
         f) Atrial fibrillation
      iv. Noncardiac causes of elevated BNP
         a) Acute pulmonary embolism
         b) Pulmonary hypertension
         c) Sepsis
         d) COPD with cor-pulmonale
         e) Hyperthyroidism[37]

G. Management
   1. Respiratory support
      a. Oxygen
      b. Noninvasive positive pressure ventilation
         i. Decreases work of breathing
         ii. Decreased need for intubation and decreased mortality[38]
         iii. Contraindicated with decreased mental status, due to aspiration risk
      c. Intubation if necessary
   2. Preload reduction
      a. Sitting upright
      b. Diuretics
         i. Furosemide is the most commonly used IV diuretic
            a) Emerging evidence points to worsening renal function and worsening

neurohormonal effects from IV furosemide that indicate a need to combine diuretics with other therapies[40-42]
   c. Nitrates
      i. Vasodilator which can lead to both preload reduction and afterload reduction (at high doses)
         a) Can be administered either as a drip or sublingually
      ii. Drips can be easily titrated to effect and blood pressure
      iii. Doses as high as 2 mg IV bolus every 3 minutes have been given safely and effectively[43]
   d. Morphine
      i. Decreases pulmonary congestion by vasodilation
         a) Secondary to morphine's histamine effects
      ii. Anxiolysis by blocking sympathetic stimulation
   e. Niseritide
      i. Niseritide is recombinant b-natriuretic peptide
      ii. Indicated for diuresis in patients in pulmonary edema
      iii. Controversial treatment
         a) Shown in the VMAC trial to be better than IV nitroglycerin in the management of acute decompensated heart failure[44]
         b) Associated with worsening renal function and increased mortality[45]

3. Afterload reduction
   a. Theorized to be more effective in patients with primary diastolic dysfunction[43]
   b. Nitrates
      i. Nitroglycerin
      ii. Nitroprusside is a pure afterload reduction agent
   c. ACE inhibitors and ARBs
      i. Decrease cardiac afterload while increasing perfusion to the kidneys and stimulating diuresis by antagonizing the renin-angiotensin-aldosterone cascade[39]

4. Inotropic agents
   a. Increases heart contractility and forward flow
   b. Reserved for patients who do not respond to above therapy
      i. Increases rates of arrhythmia[46,47]
      ii. May decrease blood pressure
   c. Dobutamine
      i. β-Receptor agonist

d. Amrinone and milrinone
  i. Phosphodiesterase inhibitors
5. Intraaortic balloon pump (IABP)
  a. Placed in proximal aorta
  b. Inflates during diastole (increases blood flow to coronary arteries) and deflates during systole (creates negative pressure and reduces afterload)

III. Cardiomyopathy

A. Dilated cardiomyopathy
  1. Epidemiology
    a. In the United States, viral myocarditis is the most common cause
    b. Worldwide, Chagas disease is the most common cause
  2. Etiology
    a. Idiopathic
    b. Familial and glycogen storage diseases
    c. Infectious inflammatory (viral myocarditis, Chagas)
    d. Noninfectious inflammatory (connective tissue diseases, peripartum cardiomyopathy, sarcoidosis)
    e. Toxic (heavy metals, cocaine, chronic alcohol ingestion, chemotherapeutic agents)
    f. Metabolic (hypothyroidism, chronic hypocalcemia, chronic hypophosphatemia)
    g. Neuromuscular (muscular dystrophies)
  3. Symptoms and signs
    a. Symptoms
      a) Congestive heart failure as above
      b) Peripheral embolization of mural thrombi
        i) Neurologic deficits
        ii) Flank pain
        iii) Pulseless extremities
        iv) Pulmonary embolism
      c) Syncope—secondary to dysrhythmias
    b. Signs
      i. As above (see congestive heart failure)
      ii. Displaced and diffuse point of maximal impulse (PMI)
        a) The PMI is normally located over the fifth intercostal midclavicular line and palpated with no more than 1 finger-pad width
  4. Diagnosis
    a. Chest x-ray
      i. Cardiomegaly
      ii. Increased vascular markings
      iii. Cephalization
      iv. Kerley B lines

b. ECG
  i. Arrhythmias (commonly atrial fibrillation)
  ii. Signs of atrial enlargement
    a) Large P waves (biatrial enlargement)
      i) Double-humped P waves in lead II (left atrial enlargement)
      ii) Peaked P waves in lead II (right atrial enlargement)
  iii. Conduction disease
  iv. Poor R wave progression
  v. Q waves secondary to myocardial fibrosis
c. Echocardiogram
  i. Dilated ventricles with minimal hypertrophy
  ii. Decreased ejection fraction
  iii. Focal wall motion abnormalities
5. Management
  a. Supportive care
  b. Anticoagulation to prevent systemic embolization
  c. Devices
    i. Biventricular pacemaker improve morbidity and mortality[48]
    ii. Automatic implantable cardioverter defibrillator improve mortality by reducing the risk of death from ventricular fibrillation or ventricular tachycardia in patients with CHF[49]

B. Hypertrophic cardiomyopathy
  1. Also known as
    a. Asymmetric septal hypertrophy
    b. Hypertrophic obstructive cardiomyopathy (HOCM)
    c. Idiopathic hypertrophic subaortic stenosis (IHSS)
  2. Epidemiology
    a. Estimated to have a prevalence of 1/500[50]
    b. Mortality 4% per year if untreated
    c. Familial form is inherited in autosomal dominant fashion
    d. Most common cause of sudden death among young athletes[51]
  3. Etiology
    a. Genetic mutation leading to dysfunctional proteins in cardiac sarcomere and disorganized muscle hypertrophy
      i. Most pronounced in the inter-ventricular septal region leading to outflow obstruction
    b. Progressively worsening diastolic dysfunction secondary to hypertrophy

4. Symptoms and signs
   a. Dyspnea on exertion
   b. Chest pain common in adults but not in children
   c. Arrhythmias and syncope
   d. Paroxysmal nocturnal dyspnea, peripheral edema, CHF (present only with advanced disease)
   e. S_4 nearly always present
   f. Double or even triple apical impulse
   g. Harsh midsystolic murmur at lower left sternal border most commonly confused with aortic stenosis
      i. Murmur increases with decreased LV volume—standing, valsalva, vasodilators, amyl nitrate
      ii. Murmur decreases with increased LV volume—squatting, leg raise, hand grip, β-blockers
5. Diagnosis
   a. ECG
      i. LVH present in ~33% of patients' ECGs
      ii. Left atrial hypertrophy in 33% to 50% of patients' ECGs
      iii. "Septal" Q waves in inferior or lateral leads
   b. Chest x-rays may reveal left atrial enlargement
   c. Echocardiography
      i. Septal wall thickness is greater than the free wall
      ii. May show evidence of systolic outflow obstruction
      iii. Systolic anterior motion (SAM) of the mitral valve
         a) Worsens outflow obstruction
6. Management
   a. Medical
      i. β-Blockers decrease chronotropy, leading to increased diastolic filling times and decreased outflow obstruction
      ii. Verapamil is shown to have similar efficacy but has been associated with death in patients with severe outflow obstruction[52]
      iii. Disopyramide, a class Ia antiarrhythmic has been used in patients with symptoms uncontrolled with β-blockade
      iv. Diuresis can worsen symptoms by decreasing preload and left ventricular volume
      v. Avoidance of strenuous activity
   b. Invasive
      i. Automatic implantable cardioverter defibrillator (AICD)—the only treatment that decreases mortality[53]
      ii. Dual chamber pacing
      iii. Catheter-based alcohol septal ablation
      iv. Consider surgical myomectomy in patients with large outflow obstructions

IV. Pericarditis and Constrictive Pericarditis

A. Definitions
   1. Isolated inflammation of the pericardium
      a. May lead to pericardial effusion and tamponade
   2. Constrictive pericarditis occurs when the thickened fibrotic pericardium impedes diastolic filling

B. Etiology
   1. Etiology is primarily idiopathic[54] (26% to 86%)
   2. Infectious
      a. Viral: Coxsackie, echo virus (1% to 10%)
      b. Bacterial (1% to 8%)
      c. Tuberculosis (4%)
      d. Fungal
   3. Malignancy
      a. Metastatic breast or lung
      b. Lymphoma
   4. Drug-induced (procainamide)
   5. Miscellaneous: connective tissue disease or autoimmune diseases (lupus or RA), uremia, postradiation, postinfarction (Dressler syndrome), myxedema

C. Symptoms and signs
   1. Symptoms
      a. Pleuritic chest pain often radiating to the back
      b. Pain relieved by sitting up and leaning forward
      c. Dysphagia with esophageal irritation
      d. Fever, especially with bacterial pericarditis
      e. Recent myocardial infarction (Dressler syndrome)
      f. Dyspnea may be a significant complaint with constrictive pericarditis
   2. Signs
      a. Tachycardia
      b. Pericardial friction rub
         i. May be monophasic (systolic), biphasic (systolic and diastolic), or triphasic (atrial, systolic, diastolic)
         ii. Steam engine-type sound
         iii. May be transient or positional
         iv. Unlike pleural rubs, heard throughout the respiratory cycle
      c. Constrictive pericarditis may have signs similar to that of tamponade and right-sided heart failure (see tamponade below)

D. Diagnosis
1. Blood tests
   a. BUN and creatinine will diagnose uremia as a cause of pericarditis
   b. Serology may indicate connective tissue or autoimmune disorders
   c. Thyroid function tests
   d. Cardiac markers
      i. Troponin can be elevated as a result of pericarditis and be residually elevated in patients with Dressler syndrome
2. ECG—classically 4 stages
   a. Stage I
      i. PR depression especially in II, aVF, V_4 through V_6
      ii. PR elevation in aVR
      iii. Diffuse concave ST segment elevation, most prominent in the precordium
   b. Stage II: flattening of ST wave and decreased amplitude T waves
   c. Stage III: isoelectric ST segment and inverted T waves
   d. Stage IV: normalization
3. Chest x-ray
   a. Usually normal
   b. "Bottle-shaped" heart with large pericardial effusion
4. Echocardiography
   a. American College of Cardiology recommends echocardiography in all patients with pericardial disease
      i. Does not address the question of when (in the ED or as an outpatient)
      ii. Strongly consider emergent echocardiography if history of fever, history of tuberculosis, use of anticoagulation (warfarin), symptoms >1 week, immunosuppression, suspicion of metastatic cancer, positive cardiac markers, or signs of tamponade
5. High-resolution CT and MRI
   a. Pericardial thickening of >4 to 6 mm
   b. Will detect large pericardial effusions

E. Management
1. Viral pericarditis
   a. NSAIDs
2. Bacterial pericarditis
   a. Mortality rate approaches **100%** without treatment
   b. Strongly suspect in the toxic-appearing patient with fever
   c. Antibiotics
   d. **Drainage of purulent effusion**

3. Tuberculosis pericarditis
   a. Tuberculosis treatment (isoniazid, rifampin, ethambutol, pyrazinamide)
   b. Steroids controversial
4. Postinfarction
   a. Avoid NSAIDs
   b. Aspirin
   c. As per standard treatment for ACS
5. Autoimmune pericarditis
   a. Steroids and NSAIDs
6. Adjuvant medical therapies
   a. Colchicine for acute or recurrent attacks
   b. Steroid usage controversial but appears to increase recurrence rates
7. Surgical pericardiectomy
   a. Reserved for refractory cases
   b. Constrictive pericarditis
8. Disposition
   a. Well-appearing patients with pain controlled by NSAIDs may be safely discharged
   b. Admit patients with positive cardiac enzymes for telemetry as perimyocarditis and myocardial infarction may develop malignant arrhythmias
   c. Admit patients suspected bacterial/tubercular pericarditis or immunocompromise
   d. Admit patients with large effusions or tamponade
      i. Patients on anticoagulation
      ii. Patients with history of neoplasm

V. Pericardial Effusion and Pericardial Tamponade

A. Definition
1. Pericardial effusion: accumulation of fluid between the visceral and parietal pericardium
   a. Pericardial space normally contains 15 to 30 mL of fluid
2. Pericardial tamponade: collection of fluid or air that creates external cardiac pressure resulting in decreased ventricular filling and hemodynamic compromise

B. Etiology—as above with pericarditis

C. Pathophysiology
1. Rapid pericardial fluid accumulation leads to elevated intrapericardial pressure and myocardial compression
   a. The rate of accumulation rather than volume is responsible for hemodynamic instability
   b. Gradual accumulation of fluid is well tolerated as some dialysis patients chronically have up to one liter of pericardial effusion

2. Lower-right-sided pressures result in evidence of compressive effects on the right heart first

D. Symptoms and signs (in addition to those seen with pericarditis)
1. Beck triad
   a. Hypotension
   b. Jugular venous distension
   c. Diminished heart sounds
2. Pulsus paradoxus
   a. Exaggerated decrease in systolic blood pressure (>10 mm Hg) with inspiration
   b. Also occurs with asthma, constrictive pericarditis, pulmonary embolism, and COPD
3. Kussmaul sign
   a. Paradoxical jugular venous distension with inspiration

E. Diagnosis
1. ECG
   a. Can show signs of pericarditis (see Diagnosis of Pericarditis and Constrictive Pericarditis above)
   b. May show signs of pericardial fluid accumulation
      i. Low voltage QRS
      ii. Electrical alternans
         a) Beat-to-beat variation in the axis of the QRS complexes
         b) Beat-to-beat variation of the axis of both the P and the QRS complexes are very specific for tamponade[55]
2. Chest x-ray
   a. Cardiomegaly/bottle shaped heart seen only after 200 mL of fluid accumulation
   b. Can show pneumomediastinum as a cause of tamponade
3. Echocardiogram
   a. Diagnostic study for detecting pericardial effusion
   b. Swinging of the heart within a pericardial effusion
   c. Can show evidence of tamponade
      i. Pericardial effusion
      ii. Collapse of the right atrium in late diastole
      iii. Collapse of the right ventricle in early diastole
      iv. Left atrial collapse is highly sensitive for tamponade

F. Management
1. Medical treatment of tamponade
   a. IV Fluid resuscitation
      i. Indicated in patients with signs of hypovolemia

      ii. May increase cardiac size and pericardial pressure and be harmful in euvolemic or hypervolemic patients[55]
   b. Inotropes
      i. Controversial
      ii. Endogenous inotropic stimulation already maximal
      iii. Supportive role until definitive treatment rendered
   c. Positive pressure ventilation
      i. Will further decrease venous return and worsen tamponade and should be avoided if possible
   d. Uremic tamponade
      i. Will often respond to emergent dialysis
2. Pericardiocentesis (see procedures section)
   a. Indicated for hemodynamic compromise if patient unstable to await pericardial window in operating room
   b. If possible, perform with ultrasound guidance
   c. Inadequate as sole treatment in patients with hemorrhagic tamponade
3. Surgical treatment
   a. Pericardial window is the definitive procedure
   b. Posttraumatic
      i. Thoracotomy may be indicated
         a) Pericardiocentesis is often unsuccessful in patients with hemorrhagic tamponade

VI. Myocarditis

A. Definition
1. Myocardial injury resulting from inflammation of the myocardium
   a. Often accompanied by pericarditis
   b. The most common long-term sequelae is dilated cardiomyopathy

B. Epidemiology
1. Major cause of sudden unexpected death in adults <40 years[56]
2. Worldwide, Chagas is the most common cause

C. Etiology
1. Most often idiopathic
2. Infectious
   a. Bacterial
      i. Rare in the immunocompetent patient
      ii. Acute rheumatic fever
   b. Viral (Coxsackie, Enterovirus, Adenovirus, HIV)
   c. Others (Fungal, spirochetal, rickettsial, parasitic)

3. Immunologic and connective tissue disorders
   a. Chagas, sarcoid, scleroderma, lupus
4. Toxic
   a. Chemotherapy, cocaine, heavy metals, radiation
5. Peripartum (1 month prior to delivery to 5 months postpartum)

D. Symptoms and signs
   1. Large range in clinical presentation
      a. May mimic MI and pericarditis
      b. Viral prodrome (fever, myalgias, weakness)
      c. Symptoms of acute congestive heart failure
   2. Tachycardia and arrhythmias
   3. Syncope or sudden death
   4. Signs of decreased cardiac output and shock

E. Diagnosis
   1. ECG
      a. May present with global or segmental ST elevation that makes this entity extremely difficult to differentiate from acute coronary syndrome
      b. Nonspecific ST and T wave changes
      c. Premature ventricular contractions and arrhythmias
      d. Conduction delays
   2. Chest x-ray
      a. Usually normal
      b. May present with CHF
      c. Dilated cardiomyopathy may develop late in course of disease
   3. Echocardiography
      a. Classically shows global hypokinesis but segmental motion abnormalities common
      b. Pericardial fluid can be seen with concomitant pericarditis
      c. Mural thrombus visualized in >10%
   4. Cardiac enzymes
      a. Creatinine kinase and troponin are often elevated
   5. Serology
      a. Can indicate autoimmune disease as a potential etiology
   6. Cardiac catherization may be necessary to rule out acute coronary syndrome

F. Management
   1. Medical
      a. Focus on supportive and symptom treatment
      b. Management as per CHF
      c. Treat identifiable causes
      d. Immunoglobulin is a controversial treatment
   2. Surgical
      a. Consider transplantation for severe cases
      b. Syncope, LBBB, and low-ejection fraction are poor prognostic indicators

VII. Valvular Heart Disease (Table 5–2)

A. Epidemiology
   1. Worldwide, rheumatic heart disease is the most common cause
   2. Aortic stenosis is the most common cardiac-valve lesion in the United States[57]
   3. Bicuspid aortic valve is the most common congenital valvulopathy

B. Mitral valve prolapse
   1. Epidemiology
      a. Incidence is between 5% and 15% of the population[58]
      b. Increased incidence of endocarditis and dysrhythmias
      c. More common in females with thin body habitus[58]
   2. Etiology
      a. Primarily idiopathic
      b. May be associated with connective tissue disorders
   3. Symptoms and signs
      a. Most patients are asymptomatic
      b. Atypical chest pain
      c. Palpitations
      d. Mid-to-late systolic click(s) with tensing of loose chordae as the mitral leaflet reaches maximal prolapse
      e. Late systolic murmur
         i. Decreasing LV volume causes earlier prolapse (earlier click, earlier and louder murmur)
            a) Valsalva
            b) Standing
            c) Vasodilators
         ii. Increasing LV volume causes "more appropriate" cordae length (and less and later click, softer or absent murmur)
            a) Squatting
            b) Isometric hand-grip
            c) β-Blockers or calcium channel blockers
   4. Diagnosis
      a. ECG
         i. Normal or nonspecific with ST and T wave changes
         ii. Rarely nonsustained ventricular tachycardia
      b. Chest x-ray
         i. Normal
         ii. Chronic mitral regurgitation may result in left atrial enlargement
      c. Echocardiography

TABLE 5–2. Valvular Disease

VALVE	SYMPTOMS	MURMUR	TREATMENT
MS	Dyspnea PND Orthopnea **Hemoptysis (especially in pregnancy)** Systemic embolization Palpitations	**Diastolic** First heart sound loud Low-pitched, rumbling, crescendo at the apex Best heard in left decubitus position Often missed	Rate control exertion Valve replacement surgery
MR	*Chronic* Relatively asymptomatic until development of CHF *Acute* Acute dyspnea Acute pulmonary edema Cardiogenic shock	**Systolic** Holosystolic murmur heard at the lower left sternal border or apex and radiates to left axilla Harsh murmur may be very loud S_4 especially if ventricular hypertrophy S_3 if CHF	*Chronic* Anticoagulation Symptomatic CHF treatment (lasix, digoxin) After-load reduction Valve replacement surgery *Acute* Rapid, oxygen, diuretics, and after-load reduction (nitroprusside) Intraaortic balloon pump if cardiogenic shock Emergent surgery may be life-saving
AS	Angina Syncope Left-sided CHF symptoms	**Systolic** Coarse crescendo–decrescendo at upper right sternal border Radiates to the carotids and sometimes to the apex May have early systolic opening snap or click	Valve replacement Endocarditis prophylaxis Caution: Blood pressure may drop with exercise or use of vasodilators Diuretics may reduce cardiac output
AR	*Chronic* Usually asymptomatic Palpitations Chest wall pain CHF after years of progression *Acute* Acute dyspnea and left ventricular failure Tachypnea, chest pain	**Diastolic** *Chronic* High-pitched, blowing, decrescendo murmur along the right sternal border Late diastolic rumble (Austin-Flint) *Acute* Usually soft and short duration	*Chronic* CHF treatment with diuretics and after-load reduction Valve replacement indicated before CHF occurs *Acute* Afterload reduction most beneficial (nitroprusside) Intraaortic balloon pump may **not** be helpful Valve replacement surgery
TS	Right-sided heart failure Peripheral edema and ascites	**Diastolic** Rumbling Left lower sternal border Radiates to xyphoid	Diuretics Valve replacement surgery
TR	Peripheral edema and ascites	**Systolic** High-pitched pan-systolic	Diuretics Valve replacement surgery
PS	Asymptomatic until right-sided congestive failure	**Systolic** Murmur at upper left sternal border radiates to left clavicle Wide split S_2	Symptomatic CHF treatment
PR	Asymptomatic until right ventricular failure Symptoms often caused by presence of pulmonary hypertension (dyspnea, fatigue, syncope)	**Diastolic** Brief crescendo then decrescendo murmur loudest at second left intercostal space May have brief midsystolic ejection murmur caused by increased flow through pulmonary valve	Treatment of right-sided failure with diuretics Valve replacement rarely indicated

5. Management
    a. β-Blockers
        i. May reduce dysrhythmias
        ii. May reduce incidence of atypical chest pain
        iii. Endocarditis prophylaxis no longer indicated even with regurgitation

C. Mitral regurgitation
    1. Acute mitral regurgitation
        a. Etiology
            i. Rupture of chordae or papillary muscle caused by infarction of the posterior descending artery
            ii. Endocarditis
            iii. Inflammatory states
            iv. Myxomatous degeneration
            v. Trauma
        b. Pathophysiology
            i. Acute regurgitation into small, nondistensible atrium
            ii. Ventricular ejection split through the mitral valve and the aortic valve, increasing stroke volume but decreased forward stroke volume
        c. Symptoms and signs
            i. Symptoms
                a) Acute and sudden dyspnea
                b) Dizziness
                c) Chest pain
            ii. Signs
                a) Murmur
                    i) Holosystolic murmur loudest at the apex, radiating to the axilla
                    ii) With acute rupture, the murmur may be heard best in the right upper sternal border
                b) Tachycardia
                c) Tachypnea
                d) Jugular venous distention
                e) Apical thrill
        d. Diagnosis
            i. Echocardiography
            ii. ECG
                a) Rule out myocardial ischemia
            iii. Chest x-ray
                a) May reveal pulmonary edema
        e. Management
            i. Afterload reduction to increase forward flow through the aortic valve
            ii. Emergent surgical valve repair
            iii. Intraaortic balloon pump for cardiogenic shock

D. Aortic stenosis
    1. Epidemiology
        a. A disease of the elderly primarily presenting in the sixth, seventh, and eighth decades of life[59]
        b. Rheumatic heart disease is the most common cause worldwide
        c. Most common cardiac-valve lesion in the United States[57]
        d. Mortality increases dramatically once patient symptomatic
            i. 50% with angina die within 5 years, without a valve replacement
            ii. 50% with syncope die within 3 years, without a valve replacement
            iii. 50% with dyspnea die within 2 years, without a valve replacement
        e. 10-year survival of patients with aortic valve replacement approaches that of the general population[6,60]
    2. Etiology
        a. Primarily idiopathic
        b. Congenital bicuspid aortic valves more likely to stenose and presents at an earlier age
    3. Pathophysiology
        a. Normal aortic valve 2 to 3 cm^2 valve area
            i. Symptomatic when <0.8 cm^2 **or** when pressure across valve >50 mm Hg
        b. As stenosis worsens, the left ventricle hypertrophies to overcome the outflow obstruction
        c. Ventricular hypertrophy leads to
            i. Decreased coronary blood flow reserve
            ii. Diastolic dysfunction
        d. Worsening stenosis and cardiac output leads to
            i. **Exercise intolerance and syncope**
            ii. **Extreme sensitivity to vasodilators**
        e. Diastolic dysfunction leads to
            i. Sensitivity to atrial fibrillation
            ii. Risk for flash pulmonary edema
            iii. Signs and symptoms of left-sided congestive heart failure
            iv. **Sensitivity to hypovolemia and diuretics**
    4. Symptoms and signs
        a. Angina
        b. **Exertional syncope**
        c. Decreased exercise tolerance
        d. Congestive heart failure
        e. Murmur
            i. Coarse systolic murmur
            ii. Crescendo—decrescendo at upper right sternal border
            iii. Radiates to the carotids and sometimes to the apex

iv. May have early systolic opening snap or click

v. Often mistaken for mitral valve prolapse (unlike MVP, murmur of AS decreases with valsalva)

f. Pulse pressure narrows (difference between systolic and diastolic)

g. Parvus et tardus

  i. Slow carotid upstroke and diminished amplitude

h. Apical cardiac impulse enlarged, sustained, and laterally displaced (caused by left ventricular hypertrophy)

i. S_4 nearly always present

j. Anemia and gastrointestinal bleeding from gastrointestinal angiodysplasia (Hyde syndrome)

5. Diagnosis

a. Echocardiography

b. Chest x-ray

  i. Can show signs of left ventricular enlargement

  ii. Can show signs of pulmonary congestion

c. ECG

  i. May show left ventricular hypertrophy often with "strain pattern"

6. Management

a. Vasodilators and diuretics can cause a precipitous drop in blood pressure caused by fixed cardiac output and diastolic dysfunction

b. Management of CHF with aortic stenosis very difficult

c. Valve replacement

  i. Only treatment shown to have a mortality benefit

E. Aortic regurgitation

1. Chronic aortic regurgitation

a. Etiology

  i. Destruction of aortic leaflets

    a) Rheumatic heart disease

    b) Myxomatous degeneration

    c) Endocarditis

    d) Rheumatic heart disease

  ii. Dilated aortic root

    a) Marfan syndrome

    b) Syphilis

    c) Ankylosing spondylitis

b. Pathophysiology

  i. Regurgitation leads to

    a) Increased left ventricular end diastolic volume

    b) Increase in stroke volume

    c) Increased systolic pressure, which leads to increase afterload

    d) Decreased diastolic pressure

  ii. Pressure transmitted to left atrium and pulmonary vasculature

  iii. Because regurgitant flow occurs during diastole and bradycardia prolongs diastole, patients do not tolerate bradycardia

c. Symptoms and signs

  i. Usually asymptomatic

  ii. Palpitations (sense of "pounding" heart)

  iii. Chest wall pain

  iv. CHF only after years of progression

  v. Vital signs

    a) Widened pulse pressure

    b) Elevated systolic blood pressure

  vi. Displaced point of maximal impulse (PMI)

  vii. "Bounding" pulses

  viii. Murmur

    a) Right sternal border

    b) Diastolic

    c) High-pitched

    d) Decrescendo

    e) Late diastolic rumble (Austin-Flint)

  ix. Duroziez sign

    a) To-and-fro murmur heard over the femoral artery

  x. Corrigan pulse

    a) Bounding full carotid pulse with a rapid downstroke

  xi. Quincke pulse

    a) Systolic plethora and diastolic blanching in the nail bed while gentle pressure is applied

  xii. Musset sign

    a) Head bobbing with the pulse

  xiii. Hill sign

    a) Systolic blood pressure in the leg >30 mm Hg than in the arms

d. Diagnosis

  i. Chest x-ray

    a) Left ventricular enlargement

  ii. ECG

    a) LVH with strain

  iii. Echocardiogram

c. Management

  i. Afterload reduction to increase forward flow

  ii. Treat symptoms of pulmonary congestion

  iii. Valve replacement

2. Acute aortic regurgitation

a. Etiology

  i. Valve destruction from endocarditis, rheumatic fever

  ii. Valve or perivalvular leak caused by trauma or **aortic dissection**

b. Pathophysiology
    i. Valve incompetence leads to regurgitant flow back into the left ventricle and decreased systemic flow
    ii. Ventricular diastolic pressures increase secondary to the increased volume
    iii. Pulmonary congestion develops
    iv. Cardiogenic shock develops if the left ventricular flow cannot overcome the regurgitant flow
c. Symptoms and signs
    i. Sudden onset of dyspnea (discriminates acute from chronic)
    ii. Chest pain
    iii. Tachypnea and tachycardia
    iv. Diastolic pressures may rise, pulse pressures normal
    v. Apical impulse normal
    vi. Cardiac auscultation
        a) Murmur is soft and of short duration caused by early equalization of the pressures in left ventricle and aorta
        b) Soft first heart sound
d. Diagnosis
    i. Chest x-ray
        a) normal cardiac size
        b) Pulmonary congestion
        c) Widened mediastinum with aortic dissection
    ii. ECG
        a) Normal or nonspecific changes
    iii. Echocardiogram
e. Management
    i. Afterload reduction most beneficial (nitroprusside)
    ii. Intraaortic balloon pump may not be helpful because it will increase regurgitant flow as aortic balloon inflates during diastole
    iii. A surgical emergency

VIII. Conduction Disease

A. Normal conduction system
    1. Normal sinus rhythm
        a. Originates in the sinoatrial node
        b. Travels along the intranodal fibers
        c. Enters the atrioventricular node
        d. Travels through the bundle of His
        e. Bundle of His splits into the
            i. Right bundle
            ii. Left bundle
                a) Left anterior fascicle
                b) Left posterior fascicle

B. Bundle branch and fascicular blocks
    1. Right bundle branch blocks (RBBB)
        a. ECG criteria
            i. Widened QRS (>0.12 seconds, but usually <0.16 seconds) because of delayed depolarization of the right ventricle
            ii. R wave larger than S wave in V_1
            iii. Abnormal QRS complexes in right precordial leads (V_1 and V_2)
                a) rSR' or rabbit ear complex
                b) qR
                c) Large-notched R wave
            iv. Deep and wide S wave in left precordial leads (V_5-V_6)
        b. ST and T wave changes
            i. The T wave, in the right precordial leads (V_1, V_2) are discordant with the terminal deflection of the QRS leading to inverted T waves
            ii. Concordant ST and T waves (in the same direction as the terminal deflection of the QRS) can indicate myocardial ischemia or can be a sign for the Brugada syndrome
        c. Incomplete right bundle branch block
            i. Right bundle branch block morphology with a normal QRS width
            ii. Common finding in children and young adults
    2. Left bundle branch blocks (LBBB)
        a. ECG criteria
            i. Wide QRS (>0.12 seconds, but usually <0.16 seconds)
            ii. Abnormal QRS morphology
                a) RR' or large wide R wave in left leads (I, V_5, and V_6)
                b) Abnormal repolarization in leads with the RR' complex (I, V_5, and V_6)
            iii. QS or RS pattern in the right precordial leads (V_1, V_2)
    3. Left anterior fascicular block (LAF)
        a. Is the more common of the two hemiblocks (left coronary artery blood supply)
        b. Leads to loss of synchronous depolarization of the left ventricle, starting from the posterior portion of the left ventricle, moving anterior
        c. ECG criteria
            i. Left axis deviation
            ii. QRS widening but narrower than 120 milliseconds
            iii. QR pattern in the left-facing limb leads (I, aVL)
            iv. RS pattern in the inferior facing limp leads (II, III, aVF)
    4. Left posterior fascicular block (LPF)
        a. Is the less common of the hemiblocks (dual coronary artery blood supply)

b. Leads to loss of synchronous depolarization of the left ventricle, starting from the anterolateral portion of the left ventricle and moving posterior

c. ECG criteria (changes are the inverse of the LAF)

   i. Right axis deviation

   ii. QRS widening but narrower than 120 milliseconds

   iii. RS pattern in the left-facing limb leads (I, aVL)

   iv. QR pattern in the inferior-facing limb leads (II, III, aVF)

5. Bifascicular block

a. The most common combination is the left anterior fascicular block with a right bundle branch block (LAF + RBBB)

b. Is a marker of advanced cardiac disease

C. Heart blocks

1. Anatomy

a. Blocks can be in the AV node, or the SA node

b. SA node derives its blood supply from the sinus node artery arising from the right coronary (65%) circumflex (25%) and both (10%)

c. AV node derives its blood supply from the AV nodal artery arising from the posterior descending artery (right coronary artery 90%)

2. Sinus nodal block and sick sinus syndrome (also sinus pause, sinus arrest, tachy-brady syndrome)

a. Definition: failure of impulse formation or conduction that results in complete lack of sinus activity

   i. Absence of entire P and QRS, and T cycles

   ii. Ventricular activity is dependent on an escape rhythm

b. Patients are predisposed to developing atrial tachyarrhythmias

c. Management: pacemaker plus a medication to suppress tachydysrhythmias

3. Atrioventricular block (AV node block)

a. First-degree AV block

   i. Definition: conduction **delay** through the atrioventricular node

     a) Not progressive except in the setting of Lyme disease

   ii. ECG criteria

     a) P waves and QRS normal

     b) PR prolonged (>0.12 second)

b. Second-degree heart block

   i. Definition: intermittent loss of conduction between the atria and the ventricle

     a) Conduction failure can occur at regular or variable atrial:ventricular ratio

   ii. Types: Mobitz I (Wenckebach) and Mobitz II

    a) Mobitz I

     i) Definition: ECG criteria

      (a) PR interval increases with each beat until a dropped beat

      (b) PR interval returns to normal after the dropped beat

      (c) Appears as groups of beats with spaces between (dropped beat)—"grouped" beating

      (d) Although PR intervals increase, they increase by less each time, leading to progressively shortened RR intervals

     ii) Management: generally does not require emergency treatment

    b) Mobitz II

     i) Definition: ECG criteria

      (a) P waves normal but QRS usually wide

      (b) PR same beat to beat with an occasional abrupt dropped beat

      (c) Appears as groups of beats with spaces between (dropped beat)—"grouped" beating

      (d) Considered to be a high degree if there are 2 or more blocked P waves

     ii) Management: immediate transcutaneous pacer pad placement—**can progress to complete heart block**

c. Third-degree AV block

   i. Definition: complete lack of conduction through the AV node

     a) Ventricular rate depends on the junctional escape rhythm

     b) Atria and ventricles beat independently

   ii. ECG criteria

     a) No association of P waves to QRS complexes

     b) P waves fire at a regular rate

     c) QRS rate bradycardic, but regular

     d) QRS firing occurs as a result of a junctional escape

     e) P waves "march through" while the QRS occur at a slower rate—may be mistaken for variable PR interval or PR prolonging

f) If complete heart block occurs with atrial fibrillation, the ECG will show a baseline of atrial fibrillation with a regular QRS rate

iii. Management: temporary placement of transcutaneous pacer pads until placement of permanent pacemaker

IX. Bradydysrhythmias

A. Sinus bradycardia
   1. Anatomy: rhythm originates in the sinus node at a rate of <60 beats per minute
   2. Etiology
      a. High vagal tone
         i. Well-trained athletes
         ii. Pain
         iii. Intraperitoneal bleeding
         iv. Inferior wall myocardial infarction
      b. Medications: especially β-blockers and calcium channel blockers
      c. Medical conditions with decreased sympathetic tone
         i. Hypothyroidism
   3. Symptoms and signs
      a. Generally asymptomatic
      b. Signs of hypoperfusion
         i. Dizziness and lightheadedness
         ii. Syncope
         iii. Confusion
   4. Management
      a. Direct towards the degree of patient symptoms
      b. Atropine
      c. Transcutaneous pacing
      d. Vasopressors

B. Nodal blocks (see Heart Blocks above)
   1. Mechanism: slow atrial rate, high ratio of blocked complexes, or both
   2. Management
      a. Atropine
         i. If heart block is secondary to AV nodal dysfunction, atropine is unlikely to improve the ventricular response and may potentiate ventricular dysrhythmia[61]
         ii. Patients with complete heart block from high vagal tone from an inferior wall infarction may improve with atropine[62]
      b. Patients with Mobitz II and complete heart block should be prepared for immediate transcutaneous pacing

C. Escape rhythms
   1. Etiology: loss of ventricular stimulation caused by sinus nodal disease or conduction disease resulting in activity of backup pacemakers within the heart
      a. The rate of the escape rhythm decreases and the width of the QRS increases as the pacemaker is located more distally
   2. Types
      a. AV junctional escape rhythm
         i. Pacemaker is located in the AV node
         ii. QRS is narrow
         iii. Rate is usually 40 to 55 beats per minute
         iv. Patients are usually asymptomatic
      b. Idioventricular escape rhythm
         i. Pacemaker is located in the His-Purkinje system
         ii. QRS is wide
         iii. Rate is 20 to 40 beats per minute
         iv. Patients are usually symptomatic
         v. Patients should be prepared for immediate pacing
            a) Avoid medications that suppress ventricular rhythms (lidocaine, amiodarone)

D. Atrial tachycardia with slow ventricular response
   1. Etiology: high degree of AV node suppression in the face of an atrial tachycardia
   2. Types
      a. Atrial fibrillation
      b. Atrial flutter
      c. Atrial tachycardia
      d. Multifocal atrial tachycardia
   3. Most commonly an iatrogenic bradycardia from too much AV nodal suppression with medication (digoxin)

E. Premature atrial contractions (PAC)
   1. Etiology: impulse originating in the atria (outside the SA node) resulting in ectopic atrial contractions that depolarize and resets the SA node
      a. Leads to a noncompensatory pause
   2. ECG findings
      a. P wave morphology will change, while the QRS morphology unchanged
      b. PR interval may be shorter than sinus rhythm
      c. Noncompensatory pause
      d. PAC may be blocked—AV node refractory and impulse not conducted to the ventricles (P wave not followed by QRS)

F. Premature ventricular contractions (PVC)
   1. Definition: impulse originating in the cardiac myocytes of the ventricle

2. Etiology: idiopathic, or can be associated with "irritable" myocardium in the setting of ischemia or hyperadrenergic states
   a. Increased frequency of may indicate impending ventricular dysrhythmias
   b. Not pathologic in isolation
3. ECG findings
   a. QRS morphology is wide and "bizarre"
   b. No association to atrial activity
   c. Compensatory pause

X. Tachycardic Rhythms (Table 5–3 and Table 5–4)

A. Narrow complex tachycardias
   1. Atrial flutter
      a. Definition: rapid and regular atrial rhythm at a rate of 280 to 340 per minute
         i. Ventricular response is determined by AV node conduction
            a) Usually 2 flutter waves to 1 QRS complex
            b) Rhythm at rate of ~140 to 160 per minute most likely atrial flutter with 2:1 conduction
            c) Block may be variable (2:1, 3:1, 4;1) leading to irregular QRS
      b. ECG
         i. Baseline reveals flutter waves
         ii. Rhythm is regular if the AV-block is fixed
         iii. QRS is narrow unless a fixed or rate related bundle branch block exists
      c. Management
         i. Unstable patients
            a) Immediate synchronized cardioversion
         ii. Stable patients
            a) Rate control with AV nodal blocking agents, calcium channel blockers, β-blockers
               b) Amiodarone
               c) Digoxin
         iii. Cardioversion is less likely to be successful in patients who are chronically in atrial flutter
         iv. The longer that a patient has been in atrial flutter, the higher the risk of post-cardioversion thromboembolism
   2. Atrial fibrillation
      a. Definition: disorganized electrical activity originating from the atrium that results in a lack of organized atrial contraction and irregular conduction to the ventricles
      b. Etiology: often heart disease leading to atrial enlargement
      c. ECG
         i. P waves absent
         ii. Baseline with a wavy appearance
         iii. QRS complexes are irregularly irregular
      d. Management
         i. Unstable patients
            a) Immediate synchronized cardioversion
               i) Cardioversion is less likely to be successful in patients who are chronically in atrial fibrillation
               ii) The longer that a patient has been in atrial fibrillation, the higher the risk of post-cardioversion thromboembolism
         ii. Stable patients
            a) Rate control with AV nodal blocking agents
               i) Calcium channel blockers—diltiazem, verapamil
               ii) Cardioselective β-blockers—metoprolol, atenolol
               iii) Digoxin
               iv) Amiodarone

TABLE 5–3.   Tachycardic Rhythms

TACHYCARDIAS	NARROW QRS	WIDE QRS
Regular	Sinus tachycardia SVT Atrial flutter	Ventricular tachycardia Sinus tachycardia with BBB WPW SVT with BBB A flutter with BBB
Irregular	Atrial fibrillation (A Fib) MAT A flutter with variable block	A Fib with BBB MAT with BBB A flutter with variable block and aberrancy

TABLE 5–4. Classification of Antidysrhythmic Agents

CLASS	EXAMPLES	EFFECT ON PR	EFFECT ON QRS	EFFECT ON QT
Sodium channel blockers				
Ia	Diisopyramide	+/–	↑	↑
	Procainamide			
	Quinidine			
Ib	Lidocaine			
	Phenytoin	+/–	+/–	+/–
	Mexiletine			
	Tocainide			
Ic	Encainide			
	Flecainide	↑	↑	↑↑
	Propafenone			
	Moricizine			
β-Blockers				
II	Propranolol			
	Atenolol	↑	+/–	+/–
	Esmolol			
	Metoprolol			
	Timolol			
Potassium channel blockers				
III	Amiodarone			
	Bretylium	↑	+/–	↑
	Sotalol			
Calcium channel blockers				
IV	Verapamil			
	Diltiazem	↑	+/–	+/–
	Nifedipine			
	Nicardipine			

b) Anticoagulation to protect against embolic stroke
   i) Aspirin
   ii) Low-molecular-weight or unfractionated heparin
3. Multifocal atrial tachycardia (MAT)
   a. Etiology: usually secondary to chronic lung disease (COPD), with hypoxia and pulmonary hypertension
   b. Diagnosis: ECG
      i. At least 3 different P wave morphologies, rate 100 to 180
      ii. Irregular because the rhythm originates at multiple different atrial sites
      iii. Commonly mistaken for atrial fibrillation
      iv. Variable PR, PP intervals because of varying distance from multiple ectopic atrial sites to AV node
   c. Management
      i. Oxygen and treatment of underlying lung disease
      ii. Rate control: calcium channel blocker (diltiazem, verapamil)

4. Supraventricular tachycardia (SVT)
   a. Definition
      i. A strict interpretation refers to a tachycardia whose impulse originates above the ventricles such as sinus tachycardia
      ii. In common speech this term is understood to refer to **paroxysmal, reentry or preexcitation** tachycardias
   b. Reentry SVT
      i. Etiology
         a) AV nodal reentry (AVNRT), atrioventricular reentry, or atrial reentry
         b) Reentry circuits require the presence of at least 2 different conduction pathways with differential refractory times
         c) Abrupt onset and termination of tachycardia distinguishes it from sinus tachycardia, which has gradual changes in rate
         d) Precipitated by a premature atrial or ventricular contraction or hyperadrenergic state

ii. ECG
a) Regular, fast rhythm
b) P waves are absent
c) QRS-most commonly narrow
iii. Management
a) Unstable patients
i) Immediate synchronized cardioversion
b) Stable patients
i) Vagal maneuvers
ii) Adenosine
(a) Used both therapeutically and diagnostically
(b) Given as rapid bolus
(c) Relatively contraindicated in patients with severe asthma
(d) Use with extreme caution in patients with heart transplant because of the possibility of extremely prolonged drug effect
iii) AV nodal blocking agents (β-blockers, calcium channel blockers)
iv) Procainamide, flecainide, propafenone, ibutilide
c. Preexcitation syndromes
i. Definition
a) Syndromes in which atrial impulse reaches the ventricle through a bypass tract
i) Bypass tracts refer to any circuit that circumvents the normal route of electrical conduction (atria → AV node → His-Purkinje bundle system)
ii. WPW (Wolff-Parkinson-White) syndrome
a) Epidemiology
i) Prevalence between 0.1% and 0.3% of the population
ii) Men > women
iii) May have a genetic component
a) 10% of patients with Ebstein anomaly have WPW
b) Etiology
i) Accessory pathway (Kent bundle) connects atria directly to ventricle resulting in simultaneous conduction through AV node and the bypass tract
(a) Develop SVT by rapid reentrant circuit through the accessory pathway

(b) Accessory pathway may conduct in an orthodromic or antidromic direction
c) Orthodromic SVT
i) Definition: transmission through the AV node is in the same direction as normal conduction (SA node → atrium → AV node → His-Purkinje system → ventricle)
ii) ECG: QRS complexes are **narrow**
iii) Management
(a) Unstable patients: immediate synchronized cardioversion
(b) Stable patients: vagal maneuvers or adenosine
d) Antidromic SVT
i) Definition: transmission through the AV node in the opposite direction (SA node → Kent fibers (bypass tract) → ventricle → AV node → atrium)
ii) ECG: while conduction through reentrant loop
(a) QRS complexes are **wide** and can be indistinguishable from ventricular tachycardia
e) Diagnosis
i) ECG while conduction through AV node (or baseline, nontachycardic ECG)
(a) Short PR interval (<0.12 seconds)
(b) Results from bypassing the AV node (retards depolarization) via Kent bundle
(c) Slightly widened QRS—delta wave
(d) Although AV node slows conduction, the His-Purkinje system depolarizes more rapidly than the myocardium
(e) Direct depolarization of the slower myocardium via Kent bundle causes initial slurring of the QRS (delta wave)
(f) May have ST and T wave repolarization abnormalities
f) Management
i) Use procainamide, propafenone, ibutilide, or flecainide
ii) AV nodal blockers are contraindicated because it will allow unimpeded transmission through the bypass tract leading to worsening

tachycardia and cardiovascular collapse

    iii) Calcium channel blocker is **absolutely** contraindicated

    iv) Adenosine is relatively contraindicated

B. Wide complex tachycardia
  1. Differential diagnosis
    a. Ventricular tachycardias
      i. Monomorphic ventricular tachycardia
      ii. Polymorphic ventricular tachycardia—torsade de pointes
      iii. Bidirectional ventricular tachycardia (digoxin toxicity)
    b. Supraventricular tachycardia with aberrancy (conduction abnormality)
      i. Bundle branch blocks
    c. SVT with pre-excitation syndrome
      i. Antidromic WPW
    d. Drug toxicity
    e. Electrolyte abnormality
    f. Paced rhythm
  2. Monomorphic ventricular tachycardia
    a. Definition
      i. Tachycardia originating from a single ventricular focus
      ii. QRS is widened because ventricular depolarization does not spread through the rapid His-Purkinje system
    b. Etiology
      i. Coronary disease (acute MI, scar tissue from previous MI)
      ii. Electrolyte abnormalities
      iii. Medications
    c. Diagnosis
      i. ECG
        a) P waves are absent unless there is AV dissociation
        b) Regular rate usually >140
        c) Concordance (Precordial QRS complexes in the same direction)
        d) QRS very wide (>0.16 seconds)
      ii. ECG characteristics favoring ventricular tachycardia, versus **SVT with aberrancy**
        a) Fusion beats (QRS complexes which appears to have a combination a ventricular focus and a normal QRS complex)
        b) Capture beats—occasional sinus impulse "capturing" a narrow ventricular complex implies that a preexisting bundle branch block does not exist and that the remaining wide

QRS complexes are ventricular in origin
        c) AV dissociation
        d) History
          i) More likely to be VT if history of cardiac disease
          ii) More likely to be VT if >50 years
          iii) More likely to be SVT with aberrancy if history of a bundle branch block, and QRS complexes has the same appearance as prior ECGs
    d. Management
      i. If unsure whether VT or SVT with aberrancy, treat as though VT
      ii. Unstable
        a) With pulse: synchronized shock (cardioversion)
        b) No pulse: unsynchronized shock (defibrillation)
      iii. Stable
        a) Correct any underlying causes
        b) Amiodarone
        c) Lidocaine
        d) Procainamide
  3. Polymorphic ventricular tachycardia (torsade de pointes)
    a. Etiology
      i. Prolonged QT
        a) Congenital QT prolongation
          1) Jervell-Lange-Nielson (autosomal recessive with deafness)
          ii) Romano-Ward
        b) QT prolonging medications
          i) Class IA (procainamide, quinidine)
          ii) Class III (amiodarone, sotalol)
          iii) Tricyclics, antifungals, some quinolones
        c) Hypomagnesemia
        d) Hypocalcemia
        e) Hypokalemia
    b. ECG
      i. Wide complex rhythm at rate of 180 to 240 minutes with undulating QRS amplitude creating "sine-wave" appearance
      ii. Baseline ECG can show QT prolongation
      iii. Can show other signs of electrolyte abnormalities
    c. Management
      i. Unstable patients require defibrillation (if no pulse) or cardioversion (if patient has a pulse)
      ii. Magnesium 1 to 4 g IV
      iii. Decrease QT interval by increasing rate

a) Overdrive pacing via transvenous pacing

b) Isoproterenol

iv. Misdiagnosis and treatment as monomorphic VT (amiodarone or procainamide) can precipitate disastrous ventricular fibrillation

4. Ventricular fibrillation
   a. Etiology
      i. Arrythmogenic "irritable," ischemic, or scarred myocardium
         a) Most common cause is ischemic heart disease
         b) Can be caused by sporadic disorders such as arrythmogenic right ventricular dysplasia
   b. ECG
      i. Irregular chaotic pattern
      ii. No discernable P or QRS complex
   c. Management
      i. ACLS protocol
         a) Immediate defibrillation
         b) Vasopressors—epinephrine or vasopressin
         c) Antiarrhythmic drugs—amiodarone or lidocaine

XI. Cardiac Devices

A. Ventricular pacing
   1. Indications for emergent pacing
      a. Bradycardia with hemodynamic instability
      b. Bradycardia with significant escape rhythms unresponsive to medications
      c. Overdrive pacing to break tachydysrhythmias
      d. Should be available for standby in
         i. Stable bradycardias
         ii. Acute MI with sinus node dysfunction
         iii. Mobitz II second-degree or third-degree block (even if hemodynamically stable)
         iv. Cardiac ischemia with new LBBB or RBBB

2. Types: transcutaneous versus transvenous pacing
   a. Transcutaneous pacing
      i. Much easier to initiate
      ii. Readily available
      iii. Difficult to obtain effective pacing
         a) Requires both electrical and mechanical capture
            i) Mechanical capture is achieved when the patient has a palpable pulse matching the set rate
      iv. Limited by body habitus
      v. Painful
   b. Transvenous pacing
      i. Placed through a central line in the internal jugular vein or subclavian vein
         a) Technically difficult to perform
         b) Has the same associated risks of central line placement

3. Permanent pacemakers (Table 5–5)
   a. Principles
      i. Pacemakers consist of a generator and lead(s)
      ii. Leads have the dual purpose of sensing impulses and pacing
      iii. Pacemaker failure can occur in the generator, the lead(s) or in the myocardium
         a) Generator failure can occur as a result of device failure or battery failure
         b) Lead failure can be caused by fracture of leads, dislodgements, or migration
         c) Myocardial dysfunction secondary to electrolyte abnormalities or worsening fibrosis of myocardium
      iv. Can be a combined pacer and defibrillator
      v. Pacemaker failure often requires interrogation of the machine
   b. Indications
      i. Third-degree heart block
      ii. Sick sinus syndrome
      iii. Severe congestive heart failure

TABLE 5–5. Five-Letter Convention for Pacemaker Naming

FIRST LETTER	SECOND LETTER	THIRD LETTER	FOURTH LETTER	FIFTH LETTER
Chamber paced	**Chamber sensed**	**Response to Sensing**	**Programmed Function**	**Antitachydysrhythmia Function**
V Ventricle	**V** Ventricle	**T** Triggered	**P** Programmable rate	**P** Pacing
A Atria	**A** Atria	**I** Inhibits	**M** Multiprogramable (rate, output, etc)	**S** Shock
D Dual (both)	**D** Dual (both)	**D** Dual (both)	**C** Communication telemetry	**D** Dual
O None	**O** None	**O** None	**R** Rate modulating	**O** None
			O None	

c. ECG
  i. Reveals pacer spikes and wide QRS complexes
  ii. With AV sequential pacing you can see two different pacer spikes
  iii. Demand pacemakers may not be required to fire all the time, so it is possible to see the underlying cardiac rhythm
  iv. QRS complexes should have a left bundle pattern
d. ECG evidence of pacemaker failure
  i. Generator problem—rate paced less than preset rate
  ii. Failure to pace—absence of spikes in bradycardic patient
  iii. Failure to sense—pacemaker not inhibited by the presence of intrinsic QRS complex and fires inappropriately
  iv. Failure to capture—electrical activity without mechanical capture (no pulse)
  v. Oversensing—pacemaker not firing because it mistakenly "oversenses" sinus electrical activity and inhibits itself
  vi. Undersensing—pacemaker fires inappropriately because it "undersenses" native electrical activity and does not inhibit[63]
  vii. Battery failure—battery life is a normal parameter reported during an interrogation
    a) some models of pacemakers will "beep" as the battery is in need of replacement
e. Diagnosis: pacemaker failure
  i. ECG monitoring
  ii. Chest x-ray
    a) Assess broken or malpositioned pacemaker leads
    b) Identifies category of device with chest x-ray (single lead, dual lead, or biventricular pacemaker)
    c) Sometimes identifies manufacturer by the shape of the generator
  iii. Laboratory studies
    a) Serum electrolytes (potassium, calcium, magnesium, acidosis)
    b) Venous and arterial blood gas for acidosis or hypoxia
  iv. Pacemaker interrogation requires manufacturer specific interrogator
  v. Pacemaker magnet
    a) Magnet will switch pacemaker from demand to fixed mode

    b) Sensing of the native beats is suppressed and pacemaker fires at preset rate
    c) Application of magnet helps to rule out mechanical or battery malfunction
    d) Can be lifesaving in a patient with "runaway pacemaker" where the pacemaker paces at an inappropriately fast rate
    e) When used over a AICD, discharges will be suppressed
4. Automatic implantable cardioverter defibrillator (AICD)
  a. Principles
    i. Consists of a generator and cardiac lead(s)
    ii. The defibrillator lead sits in the apex of the right ventricle and serves the dual purpose of sensing ventricular electrical activity and producing the defibrillating shock
    iii. The generator will deliver a defibrillator shock when it senses ventricular tachycardia or ventricular fibrillation
    iv. Almost all current versions include pacemaker functions
  b. Indications
    i. Patients at high risk for dysrhythmias
    ii. Cardiomyopathy
    iii. Severe congestive heart failure
    iv. Brugada syndrome
    v. Hypertrophic cardiomyopathy
  c. Defibrillator malfunction
    i. Failure to disrupt the rhythm
      a) Failure of the generator
      b) Failure of sensing dysrhythmia
      c) Malfunction of the lead
    ii. Inappropriate discharges
      a) Error in sensing dysrhythmia
      b) May require inactivation of unit with a pacemaker magnet if patient continues to be shocked
  d. Evaluation of AICD failure
    i. Electrolytes and drug levels
    ii. Constant ECG monitoring
    iii. Chest x-ray
      a) Can identify AICD by the presence of a apical lead with two sets of coils along the wire
      b) Can identify the category of device with chest x-ray (single lead, dual lead, or biventricular pacemaker)
      c) May be able to identify the manufacturer by the shape of the generator
    iv. AICD interrogation

XII. Hypertension

A. Definition: persistent systolic blood pressure of ≥140 mm Hg or diastolic blood pressure of ≥90 mm Hg
   1. Most patients are not symptomatic from hypertension

B. Chronic hypertension
   1. Physiologic changes to compensate for elevated blood pressure
      a. Cerebrovascular circulation
         i. Arterioles in the brain maintain constant cerebral blood flow over a wide range of blood pressures
         ii. Acceptable blood pressure range shifted upwards in chronic hypertension
         iii. Brain is able to tolerate higher pressures
         iv. Chronic changes lead to an inability to dilate sufficiently for decreases in blood pressure

C. Hypertensive "urgency"
   1. Symptoms and signs
      a. Asymptomatic
      b. No evidence of end-organ injury
      c. Diastolic >130 to 140 mm Hg
   2. Management
      a. Blood pressure should be gradually reduced over 24 hours
      b. Early outpatient follow-up

D. Hypertensive emergencies
   1. Definition
      a. Hypertension with acute end-organ system injury
      b. Diastolic usually >130 mm Hg although no set number
   2. Symptoms and signs
      a. Central nervous system
         i. Hypertensive encephalopathy
            a) Hypertension overwhelms cerebral autoregulation, leading to increased blood flow and subsequent edema
            b) Presents with altered mental status/confusion with headache, nausea, and vomiting
            c) Can present with seizures or focal neurologic deficits and confused with other neurologic entities
            d) Diagnosis
               i) Fundoscopy may reveal papilledema, flame hemorrhages, and cotton wool spots
               ii) CT or MRI
            e) Management
               i) lower blood pressure gradually
         ii. Stroke
            a) Controversy exists within the neurologic literature as to the optimum blood pressure goals for ischemic and hemorrhagic stroke
            b) In both entities, blood pressure below the limit of cerebral autoregulation can lead to hypoperfusion of the ischemic area leading to worse outcome
            c) If patient is receiving TPA it is important to get the blood pressure <180/100 mm Hg
      b. Cardiac ischemia and ACS/CHF
         i. Hypertension is usually not the cause of the ischemia, initial treatment should be directed towards the underlying cause
         ii. Diagnosis
            a) ECG, troponin
         iii. Management: nitroglycerin, and reperfusion strategies
      c. Renal system
         i. Renal failure
         ii. Diagnosis: creatinine, urinalysis (protein)
   3. Management
      a. Goal is to reduce mean arterial pressure 20% to 30% in the first hour
      b. Normalize blood pressure over the next 8 to 24 hours
      c. Cerebral hypoperfusion may occur if blood pressure dropped too quickly
      d. Intravenous medications preferable (quickly titratable)
         i. Hydralazine (may cause reflex tachycardia)
         ii. Sodium nitroprusside (prolonged exposure to light results in cyanide)
         iii. Labetalol (β-blocker with minimal α-blockade)
         iv. Esmolol (very-short-acting β-blocker)
         v. Nicardipine
         vi. Nitroglycerin
         vii. Magnesium (in eclampsia)
   4. Hypertension in special circumstances
      a. Hyperadrenergic syndromes
         i. Includes stimulants such as cocaine and methamphetamines as well as pheochromocytoma
         ii. Management
            a) Avoid β-blockers because of the unopposed α effect leading to worsening hypertension
            b) Use caution with cardioversion of tachydysrhythmias since myocardium is irritable

c) Treat with benzodiazepines
d) IV phentolamine, an α-blocker, can be used to control blood pressure in patients with pheochromocytoma or cocaine toxicity

XIII. Aortic Dissection

A. Definition
1. Intimal artery tear leading to separation from the media
   a. Can progress proximally and distally
   b. Aortic dissection is distinct from aortic aneurysms (a balloon-like dilatation of all layers of the artery rather than intima-media separation)

B. Symptoms and signs
1. Pain is the most common presenting symptom (70% to 90% of patients)
   a. Starts abruptly
   b. Excruciating and maximal at the onset
   c. Migrates as the dissecting flap propagates
   d. May be located in back, epigastrium, chest, upper back, midback, lower back, flank, or the legs
2. Other symptoms may occur as aortic branch vessels are occluded by the intimal flap
   a. Focal neurologic deficit (carotid vessels)
   b. Paraplegia (spinal artery)
   c. Cold, pulseless extremity
   d. CHF, chest pain, pulmonary edema (carotid artery)
   e. Abdominal pain (mesenteric arteries, dissecting flap)
   f. Flank pain and hematuria (renal artery)
   g. Syncope
   h. Acute MI
   i. Cardiac tamponade
3. Hypertension and tachycardia
4. Clammy, diaphoretic
5. Unequal pulses (>20 mm Hg) uncommon
6. Aortic insufficiency murmur
7. Tamponade

C. Diagnosis
1. ECG: excludes MI (but MI can occur if dissection extends into the coronary arteries)
2. Chest x-ray
   a. Usually nondiagnostic
   b. Widened mediastinum
   c. Aortic border >5 mm beyond calcific intimal shadow (calcium sign)
   d. Blurred aortic knob
   e. Pleural apical cap
   f. Pleural effusion

3. Transesophageal echocardiography
   a. Sensitivity and specificity approach 100%
   b. Visualizes pericardium and aortic valve
   c. Disadvantage: requires specialized equipment and trained operators who are often not in hospital
4. Aortography
   a. Originally thought to be the "gold standard"
   b. Availability of other modalities has shown sensitivity and specificity 90% to 95%
   c. Delineates all branch vessels, aortic valve
   d. Disadvantages: invasive, specialized personnel, contrast media, cannot be performed in the ED
5. CT scan
   a. Specificity and sensitivity 95% to 98%
   b. Identifies other potential causes for chest pain, readily available
   c. Disadvantages: does not reveal aortic regurgitation or coronary artery involvement, potential for adverse effect from contrast.
6. MRI
   a. Sensitivity and specificity approach 100%
   b. Noninvasive, no contrast reactions
   c. Disadvantages: availability limited, requires very long scan times (45 to 90 minutes), many contraindications, limited monitoring during the procedure

D. Classification systems
1. Debakey
   a. Type I: ascending and descending aorta involved
   b. Type II: ascending aorta only
   c. Type III: descending aorta only
2. Stanford
   a. Type A: involves the **A**scending aorta (includes Debakey type I and type II)
   b. Type B: involves only the descending (**B**elow) aorta

E. Management
1. Control blood pressure and rate of change of the pulse pressure with each beat (dP/dt)
   a. Nitroprusside with a β-blockader or labetalol monotherapy
   b. Reduce systolic to ~90 to 100 mm Hg
   c. Consider tamponade if patient becomes hypotensive
      i. Hypotension: managed with fluid or blood products
2. Surgical management
   a. Surgical management is indicated in Stanford type A or Debakey type I and type II
   b. Medical management is indicated in Stanford type B or Debakey type III

XIV. Abdominal Aortic Aneurysm

A. Definition
1. Localized stretching and dilatation of all 3 layers of the aorta (similar to overinflation of a balloon) caused by deterioration of the elastic fibers in the aorta
   a. As the aneurysm increases in size, the risk for aortic rupture increases
   b. Vast majority abdominal and infra-renal in location
   c. Typically once the aneurysm is >3 cm, it can grow by 4 mm per year
2. Risk factors
   a. Advanced age
   b. Male
   c. Hypertension
   d. White
   e. Smoking
   f. History of atherosclerotic disease
   g. Family history of aortic aneurysm
3. Aneurysms are typically asymptomatic until they rupture

B. Symptoms and signs
1. Sudden onset of severe chest, back, abdominal, or flank pain
2. Presenting complaint can be syncope, which may be secondary to pain or from hypotension
3. May be dull in nature and radiate to groin or legs
4. Diagnosis often confused with renal stone or musculoskeletal pain
5. Pulsatile mass palpable in ~75% of patients
   a. May not be palpable if patient is hypotensive or if aneurysm is small
   b. May not be palpable in very obese patients
6. Pulses may be unequal
7. <50% are hypotensive on arrival to the ED

C. Diagnosis
1. Abdominal x-rays: not sensitive or specific, however may see calcifications in aneurismal dilated aorta (best x-ray to order is cross table lateral lumbar spine—best exposure to look at calcification)
2. Ultrasonography: nearly 100% detection of aneurysms
   a. Cannot detect whether aneurysm leaking or ruptured—aorta retroperitoneal so fluid usually not seen intraabdominally
   b. Cannot evaluate visceral or renal arteries
3. CT scan with contrast
   a. Detects aneurysm, evaluates leak or rupture in retroperitoneum
   b. Identifies visceral artery involvement
   c. Not limited by obesity or fat
   d. Evaluates other possible etiologies of abdominal pain
4. MRI
   a. Superior to CT for detection and evaluation of aneurysm
   b. Limited availability and prolonged scan times
5. Angiography
   a. May miss aneurysm with thrombus on wall (diameter of flowing blood column appears normal)
   b. Largely supplanted by other tests

D. Management
1. Treatment of a ruptured or leaking aortic aneurysm is surgical
2. Massive blood loss possible, so efforts should be taken to have sufficient blood products available and sufficient IV access
3. Early surgical consultation is warranted in cases of suspected aortic aneurysm

REFERENCES

1. www.cdc.gov/heartdisease/
2. Thom T, Haase N, Rosamond W, et al: Heart disease and stroke statistics 2006 update: a report from the American Heart Association Statistics Committee and Stroke Statistics Subcommittee. *Circ J Am Heart Assoc.* 2006;113(6):e85.
3. Abrams J: Clinical practice: chronic stable angina. *N Engl J Med.* 2005;352(24):2524.
4. Bello N, Mosca L: Epidemiology of coronary heart disease in women. *Prog Cardiovasc Dis.* 2004;46(4):287.
5. Hamm CW, Goldmann BU, Heeschen, et al: Emergency room triage of patients with acute chest pain by means of rapid testing for cardiac troponin T or troponin I. *N Engl J Med.* 1997;337(23):1648.
6. Schwarz F, Baumann P, Manthey J, et al: The effect of aortic valve replacement on survival. *Circ J Am Heart Assoc.* 1982; 66(5):1105.
7. Lange RA, Hillis LD: Cardiovascular complications of cocaine use. *N Engl J Med.* 2001;345(5):351.
8. Barbaro G: HIV infection, highly active antiretroviral therapy and the cardiovascular system. *Cardiovasc Res.* 2003;60(1):87.
9. Passalaris JD, Sepkowitz KA, Glesby MJ: Coronary artery disease and human immunodeficiency virus infection. *Clin Infect Dis.* 2000;31(3):787.
10. Friis-Moller N, Reiss P, Sabin CA, et al: Class of antiretroviral drugs and the risk of myocardial infarction. *N Engl J Med.* 2007;356(17):1723.
11. Friis-Moller N, Sabin CA, Weber R, et al: Combination antiretroviral therapy and the risk of myocardial infarction. *N Engl J Med.* 2003;349(21):1993.

12. Antman EM, Cohen M, Bernink PJ, et al: The TIMI risk score for unstable angina/non-ST elevation MI: a method for prognostication and therapeutic decision making. *JAMA.* 2000;284(7):835.

13. Wang K, Asinger RW, Marriott HJ: ST-segment elevation in conditions other than acute myocardial infarction. *N Engl J Med.* 2003;349(22):2128.

14. Sgarbossa EB, Pinski SL, Topol EJ, et al: Acute myocardial infarction and complete bundle branch block at hospital admission: clinical characteristics and outcome in the thrombolytic era. GUSTO-I Investigators. Global Utilization of Streptokinase and t-PA [tissue-type plasminogen activator] for Occluded Coronary Arteries. *J Am Coll Cardiol.* 1998;31(1):105.

15. Feigl D, Ashkenazy J, Kishon Y: Early and late atrioventricular block in acute inferior myocardial infarction. *J Am Coll Cardiol* 1984;4(1):35.

16. Sgarbossa EB, Pinski SL, Barbagelata A, et al: Electrocardiographic diagnosis of evolving acute myocardial infarction in the presence of left bundle-branch block. GUSTO-1 (Global Utilization of Streptokinase and Tissue Plasminogen Activator for Occluded Coronary Arteries) Investigators. *N Engl J Med.* 1996;334(8):481.

17. Roongsritong C, Warraich I, Bradley C: Common causes of troponin elevations in the absence of acute myocardial infarction: incidence and clinical significance. *Chest.* 2004; 125(5):1877.

18. Heidenreich PA, Alloggiamento T, Melsop K, et al: The prognostic value of troponin in patients with non-ST elevation acute coronary syndromes: a meta-analysis. *J Am Coll Cardiol.* 2001;38(2):478.

19. Jeremias A, Gibson CM: Narrative review: alternative causes for elevated cardiac troponin levels when acute coronary syndromes are excluded. *Ann Intern Med.* 2005;142(9):786.

20. Porter A, Wyshelesky A, Strasberg B, et al: Correlation between the admission electrocardiogram and regional wall motion abnormalities as detected by echocardiography in anterior acute myocardial infarction. *Cardiology.* 2000;94(2):118.

21. Theroux P, Ouimet H, McCans J, et al: Aspirin, heparin, or both to treat acute unstable angina. *N Engl J Med.* 1988;319(17):1105.

22. Cairns JA, Gent M, Singer J, et al: Aspirin, sulfinpyrazone, or both in unstable angina. Results of a Canadian multicenter trial. *N Engl J Med.* 1985;313(22):1369.

23. Lewis HD, Jr: Which role for antiplatelet and anticoagulant drugs in unstable angina pectoris? *Cardiovasc Drugs Ther.* 1988;2(1):103.

24. Sabatine MS, Cannon CP, Gibson CM, et al: Addition of clopidogrel to aspirin and fibrinolytic therapy for myocardial infarction with ST-segment elevation. *N Engl J Med.* 2005; 352(12):1179.

25. Menon V, Berkowitz SD, Antman EM, et al: New heparin dosing recommendations for patients with acute coronary syndromes. *Am J Med.* 2001;110(8):641.

26. Chen ZM, Pan HC, Chen YP, et al: Early intravenous then oral metoprolol in 45, 852 patients with acute myocardial infarction: randomised placebo-controlled trial. *Lancet.* 2005;366(9497):1622.

27. Hochman JS, Wali AU, Gavrila D, et al: A new regimen for heparin use in acute coronary syndromes. *Am Heart J.* 1999;138(2 Pt 1):313.

28. Bozovich GE, Gurfinkel EP, Antman EM: Superiority of enoxaparin versus unfractionated heparin for unstable angina/non-Q-wave myocardial infarction regardless of activated partial thromboplastin time. *Am Heart J.* 2000;140(4):637.

29. Antman EM, McCabe CH, Gurfinkel EP, et al: Enoxaparin prevents death and cardiac ischemic events in unstable angina/non-Q-wave myocardial infarction. Results of the thrombolysis in myocardial infarction (TIMI) 11B trial. *Circ J Am Heart Assoc.* 1999;100(15):1593.

30. Antman EM, Morrow DA, McCabe CH, et al: Enoxaparin versus unfractionated heparin as antithrombin therapy in patients receiving fibrinolysis for ST-elevation myocardial infarction. Design and rationale for the Enoxaparin and Thrombolysis Reperfusion for Acute Myocardial Infarction Treatment-Thrombolysis In Myocardial Infarction study 25 (ExTRACT-TIMI 25). *Am Heart J.* 2005;149(2):217.

31. Lincoff AM: Direct thrombin inhibitors for non ST segment elevation acute coronary syndromes: what, when, and where? *Am Heart J.* 2003;146(4 Suppl):S23.

32. Bittl JA, Strony J, Brinker JA, et al: Treatment with bivalirudin (Hirulog) as compared with heparin during coronary angioplasty for unstable or postinfarction angina. Hirulog Angioplasty Study Investigators. *N Engl J Med.* 1995; 333(12):764.

33. Morey SS: ACC/AHA guidelines on the management of acute myocardial infarction. American College of Cardiology and the American Heart Association. *Am Fam Physician.* 2000;61(6):1901, 4.

34. Rosamond W, Flegal K, Friday G, et al: Heart disease and stroke statistics 2007 update: a report from the American Heart Association Statistics Committee and Stroke Statistics Subcommittee. *Circ J Am Heart Assoc.* 2007;115(5):e69.

35. Jessup M, Brozena S: Heart failure. *N Engl J Med.* 2003; 348(20):2007.

36. Maisel AS, Krishnaswamy P, Nowak RM, et al: Rapid measurement of B-type natriuretic peptide in the emergency diagnosis of heart failure. *N Engl J Med.* 2002;347(3):161.

37. Felker GM, Petersen JW, Mark DB: Natriuretic peptides in the diagnosis and management of heart failure. *CMAJ.* 2006; 175(6):611.

38. Masip J, Betbese AJ, Paez J, et al: Non-invasive pressure support ventilation versus conventional oxygen therapy in acute cardiogenic pulmonary oedema: a randomised trial. *Lancet.* 2000;356(9248):2126.

39. Silvers SM, Howell JM, Kosowsky JM, et al: Clinical policy: critical issues in the evaluation and management of adult patients presenting to the emergency department with acute heart failure syndromes. *Ann Emerg Med.* 2007;49(5):627.

40. Philbin EF, Cotto M, Rocco TA, Jr, et al: Association between diuretic use, clinical response, and death in acute heart failure. *Am J Cardiol.* 1997;80(4):519.

41. Cooper HA, Dries DL, Davis CE, et al: Diuretics and risk of arrhythmic death in patients with left ventricular dysfunction. *Circ J Am Heart Assoc.* 1999;100(12):1311.

42. Mehta RL, Pascual MT, Soroko S, et al: Diuretics, mortality, and nonrecovery of renal function in acute renal failure. *JAMA.* 2002;288(20):2547.

43. Levy P, Compton S, Welch R, et al: Treatment of severe decompensated heart failure with high-dose intravenous

nitroglycerin: a feasibility and outcome analysis. *Ann Emerg Med.* 2007;50(2):144.

44. Publication committee for the VMAC Investigators: Intravenous nesiritide vs nitroglycerin for treatment of decompensated congestive heart failure: a randomized controlled trial. *JAMA.* 2002;287(12):1531.

45. Sackner-Bernstein JD, Kowalski M, Fox M, et al: Short-term risk of death after treatment with nesiritide for decompensated heart failure: a pooled analysis of randomized controlled trials. *JAMA.* 2005;293(15):1900.

46. Cuffe MS, Califf RM, Adams KF, Jr, et al: Short-term intravenous milrinone for acute exacerbation of chronic heart failure: a randomized controlled trial. *JAMA.* 2002;287(12):1541.

47. Burger AJ, Elkayam U, Neibaur MT, et al: Comparison of the occurrence of ventricular arrhythmias in patients with acutely decompensated congestive heart failure receiving dobutamine versus nesiritide therapy. *Am J Cardiol.* 2001;88(1):35.

48. Cleland JG, Daubert JC, Erdmann E, et al: The effect of cardiac resynchronization on morbidity and mortality in heart failure. *N Engl J Med.* 2005;352(15):1539.

49. Young JB, Abraham WT, Smith AL, et al: Combined cardiac resynchronization and implantable cardioversion defibrillation in advanced chronic heart failure: the MIRACLE ICD Trial. *JAMA.* 2003;289(20):2685.

50. Maron BJ, Gardin JM, Flack JM, et al: Prevalence of hypertrophic cardiomyopathy in a general population of young adults. Echocardiographic analysis of 4111 subjects in the CARDIA Study. Coronary Artery Risk Development in (Young) Adults. *Circ J Am Heart Assoc.* 1995;92(4):785.

51. Maron BJ: Sudden death in young athletes. *N Engl J Med.* 2003;349(11):1064.

52. Epstein SE, Rosing DR: Verapamil: its potential for causing serious complications in patients with hypertrophic cardiomyopathy. *Circ J Am Heart Assoc.* 1981;64(3):437.

53. Maron BJ, Shen WK, Link MS, et al: Efficacy of implantable cardioverter-defibrillators for the prevention of sudden death in patients with hypertrophic cardiomyopathy. *N Engl J Med.* 2000;342(6):365.

54. Zayas R, Anguita M, Torres F, et al: Incidence of specific etiology and role of methods for specific etiologic diagnosis of primary acute pericarditis. *Am J Cardiol.* 1995;75(5):378.

55. Spodick DH: Acute cardiac tamponade. *N Engl J Med.* 2003;349(7):684.

56. Feldman AM, McNamara D: Myocarditis. *N Engl J Med.* 2000;343(19):1388.

57. Carabello BA: Clinical practice. Aortic stenosis. *N Engl J Med.* 2002;346(9):677.

58. Freed LA, Levy D, Levine RA, et al: Prevalence and clinical outcome of mitral-valve prolapse. *N Engl J Med.* 1999; 341(1):1.

59. Carabello BA, Crawford FA, Jr: Valvular heart disease. *N Engl J Med.* 1997;337(1):32.

60. Lindblom D, Lindblom U, Qvist J, et al: Long-term relative survival rates after heart valve replacement. *J Am Coll Cardiol.* 1990;15(3):566.

61. Lazzari JO, Benchuga EG, Elizari MV, et al: Ventricular fibrillation after intravenous atropine in a patient with atrioventricular block. *Pacing Clin Electrophysiol.* 1982;5(2):196.

62. Onodera S, Ito M, Odakura H, et al: [Atrioventricular block in acute inferior myocardial infarction]. *Kokyu to junkan.* 1992;40(3):255.

63. Hayes DL, Vlietstra RE: Pacemaker malfunction. *Ann Intern Med.* 1993;119(8):828.

Chapter 6
PULMONOLOGY AND CRITICAL CARE

Gino Farina and Mityanand Ramnarine

I. Respiratory Physiology

A. Measuring oxygenation
  1. Arterial blood gas (ABG)
     a. Definition: arterial blood sample that provides direct measurement of gas levels

     $$pH/P_aCO_2/P_aO_2/HCO_3/B.E./S_aO_2$$

        i. FiO_2 = % O_2 of inspired air
        ii. P_AO_2 mm Hg = partial pressure in the alveoli
        iii. pH = activity of H^+ ions
        iv. P_aCO_2 mm Hg or PCO_2 = partial pressure of carbon dioxide in the arteries
        v. P_aO_2 mm Hg = partial pressure of oxygen in the arteries
        vi. B.E. = Base excess
        vii. S_aO_2% = oxygen saturation of hemoglobin the arteries
        viii. ABG can also provide
             a) COHb = carboxyhemoglobin
             b) MetHb = methemoglobin
             c) Lactic acid, K^+, Na^{+2}, Hgb/Hct
             d) S_vO_2 = mixed venous oxygen saturation
                i) To be drawn from subclavian or internal jugular vein
  2. A-a gradient
     a. Definition: difference between the partial pressure of oxygen in the alveoli and arterial blood
     b. **A-a gradient = $P_AO_2 - P_aO_2$**
        i. P_aO_2 obtained from ABG
        ii. P_AO_2 value from alveolar gas equation
     c. Alveolar gas equation
        i. $P_AO_2 = FiO_2 \times (760-41) - (P_aCO_2/8)$
        ii. $P_AO_2 = \mathbf{150 - (1.25 \times P_aCO_2)}$ for quick calculation at sea level and room air
     d. Normal gradient is age dependent = age/4 + 4
  3. Hypoxemia
     a. Definition: $P_aO_2 < 60$ mm Hg
     b. Etiology

        i. V/Q mismatch
           a) Definition: airspace not being perfused or perfused areas not being ventilated
           b) Etiologies: asthma, chronic obstructive pulmonary disease (COPD), pulmonary embolism, interstitial lung disease (ILD)
           c) Management: oxygen and treat underlying cause
        ii. Shunting
           a) Definition: right-sided blood is shunted past the lungs without being oxygenated
           b) Etiology: alveolar collapse, most commonly from acute respiratory distress syndrome (ARDS); also from alveolar filling—pneumonia, pulmonary edema
           c) Management: **does not respond well to oxygen**, responds better to positive end-expiratory pressure (PEEP)
        iii. Decreased diffusion
           a) Definition: decreased diffusion of oxygen
           b) Etiology: thickening of alveolar/capillary interface—commonly ILD
           c) Management: responds to oxygen
        iv. Hypoventilation
           a) Definition: lack of respiratory effort resulting in low P_aO_2 and **high P_aCO_2**, commonly from drug overdose. **Normal A-a gradient**
        v. High altitude (low FiO_2)
           a) Definition: decrease in partial pressure of available oxygen. **Normal A-a gradient**

II. Critical Care

A. ARDS
  1. Definition
     a. Acute onset alveoli edema caused by capillary membranes injury and increased permeability

  i.   Bilateral infiltrates on chest x-ray (CXR)
  ii. Pulmonary wedge pressure <18
  iii. Ratio of PaO_2/FiO_2 < 200 mm Hg
2. Etiology
   a. Sepsis, acute pulmonary infection, nonthoracic trauma, toxins, disseminated intravascular coagulation, shock lung, freebase cocaine smoking, postcoronary artery bypass grafting (especially if on amiodarone), inhalation of high-oxygen concentrations, acute radiation pneumonia
3. Symptoms and signs
   a. Respiratory distress, hypoxemia unresponsive to increasing amounts of supplemental oxygen
   b. Onset of ARDS is often within the first 2 hours after an inciting event, but can be delayed as long as 1 to 3 days
4. Management
   a. 35% to 50% mortality
   b. Treat underlying disease
   c. Mechanical ventilation with PEEP
      i.   Shunt physiology so high FiO_2 not helpful
      ii. Use low tidal volumes to prevent barotraumas (6 mL/kg)
      iii. Use PEEP
   d. Maintenance of adequate nutrition
   e. Hemodynamic monitoring (Swan-Ganz catheterization) to guide intravenous (IV) fluid management; may also be used to confirm diagnosis
   f. Steroids **not** shown to be beneficial

B. Sepsis syndromes
1. Systemic inflammatory response syndrome (SIRS)
   a. Temperature ≥38°C or <36°C
   b. Heart Rate >90 beats per minute
   c. Respiratory rate >20 breaths per minute or
   d. PCO_2 <32 mm Hg
   e. WBC >12,000 per cubic mm or <4000 per cubic mm or the presence of >10% immature band forms
2. Sepsis
   a. SIRS with a suspected or proven infection
3. Severe sepsis
   a. Sepsis with organ dysfunction (hypotension, hypoxemia, oliguria, metabolic acidosis, thrombocytopenia, and/or obtundation)
4. Septic shock
   a. Severe sepsis with hypotension despite adequate fluid resuscitation
   b. Management
      i. **Early goal-directed therapy**
         a) IV fluids to achieve a central venous pressure of 8 to 12 mm

      b) If mean arterial pressure persists <65 mm Hg, administer vasopressors
      c) If the S_VO_2 < 70% (obtained from central venous line), red cells transfusion is given to achieve a hematocrit of at least 30%
      d) If S_VO_2 remains <70% despite above efforts, consider dobutamine administration

III. Disorders of Pleura, Mediastinum, and Chest Wall

A. Mediastinitis
1. Definition: inflammation of the mediastinum
2. Etiology
   a. Mixed organisms but most commonly *Streptococcus* and *Bacteroides* species
   b. Esophageal rupture most common cause
      i. Foreign body ingestion or stuck fish bone may accompany history of esophageal injury
   c. Consider tracheal rupture
   d. Head and neck infections may lead to descending mediastinitis
      i. Preceded by oropharyngeal infection or surgery
3. Risk factors
   a. Immunocompromise and diabetes
   b. Drug abuse
4. Symptoms and signs
   a. Fever, dyspnea, and pleuritic, retrosternal chest pain radiating to the neck or interscapular pain, neck swelling
   b. Ill appearing
   c. Subcutaneous emphysema of neck and chest
5. Diagnosis
   a. A CXR may show a widened mediastinum
   b. Soft tissue x-ray of the neck may show precervical or retropharyngeal air/edema
   c. Computed tomography (CT) should be performed to further evaluate soft tissue spaces to determine treatment
6. Management
   a. Broad-spectrum antibiotic therapy
   b. ENT and cardiothoracic surgery consult

B. Pneumomediastinum
1. Etiology
   a. Spontaneous (extremely rare), blunt chest trauma (disruption of bronchial tree, esophageal rupture), endoscopy, obstructive lung disease
   b. Consider Boerhaave syndrome if history of vomiting

    c. Valsalva maneuver (ie, forceful cough against a closed glottis, constipation)

       i. Observed in crack cocaine users

2. Symptoms and signs

    a. Symptoms: chest pain and dyspnea

    b. Signs: subcutaneous emphysema and Hamman sign (crunching, rasping sound, synchronous with heartbeat)

    c. Decreased cardiac output if tension pneumomediastinum is present

3. Diagnosis

    a. CXR

       i. Reveals free air within the mediastinum outlining the contained organs

       ii. "Ring around the artery" highlighting the right pulmonary artery

       iii. Continuous diaphragm sign (PA film)

       iv. Air posterior to sternum and posterior to the heart on lateral film

    b. Esophagogram

       i. Perform with patient in right lateral decubitus position

       ii. Initially use a water-soluble contrast agent (Gastrografin)

       iii. If clinical suspicions remains high and the initial study is negative, repeat study with oral barium contrast

         a) Higher sensitivity for small perforations

         b) Barium is not used initially because of its irritating effect on the mediastinum

    c. Esophagoscopy for suspected esophageal rupture in acute traumatic rupture

       i. Should not perform if small mucosal tears are suspected since air used during procedure may dissect through disrupted tissue

    d. Bronchoscopy for suspected bronchotracheal tree rupture

4. Management

    a. Patients with pneumomediastinum should be admitted and observed for signs of serious complications (eg, pneumothorax, tension pneumothorax, and mediastinitis)

    b. Broad-spectrum antibiotics for suspected esophageal rupture

    c. Use smallest pressures and tidal volumes possible if patient requires mechanical ventilation

C. Pleural effusion—collection of fluid within pleural space

1. Epidemiology

    a. Congestive heart failure (CHF) is most common cause followed by malignancy, bacterial pneumonia, and pulmonary embolism

    b. Tuberculosis is most common etiology of pleural effusion in developing countries

2. Etiology

    a. Transudative—CHF (more commonly right-sided), cirrhosis with ascites, nephrotic syndrome, pulmonary embolism

    b. Exudative—cancer, infectious (pneumonia, empyema, abscess, TB), inflammatory (SLE, pancreatitis, rheumatoid arthritis), and pulmonary embolism (can give both)

3. Symptoms and signs

    a. Dyspnea and pleuritic chest pain

    b. Decreased breath sounds on auscultation

    c. Dullness to percussion

4. Diagnosis

    a. CXR

       i. AP CXR demonstrates effusion when pleural fluid volume approaches 150 cc

       ii. 10 mm strip of fluid on lateral decubitus = significant effusion

    b. CT or ultrasound are most sensitive

    c. Thoracentesis necessary when etiology still unclear

       i. Light criteria: a single positive criterion is enough to classify the fluid as an exudate (Table 6–1)

       ii. Glucose: few conditions can cause very low pleural fluid glucose levels (<25 mg/dL), eg, rheumatoid arthritis, tuberculosis, empyema, and malignancies with extensive pleural involvement

       iii. pH: low pH seen with inflammatory and infiltrative processes such as infected parapneumonic effusions, empyema, malignancies, collagen vascular disease, tuberculosis, and esophageal rupture

       iv. Amylase: a high pleural amylase level (>200 U/dL) usually indicates pancreatitis, malignancy, or esophageal rupture

    d. Diagnosis of empyema

       i. Positive pleural fluid culture

       ii. pH <7.2

       iii. Glucose <60

       iv. WBC >50,000

       v. Grossly purulent fluid

TABLE 6–1. Light Criteria

LIGHT CRITERIA	TRANSUDATE	EXUDATE
Pleural and serum protein	<0.5	>0.5
Pleural and serum LDH	<0.6	>0.6
Pleural LDH	<200 IU/mL	>200 IU/mL

5. Management
   a. Treat underlying cause
   b. Therapeutic thoracentesis for patients dyspneic at rest
   c. Thoracostomy tube placement for empyema

D. Pneumothorax—simple, tension, open
   1. Etiology
      a. Spontaneous—no underlying lung disease
         i. Male:female 6:1
         ii. Young, tall, thin male
         iii. Smoking (20:1)
         iv. Valsalva
         v. Ruptured bleb
         vi. Many recur (20% to 50%)
      b. Secondary—caused by underlying disease
         i. Asthma, COPD, neoplasm
         ii. Marfan, Ehlers Danlos, cystic fibrosis (CF)
         iii. Pneumonia especially with abscess or cavitation
         iv. HIV-PCP
         v. Catamenial—endometriosis, associated with menstruation
      c. Tension pneumothorax
         i. Pleural defect creates one way valve
         ii. Increase in pleural pressure resulting in mediastinal shift and kinking of the SVC or collapse of the right ventricle
   2. Symptoms and signs
      a. Dyspnea and pleuritic chest pain
      b. Decreased breath sound and hyperresonace to percussion
      c. JVD and hypotension
      d. Tracheal deviation away from affected side
   3. Diagnosis
      a. Pneumothorax
         i. CXR for simple pneumothorax
            a) End expiratory for highest sensitivity
            b) Overall sensitivity of 80%
            c) Supine AP films are notoriously inaccurate
            d) "Deep sulcus sign" refers to an especially deep costovertebral sulcus suggestive of pneumothorax
         ii. CT very sensitive and test of choice for the supine trauma patient
         iii. Preliminary evidence with experienced ultrasonographers shows sensitivities approaching 100%
         iv. T-wave inversions on ECG
      b. Tension pneumothorax
         i. Clinical diagnosis

            a) Tracheal deviation away from affected lung
            b) Hypotension
         ii. Do **not** wait for x-rays before treating
   4. Management
      a. Small stable pneumothorax (arbitrarily <10%)
         i. 100% O$_2$
            a) Creates nitrogen/oxygen gradient
            b) Reabsorb 5% to 7% per day
         ii. Stable patients with a small pneumothorax can be discharged with next-day follow-up after 6 hours observation and stable x-ray
      b. Large pneumothorax
         i. 100% O$_2$
         ii. Tube thoracostomy (see Procedure chapter)
      c. Tension pneumothorax
         i. Immediate needle decompression followed by chest tube
      d. Be wary of reexpansion pulmonary edema
         i. Especially if pneumothorax present >3 days

II. Noncardiogenic Pulmonary Edema

A. Definition
   1. Radiographic evidence of alveolar fluid accumulation without hemodynamic evidence of a cardiogenic etiology (ie, pulmonary capillary wedge pressure <18 mm Hg)

B. Etiology
   1. ARDS (see Critical Care section)
   2. High-altitude pulmonary edema (see Environmental chapter)
   3. Reexpansion pulmonary edema
      a. Risk factors
         i. Large volume thoracentesis (>1 L)
         ii. Rapid lung re-expansion of pneumothorax, especially when it has been collapsed for >3 days
   4. Drug induced
      a. Mnemonic for drug-induced noncardiogenic pulmonary edema is **MOPS** (meprobate, opioids/naloxone, PCP, salicylates)
         i. Meprobamate
            a) Precursor anxiolytic of currently used benzodiazepines
            b) May form GI concretions
         ii. Opiate overdose
            a) Etiology
               i) Hypothesized to result from a combination of direct drug toxicity,

hypoxia, and acidosis secondary to hypoventilation
    b) Management
       i) Hyperventilation, resolution of hypoxia, and assisted ventilation
  iii. Naloxone induced pulmonary edema
    a) Pathophysiology: unknown
    b) Management: supportive
  iv. PCP (see Toxicology chapter)
  v. Salicylate toxicity associated pulmonary edema
    a) More likely with chronic poisoning
    b) Sodium bicarbonate administration to treat overdose may complicate pulmonary edema
    c) Indication for hemodialysis

III. Obstructive Lung Disease

A. Asthma and reactive airway disease (RAD)
  1. Definition
    a. Chronic inflammatory disorder of the small airways characterized by reversible obstruction
  2. Etiology and pathophysiology
    a. Airway inflammation/bronchial wall edema leading to decreased airway diameter
    b. Airway hyperreactivity, smooth muscle contraction
    c. Secretions forming mucous plugs
    d. Chronic inflammation leads to lung remodeling
  3. Symptoms and signs
    a. History associated with higher mortality
      i. > 2 hospitalizations during past year
      ii. > 3 ED visits during past year
      iii. Prior intubation or ICU admission
      iv. Use of 2 or more adrenergic canisters per month
      v. Current use of systemic steroids or recent withdrawal
      vi. Low socioeconomic class
    b. Dyspnea with or without productive cough
    c. Prolonged expiratory phase with predominantly expiratory wheezing
    d. Severe exacerbations may present with absence of wheezing, inability to speak, pulses paradoxus >20, normal to elevated CO_2, and hypoxia
  4. Diagnosis
    a. Bedside spirometry—peak flow to monitor response to β-agonist treatment and assist disposition
      i. Peak flow <50% indicates severe exacerbation
    b. Pulse oximetry—no role in predicting clinical outcome

    c. Arterial blood gas—used during severe attacks solely to assess hypoventilation/fatigue and PCO_2 levels
      i. Debatable utility in the management of asthma
    d. CXR may reveal hyperinflation or concurrent pneumonia
  5. Treatment
    a. Oxygen to keep O_2 saturation >88%
    b. β agonists
      i. Stimulation through β-adrenergic receptors activates adenyl cyclase responsible for conversion of ATP to **cyclic AMP**
        a) Increased cyclic AMP levels are associated with relaxation of bronchial smooth muscle and inhibition of release of mediators of immediate hypersensitivity from cells, especially from mast cells
      ii. Epinephrine (1:1000) is reserved for severe exacerbations, is administered SC, 0.3 mg every 20 to 30 minutes for up to 3 doses
      iii. Terbutaline (1 mg/cc) is also reserved for severe exacerbations is given SC, 0.25 mg every 20 to 30 minutes for up to 3 doses
        a) More $β_2$ selective with a longer duration of action than epinephrine
    c. Anticholinergics
      i. Ipratropium bromide targets muscarinic receptors and inhibits bronchoconstriction caused by vagal tone
    d. Corticosteroids—used in both acute and chronic setting to prevent late phase inflammatory response
      i. Inhibiting inflammatory cells
      ii. Decreases production of cytokines
      iii. Decreases revisits to ED
      iv. Oral dosing as effective as intravenous administration
    e. Magnesium
      i. Benefit in severe exacerbation
    f. Methylxanthines
      i. Should be administered if patient presents with severe exacerbation and subtherapeutic theophylline level
      ii. GI upset and seizures are potential side effects
    g. Mechanical ventilation
      i. Avoid air-trapping or auto-peep
        a) Smaller tidal volumes
        b) Keep rate low

c) Consider increasing peak inspiratory flow thereby allowing longer expiratory time

d) Early benzodiazepine use to calm the agitated patient overbreathing the set vent rate

h. Treating pregnant asthmatics

　i. Fetus more susceptible to hypoxia than mother

　ii. No contraindications to use of β agonists, corticosteroids, and anticholinergics although chronic steroids may result in lower birth weights

　iii. Epinephrine is teratogenic during first trimester and associated with preterm delivery

B. COPD

1. Definitions

a. Progressive partially reversible limitation of airflow

b. Airflow limitation is caused by two processes; chronic bronchitis and emphysema, which occur together in most patients

c. Emphysema: abnormal permanent enlargement and destruction of air spaces distal to terminal bronchioles

d. Chronic bronchitis: excess mucous secretion in the bronchial tree with chronic productive cough occurring on most days for at least 3 months in a year for 2 consecutive years

2. Epidemiology

a. The single most important risk factor for COPD is smoking

b. Congenital α_1-antitrypsin (AT) deficiency

　i. Accompanied by liver disease secondary to deposition of abnormal α_1-AT protein

3. Etiology

a. 80% of acute COPD exacerbations are of infectious origin

　i. *Streptococcus pneumoniae, Haemophilus influenzae,* or *Moraxella catarrhalis*

　ii. Less commonly by *Chlamydia pneumoniae* and viral pathogens

b. Noninfectious factors: irritants

　i. Pollutants, allergic reactions, GERD, post-nasal drip, sinusitis

4. Symptoms and signs

a. Dyspnea on exertion, tachypnea, cyanosis, agitation, apprehension, and hypertension are indicative of hypoxia

b. Wheezing, rales, rhonchi, prolonged expiratory phase, pursed-lip breathing, and clubbing of digits

5. Diagnosis

a. Elevated hematocrit secondary to chronic hypoxia

b. ABG: mild-to-moderate hypoxemia without hypercapnea in early stages

　i. Hypoxemia and hypercapnea become more pronounced as disease progresses

c. Measure α_1-AT level in patients with strong family history presenting <40 years old

d. CXR: hyperinflation, flattened diaphragms, long narrow heart shadow

e. ECG

　i. Atrial fibrillation

　ii. Multifocal atrial tachycardia (MAT)

　iii. Cor-pulmonale—right atrial enlargement evidenced by tall P waves

　iv. Right axis deviation and right ventricular hypertrophy

6. Management

a. Supplemental oxygen reduces mortality in patients with advanced COPD with room air oxygen saturation <88% to 90%

b. Nebulized anticholinergics

c. Bronchodilators

　i. β agonists

　ii. Epinephrine

　iii. Terbutaline

d. Antibiotics

　i. First-line choices include amoxicillin, cefaclor, fluoroquinolones or trimethoprim/sulfamethoxazole

　ii. Gram-negative infections more likely in those with frequent exacerbations and need a third-generation cephalosporin or augmented penicillin in combination with a fluoroquinolone or aminoglycoside

e. Corticosteroids

　i. Short courses of systemic corticosteroids may be used to manage an acute exacerbation of COPD.

　ii. Methylprednisolone 125 mg IV

C. CF

1. Epidemiology

a. 1 in 2500 children

b. Most common in Europeans and Ashkenazi Jews

2. Etiology

a. Autosomal recessive mutation in the cystic fibrosis transmembrane conductance regulator (CFTR)

　i. Leads to abnormalities in chloride transport in exocrine tissues leads to multiorgan involvement

　　a) Thick, viscous secretions in lungs, intestine, pancreas, reproductive tract

3. Symptoms and signs
    a. Respiratory manifestations
        i. Most common presentation
        ii. Often with infectious etiology
        iii. Exacerbations characterized by increased cough, sputum production, decreased lung function
    b. Undiagnosed patients may present with
        i. Failure to thrive
        ii. Chronic cough
        iii. Repeated pulmonary or sinus infections
        iv. Chronic diarrhea resulting from pancreatic insufficiency
    c. Alternative presentations
        i. Increased salt content in sweat gland secretion
        ii. Meconium ileus in neonates
        iii. Rectal prolapse
        iv. Steatorrhea from pancreatic enzyme insufficiency
        v. Intestinal obstruction
        vi. Spontaneous pnuemothorax
        vii. Chronic pancreatitis
        viii. Hepatobiliary disease: focal biliary cirrhosis, cholelithiasis
        ix. Infertility
4. Diagnosis
    a. Electrolytes: hyponatremia and alkalosis
    b. CXR: bronchiolar thickening, hyperinflation, and patchy, diffuse infiltrates
    c. Newborn screening
    d. Chloride sweat testing or genetic testing
5. Management
    a. Broad-spectrum antibiotics to cover *Staphylococcus aureus, Haemophilus influenzae,* and double cover *Pseudomonas aeruginosa*
        i. Chronic colonization with pathologic bacteria and chronic antibiotic use leads to resistant organisms requiring intravenous vancomycin, tobramycin, meropenem, ciprofloxacin, and piperacillin
    b. Mucolytics, such as dornase alfa, an enzyme that hydrolyses the DNA, are used in patients with CF to improve airway clearance
    c. Bronchodilators
    d. Aggressive chest physiotherapy
    e. Provide oxygen to all patients initially
    f. Consultation with a pulmonologist

IV. Restrictive Lung Disease—loss of lung compliance resulting in volumes loss

A. ILD
    1. Diverse group of restrictive pulmonary dysfunctions with the common end-point of interstitial collagen deposits and scarring

2. Idiopathic pulmonary fibrosis
    a. Epidemiology: 50% of ILDs
    b. Etiology: unknown, likely autoimmune
    c. Pathophysiology: damage to capillary endothelium leads to alveolar edema macrophage infiltration and proinflammatory mediator release >alveolar wall fibrosis
    d. Symptoms and signs
        i. Dyspnea, cough
        ii. Fine dry crackles, clubbing of fingers
    e. Diagnosis
        i. CXR: honeycombed lungs
        ii. CT: ground glass opacity
    f. Management
        i. Corticosteroids
        ii. Immune modulators with pulmonary consultation
        iii. Lung transplant

B. Sarcoidosis
    1. Epidemiology
        a. African Americans > whites
        b. Females > males
    2. Etiology
        a. Typical finding includes non-caseating granuloma, which is composed of T-helper cells and other inflammatory cells (macrophages, B cells)
    3. Symptoms and signs
        a. Most patients are asymptomatic
        b. Disease fatal in 10% of patients because of extensive organ involvement
        c. Constitutional symptoms (eg, fever, fatigue, weight loss, polyarthritis, myositis)
        d. Pulmonary symptoms (eg, cough, hemoptysis, shortness of breath with exertion)
        e. Neurologic symptoms (eg, Bell palsy, peripheral neuropathies, seizures)
        f. Skin lesions (eg, plaques, subcutaneous nodules, erythema nodosum, or lupus pernio [violaceous lesions on face and/or extremities])
        g. Cardiac symptoms (eg, arrhythmias or CHF)
        h. Lymphadenopathy
        i. Ophthalmologic symptoms (eg, uveitis or conjunctivitis)
    4. Diagnosis
        a. CXR
            i. Stage 0: no findings
            ii. Stage 1: Hilar adenopathy
            iii. Stage 2: Hilar adenopathy and parenchymal involvement
            iv. Stage 3: parenchymal involvement without adenopathy
            v. Stage 4: pulmonary fibrosis

b. Lab studies
   i. Leukocytosis (possibly with eosinophilia)
   ii. Elevated ESR or serum ACE
   iii. Hypercalcemia or hyperphosphatemia
   iv. Elevated CK and CK-MB with cardiac involvement
c. Gallium 67 scanning is used to detect extrapulmonary sarcoidosis
d. Biopsy of involved organ most useful for diagnosis

5. Management
   a. Cardiac monitoring for cardiac involvement
   b. Consider steroids or cytotoxic medications
   c. Lung transplantation for patients with severe refractory disease

V. Thromboembolic Disease

A. Deep venous thrombosis (DVT)
1. Risk factors
   a. Previous thrombosis
   b. Vascular endothelial damage
      i. Trauma
      ii. Surgery—especially orthopedic
      iii. Smoking
   c. Hypercoagulability
      i. Protein C or S deficitiency
      ii. Factor V Leiden
         a) Epidemiology—most common hereditary hypercoagulability disorder
         b) Pathophysiology—factor V variant that cannot be inactivated by protein C
      iii. Antithrombin III deficiency
      iv. Prothrombin mutation
      v. Homocytinuria
      vi. Anticardiolipin and antilupus antibodies
      vii. Oral contraception or third trimester pregnancy
   d. Immobilization or low cardiac output
      i. Long periods of sitting—long plane or car ride
      ii. CHF
2. Symptoms and signs
   a. Pain, warmth, and edema
   b. Discoloration of affected extremity
   c. Palpable cord of a thrombosed vein
   d. Severe occlusion can lead to phlegmasia alba dolens (PAD) and ultimately phlegmasia cerulea dolens (PCD)
      i. Occlusion of ileofemoral veins
      ii. Phlegmasia cerulea dolens is the more extreme form where even the collateral veins are occluded leading to ischemia and limb gangrene

3. Diagnosis
   a. Venograms uncommonly performed
   b. Doppler ultrasonography
      i. May require serial studies to rule out DVT in a high probability patient
      ii. Limitations
         a) Operator dependent
         b) Cannot distinguish between old and new clot
         c) Not accurate in detecting DVT in the pelvis or the small vessels of the calf
   c. CT angiography
      i. Benefits include CT angiography of the chest and lower extremity CT venography in one study
4. Management
   a. Anticoagulation
      i. Unfractionated low-molecular-weight heparin
      ii. Warfarin therapy
   b. Filter placement for patients with failure (recurrent thrombus) of anticoagulation or contraindications to anticoagulation
   c. Thrombectomy performed for with massive ileofemoral vein thrombosis (phlegmasia cerulea dolens) when limb viability is at risk

B. Pulmonary embolus (PE)
1. Risk factor are the same as for DVT
   a. 60% of patients with a DVT have a PE
2. Symptoms and signs
   a. Sudden-onset dyspnea, tachypnea, tachycardia, pleuritic, hemoptysis, syncope, cough, and wheeze
3. Diagnosis
   a. ECG
      i. Nonspecific ST-T-wave changes and/or sinus tachycardia are most commonly seen
      ii. Right heart strain (new RBBB, tall R in aVR), right axis deviation
      iii. S_1Q3T3
      iv. Precordial flipped T waves
   b. CXR
      i. Findings are usually abnormal but nonspecific
      ii. Pleural effusion
      iii. Elevated hemidiaphragm secondary to atelectasis and noninfectious infiltrates
      iv. Westermark sign—abrupt cut-off of vascular markings
      v. Hampton hump—pleural based wedge-shaped infarct
      vi. Used to interpret results of VQ scan

c. CT pulmonary angiography (CTPA) used increasingly as test of choice
   i. Sensitivity and specificity are comparable to that of contrast pulmonary angiography
   ii. May diagnose alternative lung pathology
   iii. Used in conjunction with CT venogram of lower extremities
d. Ventilation-perfusion scan (VQ scan)
   i. Useful in patients who have severe contrast allergies
   ii. Defects in radioactive tracer uptake from ventilated and perfused areas of the lungs are reported as normal, nearly normal, or indicating a low, intermediate, or high probability of embolus
   iii. A high-probability VQ scan in a high pretest probability patient provides sufficient evidence for the initiation of treatment for PE
   iv. A normal scan sufficient to exclude PE in patient with low pretest probability of disease
   v. Many inconclusive studies
      a) Treatment relies on pretest probability
      b) Require further diagnostic testing
         i) Lower extremity Doppler
         ii) Pulmonary angiography
e. Pulmonary angiography—the gold standard for diagnosing PE. It is used infrequently because of wider acceptance of noninvasive CT scans
f. Echocardiogram
   i. May reveal evidence of right heart strain
   ii. May guide thrombolytic administration if right heart strain demonstrated
   iii. May help differentiate cardiac etiology of dyspnea and chest pain
4. Management
   a. Supplemental oxygen
   b. Hemodynamic support
   c. Anticoagulation
   d. Thrombolytic
      i. Indicated in patients with associated hemodynamic instability
      ii. May have role in patients demonstrated to have new right heart strain as evidenced by ECG and/or echocardiogram
      iii. Thrombolytics directly into the thrombus by catheter has been described but has not been shown to be superior to peripheral infusion
   e. Surgical embolectomy
   f. IVC filters for anticoagulation failure or contraindication.

VI. Pulmonary Infections

A. Bacterial pneumonia
   1. Epidemiology
      a. In 2005 the CDC reports that influenza and pneumonia combined were the eighth leading causes of death in the United States
         i. These are combined since fatal bacterial pneumonia often follows an influenza virus infection
      b. Decreased mortality from pneumonia and influenza owing to vaccinations for the elderly and immunocompromised
   2. Etiology
      a. Typical pneumonia is caused by *S. pneumoniae*, *H. influenzae*, and *Staphylococcus* species
         i. *S. pneumoniae* is the most common cause of bacterial pneumonia
      b. Atypical pneumonia is usually caused by the influenza virus, mycoplasma, *Chlamydia*, *Legionella*, and adenovirus
         i. *Legionella* is associated with air travel and infected water supplies
      c. *S. aureus* is prevalent among IV drug abusers
      d. *K. pneumoniae* is associated with alcoholism, diabetes, and COPD
      e. *H. influenzae* associated with COPD and asthmatics
      f. Hospital-acquired pneumonia—pneumonia developing >72 hours after admission
         i. *Pseudomonas aeruginosa* is most common organism
         ii. Often a result of aspiration and so must consider Gram-negative rods, anaerobes, and *S. aureus*
   3. Symptoms and signs
      a. Chest pain
      b. Productive cough
         i. *Klebsiella*—currant jelly
         ii. *S. pneumoniae*—bloody or rusty-colored
         iii. Aspiration—foul-smelling sputum
         iv. *Chlamydia*—staccato cough
      c. Rigors particularly associated with *S. pneumoniae*
      d. Diarrhea and GI upset with *Legionella pneumophila*
      e. Bullous myringitis with *Mycoplasma pneumoniae*
      f. Pleural rubs
   4. Diagnosis
      a. Auscultation
      b. Chest radiography
         i. May reveal a lobar consolidation with air bronchogram

ii. Bilateral diffuse infiltrates consistent with atypical infections (*M. pneumoniae, P. carinii, C. psittaci*)

iii. Abscess and bulging lung fissures are indicative of infections caused by *Klebsiella* and *S. aureus*

iv. Bronchiectasis may occur with *S. aureus* and *Klebsiella*

v. The presence of pleural effusions and empyema associated with cavitary lesions are seen with *S. aureus* and *M. tuberculosis*

vi. Upper lung fields—*K. pneumoniae*

vii. Lower lung fields—*L. pneumophila*

viii. Miliary pattern—*M. tuberculosis*

c. Laboratory studies

i. CBC, chemistry—help to determine management

a) Hyponatremia and hypophosphatemia associated with *L. pneumophila*

b) Increased leukocyte count

ii. 2 sets of blood cultures (50% yield)

iii. Sputum samples for Gram stain and culture are accurate ~50% of the time

a) Adequate sputum contains <10 epithelial cells, >25 WBC per low-power field and remain uncontaminated from oral flora

iv. Urine *Legionella* antigens

v. *Mycoplasma* and *Chlamydia* immunoglobulin M antibodies—a rise in antibody titer of 1:128 confirms the diagnosis

5. Management

a. Community-acquired pneumonia

i. Pneumonia severity index score helps determine risk (Table 6–2)

ii. Admit if total score >90 points and consider ICU evaluation for >130 points

iii. Conservative use of new fluoroquinolones (levofloxacin, gatifloxacin, moxifloxacin) is recommended to minimize resistance patterns

b. Treatment of hospital-acquired pneumonia

i. Double-drug coverage for *Pseudomonas*

ii. Optimal combinations include cefipime plus levofloxacin, aztreonam, meropenem, or aminoglycoside

c. Treatment of aspiration pneumonia

i. Intubation should be considered in any patient who is unable to protect his or her airway

ii. Add anaerobic coverage

6. Types

a. Bordetella pertussis (whooping cough)

i. Epidemiology

TABLE 6–2. Pneumonia Severity Index for Community-Acquired Pneumonia

Total severity index score determines risk.

Demographics		**Physical examination findings**	
Men:		Altered mental status	+20
Age (years)	+Age	Respiratory rate ≥30 bpm	+20
Women:		Pulse rate ≥125 bpm	+20
Age (years)	+Age-10	Systolic blood pressure <90 mm Hg	+15
Nursing home resident	+Age+10	Temperature <95°F or ≥104°F	+10
Comorbidities		**Laboratory and radiographic findings**	
Cancer	+30	Arterial pH <7.35	+30
Liver disease	+20	Blood urea nitrogen >30 mg/dL	+20
Heart failure	+10	Na <130 mmol/L	+20
CVA	+10	PaO_2 <60 mm Hg	+10
Renal failure	+10	Glucose ≥250 mg/dL	+10
		Hematocrit <30%	+10
		Pleural effusion	+10

Prediction of Mortality from Pneumonia

CLASS	POINTS	MORTALITY, %	TREATMENT RECOMMENDATION
I	No predictors	0.1	Outpatient
II	<70	0.6	Outpatient
III	71–90	2.8	Inpatient (briefly)
IV	91–130	8.2	Inpatient
V	>130	29.2	Inpatient

a) Infants present with more severe illness

b) Summer and fall months

c) Neither active disease nor vaccination provides lifelong immunity

ii. Etiology

   a) *Bordetella pertussis* and > *B. parapertussis*

   b) Gram-negative pleomorphic bacilli

   c) Spread via aerosolized droplets

iii. Symptoms and signs: 3 stages, each lasting ~2 weeks

   a) Catarrhal

     i) Most infectious during this time

     ii) Symptoms indistinguishable from an upper respiratory infection (sneezing, coughing, rhinorrhea)

   b) Paroxysmal

     i) Coughing episodes followed by an inspiratory "whoop," caused by passage of air through a partially closed airway

     ii) Post-tussive exhaustion and emesis

   c) Convalescent

     i) Chronic cough that can last several months

     ii) Complications include mucous plug, secondary bacterial infection, ruptured diaphragm, hernia, and rectal prolapse

iv. Diagnosis

   a) Degree of lymphocytosis correlates with severity of disease

   b) Definitive diagnosis is made via nasopharyngeal culture on Regan-Lowe or Bordet-Gengou agar

   c) Culture results return in about 1 week

v. Treatment

   a) Erythromycin × 14 days

   b) Alternatively azithromycin or bactrim

   c) Consider prophylaxis with erythromycin for close contacts

   d) Consider hospitalization for infants <6 months; premature infants; and those with significant comorbidities

b. Mycoplasma pneumonia

  i. Most common atypical

  ii. 14-day incubation period

  iii. More common in young adults

  iv. Associations

   a) Bullous myringitis

   b) Meningitis and encephalitis

   c) Erythema multiforme

   d) Guillain-Barré

  v. CXR may show interstitial pattern or patchy infiltrate

vi. CXR classically looks worse than the patient

vii. Treat with macrolide antibiotic

c. Chlamydia pneumonia

  i. Obligate intracellular parasite

  ii. Infants

   a) Acquired at birth

   b) 50% conjunctivitis

   c) Tachypnea

   d) May be afebrile

   e) CXR shows hyperinflation and diffuse infiltrates

  iii. Common in young adults complaining of hoarseness, cough, and persistent malaise

  iv. Staccato cough

  v. Treat with macrolide

d. *Legionella* pneumonia

  i. Epidemiology

   a) Epidemics in summer and fall

  ii. Etiology

   a) Airborne and associated with water sources

   b) Classically associated with recent **air travel**

   c) Tourists contract *Legionella* in spas or saunas and spread it onboard a flight with limited ventilation

   d) No person-to-person transmission

  iii. Symptoms and signs

   a) Pleuritic chest pain

   b) Relative bradycardia

   c) Gastrointestinal symptoms prominent

  iv. Diagnosis

   a) Labs may reveal **hyponatremia** and hypophosphatemia

   b) CXR may show alveolar infiltrates or consolidation that may progress to hilar adenopathy and pleural effusion

   c) Predilection for lower lung fields

  v. Management

   a) Treat with erythromycin for 3 weeks

B. Tuberculosis (see Infectious Diseases chapter)

C. Viral pneumonia

  1. Types

   a. Influenza

    i. Epidemiology: epidemics occur in winter months with the immunocompromised (elderly and those with cardiopulmonary comorbidities) more at risk for complications

    ii. Often associated with bacterial superinfection (*S. aureus*)

    iii. Diagnosis: nasopharyngeal swab culture for influenza aid diagnosis

        a) CXR shows diffuse bilateral infiltrative

b. Varicella

    i. Symptoms and signs: pneumonia may present with chest pain and hemoptysis preceded by a rash

        a) More severe in adults

    ii. Management: mandates admission for treatment with acyclovir

c. Cytomegalovirus

    i. Epidemilogy: most common in solid organ transplant and bone marrow transplant recipients

        a) Often presents simultaneously with pneumocystis pneumonia

    ii. Symptoms and signs: fever, nonproductive cough and dyspnea

    iii. Diagnosis: CXR

        a) Bilateral interstitial pattern

        b) Uncommonly, a miliary pattern on CXR

    iv. Management: intravenous ganciclovir or foscarnet plus immunoglobulin therapy

d. Hantavirus

    i. Epidemiology: aerosolized contaminated material from rodent feces or urine

        a) Southwest United States

    ii. Symptoms and signs: flu-like symptoms that progress to respiratory distress and shock

    iii. Diagnosis: CXR reveals bilateral infiltrates

D. Fungal pneumonia

    1. Etiology: *Histoplasma capsulatum, Blastomyces dermatitides,* and *Coccidioides immitis* present in the soil in various geographic areas of the United States

    2. Epidemiology

      a. *Histoplasma capsulatum* in the Mississippi and Ohio River valleys

      b. *Blastomyces dermatitides* in a poorly defined area extending beyond that of *H. capsulatum*

      c. *Coccidioides immitis* in desert areas of the Southwest

    3. Symptoms and signs: vary from acute or chronic pneumonia to asymptomatic granulomas on CXR

    4. Diagnosis: hilar adenopathy

BIBLIOGRAPHY

Cunha BA: The atypical pneumonias: clinical diagnosis and importance. *Clin Microbiol Infect.* 2006 May;12Suppl 3:12.

Tintinalli JE, Kelen GD, Stapczynski JS, Ma OJ, Cline DM: *Emergency Medicine: A Comprehensive Study Guide.* 6th ed. New York, NY: McGraw-Hill Professional; 2003.

Ferguson GT, Cherniack RM: Management of chronic obstructive pulmonary disease. *N Engl J Med.* 1993 Apr; 8;328(14):1017.

Kollef MH, Schuster DP: The acute respiratory distress syndrome. *N Engl J Med.* 1995 Jan 5; 332(1): 27.

Light RW: Clinical practice. Pleural effusion. *N Engl J Med.* 2002 Jun 20; 346(25):1971.

Lutfiyya MN, Henley E, Chang LF: Diagnosis and treatment of community-acquired pneumonia. *Am Fam Physician.* 2006 Feb 1;73(3):442.

McFadden ER Jr, Hejal RB: The pathobiology of acute asthma. *Clin Chest Med.* 2000 Jun; 21;(2):213.

National Asthma Education and Prevention Program: Expert Panel Report 2: Guidelines for the diagnosis and management of asthma. NIH Publication No. 97-4051. Bethesda, MD: National Institutes of Health; 1997.

Niederman MS, Bass JB, Campbell GD: Guidelines for the initial management of adults with community-acquired pneumonia: diagnosis, assessment of severity, and initial antimicrobial therapy. American Thoracic Society. Medical Section of the American Lung Association. *Am Rev Respir Dis.* 1993 Nov; 148(5):1418

Papi A, Luppi F, Franco F: Pathophysiology of exacerbations of chronic obstructive pulmonary disease. *Proc Am Thorac Soc.* 2006 May; 3(3):245.

Ramzi DW, Leeper KV: DVT and pulmonary embolism. Diagnosis, treatment and prevention. *Am Fam Physician.* 2004 Jun 15;69(12):282.

Chapter 7
ENVIRONMENTAL EMERGENCIES

Susi Vassallo and Dimitrios Papanagnou

I. Submersion

A. Definitions
1. Drowning: asphyxiation caused by submersion in a liquid that causes interruption of the body's oxygen absorption
2. Near-drowning: a term formerly used to describe victim's survival at least 24 hours after submersion[1]
3. Fluid type: salt versus fresh water is no longer emphasized as degree of pulmonary insult is determined by quantity aspirated[2]

B. Epidemiology
1. 8000 deaths per year in the United States
   a. 20% to 25% are children

C. Pathophysiology
1. Wet drowning
   a. Aspiration of water into airways and lungs (85%)
      i. 1 to 3 cc of aspirated water will lead to destruction of surfactant, alveolar instability, noncardiogenic pulmonary edema, and impaired gas exchange
2. Dry drowning
   a. Severe parasympathetically mediated laryngospasm (15%)
3. Both types result in common pathway of hypoxia which leads to acidosis, cardiac arrest, and brain death

D. Risk factors
1. Drug and alcohol intoxication
2. Cardiac arrest
3. Hypoglycemia
4. Seizure
5. Suicidal or homicidal behavior
6. Child abuse

E. Symptoms and signs
1. Hypoxia
   a. Key factors predicting outcome are **duration** and **severity** of hypoxia

2. Vomiting
   a. 66% of victims who receive rescue breaths vomit
   b. 86% of victims who require chest compressions and ventilations vomit
3. Mental status changes, tachycardia, cardiac dysrhythmias, tachypnea, wheezing, pulmonary edema, cyanosis, apnea
4. Diving injuries
   a. Potential head or cervical spine injury must be considered

F. Diagnostic studies[3]
1. Arterial blood gas (ABG)—hypoxemia may be out of proportion to patient's clinical presentation
2. Electrolyte panel
3. Chest x-ray (CXR)

G. Management
1. Routine stabilization of cervical spine unnecessary unless
   a. History of diving
   b. Use of water slide
   c. Signs of injury
   d. Signs of alcohol intoxication
2. Rescue breathing
   a. No need to clear airway of aspirated water as it does not obstruct the trachea
      i. Heimlich maneuver or abdominal thrusts to remove water is **unnecessary**
3. Airway management
   a. Endotracheal intubation as necessary
   b. Noninvasive ventilatory support as necessary
   c. Serial ABGs traditionally used to guide need for ventilatory support

II. Extremes of Body Temperature

A. Thermoregulation
1. Definition: ability to maintain normal body temperature physiologic levels despite external environmental temperature

2. Mechanism
   a. Heat conservation
      i. Shivering, vasoconstriction, and piloerection
   b. Cooling
      i. Radiation (60%)
         a) Transfer of heat via electromagnetic waves from body to cooler air
         b) Greatest source of heat loss
      ii. Evaporation (30%)
         a) Heat loss by perspiration, breathing, saliva
         b) Acetylcholine regulates sweat glands and is impaired by anticholinergic drugs
      iii. Convection (8%)
         a) Transfer of heat from body to fluid, surrounding air or water vapor
         b) Wind or "wind chill" is an example
      iv. Conduction (2%)
         a) Direct transfer of heat via physical contact

B. Hypothermia
   1. Definition
      a. Normal: 97.7°F to 98.6°F (36.5°C to 37°C)
      b. Mild: 93.2°F to 96.8°F (34°C to 36°C)
      c. Moderate: 86°F to 93.2°F (30°C to 34°C)
      d. Severe: <86°F (<30°C)
   2. Etiology
      a. Environmental exposure
      b. Toxicologic—mnemonic **COOLS**
         i. **C**arbon monoxide, **o**ral hypoglycemics, **o**pioids, **l**iquors, **s**edatives (eg, benzodiazepines)
         ii. Alcohol intoxication may lead to impaired decision making and prolonged environmental exposure
      c. Systemic
         i. Sepsis, hypothyroid, hypoadrenalism, malnutrition, central nervous system (CNS) injury
   3. Symptoms and signs
      a. Mild hypothermia 93.2°F to 96.8°F (34°C to 36°C)
         i. Shivering
      b. Moderate hypothermia 86°F to 93.2°F (30°C to 34°C)
         i. Confusion
         ii. Poor judgment
         iii. Paradoxical undressing
            a) Prolonged vasoconstriction becomes overwhelmed and vasodilates, causing the skin to feel "hot"
         iv. Tachycardia and tachypnea
         v. Dilated pupils
         vi. "Shivering" reflex no longer present at 86°F (30°C)
         vii. Cold diuresis

   c. Severe hypothermia <86°F (<30°C)
      i. Bradycardia and slow atrial fibrillation
      ii. <82°F (<28°C)—patient may appear dead (unresponsive, fixed pupils, apneic)
         a) Asystole and ventricular fibrillation common
4. Complications
   a. Pancreatitis
   b. Acute tubular necrosis
   c. Rhabdomyolysis
   d. Disseminated intravascular coagulopathy (DIC)
   e. Acute respiratory distress syndrome
5. Diagnosis
   a. Temperature
      i. Rectal probe for continuous temperature monitoring
      ii. Warm patients to normal or near normal body temperature before declaring them dead
   b. Laboratory tests
      i. ABG
         a) Elevated pH
         b) PCO_2 decreased
      ii. Complete blood count (CBC)
         a) Hematocrit levels rise 2% for every 1°C drop in temperature
         b) False hemoconcentration such that a normal hematocrit could represent severe anemia
      iii. Coagulation profile prolonged
      iv. Evidence of DIC (low fibrinogen, elevated split products, abnormal coagulation profile)
      v. Creatinine kinase may be elevated with rhabdomyolysis
      vi. Amylase or lipase may be elevated with pancreatitis
   c. ECG: Osborn waves (Figure 7–1)
      i. Size of the wave correlates with degree of hypothermia
      ii. Usually resolves with rewarming
      iii. No prognostic value
6. Management[4]
   a. Rewarming methods
      i. All patients
         a) Remove wet and cold garments
         b) Cover with warm blanket
         c) Cardiac monitoring
         d) Handle gently as hypothermic heart is irritable and prone to unstable dysrhythmias
      ii. Rewarming techniques
         a) Passive rewarming
            i) Cover with blanket
         b) Active **external** rewarming
            i) Forced hot air, warming blanket
            ii) Rewarm trunk

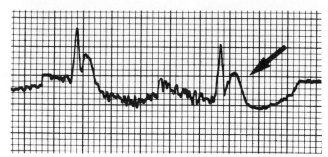

FIGURE 7–1. Osborn waves. The arrows in the above 12-lead ECG denote Osborn waves, extra deflections at end of QRS complex. (Reproduced, with permission, from Tintinalli JE, Kelen GD, Stapczynski JS: *Tintanelli's Emergency Medicine: A Comprehensive Study Guide,* 6th ed. Copyright © 2004, New York: McGraw-Hill.)

    c) Active **internal** rewarming
      i) Warm IV fluids to 115°F (45°C)
      ii) Warm humidified oxygen
      iii) Peritoneal lavage
      iv) Bladder lavage
      v) Extracorporeal rewarming
        a. Cardiopulmonary bypass
  iii. Prevent after-drop of core temperature
    a) Active rewarming of extremities leads to vasodilation and return of cold blood to core from periphery
    b) Potentially initiates or exacerbates dysrhythmias
  b. Stable patients
    i. Mild hypothermia 93.2°F to 96.8°F (34°C to 36°C)
    a) Passive rewarming
    b) Active external rewarming
    ii. Moderate hypothermia 86°F to 93.2°F (30°C to 34°C)
    a) Passive rewarming
    b) Active external rewarming
    iii. Severe hypothermia 86°F (<30°C)
    a) Passive and active external rewarming
    b) Active internal rewarming until core temperature >95°F (35°C)
  c. Unstable patients
    i. Start CPR
    ii. Defibrillate ventricular tachycardia and fibrillation
    iii. Intubation with warm humidified oxygen
    iv. Warm IV fluids
    v. Mild or moderate hypothermia
    a) As per ACLS protocol
    vi. Severe hypothermia
    a) Withhold IV medications
    b) Active internal rewarming

  d. Advanced cardiac life support (ACLS) in the hypothermic patient
    i. The cornerstone of ACLS in the severely hypothermic patient is active rewarming
    ii. Hypothermic bradycardia is not caused by increased vagal tone but rather slowing of automaticity, and unlikely to respond to atropine
    iii. Medications ineffective until patient is 82°F (>28°C) and may accumulate to toxic levels if given indiscriminately
    iv. Current 2005 ACLS recommendations for defibrillation
    a) 86°F to 88°F (30°C to 32°C): defibrillate once, then resume CPR and rewarming
    b) No additional attempts to defibrillate should be made until the patient is >86°F to 88° F (30°C to 32°C)

C. Hyperthermia
  1. Epidemiology
    a. The elderly, very young, or chronically ill are most vulnerable to hyperthermia
    b. Exertional heat stroke is the second leading cause of sports-related mortality (secondly only to spinal cord injuries)
  2. Etiology
    a. Loss of radiation
      i. Radiation account for 60% of heat loss
      ii. Radiation of heat becomes less efficient with increasing ambient temperature
      iii. Ceases when ambient temperature ≥body temperature
    b. Inefficient evaporation
      i. Normally accounts for 30% of heat loss
      ii. Less efficient with increasing ambient humidity
      iii. Ceases when humidity approaches 100%
      iv. Lack of acclimatization (individual not used to hot climate) results in inefficient perspiration until days 7 to 10
      v. Impaired sweating
      a) Anticholinergics
      b) Skin disorders—scleroderma, psoriasis, burns
      c) Autonomic disorders—diabetes
    c. Toxicologic
      i. Sympathomimetics (amphetamine, cocaine)
      ii. Neuroleptic malignant syndrome, serotonin syndrome, malignant hyperthermia
      iii. Anticholinergics
      iv. Salicylate poisoning
    d. Systemic conditions
      i. Hyperthyroid, infection, pheochromocytoma

3. Symptoms and signs
   a. Continuum of illness ranging from heat cramps and heat exhaustion to heat stroke
   b. Heat cramps
      i. Etiology: inadequate intake of fluids and electrolytes
      ii. Symptoms and signs: muscle cramping usually affecting the calves and abdomen
   c. Heat exhaustion
      i. Nonspecific weakness, headache, nausea and vomiting caused by dehydration
      ii. Temperature <106°F (41°C) or normal
   d. Heat stroke
      i. Temperature >106°F (41°C)
      ii. Organ damage (Table 7–1)
      iii. Mental status change (irritability to coma)
         a) Presence of CNS dysfunction differentiates head exhaustion from heat stroke
      iv. Anhidrosis (not universal)
4. Complications
   a. Rhabdomyolysis
   b. Compartment syndrome
   c. Liver failure
   d. Seizure
   e. Dysrhythmias
   f. Pulmonary edema and acute respiratory distress syndrome (ARDS)
   g. Acute renal failure
   h. DIC
5. Diagnosis
   a. Laboratory testing
      i. CBC, CPK, glucose, BUN/creatinine, and LFTs
         a) Hypoglycemia is a common occurrence
         b) Abnormal liver function tests almost universal with heat stroke
   b. CXR to rule out pulmonary edema
   c. Head CT and lumbar puncture may be required to differentiate encephalitis/meningitis from heat stroke
6. Management
   a. Hydration, but excessive fluids should be avoided to avoid pulmonary edema
   b. Rapid cooling
      i. Temperature 106°F (>41°C) requires immediate management
      ii. Cool to a target of 102°F (39°C) within 10 to 20 minutes
   c. Mechanical cooling
      i. Remove clothing
      ii. Cool mist and fan (augments heat transfer via convection, radiation, and evaporation)
      iii. Ice water immersion advocated by some
   d. Pharmacologic
      i. Antipyretics (NSAIDs and acetaminophen) have **no** role in environmental heatstroke
         a) Acetaminophen may be harmful with fulminant liver failure
      ii. Benzodiazepines to manage agitation and shivering

III. Thermal Injuries

A. Frostbite
   1. Definition
      a. Frostbite: tissue injury due to prolonged exposure to below freezing temperatures (<32°F, 0°C)

TABLE 7–1. Clinical Effects of Heat Stroke

Systemic inflammatory response	Inflammatory mediators (ie, leukotrienes) released, triggering inflammatory cascade
Cardiac	Nonspecific electrocardiographic changes
	Myocardial enzyme elevations possible
Neurologic	Mental status alteration
	Outcome related to time with elevated temperature
	Permanent cerebellar injury may result
Renal	Acute renal failure in 10%
	Injury is secondary to myoglobinuria, direct injury to tubules, and volume depletion
Skeletal muscle	Rhabdomyolysis
	Elevated CPK
	Hyperkalemia when myocytes destroyed
	Hypocalcemia
Gastrointestinal	Vomiting
	Diarrhea
Coagulation	Direct injury to clotting factors
	Disseminated intravascular coagulation (DIC)
	Acute liver injury, often delayed
	Thrombocytopenia

2. Differential
   a. Frost nip: mild, reversible superficial cold injury without tissue destruction or crystal formation
   b. Trench foot: prolonged **wet,** cold but nonfreezing exposure causing reversible neurovascular injury
   c. Chilblain (pernio): skin injury consisting of painful edema, erythema, and plaques caused by repeated **dry,** cold but nonfreezing exposure
3. Pathophysiology
   a. Vasoconstriction leads to decreased delivery of warm blood to extremities and formation of ice crystals in tissue
   b. Leads to sludging at capillary level and microvascular thrombosis [5]
   c. Reperfusion injury occurs when frozen tissue thaws
4. Symptoms and signs
   a. Numbness followed by anesthesia is suggestive of frostbite
   b. First-degree frostbite
      i. Definition injury is confined to the epidermis (cornified epithelial cells)
      ii. Symptoms and signs: erythema and edema
   c. Second-degree frostbite
      i. Definition: injury to epidermis and dermis (middle layer containing capillaries, nerve endings, hair follicles)
      ii. Symptoms and signs: hard edema and clear blisters
   d. Third-degree (full thickness) frostbite
      i. Definition: injury through and involving the hypodermis (connective tissue and adipose connecting dermis to underlying structures)
      ii. Symptoms and signs: hemorrhagic bullae, pale grey extremity
         a) Severe pain with rewarming
   e. Fourth-degree frostbite
      i. Definition: injury through to and involving the skin, muscles, tendons, bones
         a) Painless during rewarming
5. Management
   a. Rewarming
      i. Thawing in warm water 104°F to 108°F (40°C to 42°C)
      ii. Do not use dry heat such as a hair dryer
      iii. Do not rewarm if risk of refreezing exists as subsequent injuries worsen prognosis
      iv. Thawing requires 20 to 40 minutes for superficial injuries and up to 1 to 2 hours for deep injuries (third- and fourth-degree frostbite)
      v. Inadequate thawing often due to early stoppage because of inadequate analgesia
      vi. Endpoint of thawing is a warm and soft extremity
   b. Wound care
      i. Unroof clear blisters rich in injurious thromboxane
      ii. Do not unroof hemorrhagic blisters
      iii. Topical aloe vera over all affected areas
      iv. Update tetanus status
      v. Antibiotics if infection or penetrating wound
   c. Consultation with surgery since tissue requires 6 to 8 weeks to determine need for amputation

B. Thermal burns
   1. Classification (Table 7-2)
   2. Diagnosis
      a. Carbon monoxide levels for all patients involved in a fire
      b. Cyanide toxicity should be suspected in industrial fires

TABLE 7–2.   Classification of Burn Depth and Physical Findings

DEGREE OF BURN	THICKNESS	EXAMINATION
First	Epithelial damage of epidermis	Erythema, tenderness, pain Sunburn No blisters
Second	Epidermis and dermis Superficial partial thickness Deep partial thickness	Very painful unless deep second-degree burn Skin is red and blanches with pressure Blisters, which usually rupture Deep second-degree burn can transform into third-degree burn if not promptly cared for
Third	All skin layers Full thickness	Pale, leathery appearance Insensate secondary to destruction of nerve endings and blood supply
Fourth	Full thickness destruction of skin, as well as of underlying fascia, tendon, muscle, bone	Correlated to the severity and the extent of involvement of underlying subcutaneous tissue

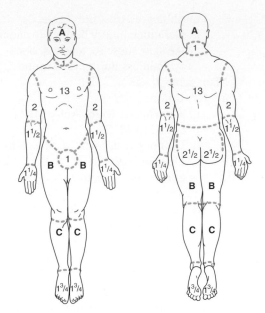

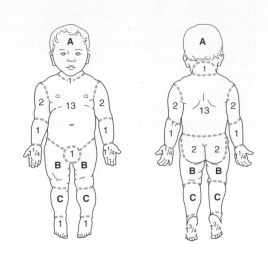

Relative Percentages of Areas Affected by Growth

	Age		
Area	**10**	**15**	**Adult**
A = half of head	5 $\frac{1}{2}$	4 $\frac{1}{2}$	3 $\frac{1}{2}$
B = half of one thigh	4 $\frac{1}{4}$	4 $\frac{1}{2}$	4 $\frac{3}{4}$
C = half of one leg	3	3 $\frac{1}{4}$	3 $\frac{1}{2}$

Relative Percentages of Areas Affected by Growth

	Age		
Area	**0**	**1**	**5**
A = half of head	9 $\frac{1}{2}$	8 $\frac{1}{2}$	6 $\frac{1}{2}$
B = half of one thigh	2 $\frac{3}{4}$	3 $\frac{1}{4}$	4
C = half of one leg	2 $\frac{1}{2}$	2 $\frac{1}{2}$	2 $\frac{3}{4}$

FIGURE 7–2. The rule of nines. (Reproduced, with permission, from Doherty GM, Way LW: *Current Surgical Diagnosis and Treatment,* 12th ed. Copyright © 2006, New York: McGraw-Hill.)

    i. Sources of cyanide include insecticides, internal combustion engines, tobacco smoke, plastics made from acrylonitrite

  c. Estimation of body surface area (BSA) involved

    i. Rule of nines (Figure 7–2)

      a) Pediatric version: patient's palmar surface is 1% of BSA

      b) Note that the head is the highest percentage in pediatric patients

3. Management

  a. First-degree burns do not require more than simple analgesia

  b. Fluid management

    i. Parkland formula: 4 mL/kg × % total BSA burned (in pediatrics give 3 mL/kg)

      a) 50% given in the first 8 hours and remainder over 16 hours

      b) Ringer lactate is preferred IV fluid [6]

    ii. Maintain urine output at a minimum of 1 mL/kg/h

  c. Wound management

    i. Blisters should be left intact (controversial)

    ii. Apply silver sulfadiazine or triple antibiotic ointments to burned areas

    iii. Deep burns require sterile management

    iv. Silver sulfadiazine should not be used on cartilaginous areas (eg, nose, ears) because of dark silver staining

    v. Open wounds should be covered with sterile saline-soaked gauze as there is an increased risk of infection

    vi. Update tetanus status

  d. Consider escharotomy for circumferential and full-thickness burns

    i. Circumferential full thickness burns may cause vascular insufficiency in limbs and digits

    ii. Circumferential full thickness burns involving the chest may cause respiratory compromise

  e. Consider securing airway if inhalation injury suspected

    i. Suspect inhalation injury if:

      a) Sore throat and dyspnea

      b) Stridor with airway edema

      c) Soot or burns to the nasopharynx

      d) Singed facial or nasal hair

      e) Carbonaceous sputum

    ii. Patient's airway can unexpectedly and suddenly obstruct secondary to edema

iii. Strongly consider prophylactic intubation as it is difficult to predict which patients will deteriorate

iv. Consider fiberoptic laryngoscopy in patients with low suspicion for significant inhalation injury

f. Transfer to burn center if [5]

i. >10% BSA of partial thickness degree burns

ii. Third-degree burn (guidelines do not specify BSA)

iii. Second- or third-degree burns of hands, feet, genitalia, perineum, or over joints

iv. Electrical, chemical, or inhalation injury

v. Significant comorbid conditions

IV. Electrical Injuries

A. Definitions
1. Direct current (DC)
   a. Current of electrons flows in one direction
   b. Examples of DC power sources include simple batteries
2. Alternating current (AC)
   a. Current of electrons flows in a back-and-forth direction
   b. Unlike DC, the magnitude and direction of AC has a frequency (60 Hz)
   c. Household outlets provide AC power
   d. In general, **more dangerous** than DC
3. High voltage
   a. Defined in terms of patient care and disposition as anything >500 V
   b. Household outlets typically provide 110 V, and occasionally 220 V for larger appliances such as washers and dryers
   c. High-voltage current can "arc" several feet through air

B. Mechanism of injury
1. Thermal injury
   a. Heat generated by resistance to current causes internal burns and edema
   b. Nerves and muscles have least resistance while bone and fat have the highest resistance
2. Mechanical injury
   a. Contractions of muscles can result in fractures and dislocations
   b. Electrical injuries associated with trauma (eg, fall from ladder while installing light fixture)
3. Disruption of depolarization
   a. Pathway of current through brain can cause seizures
   b. Current traversing the chest can lead to arrhythmias

4. Degree of injury directly related to voltage **and** duration of exposure (eg, "static shock" consisting of 5 to 10000 V over a split second is benign, while prolonged exposure to household outlets powered with 110 V can be dangerous)

C. Symptoms and signs
1. Cutaneous
   a. Skin burns (arc burns, flashover)
   b. Entry and exit wounds
   c. "Kissing burns" as tetanic contractions cause opposition of skin creases (eg, burn as hand grips live wire)
2. Musculoskeletal
   a. DC
      i. Single powerful muscle spasm can cause fractures
         a) DC more likely than AC to result in traumatic **fractures** as patient is thrown from source
   b. AC
      i. Causes sustained contractions (typical household is transmitted at 60 Hz resulting in 60 cycles per second of contractions)
      ii. Flexor muscles are more powerful than extensors—causes patient to draw himself closer to electrical source thus prolonging the contact
      iii. Internal rotators are more powerful than external rotators—may cause **posterior shoulder dislocations**
3. Vascular
   a. Venous thrombosis
      i. Venous injury more common as flow is slower than arterial and therefore less able to dissipate heat
   b. Delayed arterial thrombosis
      i. May be difficult to clinically differentiate from compartment syndrome
      ii. Mesenteric artery thrombosis
4. CNS
   a. Seizures
   b. Loss of consciousness and amnesia
   c. Median nerve injury common
   d. Autonomic dysfunction
      i. Do not cease resuscitation based solely on fixed and dilated pupils
5. Cardiac
   a. DC injury can cause asystole
   b. AC injury can cause ventricular fibrillation

D. Complications
1. Compartment syndrome
2. Cataracts
3. Rhabdomyolysis

4. Labial artery bleeding in child who bites electrical cord (see Pediatrics chapter)
5. Depression
6. Delayed neurologic symptoms mimicking amyotrophic lateral sclerosis (ALS) and transverse myelitis
7. Delayed lower extremity weakness

E. Diagnosis
   1. ECG
   2. Laboratory testing (CPK, chemistry panel, cardiac enzymes)
   3. Urinalysis for myoglobin
   4. Imaging as indicated to assess trauma
   5. Compartment pressure measurements as indicated

F. Management
   1. Cardiac monitoring
   2. Fluid management
      a. Difficult to assess degree of volume loss as majority of injury is unseen
      b. Keep urine output at 1 cc/kg/h
      c. Urine alkalinization and diuretics may benefit myoglobinuria and prevent renal failure
   3. Fasciotomy or carpal tunnel release if necessary
   4. Disposition
      a. Admit if:
         i. Abnormal ECG
         ii. Loss of consciousness
         iii. Admit all patients with path of current potentially traversing the heart
         iv. Admit all high-voltage (>500 V) injuries regardless of path of current
         v. Transfer significant electrical injuries to a burn center
      b. Discharge
         i. After 6-hour monitoring for most low-voltage injuries without loss of consciousness

V. Lightning Injury

A. Definition
   1. Neither AC or DC
   2. Massive "unidirectional current"

B. Epidemiology
   1. Mortality rate from lightning injuries 30%
   2. Up to 70% of survivors sustain significant morbidity

C. Symptoms and signs
   1. Flashover burns are common with lightning, although patients may sustain various types of burns after a lightning exposure

      a. Electricity passes over body
      b. **Ferning** pattern or Lichtenberg sign
   2. Deep thermal tissue damage uncommon and therefore, myoglobinuria, rhabdomyolysis, and renal failure uncommon
   3. Patients may be thrown significant distances from single powerful muscle contractions causing traumatic injury from falls
   4. Shock wave from rapid expansion and contraction of superheated air causes trauma and **tympanic membrane** rupture (>50%)
   5. Cataract formation within days of injury is common
   6. Most common complications are related to depolarization abnormalities such as loss of consciousness, seizures, and cardiac arrhythmias
   7. Death caused by ventricular fibrillation or asystole

D. Management
   1. Management for lightning injuries distinct from that indicated for typical high-voltage injuries
      a. Massive fluid boluses and urine alkalinization not required as internal tissue necrosis occurs infrequently
   2. Good prognosis if there is no respiratory or cardiac arrest
   3. Unlike the management of most mass casualty events, the highest **priority** should be given to those in cardiac and respiratory arrest who would otherwise be "black tagged"
   4. Continue resuscitation even if victims appear dead as patients may be unresponsive and pupil fixed and dilated
   5. Use autonomic external defibrillator to restore rhythm

VI. High-Altitude Illness

A. Acute mountain sickness (AMS)
   1. Etiology
      a. Caused by hypoxia
      b. Decreased oxygen pressure increases cerebral blood flow causing cerebral edema
   2. Symptoms and signs
      a. Headache
      b. Nausea and vomiting
      c. Insomnia
      d. Decreased urination
      e. Peripheral or facial edema
      f. Retinal hemorrhage (uncommon)
   3. Management
      a. Halt ascent
      b. Acetazolamide (diamox) aids acclimatization
         i. Carbonic anhydrase inhibitor

ii. Taken 12 to 24 hours before ascent as prophylaxis for unavoidable rapid ascent (not routinely recommended)

iii. Bicarbonate diuresis (metabolic acidosis) stimulates compensatory ventilation

iv. Acetazolamide contraindicated in sickle cell patients and patients with sulfa allergies

c. Steroids alleviate symptoms by decreasing brain edema

d. Descent for refractory cases

B. High-altitude cerebral edema (HACE)

1. Symptoms and signs

a. Global cerebral dysfunction; most severe manifestation of AMS

b. Ataxia, confusion, altered mental status

c. Retinal hemorrhages common

d. Death usually secondary to brain-stem herniation

e. All patients with AMS should be observed for ataxia, which is an early sign of HACE

2. Management

a. Descent

b. Oxygen

c. Acetazolamide (Diamox)

d. Steroids

e. Portable hyperbaric chamber if descent not possible

C. High-altitude pulmonary edema (HAPE)

1. Epidemiology

a. Most common cause of death from high-altitude illness

2. Etiology

a. Hypoxia-induced pulmonary vasoconstriction

3. Symptoms and signs

a. Occurs a few days after ascent

b. Symptoms worse in the evening

c. Cough, decreased exercise tolerance

d. Low-grade fever

e. Tachypnea, tachycardia

f. Rales, rhonchi

4. Management

a. Immediate descent

b. Oxygen

c. Calcium channel blockers (eg, nifedipine)

d. Acetazolamide **not** useful in the acute management of HAPE but may be useful for prophylaxis

e. Portable hyperbaric chamber if descent not possible

VII. Diving Dysbarism

A. Definition

1. Pathology related to the increases and decreases of external pressure on the human body

B. Pathophysiology

1. Pressure and volume changes as a function of depth

2. Boyle law: pressure × volume = k (constant)

a. At a set temperature, pressure and volume are inversely related (ie, if pressure doubles, volume halves)

b. Law governs all gases under pressure

3. Atmospheric pressure roughly doubles every 33 ft underwater

4. Clinical scenarios involve pressure changes caused by diving or air flight

C. Systems most commonly effected

1. HEENT

a. Middle ear

i. Most commonly affected organ due to eustachian tube dysfunction

ii. Eustachian tube functions to equalize pressures in middle ear to external environment

iii. On descent, patients with eustachian tube dysfunction can develop pain, hematoma, tympanic rupture, and vertigo

iv. On ascent, rapidly expanding air causes outward pressure on the tympanic membrane resulting in similar symptoms and signs

v. Treat with decongestants

b. Inner ear

i. Rapid ascent may cause rupture of **round window**

ii. May result in sudden hearing loss, vertigo, and tinnitus

iii. Requires ENT consultation and surgical repair

c. Sinus squeeze

i. Frontal sinus most commonly affected

ii. Normally, sinuses drain into nasal cavity via small openings called ostia

iii. Inflammation or blockage of ostia because of allergies or upper respiratory infections cause problems

iv. On descent, air in sinuses contract and place negative pressure on sinus mucosa, leading to edema, hemorrhage, and pain

v. On ascent, expanding gas places pressure on noncompressible and nonexpandable sinuses

vi. Treat with decongestants, steroids, and antibiotics if infected

d. Dental pain

i. Trapped air in cavity fillings may cause severe dental pain on descent and ascent

2. Pulmonary

a. Volume of air equalized by inhaling or exhaling as necessary

b. Complications of rapid descent
   i. Hemoptysis (rare)
c. Complications of rapid ascent
   i. Caused by failure to adequately exhale during ascent
      a) Lung volume doubles every 33 ft and needs to be exhaled to avoid injury
      b) Inexperienced divers mistakenly hold their breath during ascent in order to conserve oxygen
   ii. Pneumothorax, pneumomediastinum, subcutaneous emphysema
   iii. Hypotension may result from tension pneumothorax
   iv. Arterial gas embolism (see Air Embolism below)
d. Management
   i. Care for underlying pneumothorax
   ii. Hyperbaric treatment

D. Air embolism
1. Rupture of air or nitrogen into pulmonary vein may lead to systemic microgas emboli as it bypasses filtration of the lungs or via atrial septal heart defects
2. Suspect in any diver who comes up unconscious
3. Pulmonary air embolus may present with pulmonary embolism like symptoms and signs (dyspnea, hemoptysis, chest pain)
4. Air embolus into coronary artery can cause myocardial infarction
5. Air embolus to brain can cause stroke like symptoms
6. Requires **immediate** hyperbaric treatment and supportive care

E. Decompression sickness
1. Definition
   a. Dysbarism due to the reformation of dissolved nitrogen into gas bubbles in tissue (brain, lungs, muscle, skin, etc.)
2. Pathophysiology
   a. During descent, oxygen and nitrogen is compressed as per Boyle law
      i. Example: at 33 ft or 2 atm of pressure, twice as many oxygen and nitrogen particles exist in the same volume in comparison with sea level atmosphere
   b. Oxygen continues to be consumed by the body while nitrogen accumulates in body
   c. During ascent, nitrogen bubbles form in tissue, joints, and lungs that obstruct vessels
3. Risk factors
   a. Increasing depth of dive and rapidity of ascent
   b. Multiple dives within same day (nitrogen lasts 12 hours in the body)
   c. Air flight soon after dive
   d. Obesity (nitrogen is fat soluble)
   e. Older age, poor conditioning, strenuous exertion under water
4. Symptoms and signs
   a. Onset usually within 6 hours
   b. Musculoskeletal
      i. "The bends": joint pain
   c. Pulmonary
      i. "The chokes": dyspnea, chest pain, and cough
   d. Neurologic
      i. "The staggers": vertigo, hearing loss, and nausea resulting from inner ear involvement
      ii. Spinal cord: "pins and needles" sensation
      iii. Cerebral: visual disturbances and headache
   e. Dermatologic
      i. "Skin bends": pruritis and burning of skin
      ii. Mottling: purpura marmorata
      iii. Erysipelas-like rash over fatty areas
5. Diagnosis
   a. Clinical diagnosis
   b. Severe decompression illness and arterial gas embolism (AGE) may be difficult to differentiate
      i. AGE presents suddenly within 10 to 20 minutes of ascent
      ii. AGE affects only the brain and spares the spinal cord unlike decompression illness
      iii. AGE can occur with short and shallow dives while long and deep dives can cause decompression injury
6. Management
   a. Administer 100% oxygen
   b. IV hydration
   c. Aspirin if not bleeding
   d. "Recompression" with hyperbaric treatment for any but the mildest symptoms (pain or rash only)
   e. Prevention
      i. Slows ascent with "stops"
      ii. Limit depth or time of dives
      iii. No flying for 12 to 24 hours

F. Breathing gases under high pressure
1. Pathophysiology
   a. Breathing oxygen or nitrogen at high partial pressures is neurotoxic
2. Oxygen toxicity
   a. Risk begins at ~200 ft
   b. Tingling, focal seizures
   c. Vertigo, nausea, and vomiting
   d. Loss of consciousness can result in drowning
3. Nitrogen narcosis—"rapture of the deep"
   a. Risk begins at 100 ft and incapacitation at 300 ft

b. Resembles alcohol intoxication
  i. Euphoria
  ii. Poor judgment—failure to ascend
4. Prevention
  a. Deep divers use special gas mixtures lower in oxygen and mixed with either helium or hydrogen instead of nitrogen
5. Management
  a. Ascent
  b. Condition is rapidly reversible

VIII. Radiation Injuries

A. Definition: energy emitted from higher energy state to lower energy state in the form of atomic particles or waves

B. Ionizing versus nonionizing radiation
  1. Ionizing
    a. Energy created from particles released from unstable atoms as they decay to a more stable state
    b. Able to break chemical bonds and form ion pairs
    c. Causes cellular injury by cleaving DNA strands and producing free radicals
    d. Most clinically significant type of radiation by inducing genetic mutations and inducing cancer
    e. May be in the form of electromagnetic radiation or particulate radiation
  2. Nonionizing
    a. All forms of electromagnetic radiation, except high-energy ultraviolet, x-ray, and gamma ray radiation
    b. Includes (in increasing energy) radio wave, microwave, infrared visible light and low-energy ultraviolet radiation
    c. Can cause thermal burns

C. Electromagnetic versus particulate radiation
  1. Electromagnetic radiation
    a. Self-propagating waves of energy with an electric and magnetic component
    b. May be ionizing or nonionizing
      i. Ionizing electromagnetic radiation includes ultraviolet (UV) rays, x-rays, and gamma rays
    c. UV radiation
      i. Wavelength just below visible light
        a) High-frequency UV is ionizing while low-frequency is nonionizing
    d. X-ray
      i. High-energy, high-penetration waves
      ii. Created by the sudden deceleration of electrons or when electrons transition between atomic energy levels

    e. Gamma
      i. Gamma rays come from the radioactive decay of an atom's nucleus
  2. Particulate radiation—have mass and kinetic energy
    a. Alpha
      i. Consists of 2 neutrons and 2 protons
      ii. Low penetrating
        a) Cannot penetrate skin
      iii. Dangerous if internalized (ie, if ingested or inhaled) as they decay when trapped inside the body
    b. Beta
      i. High-energy electrons
      ii. More penetrating than alpha particles
        a) Can penetrate skin and cause burns
      iii. Heavy clothing can prevent penetration
      iv. Internalization is dangerous
    c. Neutrons
      i. Usually arise from nuclear explosions
      ii. Very damaging to tissue
      iii. Primary product known as "nuclear fallout"
      iv. Penetrate tissue due to lack of electrical charge
      v. Cause radioactivity as they penetrate and become absorbed by other nuclei

D. Symptoms and signs
  1. Early vomiting correlates with radiation exposure
    a. 1 Gray (Gy) = 100 rads
    b. LD 50/30 (lethal dose causing 50% mortality at 30 days is 4.5 Gy)
    c. No documented survival with >10 Gy exposure
  2. Dermatologic
    a. Localized exposure results in cutaneous burns
    b. Delayed blistering and peeling weeks later
  3. Hematopoietic syndrome (2 to 5 Gy exposure)
    a. Destruction of bone marrow
    b. Pancytopenia resulting in anemia, bleeding, and infections
  4. Gastrointestinal syndrome (5 to 12 Gy exposure)
    a. Prodrome of nausea, vomiting, and diarrhea
    b. Symptoms worsen after 1 week with dehydration, bloody diarrhea, and sepsis
    c. Death typically within 3 to 10 days
  5. CNS syndrome (with massive exposure)
    a. Nausea, vomiting, ataxia
    b. Seizures, mental status change
    c. Rapid death within hours to days

E. Diagnosis
  1. CBC
    a. Lymphocyte count at 48 hours is prognostic
    b. Good prognosis if >1500/mm^3
    c. Poor prognosis if <1500/mm^3

F. Management
  1. Decontamination
     a. Removal of clothing, showers, soap and water, etc.
  2. Blocking agents to reduce amount of radiation absorbed
     a. Potassium iodide as quickly as possible to prevent absorption by the thyroid gland
     b. Close wound early to decrease infection in those exposed to higher dose of whole-body radiation
  3. Supportive care
     a. IV fluids
     b. Antiemetics
     c. Leukocyte poor blood transfusion if necessary
     d. Antibiotics and antivirals if neutropenic

IX. Animal Bites

A. Human
  1. Etiology
     a. Direct bite (fingers, ears, scalp)
     b. "Fight bite"
  2. Symptoms and signs
     a. "Fight bite": laceration over the knuckle (metacarpophalangeal joint) due to contact with teeth
  3. Diagnosis
     a. Radiograph
        i. Film of closed fist injuries as fractures may require inpatient antibiotics (open fracture)
        ii. Rule out foreign body (tooth)
  4. Management
     a. Fight bites
        i. Wound irrigation and exploration in full range of motion particularly in clenched-fist position
        ii. Admit all infected fight bites
        iii. Consider admitting uninfected fight bites or ensure close follow-up
        iv. **Antibiotics** for all wounds with or without infection
     b. Treat infections
        i. Cover skin flora, particularly *Staphylococcus, Streptococcus,* and oral flora, particularly anaerobes (eg, *Eikenella corrodens*)
        ii. Amoxicillin/clavulanate is recommended
        iii. Options include either clindamycin or erythromycin **plus** dicloxicillin, cephalexin, or cefuroxime
        iv. Wounds on extremities should **not** undergo primary repair; they can be closed by secondary intention or delayed primary closure
     c. Communicable diseases
        i. Consider prophylaxis if contact with saliva mixed with blood

B. Cat and dog bites
  1. Pathophysiology
     a. Dogs and large animals have powerful jaws that cause **crush** injuries
        i. Impressive wounds.
        ii. Underlying fractures common
        iii. Underlying muscle, tendon, nerve injury common
     b. Cats and smaller animals cause **puncture** injuries
        i. Wounds appear benign
        ii. Puncture wounds are at a higher risk for infection[7]
  2. Infection (in decreasing order of frequency)
     a. Dogs
        i. *Staphylococcus, Streptococcus, Eikenella, Pasteurella*
     b. Cats
        i. ***Pasteurella,*** *Actinomyces, Bacteroides, Fusobacterium*
        ii. Infection rates 50% to 80% with cat bites
  3. Management
     a. Treat underlying wound, fracture, nerve injury
        i. Careful neurovascular examination
        ii. Tendon evaluation
     b. Be wary of dog bites to the head of young children
        i. Neurosurgery consultation and admission if skull penetration suspected
     c. Update tetanus status
     d. Assess for risk for rabies; reporting per state regulations (see Infectious Disease section)
     e. Antibiotics
        i. Most cat bites should be treated with antibiotics
        ii. Antibiotics for dog bites on a case-by-case basis
        iii. Regimens
           a) Amoxicillin/clavulanate
           b) Clindamycin and ciprofloxacin
           c) Clindamycin and bactrim

X. Snake Envenomations

A. 25 poisonous species of 2 major families (Viperidae and Elapidae) are native to North America

B. Viperidae family (subfamily crotalids or pit vipers) include rattlers, cottonmouths, copperheads, and the western diamondbacks
  1. Epidemiology
     a. 98% of all envenomations in United States
  2. Identification
     a. Triangular-shaped head
     b. Nostril pits (heat-sensing organ) anteroinferior to eye

    c. Elliptical pupils
    d. Single row of plates at distal tail
  3. Symptoms and signs
    a. Most bites are "dry"
    b. Systemic effects
       i. Weakness, paresthesias
      ii. Metallic taste
     iii. Chest pain, dyspnea
    c. Local effects
       i. Very painful
      ii. Edema, erythema, bullae
     iii. Rhabdomyolysis
     iv. Compartment syndrome
    d. Hematologic consequences
       i. Coagulopathy, thrombocytopenia, bleeding
  4. Diagnosis
    a. CBC, coagulation studies, urinalysis
    b. CPK to exclude rhabdomyolysis
    c. Compartment pressure measurement
    d. Radiographs to rule out foreign body (fangs)
  5. Management
    a. Antivenin
       i. Crotalidae polyvalent immune Fab (CroFab)
         a) Sheep product with few allergic manifestations
         b) Administer to most patients as allergic reactions are uncommon
      ii. Antivenin (Crotalidae) polyvalent
         a) Older formulation from horse serum
         b) Greater risk of anaphylaxis and serum sickness (type III hypersensitivity reaction) in comparison with CroFab
         c) Administer only for moderate to severe envenomations
    b. Consider fasciotomy for compartment syndrome
    c. Disposition
       i. Observe "dry bites" for 8 hours prior to discharge with good instructions
      ii. Admit all true envenomations

C. Elapidae family includes coral snakes, cobras, and mambas (only coral snakes native to United States)
  1. Identification of coral snakes
    a. Round pupils
    b. Double row of plates at distal tail
    c. Brightly colored
       i. Axiom identifies poisonous snake: "black on yellow kill a fellow, red on black venom lack"
      ii. Applies only to **domestic** coral snake as many individuals illegally obtain exotic snakes as pets
  2. Symptoms and signs
    a. Delayed symptoms for up to 13 hours
       i. Patient may look deceptively well early on

    b. Local symptoms
       i. Unlike pit viper envenomations, pain and edema may be limited
    c. **Neurotoxicity** predominates
       i. Blurred vision, ophthalmoplegia, ptosis, fasciculations, paresthesias, and hypersalivation
      ii. Late symptoms: paralysis of face, palate, jaws, vocal cords
    d. Respiratory failure from neuromuscular blockade
  3. Management
    a. Do not underestimate degree of envenomation because of lack of initial symptoms
    b. All Eastern and Texas coral snake bites should be treated with antivenin
       i. Micrurus fulvius antivenin
      ii. Completely reversible with antivenin
    c. Admit all coral snake bites

XI. Spiders: Black Widow and Brown Recluse

A. Black widow (*Lactrodectus mactans*)
  1. Identification
    a. Red hourglass shape on ventral abdomen (memory jog: It was just a matter of *time* before she killed him)
  2. Symptoms and signs
    a. Systemic
       i. Autonomic instability
      ii. Hypertension and tachycardia
     iii. Nausea, vomiting
    b. Neurologic
       i. Muscle cramps
      ii. Severe abdomen pain (rigid abdomen mimicking surgical pathology)
     iii. Fasiculations
     iv. Ptosis
      v. Headache
  3. Management
    a. Most managed with supportive care alone
       i. Analgesia
      ii. Treat cramps with benzodiazepines
     iii. Intravenous calcium discouraged
    b. Antivenin only for severe symptoms
       i. Horse-derived
      ii. Anaphylaxis and serum sickness may occur

B. Brown recluse (fiddlestick spider) (*Loxosceles recluse*)
  1. Identification
    a. Violin-shaped markings on back (memory jog: The lonely recluse played sad violin music)
  2. Symptoms and signs
    a. May cause fever, chills, malaise, and hemolysis
    b. "Bull's eye" lesion: red and white, with a necrotic center

    c. Cutaneous manifestation may become quite severe requiring plastic surgery consultation

    d. Rarely, hemolysis and renal failure result in mortality

  3. Diagnosis

    a. Check labs for systemic loxoscelism (rare)

      i. Hemolysis, renal failure, and DIC

      ii. CBC, metabolic panel, coagulation studies

  4. Management

    a. Consider anthrax in the differential

    b. Local wound care

    c. Some evidence for dapsone, but beware of adverse effects (ie, methemoglobinemia)

    d. Supportive care

XII. Scorpion Stings

A. The "bark scorpion" (*Centuroides exilicauda*) is the only potentially lethal scorpion species in the United States

  1. Found in Arizona, New Mexico, and Colorado

B. Symptoms and signs

  1. Rarely cause more than local pain and inflammation

  2. Neurotoxic

    a. Roving eye movements

    b. Opisthotonic posturing

    c. Paresthesias

C. Treatment

  1. Antivenin is available for severe symptoms due to bark scorpion stings

  2. Supportive care

XIII. Lethal Jellyfish Stings

A. Classification

  1. Box jellyfish

  2. Portugese man-of-war

B. Symptoms and signs

  1. Box jellyfish carry the most lethal marine toxin

    a. Over 5000 deaths reported worldwide

    b. Severe pain and spasms

    c. Parasympathetic overstimulation leads to cardiac arrest

    d. Paralysis, respiratory weakness, and drowning

  2. Portugese man-of-war

    a. Severe pain likened to being struck by lightening

    b. Rarely deadly

C. Management

  1. Remove and prevent unfired nematocysts

    a. Wash with **sea water** if sterile saline water not available (fresh water can cause discharge)

    b. Fix nematocyst (keeps undischarged nematocysts from firing) with household vinegar (ie, acetic acid)

    c. Remove tentacles with gloves, forceps

    d. Coalesce nematocyst using talcum powder or shaving cream, then scrape off skin with a knife

    e. Apply topical anesthetic, antihistamines, and/or corticosteroids if local reaction occurs

    f. Update tetanus as necessary

    g. Alcohol and urine, common folk remedies, may cause massive discharge

  2. Antivenin exists for box jellyfish from Australia but ineffective after start of symptoms

  3. Local wound care

  4. Supportive care

REFERENCES

1. American Heart Association European Resuscitation Council. ILCOR Advisory Statements: Recommended guidelines for uniform reporting of data from drowning. *Circulation*. 2003; 108:2565.

2. Orlowski JP, Szpilman D: Drowning: rescue, resuscitation, and reanimation. *Pediac Clin North Am*. 2001;48:627.

3. Modell JH, Davis JH: Electrolyte changes in human drowning victims. *Anesthesiology*. 1969;30:414.

4. Shields CP, Sixsmith DM: Treatment of moderate-to-severe hypothermia in an urban setting. *Ann Emerg Med*. 1990;19:1093.

5. American College of Surgeons Committee on Trauma. Resources for optimal care of the injured patient. Chicago: American College of Surgeons, 2006.

6. Monafo WM: Initial management of burns. *N Engl J Med*. 1996;335:21.

7. Dire DJ: Cat bite wounds: risk factors for infection. *Ann Emerg Med*. 1991;20:973.

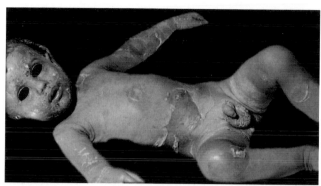

FIGURE 17–3. SSSS. (Reproduced, with permission, from Wolff K, Johnson RA, Suurmond D: *Fitzpatrick's Color Atlas and Synopsis of Clinical Dermatology,* 5th ed. Copyright © 2005, New York: McGraw-Hill.)

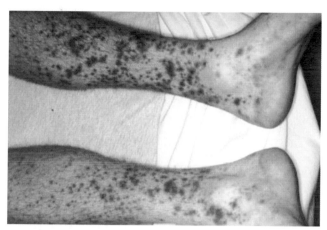

FIGURE 17–5. Rocky Mountain spotted fever. (Reproduced, with permission, from Kasper DL et al: *Harrison's Principles of Internal Medicine,* 16th ed. Copyright © 2005, New York: McGraw-Hill).

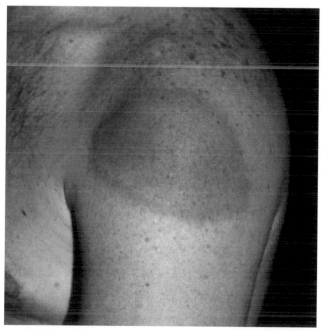

FIGURE 17–4. Erythema migrans. (Reproduced, with permission, from Wolff K, Johnson RA, Suurmond D: *Fitzpatrick's Color Atlas and Synopsis of Clinical Dermatology,* 5th ed. Copyright © 2005, New York: McGraw-Hill.)

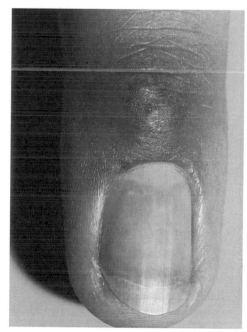

FIGURE 17–7. Septic embolus. (Reproduced, with permission, from Wolff K, Johnson RA, Suurmond D: *Fitzpatrick's Color Atlas and Synopsis of Clinical Dermatology,* 5th ed. Copyright © 2005, New York: McGraw-Hill.)

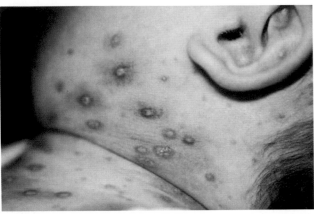

FIGURE 17–13. Chicken pox. (Courtesy of Lawrence B. Stack, MD as reproduced, with permission, from Knoop KJ, Stack LB, Storrow AB. *Atlas of Emergency Medicine*, 2nd ed. New York: McGraw-Hill, 2002.)

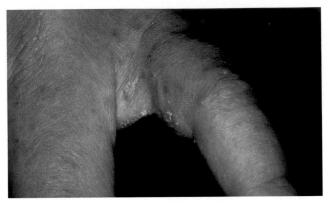

FIGURE 17–18. Scabies. (Reproduced, with permission, from Wolff K, Johnson RA, Suurmond D: *Fitzpatrick's Color Atlas and Synopsis of Clinical Dermatology*, 5th ed. Copyright © 2005, New York: McGraw-Hill.)

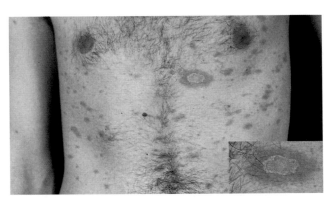

FIGURE 17–15. Pityriasis rosea. (Reproduced, with permission, from Wolff K, Johnson RA, Suurmond D: *Fitzpatrick's Color Atlas and Synopsis of Clinical Dermatology*, 5th ed. Copyright © 2005, New York: McGraw-Hill.)

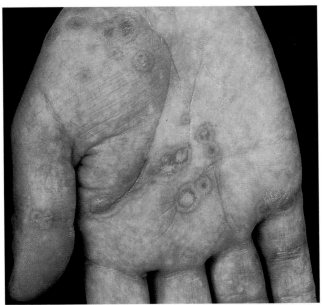

FIGURE 17–22. Erythema multiforme. (Reproduced, with permission, from Wolff K, Johnson RA, Suurmond D: *Fitzpatrick's Color Atlas and Synopsis of Clinical Dermatology*, 5th ed. Copyright © 2005, New York: McGraw-Hill.)

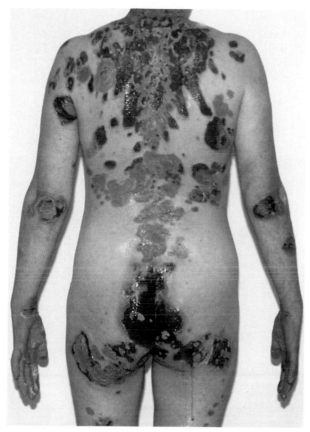

FIGURE 17–25. Pemphigus vulgaris. (Reproduced, with permission, from Wolff K, Johnson RA, Suurmond D: *Fitzpatrick's Color Atlas and Synopsis of Clinical Dermatology*, 5th ed. Copyright © 2005, New York: McGraw-Hill.)

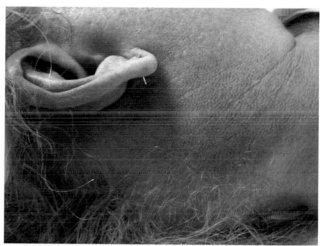

FIGURE 24–1. Battle's sign. (*Courtesy of Adam Rosh, MD.*)

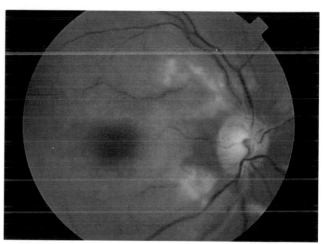

FIGURE 24–4. (Reproduced, with permission, from Tintanalli JE, Kelen GD, Stapczynski JS: *Tintinalli's Emergency Medicine: A Comprehensive Study Guide*. 6th ed. Copyright © 2004, New York: McGraw-Hill.)

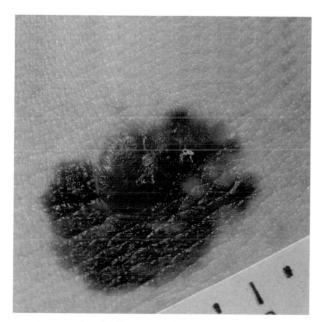

FIGURE 17–29. Melanoma. (Reproduced, with permission, from Wolff K, Johnson RA, Suurmond D: *Fitzpatrick's Color Atlas and Synopsis of Clinical Dermatology*, 5th ed. Copyright © 2005, New York: McGraw-Hill.)

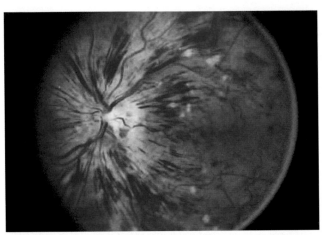

FIGURE 24–5. (Reproduced, with permission, from Knoop KJ, Stack LB, Storrow AB: *An Atlas of Emergency Medicine.* 2nd ed. Copyright © 2002, New York: McGraw-Hill.)

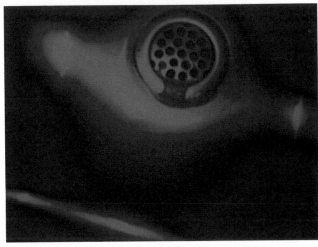

FIGURE 24–7. (*Courtesy of Adam Rosh, MD.*)

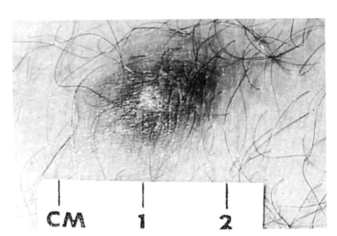

FIGURE 24–6. (Reproduced, with permission, from Kasper DL, Braunwald E, Fauci AS, et al: *Harrison's Principles of Internal Medicine,* 16th ed. Copyright © 2005, New York: McGraw-Hill.)

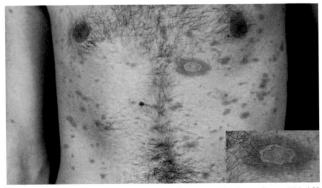

FIGURE 24–8. (Reproduced, with permission, from Wolff K, Johnson RA, Suuromond D: *Fitzpatrick's Color Atlas and Synopsis of Clinical Dermatology,* 5th ed. Copyright © 2005, New York: McGraw-Hill.)

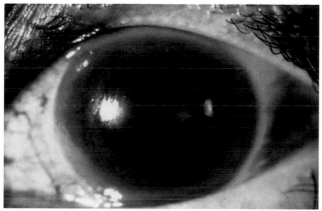

FIGURE 24–9. (Reproduced, with permission, from Knoop KJ, Stack LB, Storrow AB: *An Atlas of Emergency Medicine*. 2nd ed. Copyright © 2002, New York: McGraw-Hill.)

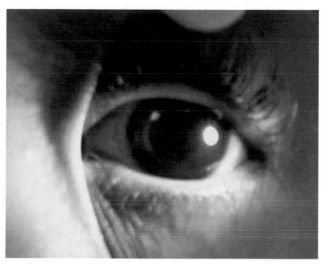

FIGURE 24–13. Hyphema (*Courtesy of Ami Dave, MD.*)

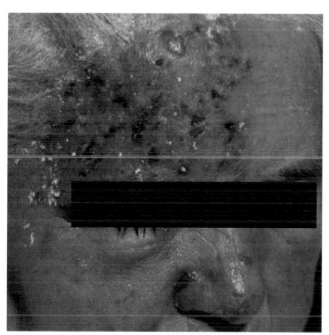

FIGURE 24–11. (Reproduced, with permission, from Wolff K, Johnson RA, Suurmond D: *Fitzpatrick's Color Atlas and Synopsis of Clinical Dermatology,* 5th ed. Copyright © 2005, New York: McGraw-Hill.)

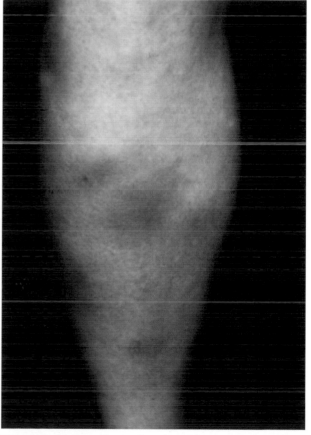

FIGURE 24–14. (Reproduced, with permission, from Wolff K, Johnson RA, Suurmond D: *Fitzpatrick's Color Atlas and Synopsis of Clinical Dermatology,* 5th ed. Copyright © 2005, New York: McGraw-Hill.)

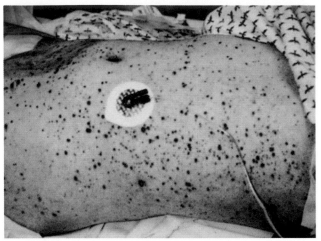

FIGURE 24–16. (Reproduced, with permission, from Knoop KJ, Stack LB, Storrow AB: *An Atlas of Emergency Medicine.* 2nd ed. Copyright © 2002, New York: McGraw-Hill.)

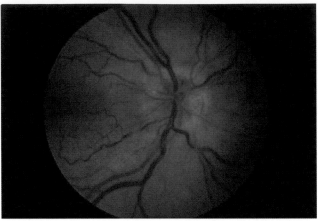

FIGURE 24–20. (Reproduced, with permission, from Knoop KJ, Stack LB, Storrow AB: *An Atlas of Emergency Medicine.* 2nd ed. Copyright © 2002, New York: McGraw-Hill.)

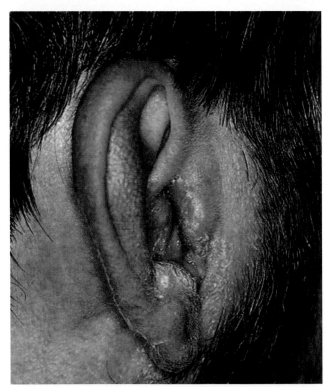

FIGURE 24–18. (*Courtesy of Frank Birinyi, MD.*)

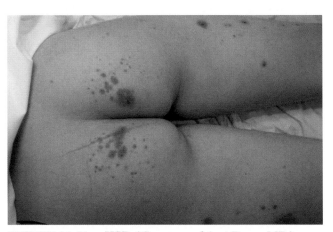

FIGURE 24–21. HSP. (*Courtesy of Ami Dave, MD.*)

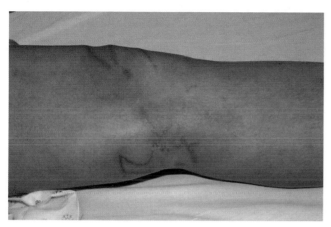

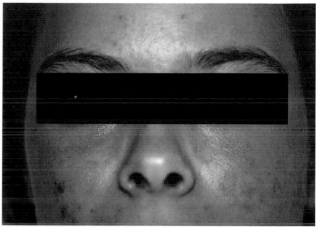

FIGURE 24–22. Jellyfish sting. (*Courtesy of Corey Long, MD.*)

FIGURE 24–25. (Reproduced, with permission, from Wolff K, Johnson RA, Suurmond D: *Fitzpatrick's Color Atlas and Synopsis of Clinical Dermatology,* 5th ed. Copyright © 2005, New York: McGraw-Hill.)

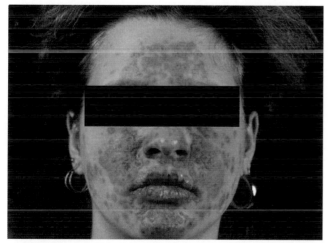

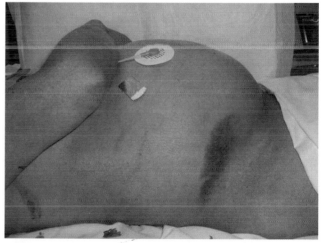

FIGURE 24–24. (Reproduced, with permission, from Wolff K, Johnson RA, Suurmond D: *Fitzpatrick's Color Atlas and Synopsis of Clinical Dermatology,* 5th ed. Copyright © 2005, New York: McGraw-Hill.)

FIGURE 24–26. Grey-Turner sign. (*Courtesy of Ami Dave, MD.*)

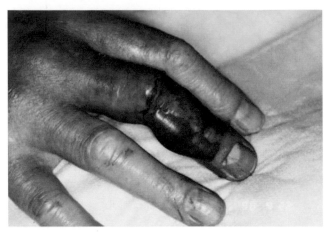

FIGURE 24–28. (Reproduced, with permission, from Knoop KJ, Stack LB, Storrow AB: *An Atlas of Emergency Medicine.* 2nd ed. Copyright © 2002, New York: McGraw-Hill.)

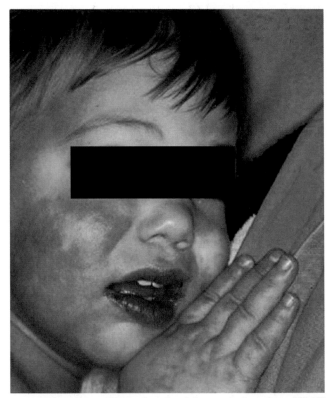

FIGURE 24–30. (Reproduced, with permission, from Wolff K, Johnson RA, Suurmond D: *Fitzpatrick's Color Atlas and Synopsis of Clinical Dermatology,* 5th ed. Copyright © 2005, New York: McGraw-Hill.)

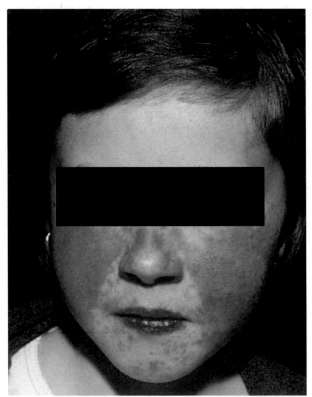

FIGURE 24–31. (Reproduced, with permission, from Wolff K, Johnson RA, Suurmond D: *Fitzpatrick's Color Atlas and Synopsis of Clinical Dermatology,* 5th ed. Copyright © 2005, New Yok: McGraw-Hill.)

Chapter 8

GYNECOLOGIC AND OBSTETRIC EMERGENCIES

Christopher McStay and Kevin Tao

I. Vaginal Disorders

A. Candidiasis
1. Etiology: most commonly *Candida albicans*
2. Risk factors
   a. Recent antibiotics, pregnancy, diabetes mellitus, immunocompromise, oral contraception use
3. Symptoms and signs
   a. Itching, dysuria, dyspareunia, "cottage-cheese" discharge, erythema, white plaques
4. Diagnosis
   a. Yeast buds and pseudohyphae demonstrated on wet-mount with potassium hydroxide
   b. Culture is considered gold standard but rarely sent
5. Management
   a. Fluconazole
      i. Topical suppositories or creams (safe in pregnancy)
      ii. Oral fluconazole 150 mg PO × 1
         a) As effective as topical[1]
         b) Contraindicated in pregnancy
   b. Complicated infections: ≥4 episodes year
      i. Require longer treatment and maintenance
         a) Acute episode
            i) 7 to 14 days of topical or
            ii) Oral fluconazole every 3 days × 3 doses
         b) Maintenance: oral fluconazole weekly for 6 months
         c) Consider ruling out diabetes or immunosuppression

B. Bacterial vaginosis (BV)
1. Epidemiology: most common cause of vaginal discharge and malodor
2. Etiology: change of normal vaginal flora from predominantly *Lactobacillus* to polymicrobial growth of anaerobes, *Gardenella vaginalis*, *Mobiluncus sp.*, and *Mycoplasma hominis*
3. Risk factors
   a. Vaginal pH >4.5, frequent douching, pregnancy, intrauterine device
4. Symptoms and signs
   a. White or grey, thin, malodorous discharge
5. Diagnosis
   a. Amsel criteria: 3 out of 4 of the following criteria
      i. Thin, white, homogeneous discharge
      ii. Presence of **clue cells** (epithelial cells stippled with bacteria)
      iii. Vaginal pH >4.5
      iv. Fishy odor before or after 10% KOH (**whiff test**)
   b. Gram stain showing predominance of and *Mobiluncus sp.*
   c. Culture not helpful as *G. vaginalis* colonizes >50% healthy women
6. Management
   a. Treat symptomatic patients to reduce upper genital tract infection
   b. Metronidazole
      i. 500 mg PO bid × 7 days or topical gel 0.75% daily × 5 days have similar efficacy
      ii. 2 g PO × 1 no longer recommended because of decreased efficacy
   c. Clindamycin
      i. 300 mg PO bid × 7 days **or**
      ii. Cream 2% qhs × 7 days
   d. Pregnant, symptomatic women should be treated with oral regimen

C. Other etiologies of vulvovaginitis
1. Allergic and chemical
2. Douches, soaps, latex condoms
3. Atrophic vaginitis

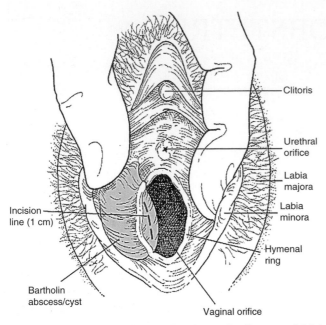

FIGURE 8–1. Bartholin cyst. Large, tender fluctuant labial abscess. (Reproduced, with permission, from Reichman EF, Simon RR: *Emergency Medicine Procedures*. New York: McGraw-Hill, 2004:1086.)

a. Postmenopausal women secondary to estrogen deficiency

b. Treatment: topical or oral estrogen replacement therapy

D. Bartholin cyst and abscess (Figure 8–1)
  1. Etiology
    a. Obstruction of duct leading to Bartholin glands located inferiorly on either side of the vaginal introitus
    b. Leads to mucous-filled cyst → polymicrobial infection → abscess
    c. Often caused by normal vaginal flora: *S. aureus, Streptococcal sp., E. coli* or sexually transmitted diseases (STDs) (*N. gonorrhea* or *Chlamydia trachomatis*)
  2. Symptoms and signs
    a. Painful labial swelling
  3. Management
    a. Incision and drainage of mucosal surface
    b. Gauze packing or Word catheter for 6 to 8 weeks
    c. Sitz baths
    d. Antibiotic coverage for *N. gonorrhea* or *Chlamydia trachomatis*
    e. Recurrent abscess: marsupialization or excision in the OR

E. Vaginal foreign body
  1. Symptoms and signs: foul-smelling or bloody discharge
    a. Superabsorbent or forgotten tampons can cause toxic shock syndrome (see Infectious Disease chapter)
  2. Management: removal of foreign body

II. Uterine Disorders

A. Dysfunctional uterine bleeding (DUB)
  1. Definition: abnormal bleeding occurring in the absence of organic pathology
  2. Epidemiology
    a. Most common cause of abnormal vaginal bleeding in reproductive women
    b. Most commonly occurs in adolescence or perimenopausal period
  3. Etiology: classically categorized as anovulatory or ovulatory
    a. Anovulatory bleeding (90%)
      i. Pathophysiology- failure of corpus luteal cyst formation
        a) Corpus luteal cyst normally secretes progesterone which organizes endometrial tissue
        b) Without progesterone, unopposed estrogen stimulation leads to continued endometrial proliferation resulting in bleeding and necrosis when endometrium outgrows vascular supply
      ii. Etiology of ovulatory failure
        a) Oral contraception
        b) Polycystic ovarian syndrome
          i) Obesity, insulin resistance, excess androgens (hirsutism, acne), oligomenorrhea, large cystic ovaries, difficulty with conception
        c) Thyroid disease
        d) Hyperprolactinemia
        e) Weight loss or eating disorders
        f) Stress
      iii. Symptoms and signs
        a) **Unpredictable** bleeding
        b) Intermittent spotting
        c) Heavy bleeding uncommon
    b. Ovulatory bleeding (10%)
      i. Pathophysiology less well understood
      ii. Etiology
        a) Bleeding disorder (von Willebrand disease common)
        b) Medications: warfarin, aspirin, NSAIDs

3. Symptoms and signs: n[
   a. Ovarian or pelvic m[
   b. Abdominal pain or b[
   c. Ascites
   d. Weight gain (from n[
4. Diagnosis
   a. Any woman with first[
      a gynecologic maligna[
   b. Complete gynecolog[
   c. Abdominal compute[
   d. Diagnostic paracent[
   e. Ovarian antigen CA[
      ing treatment respon[
5. Management: surgery,[
   radiation therapy

C. Gestational trophoblastic di[
   1. Definition: class of tum[
      mal trophoblastic (plac[
      and proliferate within th[
   2. Symptoms and signs
      a. Painless vaginal ble[
         fifth month of pregna[
      b. Persistent hyperemes[
      c. Symptoms of hypert[
         i. TSH and β-hCG[
            structures
      d. Early preeclampsia
      e. Larger than expected[
      f. Enlarged ovaries
   3. Classification
      a. Hydatidiform mole
         i. Types (Table 8–1[
            a) Complete mo[
               i) Develops f[
                  izing an e[
               ii) Results ir[
                  chorionic [
                  fetal tissue[

TABLE 8–1. **Complete**

	COMP[
Symptoms	Vaginal[
	Uterine[
	Hypere[
	Preecla[
	Hyperth[
	Trophol[
	Absent[
Diagnosis	Ultrasou[
	coupl[

Reprinted, with permission[
McGraw-Hill, 2004.

iii. Symptoms and signs (contrast with anovulatory DUB)
   a) Presence of premenstrual symptoms (breast tenderness, bloating)
   b) Dysmenorrhea: uterine pain during menstruation
   c) Menorrhagia: abnormally heavy and prolonged menstrual period
   d) Regular cycles
   e) **Predictable** bleeding
4. Diagnosis
   a. Diagnosis of exclusion
   b. Rule out pregnancy
   c. Detailed workup beyond scope of ED visit
   d. Consider outpatient TSH, FSH, prolactin, DHEAS levels
5. Management
   a. Unstable patients
      i. Resuscitation
      ii. IV estrogen stabilizes bleeding but does not address underlying cause
      iii. Tamponade bleeding by inflating pediatric Foley in cervix
      iv. Immediate ob-gyn consultation
         a) Dilation and curettage or hysterectomy (rarely required)
   b. Stable patients
      i. Oral estrogens and/or progesterone
      ii. Gynecologic follow-up

B. Endometriosis
   1. Definition: ectopic endometrial-like tissue
      a. Usually found in posterior cul de sac, fallopian tubes, or ovaries
   2. Epidemiology: effects 6% to 8% of women
   3. Anatomy: most commonly exists in the most posterior aspect of the female pelvis
   4. Symptoms and signs
      a. Nonspecific complaints of abdominal/pelvic/rectal pain, bloating, back pain
      b. Dyspareunia
      c. Symptoms worse with menstruation
      d. Infertility
      e. Vaginal bleeding
   5. Diagnosis
      a. Consider in any patient with pelvic pain
      b. Laparoscopy is the only definitive study
      c. Imaging typically not useful
   6. Management
      a. Pain management with NSAIDs
      b. Medical
         i. Interruption or suppression of the menstrual cycle is the mainstay of treatment

a) Most commonly accomplished with oral contraception although issues with fertility not resolved
   ii. Danazol and GnRH agonists for moderate-to-severe symptoms
   c. Surgical management
      i. Laparoscopic removal
         a) 20% recurrence
         b) Superior with respect to fertility and pain management
      ii. Bilateral oophorectomy and hysterectomy in patients with intractable pain and no desire for pregnancy

C. Uterine prolapse
   1. Definition
      a. Herniation of uterus into or beyond the vagina
      b. One of many "pelvic organ" prolapse syndromes
         i. Cystocele (bladder herniation and bulging into posterior vagina)
         ii. Rectocele (rectum herniation)
         iii. Enterocele (sigmoid and small bowel herniation)
   2. Etiology
      a. Vaginal wall weakness caused by age, multiparity, decreasing estrogen levels, pelvic trauma
   3. Symptoms and signs
      a. Pelvic pressure or pain
      b. Protrusion of tissue
      c. Constipation
      d. Back pain
   4. Diagnosis
      a. Gynecological examination
      b. Sim speculum (double-duck-billed vaginal speculum) or use of posterior blade of standard speculum while patient bears down
         i. Uterine prolapse grades
            a) Grade 1: cervix within vagina
            b) Grade 2: cervix protrudes beyond introitus
            c) Grade 3: entire uterus outside vulva
   5. Management: depends on grade, age, and patient preferences
      a. Digital reduction
      b. Kegel (pelvic floor strengthening exercises)
      c. Estrogen
      d. Pessary
      e. Grade 3 prolapse often requires surgery

III. Ovarian Disorders

A. Ovarian cyst pain
   1. Definitions

a. Cyst: thin-walled flu
within the ovary
b. Functional cysts: cysts f
ovulation
c. Types
  i. Graafian cyst: midc
  developing follicle
    a) Pain from midcy
    lar cysts is know
  ii. Corpus luteum cyst
  transformed into the
  ing copus luteum af
  oocyte. Cyst resu
  corpus luteum with
  iii. Hemorrhagic cyst: b
  that results from a s
  into a cyst
2. Symptoms and signs:
  a. Unilateral pelvic pain
  b. Pelvic mass on examina
  c. Cervical motion tenderr
  d. Often result from cyst r
    i. Cyst rupture may o
    or strenuous activity
    ii. May result in perito
    iii. Ruptured hemorrha
    hypotension
3. Diagnosis
  a. Pelvic ultrasound
    i. Simple cysts with
    unlikely neoplastic
    ii. Suspect neoplasm i
    and thick or intern
    plex cysts)
4. ED Management
  a. Rule out ectopic pregnar
  b. Rule out neoplasm
  c. Pain control
  d. OB-gyn referral

B. Ovarian torsion
1. Definition: a twisting of th
lar pedicle which results in
2. Risks factors[2]
  a. Ovarian masses or cyst
  b. Previous pelvic surgery
  c. Ovarian stimulation (fe
  d. Pregnancy
3. Symptoms and signs
  a. Sudden onset, severe u
  b. Can be dull with intern
  c. Onset during strenuous
  d. Nausea and vomiting v
  e. Right ovary involved in

  iv. Vaginal bleeding may be **absent**
  v. Physical findings variable
    a) May have relative bradycardia secondary to vagal effects
    b) May have normal pelvic examination
d. Diagnosis
  i. β-hCG
    a) Levels may decrease, double slowly, or increase normally early in pregnancy
    b) Decreased rates of doubling should raise suspicion for an abnormal or ectopic pregnancy
  ii. Ultrasound
    a) Ectopic effectively excluded when ultrasound reveals an IUP, no other abnormalities present and patient is low risk for heterotopic pregnancy (combined IUP and ectopic)
      i) Patients who use assisted reproductive techniques are at risk for heterotopic pregnancy
    b) Findings suggestive of ectopic pregnancy
      i) Ectopic fetal heart beat
      ii) Free fluid + absent IUP
      iii) Adnexal mass + absent IUP
    c) If absent IUP and no findings suggestive of ectopic then use β-hCG quantitative levels and the discriminatory zone (see Normal Pregnancy above)
      i) β-hCG >discriminatory zone + no IUP suggests ectopic pregnancy
      ii) β-hCG <discriminatory zone + no IUP is indeterminate
    d) Ectopic pregnancies can occur at very low β-hCG levels so ultrasound should always be performed despite the β-hCG level
    e) If ultrasound is indeterminate and the patient is stable then follow serial β-hCG levels
  iii. Dilatation and curettage
    a) Confirms IUP when chorionic villi obtained from uterus
    b) Confirms ectopic if only deciduas is obtained (maternal uterine lining formed under the influence of progesterone)
  e. Management
  i. Surgical
    a) Laparoscopy versus laparotomy
    b) Salpingostomy versus salpingectomy
  ii. Medical: methotrexate
    a) Inhibits cell division in rapidly growing tissue

    b) Indications
      i) Hemodynamically stable
      ii) No free fluid seen on ultrasound
      iii) Mass <4 cm
    c) Common side effects include
      i) Abdominal pain: further evaluation and observation needed to rule out ruptured or persistent ectopic pregnancy
      ii) Flatulence
    d) Risk factors for methotrexate failure include[4]
      i) High initial β-hCG level
      ii) Presence of fetal heart beat
  iii. RhoGAM for Rh-negative patients
3. Abruptio placentae
  a. Definition: separation of placenta from uterine wall
  b. Epidemiology: occurs in 1% of all pregnancies
  c. Risk factors
    i. Hypertension
    ii. Trauma
    iii. Increasing maternal age
    iv. Multiparity
    v. Smoking
    vi. Cocaine
    vii. Previous abruption
  d. Symptoms and signs
    i. **Painful** vaginal bleeding
      a) Vaginal bleeding is **not** always present
    ii. Uterine tenderness
    iii. Uterine contractions
    iv. Rising fundus (indicating active bleeding)
    v. Fetal distress
    vi. DIC
  e. Diagnosis
    i. Based on clinical suspicion
    ii. Ultrasound insensitive to abruption as echogenicity of blood similar to placenta
    iii. 50% of patients will have laboratory evidence of coagulopathy
    iv. Never perform a digital or speculum examination until placenta previa is ruled out as it could precipitate severe hemorrhage
  f. Management
    i. IV fluids
    ii. Fresh frozen plasma to correct coagulopathy
    iii. Emergent obstetrical consultation
    iv. Fetal monitoring
    v. Emergent delivery if
      a) Fetus is mature
      b) Fetus or mother are in distress

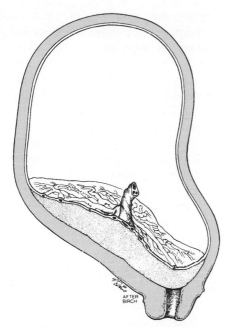

FIGURE 8–2. Placenta previa. (Reproduced, with permission, from Cunningham FG, Leveno KL, Bloom SL, Hauth JC, et al: *Williams Obstetrics,* 22nd ed. New York: McGraw-Hill, 2005:819.)

4. Placenta previa
   a. Definition- implantation of the placenta over the cervical os (Figure 8–2)
   b. Risk factors
      i. Multiparity
      ii. Previous cesarean section
      iii. Advanced maternal age
      iv. Smoking
   c. Symptoms and signs
      i. **Painless**, bright, red vaginal bleed
   d. Diagnosis
      i. Transvaginal ultrasound ~95% sensitive
      ii. When placenta previa suspected, never perform a digital or speculum examination, as it could precipitate severe hemorrhage
   e. Management
      i. Stabilization of mother
      ii. Urgent obstetrical consultation
      iii. Fetal monitoring
5. Vasa previa
   a. Definition
      i. Fetal intramembranous vessels traverse the internal os ahead of the fetal presenting part
      ii. Rupture of vessels can occur with or without rupture of membranes and lead to fetal exsanguinations
   b. Symptoms and signs
      i. Painless vaginal bleed antepartum or during rupture of membranes

   c. Diagnosis
      i. Fetal blood in vagina
         a) Add 5% KOH to vaginal blood will lyse maternal blood turning serum yellow. Fetal blood remains stable
      ii. Doppler ultrasound
   d. Management
      i. Emergent C-section
      ii. If vasa previa is diagnosed prenatally, patient should be monitored at 32 weeks, C-section at ~35 weeks or as indicated

B. Hypertensive disorders of pregnancy
   1. Epidemiology: second most common cause of maternal death
   2. Types
      a. Chronic hypertension[5]
         i. 90% caused by essential hypertension
         ii. Elevated blood pressure ≥140/90 mm Hg <20 weeks' gestation
      b. Pregnancy-induced hypertension (PIH) and gestational hypertension
         i. Definition: spectrum of hypertensive disorders occurring in women >20 weeks' gestation
            a) Includes hypertension to preeclamsia and finally eclamsia
         ii. Gestational hypertension
            a) Bood pressure ≥140/90 mm Hg or a 20 mm Hg rise in systolic or 10 mm Hg rise in diastolic from baseline occurring >20 weeks' gestation
         iii. Preeclampsia
            a) Hypertension (systolic blood pressure ≥140 mm Hg or diastolic ≥90 mm Hg **or** increase in systolic by 20 mm Hg or diastolic by 15 mm Hg) **and** proteinuria (300 mg/24 h or 1 g/mL) >20 weeks' gestation ± peripheral edema
            b) Symptoms and signs
               i) Headache
               ii) Vision changes, scintillating scotoma
               iii) Peripheral edema
               iv) Abdominal pain
            c) May occur during second or third trimester **and** up to **6 weeks after** delivery
            d) Consider molar pregnancy if <20 weeks' gestation (see above)
         iv. Severe preeclampsia
            a) Systolic blood pressure ≥160 mm Hg or diastolic ≥110 mm Hg

b) Proteinuria ≥5 g 24 hours

c) Microangiopathic hemolysis

d) Thrombocytopenia

e) Elevated transaminase levels

f) Uterine growth restriction

g) Symptoms of end-organ involvement

v. HELLP syndrome (acronym for **H**emolysis, **E**levated **L**iver enzymes, and **L**ow **P**latelets)

a) Variant of preeclampsia

b) Consider diagnosis in any gravid patient with abdominal pain

vi. Eclampsia

a) Definition: preeclampsia + seizures

3. Management

a. Uric acid may be elevated in preeclampsia and may be followed to watch for resolution of symptoms

b. Chronic hypertension and PIH

i. Rule out preeclampsia

ii. Monitor for worsening hypertension

iii. There is no clear benefit to antihypertensive drug therapy for mild PIH or preeclampsia

c. Severe preeclampsia and eclampsia

i. Magnesium sulfate 4 to 6 g IV over 20 minutes then infusion of 2 g/h

a) Magnesium toxicity can lead to decreased deep tendon reflexes followed by respiratory depression and eventual respiratory paralysis

b) Treat seizures with magnesium followed by benzodiazepines if seizures refractory

ii. Admit for observation and serial blood pressure checks

d. Antihypertensives

i. Hydralazine

ii. Nimodipine or labetolol

C. Hyperemesis gravidarum

1. Epidemiology

a. Nausea and vomiting affects 70% of pregnancies during the first 12 weeks

b. Hyperemesis gravidarum occurs in 2% of pregnancies

2. Symptoms and signs

a. Hyperemesis gravidarum characterized by intractable vomiting with

i. Weight loss

ii. Dehydration

iii. Hypokalemia

b. Ketonemia

i. There is no evidence that ketosis is harmful to the fetus

c. Abdominal pain is not characteristic of hyperemesis gravidarum and should promote further investigation

3. Diagnosis

a. Check complete blood count (CBC), electrolytes, blood urea nitrogen (BUN), creatinine, and urinalysis

4. Management

a. IV fluids with 5% dextrose in lactated ringers (LR) or normal saline (NS) to restore volume and reverse ketosis

b. Antiemetics

i. Phenothiazines: promethazine, prochlorperazine

ii. Metoclopramide

iii. Ondansetron

iv. Pyridoxine (vitamin B_6)

5. Indications for admission

a. Persistent vomiting

b. Persistent acidosis or severe electrolyte abnormalities

c. Weight loss >10% pre-pregnancy weight

d. Uncertain diagnosis

VII. Normal Labor and Delivery

A. Consider all fetuses viable at ≥22 weeks' gestational age

B. Normal delivery

1. Labor characterized by synchronous uterine contractions of increasing frequency, duration, and strength that lead to cervical dilation

a. Braxton-Hicks contractions ("false labor") are **not** associated with cervical dilation

i. Less regular

ii. Less severe

iii. Often resolve with ambulation

b. Bloody show

i. Passage of cervical mucous plug signifying commencement of cervical dilation

ii. Associated with small amount of bleeding

c. Effacement: thickness of cervix

d. Dilation: dilation of cervical os

e. Station: relation of the baby's head to the maternal ischial spines

2. Stages of labor

a. First stage: begins with slow cervical dilation, ends when cervix is fully dilated (10 cm) and effaced (paper-thin)

i. Latent phase: slow steady dilation

ii. Active phase: rapid dilation and effacement

b. Second stage: characterized by complete dilation of cervix, urge to push by mother, crowning of fetal presenting part, then delivery

c. Third stage: delivery of placenta

d. Fourth stage: postpartum

3. Diagnosis

a. Vaginal examination

i. Contraindicated in any third trimester bleeding unless placenta previa is ruled out by ultrasound

ii. Determine progression of labor, fetal presenting part

iii. If fontanel not felt, suspect fetal malposition

b. Electronic fetal monitoring to rule out fetal distress

c. Ultrasound

i. Number of fetuses

ii. Placental position, integrity

iii. Age of fetuses

iv. Cord location (prolapse)

4. Delivery of infant (Figure 8–3)

a. When crowning occurs, try to ensure controlled delivery

i. Precipitous delivery may cause lacerations

ii. Mother should not push, but pant as she delivers

iii. Modified Ritgen maneuver

a) One gloved hand used to stretch perineum while putting gentle pressure on the fetal chin, other hand puts pressure on occiput

b. After head delivered, let head rotate

c. Suction nares, oropharynx prior to delivery of shoulders

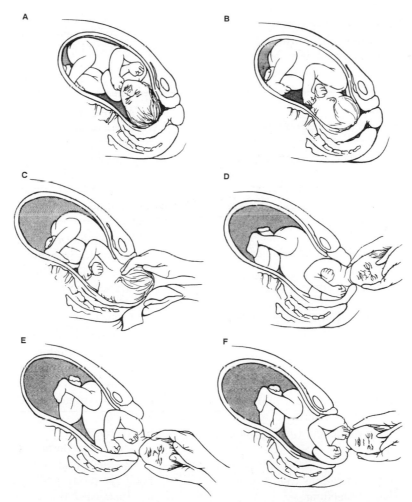

FIGURE 8–3. Movements of normal delivery. **A.** Engagement, flexion, and descent. **B.** Internal rotation. **C.** Extension and delivery of the head. After delivery of the head the infant's nose and mouth should be suctioned and check for nuchal cord. **D.** External rotation bringing the thorax into the anteroposterior diameter of the pelvis. **E.** Delivery of the anterior shoulder. **F.** Delivery of the posterior shoulder. Note that after delivery, the head is supported and used to gently guide delivery of the shoulder. Traction should be minimized. (Reproduced, with permission, from Tintinalli JE, Kelen GD, Stapczynski JS: *Tintinalli's Emergency Medicine: A Comprehensive Study Guide*, 6th ed. Copyright © 2004, New York: McGraw-Hill.)

    d. Shoulders usually deliver themselves, anterior, then posterior
        i. Lack of spontaneous delivery may represent shoulder dystocia
    e. Keep infant at level of perineum before clamping cord to promote blood flow from placenta into baby, then clamp and cut cord
    f. Episiotomies not recommended
    g. Dry infant, place in warmer while calculating Apgar score
  5. Delivery of placenta
    a. Normally expelled spontaneously within 5 to 10 minutes
    b. Uterine massage may aid
    c. No need for traction on cord
    d. Examine placenta to ensure complete delivery
    e. Examine cord anatomy (2 arteries, 1 vein)
    f. Oxytocin 10 to 40 U IV in 1 L fluid bolus after delivery of placenta to promote uterine contraction and prevent hemorrhage often considered routine management in third stage of labor

VIII. Complications of Labor

A. Premature labor
  1. Definition: uterine contractions with cervical changes <37 weeks
  2. Diagnosis
    a. Uterine contractions and cervical changes with estimated fetal weight on ultrasound <2500 g
    b. Must differentiate from false labor
  3. Management
    a. Medical tocolysis if healthy mother with viable fetus
        i. Magnesium sulfate competitively inhibits smooth muscle calcium uptake causing relaxation
        ii. β-agonists (ritodrine and terbutaline) cause smooth muscle relaxation
        iii. Prostaglandin synthetase inhibitors (indomethacin and sulindac)
        iv. Calcium channel blockers (nifedipine or nicardipine)
        v. Bed rest
        vi. Absolute contraindications to tocolysis
           a) Acute vaginal bleeding
           b) Fetal distress
           c) Lethal fetal anomaly
           d) Chorioamnionitis
           e) Preeclampsia
           f) Sepsis
           g) DIC

B. Premature rupture of membranes (PROM)
  1. Definition: rupture of membranes before actual onset of labor
    a. PROM often results in normal labor
    b. PROM occurring with fetal prematurity is associated with significant fetal morbidity and mortality
  2. Epidemiology
    a. Occurs in 3% of pregnancies
  3. Symptoms and signs
    a. Spontaneous gush of fluid
  4. Diagnosis
    a. Often clinical diagnosis based on history
    b. Sterile examination to prevent ascending infection
        i. Incidence of infection in proportion to number of examinations
    c. Moist perineum, with odorless fluid in vaginal vault
        i. Nitrazine test of fluid pH 7.2 consistent with amniotic fluid. Normal vaginal pH 3.5 to pH 6
        ii. Ferning of fluid caused by crystallization of amniotic fluid as it dries
  5. Management
    a. Admission and obstetrical consultation
    b. Corticosteroids for fetal pulmonary maturation in gestations <36 weeks
    c. Consider tocolytics in preterm PROM
    d. Assess for chorioamnionitis

C. Chorioamnionitis
  1. Definition
    a. Intra-amniotic infection commonly caused by ascending infection by normal vaginal flora (*Bacteroides, Prevotella, E. Coli*, group B streptococci)
  2. Risk factors
    a. PROM
    b. Preterm labor
    c. Prolonged rupture of membranes
    d. Multiple vaginal examinations
    e. Genital tract infections
  3. Maternal symptoms and signs
    a. Fever
    b. Tachycardia
    c. Uterine tenderness
    d. Purulent vaginal discharge
  4. Fetal symptoms and signs
    a. Tachycardia
    b. Decreased fetal activity
    c. Decreased fetal heart rate variability
    d. Abnormal biophysical profile
  5. Diagnosis
    a. Clinical diagnosis
    b. Culture cervix and vagina

6. Management
    a. Antibiotics: ampicillin plus gentamicin; add anaerobic coverage for C-sections (clindamycin or metronidazole)
    b. Fetal monitoring and emergent delivery if in distress

IX. Complications During Delivery

A. Dystocia
1. Definition: abnormal progression of labor because of
    a. Problems with pelvic architecture
    b. Size of fetus
    c. Presentation of fetus
    d. Uterine discoordination
2. Epidemiology: accounts for 50% of C-sections

B. Breech
1. Definition: buttocks first presentation
2. Epidemiology
    a. Most common dystocia occurring in 4% of deliveries
    b. 50% of term infant mortality are caused by breech deliveries
3. Symptoms and signs
    a. Neonate buttocks does not cause dilation of cervix fully, entrapping the head later in delivery
    b. Increased incidence of umbilical cord prolapse
    c. Death secondary to asphyxia
4. Diagnosis
    a. Leopold maneuvers: Series of four abdominal palpation maneuvers that aid in determining the position of the fetus
    b. Sterile vaginal examination
    c. Ultrasound
5. Management
    a. C-section unless imminent delivery
    b. Effort should be made to allow imminent delivery happen spontaneously
    c. Episiotomy

C. Shoulder dystocia
1. Definition
    a. Inability to deliver the fetal shoulder
        i. Normally shoulders traverse the pelvis sequentially, but with dystocia, both enter simultaneously usually resulting in impaction of anterior shoulder on pubic symphysis
2. Epidemiology
    a. Second most common malpresentation
    b. Occurs in 1:300 deliveries

c. Develops intrapartum and is unpredictable
d. Seen with large fetuses caused by postmaturity, maternal diabetes, obesity, erythroblastosis fetalis
3. Diagnosis
    a. Clinical diagnosis
    b. Shoulders felt in vertical axis
    c. Arrested delivery of fetal head
4. Management: goal is to disengage anterior shoulder
    a. Episiotomy
    b. Drainage of mother's bladder with Foley catheter
    c. McRoberts maneuver
        i. Leg flexion of the mother to knee-chest position disengages anterior shoulder
        ii. Suprapubic pressure
        iii. Pressure on posterior shoulder through episiotomy
    d. Wood screw maneuver
        i. Create or extend episiotomy
        ii. Apply pressure to rotate posterior shoulder clockwise
    e. Intentional clavicle fracture
    f. Zavanelli maneuver: push fetal head back into mother and deliver via C-section (last resort)
5. Complication: seen in 20% of shoulder dystocias
    a. Asphyxia
    b. Brachial plexus injury
    c. Clavicular or humeral fractures

D. Umbilical cord prolapse (Figure 8–4)
1. Definition
    a. Umbilical cord precedes delivery of fetus
    b. Pressure of presenting part (typically the occiput) on prolapsed cord causes anoxic injury
2. Epidemiology
    a. Incidence range from 1:160 to 1:600
    b. Associated with malpresentations and PROM
3. Diagnosis
    a. Sterile vaginal examination
    b. Doppler ultrasound
4. Management
    a. Emergent C-section
    b. Maneuvers to preserve cord circulation until C-section
        i. Trendelenburg position
        ii. Knee-chest position
        iii. Digitally lift presenting part until C-section
        iv. Tell mother to avoid pushing
        v. Instill 500 cc of normal saline into bladder to try to lift fetus off cord
        vi. Tocolysis

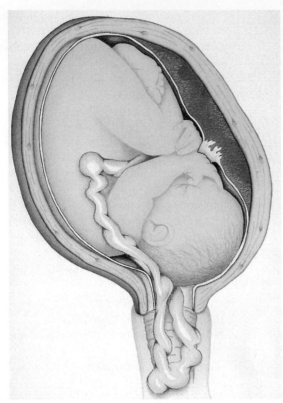

FIGURE 8–4. Umbilical cord prolapse. (Reproduced, with permission, from Knoop KJ, Stack LB, Storrow AB: *Atlas of Emergency Medicine,* 2nd ed. Copyright © 2002, New York: McGraw-Hill.)

    c. If C-section cannot be done immediately
       i. Fundal reduction: manual replacement of cord into uterus
       ii. Rapid vaginal delivery

E. Umbilical cord knots
  1. 5% of stillborns
  2. Management: rapid delivery

F. Nuchal cord
  1. Definition: long umbilical cord entangled with fetus
    a. Most commonly around the neck
  2. Epidemiology: 1:5 births
  3. Management
    a. Reduce loose nuchal cords at the perineum
    b. Body coils generally reduce spontaneously
    c. Tight coils nonreducible
      i. Cut and clamp cord
      ii. Rapid delivery
      iii. Ventilate to prevent asphyxia

X. Postpartum Complications

A. Postpartum hemorrhage (blood loss of >500 mL)
  1. Uterine atony
    a. Definition: loss of uterine muscle tone
    b. Epidemiology
      i. Most common cause of hemorrhage—50% of cases
    c. Risk factors
      i. Multiparity
      ii. Prolonged labor
      iii. Overdistention of uterus
      iv. Excessive uterine manipulation
    d. Symptoms and signs
      i. Uterus is soft and boggy
      ii. Acute hemorrhage caused by lack of uterine contraction to compress vessels and prevent bleeding
    e. Diagnosis of exclusion
    f. Management
      i. Two-handed uterine massage
      ii. Oxytocin 5 U IV bolus or 20 U in 1 L IV fluid bolus
      iii. Type and crossmatch blood as needed
      iv. Additional methods of hemostasis
        a) Uterine packing
        b) Pelvic vessel embolization: alternative to hysterectomy and preserves reproductive capability
        c) Aortic compression against anterior surface of vertebral column
        d) Hysterectomy
  2. Retained products of conception (POC)
    a. Epidemiology: accounts for 10% of postpartum hemorrhage
    b. Symptoms and signs
      i. Retained fragments prevent uterine contraction resulting in bleeding
      ii. Infection of POCs may lead to pain, fever, and discharge
    c. Diagnosis
      i. Clinical diagnosis and suspicion
      ii. Examine placenta
      iii. Ultrasound
    d. Management
      i. Removal of retained products manually or by dilation and curettage
      ii. Digital uterine exploration with blunt dissection
  3. Abnormal placental attachment
    a. Epidemiology
      i. 1:2000 to 1:7000 deliveries
    b. Types

       i. Placenta accreta: placenta adheres without deciduas basalis

      ii. Placenta increta: villi extend into myometrium

     iii. Placenta percreta: villi extend full thickness though myometrium

  c. Risk factors

       i. Multigravidity

      ii. Prior C-section

     iii. Placenta previa

     iv. Prior curettage

      v. Prior uterine infection

  d. Symptoms and signs

       i. Postpartum hemorrhage

  e. Diagnosis

       i. Digital uterine exploration

      ii. Ultrasound

  f. Management

       i. Curettage

      ii. Hysterectomy in severe cases

B. Uterine inversion

  1. Epidemiology

    a. 1:2000 deliveries

    b. Occurs spontaneously or with traction of umbilical cord during placental delivery

  2. Risk factors

    a. Primiparity

    b. Fundal implantation of placenta

    c. Fundal pressure during delivery

  3. Symptoms and signs

    a. Sudden onset severe abdominal pain

    b. Complete

       i. Palpate uterine fundus in cervical os

    c. In complete

       i. Palpating the fundal wall in the lower uterine segment

  4. Diagnosis is clinical

  5. Management

    a. If placenta still attached, do not remove

    b. Push fundus upward via the introitus before cervix contracts

    c. If cervix contracted use tocolytics

    d. After uterus repositioned begin oxytocin

C. Uterine rupture

  1. Epidemiology

    a. Increasing frequency due to increased rate of vaginal births after cesarean (VBAC)

       i. Occurs in 0.3% to 1.7% of VBAC

  2. Risk factors

    a. >3 C-sections

    b. Prior vertical uterine incision

  3. Symptoms and signs

    a. Pain, sudden termination of uterine contractions with tearing sensation, vaginal bleeding, fetal heart rate abnormalities

    b. Ranges from simple scar dehiscence to complete fetal extrusion

  4. Diagnosis

    a. Retain high clinical suspicion as pain not always present

    b. Ultrasound

  5. Management

    a. Rapid delivery via C-section

    b. Oxytocin contraindicated as it may enlarge rupture

D. Endometritis

  1. Definition: inflammation of the uterine endometrium

    a. Acute endometritis: secondary to *S. aureus* or *Streptococcal* infections

    b. Chronic endometritis: characterized by plasma cells in the stroma

    c. Often caused by chronic pelvic inflammatory disease (PID) (see STD section)

  2. Epidemiology

    a. Affects 2% to 8% of all pregnancies

  3. Risks factors

    a. C-section

    b. PROM >24 hours

    c. Stage 2 labor >12 hours

    d. High number of pelvic examinations

    e. Infection caused by Gram-negative bacteria, *Bacteroides, Streptococci*

  4. Symptoms and signs

    a. Develops in second or third day postpartum

    b. Fever

    c. Foul-smelling lochia

    d. Abdominal pain

    e. Leukocytosis

  5. Diagnosis

    a. Clinical presentation

    b. Ultrasound for retained products of conception

  6. Management

    a. Empiric antibiotics based on clinical suspicion

    b. Clindamycin + aminoglycoside **or**

    c. Second- or third-generation cephalosporins

E. Mastitis

  1. Definition: inflammation of the mammary gland

    a. Must distinguish cellulitis from abscess which requires drainage

    b. Inflammatory breast cancer may have similar presentation

2. Epidemiology: increased risk in nursing women
3. Management
   a. Anti-staphylococcus penicillin (dicloxacillin) or cephalosporin
   b. Warm compresses
   c. Continue nursing

XI. Medication Therapy During Pregnancy

A. Teratogenic risk classification according to FDA (Table 8–2)

B. Increased teratogenicity during organogenesis; days 21 to 56 of gestation

C. Drugs may effect nervous system during central nervous system (CNS) development; weeks 10 to 17

D. Commonly used drugs
   1 Acetaminophen: safe
   2. Aspirin: not recommended because of prostaglandin effects on delaying onset of labor, increasing duration of labor, effects on ductus arteriosus
   3. Opiates: considered safe during pregnancy but caution during labor as they may cause respiratory depression

4. Antibiotics
   a. Sulfonamides: near term as can cause kernicterus
   b. Chloramphenicol at term: grey baby syndrome (cardiovascular collapse of neonate)
   c. Aminoglycoside: ototoxicity, renal toxicity
   d. Tetracycline:
      i. Maternal: liver disease
      ii. Fetal: intense yellow coloration of mineralized skeleton (best seen in teeth), congenital defects
   e. Quinolones: musculoskeletal dysfunction
   f. Fluconazole (oral): associated with slight increase in craniofacial, bone, and joint abnormalities
5. Antihistamines: considered safe except for meclizine in first trimester
6. Antiemetics: dopamine antagonists and 5-HT$_3$ antagonists are considered safe
7. Oral hypoglycemics are contraindicated; insulin is safe.

TABLE 8–2. Safety of Medications During Pregnancy

CLASS	SIGNIFICANCE
A	Studies done, no risk to fetus
B	No human studies done, no evidence of risk for humans, animal studies may show risk or not
C	May engender risk, no studies done; potential benefit may outweigh potential harm
D	Studies have demonstrated risk; potential benefit may outweigh potential harm
X	Contraindicated in pregnancy

REFERENCES

1. Sobel. J, Brooker D, Stein G, et al. Single oral dose fluconazole compared with conventional clotrimazole topical therapy of Candida vaginitis. Am J Obstet Gynecol 1995; 172 (4): 1263-1268.
2. Houry D, Abbott J. Ovarian Torsion: A fifteen-year review. *Ann Emerg Med.* 2001 Aug;38(2):156.
3. Pena JE, Ufberg D, Cooney N, et al:, Usefulness of Doppler sonography in the diagnosis of ovarian torsion. *Fertil Steril.* 2001 May;75(5):1041.
4. Lipscomb G, McCord M, Stovall T, et al. Predictors of success of methotrexate treatment in women with tubal ectopic pregnancies. *N Engl J Med.* 1999; 341(26):1974-1978.
5. Sibai BM: Treatment of hypertension in pregnant women. *N Engl J Med.* 1996; 335(4):257.

Chapter 9

UROLOGIC AND RENAL EMERGENCIES

William Chiang and Jasper Schmidt

I. Male Genitourinary Diseases

A. Fournier gangrene
1. Definition: necrotizing fasciitis of the perineum
2. Etiology: polymicrobial, may include both aerobic & anaerobic organisms
   a. *E. Coli, Bacteroides fragilis*
   b. *Staphylococcus, Clostridia*, β-hemolytic *Streptococcus*
   c. Spread to multiple fascial planes, potentially involving the entire perineum and lower abdomen
3. Risk factors: immunocompromised
   a. Immune-mediating medications, chemotherapy
   b. Elderly, diabetic, alcoholic
   c. Recent trauma or instrumentation to the perineum
4. Symptoms and signs
   a. Pain out of proportion to physical findings
   b. Pain may be **absent** as underlying nerves in dermis destroyed
   c. Erythema and edema of the scrotum
   d. Fever
   e. Crepitus is a late finding
5. Diagnosis
   a. Clinical evaluation
   b. Plain films may reveal subcutaneous emphysema
   c. Computed tomographic (CT) scan
6. Management
   a. True surgical emergency
   b. Antibiotics to cover both aerobic and anaerobic organisms
   c. Immediate urology consultation for surgical debridement
   d. Intravenous fluid resuscitation
   e. Potential use for hyperbaric oxygen

B. Priapism
1. Definition
   a. Prolonged sustained erection of the penis

2. Pathophysiology
   a. Engorgement of the corpora cavernosa caused either by occlusion of corpora cavernosa (low flow priapism) or uncontrolled arterial inflow (high flow priapism) (Figure 9–1)
3. Etiology (Table 9–1)
   a. Low flow priapism (more common)
      i. Medications: sildenafil and other phosphodiesterase 3 inhibitors, papaverine, phenothiazines
      ii. Hematological disease: sickle cell disease
      iii. Malignancy: leukemia, lymphoma, bladder and prostate tumors
      iv. Neurologic: **spinal cord injury (C5)**
   b. High flow priapism (rare)
      i. Trauma: rupture of cavernous artery
      ii. Arteriovenous fistula
4. Diagnosis
   a. Clinical
   b. Blood gas aspiration from corpora cavernosa can differentiate low flow from high flow priapism
      i. Low flow priapism results in penile ischemia and has a low pH
      ii. High flow priapism does **not** result in ischemia
5. Management
   a. Low flow
      i. External compression and ice pack (unlikely to resolve by itself)
      ii. Medications
         a) Terbutaline (subcutaneous 0.25 or 0.5 mg IM or 5 mg PO)
         b) Phenylephrine (100 to 500 mcg intracavernosal)
         c) Methylene blue (50 mg intracavernosal)
      iii. Corporeal aspiration
         a) Aspirate 30 to 60 mL of blood at the 2 or 11 o'clock position of the penis (this avoids inadvertent puncture of the ventral spongiosum)

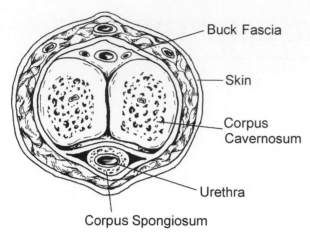

FIGURE 9–1. Cross sectional anatomy of the penis. (Reproduced, with permission, from Tintinalli JE, Kelen GD, Stapczynski JS: *Tintanelli's Emergency Medicine: A Comprehensive Study Guide,* 6th ed. Copyright © 2004, New York: McGraw-Hill.)

    iv. Miscellaneous
      a) Transfusion and exchange transfusion in sickle cell patients
  b. High flow
    i. Not a medical emergency
    ii. Identify and obliterate secondary fistulas
    iii. Penile duplex ultrasonography helps identify location of fistulae
    iv. Angiographic confirmation and embolization of the fistula follow
    v. Surgical intervention may be necessary
6. Complications: prolonged low flow priapism leads to fibrosis of the penis and erectile dysfunction

C. Testicular torsion
  1. Epidemiology
    a. Bimodal distribution, with highest risk at 1 year of age and during puberty
    b. Tenfold increase in risk with undescended testicle
    c. 50% unsalvageable due to delays in presentation and diagnosis

TABLE 9–1. Low Flow versus High Flow Priapism

	LOW FLOW	HIGH FLOW
pO_2	<60 kPa	>60 kPa
pCO_2	>70 kPa	<70 kPa
Ph	<7	>7
Arterial inflow	Low	High
Venous outflow	Closed	Open
Painful	Usually	Seldom

2. Anatomy
  a. Extravaginal: almost all neonates
    i. Twisting of the tunica vaginalis and testicle before complete descent and fusion to the scrotal wall
    ii. Bell clapper deformity (horizontally hung testicle)
  b. Intravaginal torsion
    i. Inadequate fixation of the tunica vaginalis on the spermatic cord
    ii. This allows rotation of the testicle within the scrotum
3. Pathophysiology
  a. Twisting of vessels leads to obstruction of venous return and arterial occlusion
    i. Torsion <6 hours, almost 100% salvage rate
    ii. >6 hours, loss of Leydig cells and gonad function
    iii. 24 hours, 42% to 75% salvage rate
    iv. >48 hours, 0% salvaged
4. Symptoms and signs
  a. Acute onset of pain, unilateral
  b. Previous episodes of similar pain
  c. Abdominal pain, nausea, and vomiting
  d. Swollen painful testicle
  e. More often involves the left testicle
  f. Horizontal lie of testicle
  g. Elevated testicle
  h. Lack of cremasteric reflex
5. Diagnosis
  a. Doppler ultrasound
  b. Testicular scintigraphy
    i. Radionuclide test
    ii. Highly sensitive and specific
    iii. Time-consuming and not as readily available
    iv. Better than ultrasound to evaluate small testicles of young children than ultrasound
6. Management
  a. Immediate urology consultation for surgery
  b. Manual de-torsion if delays expected
    i. Medial to lateral rotation (opening a book)
    ii. Reverse rotation direction if not working or symptoms worsen

D. Torsion of a testicular or epididymal appendage
  1. Epidemiology
    a. Most commonly seen in males aged 7 to 13 years
  2. Symptoms and signs
    a. Unilateral testicular pain
    b. Localized to the superior aspect of the testicle
    c. May see a "blue dot" sign (infracted appendage) with transillumination
    d. Cremasteric reflex intact

3. Diagnosis: differentiating from testicular torsion
   a. Clinical examination
   b. Doppler study: normal arterial flow
   c. Nuclear scan: mild increase in perfusion of the affected side, may reveal hot dot
4. Management
   a. Pain control

E. Epididymitis and orchitis
   1. Etiology
      a. Ascending infection from urethra, prostate, bladder
         i. Sexually transmitted etiology
            a) Most common etiology in sexually active males <35 years
            b) *Chlamydia trachomatis*
            c) *Neisseria gonorrhoeae*
            d) *E. coli* from insertive anal intercourse
         ii. Nonsexually transmitted
            a) *E. coli*
            b) *Enterobacteriaceae*
      b. Occasionally by hematogenous spread (*E. coli, Klebsiella*, mumps)
      c. Trauma and idiopathic are less common
   2. Symptoms and signs
      a. Antecedent urethritis
      b. Gradually increasing dull, unilateral scrotal pain
      c. Involvement of vas deferens leads to radiation of pain to the cord and lower abdomen
      d. Fever
      e. Erythematous, painful, swollen scrotum
      f. Transillumination may demonstrate a reactive hydrocele
      g. "Phren" sign: relief of pain with scrotal elevation
         i. Should **not** be relied upon to exclude torsion
   3. Diagnosis
      a. Diagnosis of exclusion
      b. Pyuria does not rule out torsion
      c. Doppler ultrasound
         i. Exclude torsion
         ii. Visualization of a swollen epididymis and testicle
         iii. Increased blood flow
   4. Management
      a. Older men and nonsexually active patients
         i. Cover for coliform bacteria
            a) Trimethoprim or sulfamethoxazole × 10 to 14 days
      b. Sexually active males
         i. Cover for *C. trachomatis*
            a) Doxycycline 100 mg PO bid × 14 days or azithromycin 1 g PO × 1

      ii. Cover for *N. gonorrhoeae* and enterics
         a) Ceftriaxone 250 mg IM × 1
      iii. May treat both with 2 g of azithromycin
      iv. Fluoroquinolones no longer recommended
   c. Scrotal support and analgesia
   d. Follow-up with urologist in 3 to 7 days
5. Complications
   a. Abscess
   b. Testicular infarction
   c. Chronic pain
   d. Infertility

F. Prostatitis
   1. Types: 4 distinct syndromes characterized by
      a. Acute bacterial prostatitis—usually with rapid presentation of symptoms
      b. Chronic bacterial prostatitis—common in those with recurrent UTI or obstruction
      c. Chronic pelvic pain syndrome—discomfort or pain in the pelvic region for at least 3 months with variable voiding and sexual symptoms and/or no demonstrable infection
      d. Asymptomatic inflammatory prostatitis—evidence of inflammation in urine, semen, or biopsy specimen
   2. Pathophysiology
      a. Reflux of urine from urethra into intraprostatic ducts
         i. Bacterial infection
            a) Primarily *E. coli*
            b) *Klebsiella, Enterococcus, Proteus, Pseudomonas*
            c) In patients <35 years, consider *Neisseria gonorrhea* and *Chlamydia trachomatis*
            d) Chemical inflammation
   3. Acute prostatitis
      a. Symptoms and signs
         i. Fever, perineal pain, low back pain
         ii. Dysuria
         iii. Urinary retention
      b. Diagnosis for acute prostatitis
         i. Tender boggy prostate
         ii. Evidence of pyuria
      c. Management
         i. Antibiotics for 4 weeks is recommended to prevent relapse
            a) Initial therapy should be directed at Gram-negative enteric bacteria
            b) Quinolones with urinary excretion or trimethoprim-sulfamethoxazole if sexually transmitted disease (STD) unlikely
            c) Cultures and sensitivities must be followed and antibiotics adjusted accordingly

d) Other considerations—cephalosporins, aminoglycosides, imipenim

ii. Outpatient versus inpatient depending on the degree of toxicity, complicating host factors, urinary obstruction

iii. Treatment may be complicated by poor antibiotic penetration into the prostate and acidic prostate pH

iv. Analgesia, stool softener, sitz bath

v. Complicated, unresolving, and chronic cases should be referred to a urologist

G. Phimosis (Figure 9–2)
   1. Definition: inability to retract foreskin behind the glans penis
   2. Etiology: inflammation or infection of the foreskin resulting in progressive scarring
   3. Definitive therapy: circumcision

H. Paraphimosis (Figure 9–2)
   1. Definition
      a. Retracted foreskin unable to be replaced over glans penis

Phimosis

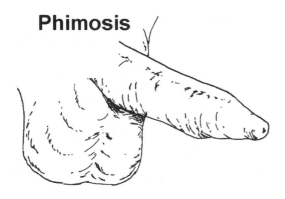

Paraphimosis

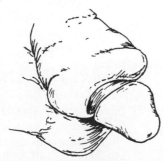

FIGURE 9–2. Phimosis versus paraphimosis. (Reproduced, with permission, from Tintinalli JE, Kelen GD, Stapczynski JS: *Tintanelli's Emergency Medicine: A Comprehensive Study Guide,* 6th ed. Copyright © 2004, New York: McGraw-Hill.)

2. Risk factors
   a. Children in which foreskin was retracted forcefully
   b. Chronic balanoposthitis (contracture of the foreskin)
   c. Iatrogenic and indwelling catheters
3. Symptoms and signs
   a. Forms a constricting band leading to vascular compromise
   b. Pain
4. Management
   a. Rule out hair tourniquet in young children
   b. Reduction of paraphimosis
      i. Ice pack
      ii. Continuous firm pressure around the glans penis for 5 to 10 minutes
      iii. Pain control, conscious sedation, or penile block
      iv. Two-hand reduction using the thumbs to push back the glans penis
      v. Dorsal slit may be required if unsuccessful
   c. Definitive treatment: circumcision

I. Penile fracture
   1. Definition
      a. Traumatic tear of the tunica albuginea of the corpus cavernosum
      b. A urologic emergency
   2. Etiology
      a. Trauma to an erect penis
   3. Symptoms and signs
      a. "Popping sound," swelling, pain
      b. Gross hematuria or blood at the meatus indicates that urethra or spongiosum is likely affected
      c. Penis deviated to one side
   4. Diagnosis
      a. Clinical diagnosis
      b. Exclude urethral injury with retrograde urethrogram
   5. Management
      a. Immediate surgical repair

J. Balanoposthitis
   1. Definitions
      a. Balanitis: inflammation of the superficial layer of the glans penis
      b. Posthitis: involvement of the distal foreskin
   2. Etiology
      a. Irritation: soap, bubble bath, detergent
      b. Infectious
         i. Candida is most common
         ii. Anaerobic, streptococcal
         iii. STDs less common
      c. Poor hygiene is the most common factor

3. Symptoms and signs
   a. Burning, pain, itching, and erythema
   b. Candida appears as eroded plaques with a whitish discharge
4. Management depends on etiology
   a. Improved hygiene
   b. Removal of potential irritants
   c. Hydrocortisone cream
   d. Antifungal cream
   e. Occasionally, antibiotics

II. Acute Renal Failure

A. Prerenal
   1. Definition
      a. Renal failure caused by underperfusion of a normal kidney
   2. Etiology[1]
      a. Volume loss: hemorrhagic shock, vomiting, diarrhea, diuretics
      b. Decreased cardiac output
      c. Renal artery stenosis and small vessel disease
      d. Afferent vasoconstriction: NSAIDs, amphotericin B
      e. Efferent vasoconstriction: ACE inhibitors, ARBs
   3. Diagnosis
      a. BUN/CR >20
      b. Urine Na <20
      c. $FE_{Na} < 1\%$
         i. $FE_{Na} = U_{Na} P_{Na} \div U_{Cr} P_{Cr}$
         ii. May also be low with intrinsic renal failure if tubular concentrating capacity is retained, as with glomerulonephritis
   4. Management
      a. Manage underlying pathology
      b. Fluid and blood administration

B. Postrenal
   1. Definition
      a. Potentially reversible renal failure due to obstruction of urine flow
   2. Etiology
      a. Neurogenic bladder
         i. Medications (anticholinergics)
         ii. Diabetes
      b. Mass or tumor
      c. Prostate enlargement or cancer
      d. Kidney stones
   3. Diagnosis
      a. Bladder catherization
      b. Bilateral renal ultrasound
      c. Noncontrast CT scan
   4. Management
      a. Bladder catherization
      b. Treat underlying obstruction

C. Intrinic-renal
   1. Definition
      a. Renal failure due to structural and functional kidney injury
   2. Etiology
      a. Tubular injury
         i. Acute tubular necrosis (ATN) is the most common cause of **intrinsic** renal failure
         ii. Ischemic and hypovolemic
         iii. Toxin-induced
            a) **Aminoglycosides**, lithium, amphotericin B
            b) Crystals from **ethylene glycol** poisoning
         iv. Inability to concentrate urine distinguishes ATN from prerenal failure
      b. Interstitial injury
         i. Infection (pyelonephritis, abscess)
         ii. Drugs penicillin [PCN], cephalosporins, proton pump inhibitors)
         iii. Systemic illness (sarcoid, lupus, lymphoma)
      c. Glomerular injury
         i. Rapidly progressing crescentic glomerulonephritis
         ii. Postinfectious (**Gram-positive A streptococcal**, coxsackie, CMV, EBM)
         iii. Vasculitis (Churg-Strauss, Wegeners, Henoch-Schonlein purpura)
   3. Diagnosis
      a. Laboratory
         i. Complete blood count (CBC) and peripheral smear may reveal hemolysis and evidence of microangiopathic vasculitis (TTP, HUS)
         ii. Creatinine that increases by >1.5 to 2 mg/dL in a 24-hour period should make one suspicious for tissue breakdown such as in rhabdomyolysis
         iii. Antistreptolysin O (ASO) positive in most patients (80%) in 1 to 3 weeks and returns to normal in 6 months
         iv. Specific tests in consultation with rheumatology and nephrology (ANCA, C-ANCA, anti-DNA antibodies, C3 and C4 complement, etc.)
      b. Urinalysis
         i. Granular muddy brown casts suggest acute tubular necrosis
         ii. Proteinuria suggests glomerulonephritis or interstitial injury
         iii. WBC or WBC casts suggest infection

iv. Uric acid crystals may suggest tumor lysis syndrome

v. **Oxalate crystals** suggest ethylene glycol poisoning

vi. **RBC casts** suggest glomerulonephritis

c. $Fe_{Na} > 1\%$ suggests acute tubular necrosis

i. Unable to concentrate urine despite oliguria

d. Renal biopsy

D. Management

1. Prerenal

a. Administer fluid and blood

b. Treat underlying etiology (pancreatitis, congestive heart failure [CHF], sepsis, etc)

2. Postrenal

a. Maintain high level of suspicion for this potentially reversible cause of acute renal failure and liberally image with bilateral renal ultrasound or CT scan

b. Bladder catherization

c. Treat underlying obstruction

3. Intrinsic renal

a. Remove offending toxin or medication

b. Treat underlying etiology (steroids for select vasculitis, fluids, and consider mannitol and bicarbonate for rhabdomyolysis, ethanol or fomepizole for ethylene glycol poisoning)

4. Dialysis

a. **Acute** indications

i. Uremia

a) Bleeding (from platelet dysfunction)

b) Encephalopathy

c) Pericarditis

ii. Electrolyte disturbances

a) Hyperkalemia

b) Acidemia

c) Hypocalcemia

d) Hyperphosphatemia

iii. Intractable fluid overload

iv. Toxic ingestions

b. Complications of hemodialysis

i. Vascular access: thrombosis, infections, atrioventricular (AV) fistula, bleeding

ii. During hemodialysis

a) Hypotension

b) Dialysis disequilibrium (nausea, vomiting, headache, seizures, coma) osmolar imbalance between the brain and serum

c) Electrolyte abnormalities

d) Allergic reaction

e) Hypovolemia from excessive fluid removal

f) Air embolism

c. Complications of peritoneal dialysis

a) Infection: soft tissue at catheter site and peritoneum

b) Fluid leaks into the surrounding tissue, often the scrotum

c) Hernias

III. Renal Transplant (see Immunology and Rheumatology chapter)

A. Primary renal complications

1. Graft failure: graft survival from living donors ~95% at 1 year and 76% at 5 years, and from cadaveric donors 89% at 1 year and 61% at 5 years

2. Renal artery thrombosis: usually immediately posttransplantation, but may present later

a. Diagnosis: color flow Doppler

3. Renal artery stenosis: a late complication

a. Symptoms and signs: uncontrolled hypertension, allograft dysfunction, and peripheral edema

b. Diagnosis: color Doppler

4. Renal vein thrombosis: an early complication

a. Symptoms and signs: graft tenderness and edema, dark hematuria, and diminished urine volume

b. Diagnosis: color Doppler

5. Urine leak and ureter obstruction: early complication

a. Symptoms and signs: fever, pain, abdominal swelling, and graft dysfunction

b. Diagnosis: ultrasonography demonstrates perigraft fluid collection

6. Infection: most common cause of first-year posttransplantation mortality and morbidity

a. Infection most commonly occurs in mucocutaneous areas (41.0%), urinary tract (17.2%), and respiratory tract (13.9%)

b. Etiology: bacterial (45.9%); viral (40.6%)—CMV, herpes simplex, and herpes zoster; fungal (12.5%); and protozoan (1%)

7. Rejection

a. Early acute rejection

i. <3 months posttransplantation

ii. Secondary to prior sensitization to donor alloantigen

b. Late acute rejection

i. >6 months posttransplantation

ii. Correlated with withdrawal of immunosuppressive therapy

c. Chronic rejection >1 year posttransplantation

i. Caused by immunologic agents and cellular and humoral factors

ii. Present with progressive loss of renal function

B. Secondary complications
1. Hypertension (75% to 85% of all renal transplant recipients)
2. Hyperlipidemia (60%)
3. Cardiovascular disease (15.8% to 23%—a tenfold increase over the general population)
4. Diabetes mellitus (16.9% to 19.9%), osteoporosis (60%), malignant neoplasm (14%)

IV. Renal Calculus and Colic

A. Epidemiology: 3% to 5% lifetime risk
1. Peak incidence 20 to 50 years of age
2. Male to female 3:1

B. Types of stones
1. Calcium oxalate: most common ~80%
2. Struvite: second most common 2% to 20%
   a. Majority of staghorn calculi
   b. Triple-phosphate stones (magnesium, ammonium, phosphate)
   c. Urine pH >7.2 and ammonia required
   d. Urease-producing bacteria as the underlying etiology
      i. *Proteus, Klebsiella, Staphylococcus*
3. Uric acid: 6% (radiolucent on x-ray)
   a. Forms in urine pH <6
4. Cystine: approximately 1% (radiolucent on x-ray)
5. Indinavir (only in individuals taking this medication to treat HIV): radiolucent on x-ray and CT

C. Symptoms and signs
1. Flank pain radiating to the groin (or lower abdominal pain)
   a. Acute, colicky
   b. Nausea, vomiting
   c. Gross or microscopic hematuria in 85% to 90%

D. Diagnosis
1. Rule out abdominal aortic aneurysm
2. Ultrasound—hydronephrosis
3. Helical CT scan (noncontrast)

E. Management
1. Determine the presence or absence of obstruction or infection
   a. No obstruction or infection: analgesics and other medical measures to facilitate passage of the stone
      i. Medical therapy includes 0.4 mg tamsulosin once daily[2] or other α-blockers[3] and calcium channel blockers may accelerate passage of small stones, although evidence is not yet conclusive[4]

      ii. Urine alkalinization to treat uric acid stones (potassium citrate)
   b. Obstruction most likely with stones >5 to 6 mm
      i. May require surgical measures and lithotripsy
   c. If both obstruction and infection are present, then emergent decompression of the upper urinary collecting system is required
2. Admission
   a. Intractable pain
   b. Infected stone or urine
   c. Unilateral functional kidney with obstruction
   d. Evidence of renal dysfunction (increase in creatinine)

V. Polycystic Kidney Disease

A. Genetic kidney disorder with growth of numerous cysts in the kidneys
1. 90% autosomal dominant—symptoms usually develop at 30 to 40 years
2. Autosomal recessive—rare and usually affects neonates and infants

B. Pathophysiology: growth of cysts results in decreased renal function and leads to renal failure

C. Complications
1. Urinary tract infections
2. Hematuria and bleeding into the cysts
3. Liver and pancreatic cysts
4. Hypertension
5. Aneurysm (brain)
6. Kidney stones
7. Renal failure

REFERENCES

1. Sinert R, Peacock PR: Acute renal failure. In: Tintanelli JE, Kelen GD, Stapczynski, eds. *Emergency Medicine: A Comprehensive Study Guide.* 6th ed. New York: McGraw-Hill. 2004;593.
2. Dellabella M, Milanese G, Muzzonigro G: Efficacy of Tamsulosin in the medical management of juxtavesical ureteral stones. *J Urol.* 2003;170(6 Pt 1):2202.
3. Ukhal M, Malomuzh O, Strashny V: Administration of doxazosine for speedy elimination of stones from lower section of ureter. XIVth Congress of the EUA, April 7-11, 1999; Stockholm, Sweden.
4. Philipraj, SJ. Bhat, S. Thomas, J: Alpha blockers for ureteral calculi. [Protocol] Cochrane Renal Group Cochrane Database of Systematic Reviews. 3, 2007.

Chapter 10
OPHTHALMOLOGIC EMERGENCIES

Ugo A. Ezenkwele and Benjamin Kavinoky

I. Acute Visual Loss (Table 10–1)

A. Retinal detachment
1. Definition: an ocular emergency in which a layer of the retina separates from underlying epithelial support tissue
2. Types
   a. Rhegmatogenous retinal detachment (most common): a defect in the retina allows accumulation of vitreous fluid and lift of the retina
      i. Etiology: aging, trauma, cataract surgery, diabetes, uveitis
   b. Exudative retinal detachment: exudative fluid accumulates under the retina resulting in detachment
      i. Etiology: tumors and inflammatory disorders
   c. Traction retinal detachments: fibrovascular tissue within the vitreous cavity creates traction on the retina resulting in detachment
      i. Etiology: proliferative diabetic retinopathy
3. Symptoms and signs
   a. Usually **painless**
   b. Flashing lights, presence of "spider webs" or "coal dust"
   c. Floaters (small spots in the vision)
4. Diagnosis
   a. Direct fundoscopy: dull, grey detached retina
   b. Indirect fundoscopy: visualization of tear
5. Management
   a. Immediate ophthalmology consult for surgical intervention, laser therapy or cryotherapy
   b. Place patient on bed rest until ophthalmology evaluation

B. Retinal artery occlusion
1. Definition: occlusion of blood flow to the retina, usually by emboli from the carotid artery or the heart

2. Risk factors: high cholesterol, heart disease, arteriosclerosis, hypertension, diabetes, glaucoma
3. Types: name refers to vessel occluded
   a. Central retinal artery occlusion (CRAO)
   b. Branch retinal artery occlusion (BRAO)
4. Symptoms and signs
   a. Central artery: sudden, **painless**, complete loss of vision in one eye
   b. Branch artery: sudden, **painless**, partial loss of vision in one eye. Area of blindness correlates to branch occluded
   c. Exam initially normal, after 2 to 3 hours → Marcus Gunn pupil (normal consensual light response followed by paradoxical dilatation with light exposure)
5. Diagnosis
   a. Rule out temporal arteritis (see Rheumatology and Neurology chapter)
   b. Decreased visual acuity
   c. Fundoscopic examination: applies to whole retina with CRAO and area of retina supplied by occluded branch in BRAO
      i. Early findings (<2 hours)
         a) Vascular stasis
         b) Retinal vessels with interruption in the column of blood giving them a boxcar appearance
      ii. Late findings (>2 hours or days)
         a) Retinal pallor and narrowing of vessels
         b) Cherry red spot on fovea (Figure 10–1)
6. Management
   a. Immediate ophthalmology consult
   b. Orbital massage—dislodge the clot
   c. Anterior chamber (AC) paracentesis (if visual loss <24 hours)
   d. Acetazolamide
   e. Hyperosmotic diuretics—mannitol
   f. Topical β-blocker—timolol
   g. Sympathomimetics
   h. Thrombolytics (experimental)

TABLE 10–1. **Common Causes of Acute and Painless Loss of Vision**

Temporal arteritis (causes headaches)
Central retinal artery occlusion
Central retinal vein occlusion
Retinal detachment
Optic Neuritis
Hysterical blindness

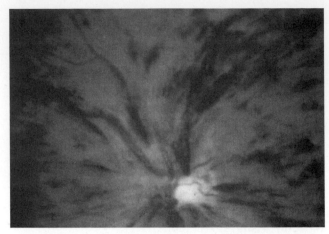

FIGURE 10–2. Retinal vein occlusion: Blood and thunder fundus. (Reproduced, with permission from Tintinalli JE, Kelem GD, Stapczynski JS: *Emergency Medicine A Comprehensive Study Guide,* 6th ed. Copyright © 2004, New York: McGraw-Hill.)

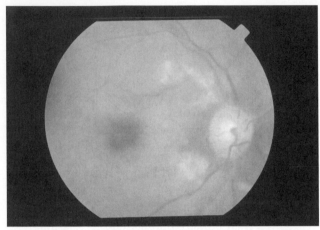

FIGURE 10–1. Central retinal artery occlusion (CRAO). (Reproduced, with permission from Tintinalli JE, Kelen GD, Stapczynski JS: *Emergency Medicine A Comprehensive Study Guide,* 6th ed. Copyright © 2004, NewYork: McGraw-Hill.)

C. Retinal vein occlusion (RVO)
  1. Definition: thrombotic obstruction of the central retinal vein as it constricts through the lamina cribrosa
  2. Etiology: abnormal blood flow or blood constituents, atherosclerosis, vessel anomalies or a combination of these factors
  3. Types
    a. Branch retinal vein occlusion (BRVO)
    b. Central retinal vein occlusion (CRVO)
      i. Non-ischemic type: mild form classified by absence of afferent pupil defect and good perfusion of the retina—can progress to ischemic type
      ii. Ischemic type: venous stasis leads to an increased vascular back-pressure that results in decreased arterial blood flow to the retina
  4. Symptoms and signs
    a. Presents with mild to severe, sudden, **painless**, monocular visual loss

    b. Slowly reactive pupil
    c. Fundoscopic examination (**blood and thunder fundus**) (Figure 10–2)
      i. Mild-to-severe hemorrhage
      ii. Cotton-wool spots in the retina indicates ischemia
    d. Ischemic type of CRVO almost always has vision of <20/100
      i. Afferent pupil defect
  5. Management
    a. Ophthalmology referral
    b. No consistently effective treatment available
    c. Non-ischemic type may benefit from systemic steroids
    d. Anticoagulation, antiplatelet agents, thrombolytics do not improve outcome
    e. Lower elevated intraocular pressure (IOP) if necessary (see acute angle closure glaucoma below)
    f. Prognosis for the non-ischemic type of CRVO is good; results in spontaneous return of flow as macular edema resolves

D. Optic neuritis (ON)
  1. Definition: optic nerve inflammation
  2. Etiology
    a. Most often idiopathic
    b. Associated with demyelinating diseases
      i. 25% to 60% of patients with optic neuritis will develop multiple sclerosis
  3. Symptoms and signs
    a. Marcus Gunn pupil
    b. Mild to severe loss of central vision; central blind spot

c. Pain with eye movement (>90% of patients)

d. Reduced color perception

e. Decreased peripheral vision

f. Fever, headache, nausea

g. Decreased vision following exercise, hot bath or shower (activities that elevate body temperature)

h. 66% of cases with normal fundus because location of inflammation is retrobulbar

4. Treatment

a. Ophthalmology and/or neurology consultation

b. Admit for intravenous steroids

E. Acute angle closure glaucoma (ACG)

1. Definition

a. Increased IOP >21 mm Hg caused by acute obstruction of aqueous drainage through Schlemm canal

2. Anatomy (Figure 10–3)

a. The anterior chamber "angle" refers to the angle formed by the cornea (externally) and the iris (internally)

b. The ciliary body produces aqueous humor and is located posterior to the iris

c. The Schlemm canal, located in the angle of the anterior chamber, drains aqueous humor in the anterior chamber

d. The trabecular meshwork is a sieve-like cover of the Schlemm canal (Figure 10–4)

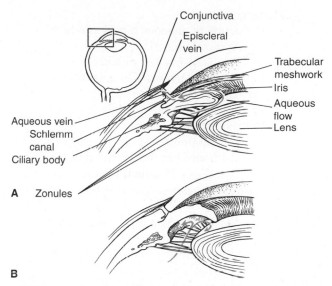

FIGURE 10–4. Anatomy of anterior chamber. (Reproduced, with permission from Tintinalli JE, Kelem GD, Stapczynski JS: *Emergency Medicine A Comprehensive Study Guide,* 6th ed. Copyright © 2004, New York: McGraw-Hill.)

3. Mechanism

a. Contact between iris and cornea (angle closure) obstructs Schlemm canal

b. Anterior movement of iris occurs because it is either pushed or pulled forward

   i. **Pushed** from behind because of increased pressure in posterior chamber

      a) Pupillary block most common mechanism—contact between iris and lens blocks aqueous flow from posterior to anterior chamber that leads to a buildup in posterior chamber pressures

      b) Pupillary dilation (adjustment to darkness, anticholinergics, Sympathomimetics and mydriatics)

   ii. **Pulled** anteriorly

      a) Inflammatory conditions (eg, sarcoidosis, Behcet syndrome, inflammatory bowel disease)

4. Symptoms and signs

a. Ocular and facial pain

b. Nausea and vomiting

c. Visual changes, unilateral blurring vision

d. Photopsiae—flashes of light in the form of colored halos around lights

e. IOP >21 mm Hg

f. Conjunctival injection

g. Corneal epithelial edema—"cloudy, steamy cornea"

h. Mid-dilated nonreactive pupil

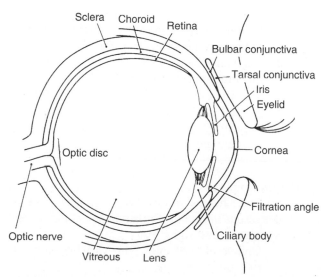

FIGURE 10–3. Anatomy of anterior and posterior segments. (Reproduced, with permission from Tintinalli JE, Kelen GD, Stapczynski JS: *Tintinalli's Emergency Medicine: A Comprehensive Study Guide,* 6th ed. New York: McGraw-Hill, 2004.)

5. Management
   a. Reduction of aqueous humor production
      i. Acetazolamide IV
      ii. Topical β-blocker (timolol)
      iii. Topical α agonist (apraclonidine)
   b. Decreasing inflammation
      i. Topical steroids (prednisolone)
   c. Reversing angle closure
      i. Topical miotic agents: pilocarpine, given at 1 hour after the initiation of treatment. Two doses 15 minutes apart
   d. Address symptoms that cause further increases in IOP
      i. Nausea and vomiting: antiemetics
      ii. Pain: analgesics
   e. Adjuncts for further reduction of IOP 2 hours after the initiation of treatment
      i. Hyperosmotic agents (IV mannitol, oral glycerol, or isosorbide)
   f. **Immediate ophthalmology consultation** (Table 10–2)
      i. Laser iridotomy

II. Infectious Disorders of the Eye

A. Cytomegalovirus (CMV) retinitis
   1. Definition
      a. Viral retinitis occurring almost exclusively in the immunocompromised
   2. Risk factors
      a. HIV, chemotherapy, immunosuppressive medications (post-transplant or for autoimmune disease)
   3. Symptoms and signs
      a. Gradual and progressive vision change (decreased visual acuity, floaters)
      b. External exam usually unimpressive
      c. Fundoscopy: "pizza pie fundus"
      d. Retinal detachment
   4. Diagnosis
      a. Check patient for immunocompromise

TABLE 10–2. Ophthalmologic Emergencies Requiring Immediate Consultation

Acute angle closure glaucoma
Herpes zoster ophthalmicus
Orbital cellulitis
Ruptured globe
Optic neuritis
Hyperacute bacterial conjunctivitis
CMV retinitis
Corneal ulcer
Central retinal artery occlusion
Retrobulbar hematoma

      i. HIV testing
      ii. CD4 count (usually <50 cells/mL)
   b. CMV antigenemia assay: detects the viral particles on the surface of white blood cells; indicates if the virus is replicating in the body or is inactive
   c. Blood or urine culture
      i. Results take as long as 3 weeks
   d. Serum DNA-PCR
   5. Management
      a. Ophthalmology consultation
      b. Admit and treat underlying disease
      c. Antiviral therapy (Ganciclovir, foscarnet, valganciclovir)
      d. Ganciclovir implants or intravitreal injection

B. Herpes zoster ophthalmicus
   1. Etiology: reactivation of latent human herpes virus 3 (varicella/zoster) in the ophthalmic division of the trigeminal nerve
   2. Symptoms and signs
      a. Eye pain, unilateral red eye, tearing, blurred vision
      b. Facial pain, fever and general malaise
      c. Involvement of the tip of the nose (**Hutchinson sign**) may be a clinical predictor of ocular involvement
      d. Unilateral vesicular rash, dermatomal pattern of the ophthalmic branch of the trigeminal nerve
      e. Fluorescein staining may reveal pseudodendrites
   3. Management
      a. Immediate ophthalmology consult
      b. Steroids only if advised by ophthalmology
      c. PO antiviral (acyclovir or famciclovir)
      d. Intravenous acyclovir
         i. Immunocompromised patients
         ii. Any evidence of retinal involvement
      e. Topical antibiotic
      f. Topical cycloplegic
      g. Oral analgesics

C. Herpes simplex keratitis
   1. Etiology: herpes simplex virus (usually HSV 1) that results in keratitis (inflammation of the cornea)
   2. Symptoms and signs
      a. Unilateral "red eye" with variable pain and irritation
      b. Pain, foreign body sensation, photophobia, tearing, visual changes
   3. Diagnosis
      a. **Dendritic** pattern on cornea with fluorescein staining (Figure 10–5)

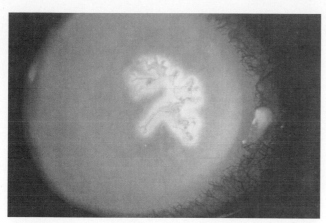

FIGURE 10–5. Dendrites. (Reproduced, with permission from Tintinalli JE, Kelen GD, Stapczynski JS: *Tintinalli's Emergency Medicine: A Comprehensive Study Guide,* 6th ed. New York: McGraw-Hill, 2004.)

4. Management
   a. Prompt ophthalmology consult
   b. Topical antiviral: trifluridine 1% given 9 times daily at 2-hour intervals
   c. Cycloplegic (homatropine)
   d. Do **not** apply topical steroids
   e. PO antivirals indictated if keratouveitis

D. Viral conjunctivitis
   1. Etiology: adenovirus (most common)
   2. Symptoms and signs
      a. Often starting in one eye with high rate of auto-inoculation to other eye
      b. 50% with systemic symptoms
      c. Lymphadenopathy
      d. Erythema, watery discharge, conjunctival swelling, tender preauricular node, foreign-body sensation
      e. Photophobia uncommon
   3. Management
      a. Supportive
      b. Cold compresses and topical vasoconstrictors may provide symptomatic relief
      c. May treat with topical antibiotics if unable to differentiate from bacterial conjunctivitis
      d. Steroids are contraindicated
      e. Prompt ophthalmology follow-up

E. Bacterial conjunctivitis
   1. Etiology: *Streptococcus pneumoniae, Haemophilus influenzae,* and *Staphylococcus aureus*
   2. Symptoms and signs
      a. Redness, burning, irritation, tearing, purulent discharge
      b. Copious purulent discharge, often unilateral
      c. Conjunctival chemosis: thickened, edematous conjunctiva
      d. White ulcer at lid margins
      e. Preauricular adenopathy
   3. Management
      a. Topical antibacterial agents × 5 to 7 days, every 4 to 6 hours
      b. Warm compress
      c. Ophthalmology follow-up

F. *Neisseria gonorrhea*
   1. Symptoms and signs
      a. Marked conjunctival injection, chemosis, lid swelling, and tender preauricular adenopathy
      b. Abrupt onset characterized by copious yellow-green purulent discharge
   2. Diagnosis
      a. Gram-stain and culture
   3. Management
      a. Ophthalmology consultation
      b. **Admit** for intravenous and topical antibiotics
         i. Intravenous penicillin G for neonatal gonorrhea infections
         ii. Third-generation cephalosporins for adult gonorrhea infections
      c. Treat for coinfection with chlamydia
      d. Frequent ocular irrigation

G. *Chlamydia trachomatis*
   1. Definition
      a. Infection with obligate intracellular bacterium that results in **3 distinct** conjunctivitis syndromes (trachoma, adult inclusion conjunctivitis, and neonatal inclusion conjunctivitis)
   2. Trachoma
      a. Epidemiology
         i. Most common cause of worldwide preventable blindness
         ii. Not a sexually transmitted disease unlike inclusion conjunctivitis
         iii. Children <10 years most commonly infected
      b. Transmission
         i. Direct contact of infected eye, nasal, and throat secretions
            a) Infected towels or clothing
            b) Spread from child to child in day care
            c) Spread among family members
         ii. Associated with poor hygiene
      c. Mechanism
         i. Repeated infections causing inversion of eyelashes

      ii. Repeated irritation and scarring of cornea by eyelashes causes vision loss in adulthood

   d. Symptoms and signs

      i. Chronic bilateral conjunctivitis

      ii. Various degrees of upper tarsal inflammation and thickening

      iii. Inversion of eyelashes

      iv. Various degrees conjunctival scarring

      v. Corneal opacification

   e. Diagnosis

      i. Clinical suspicion

      ii. Polymerase chain reaction, enzyme immunoassay (EIA), or cultures of conjunctival smears

   f. Management

      i. Prevention with improved personal hygiene

      ii. May need to treat entire families

      iii. World Health Organization (WHO) recommends either oral azithromycin or topical tetracycline eye ointment

      iv. Monitor for reinfection

  3. Adult inclusion conjunctivitis

   a. Etiology

      i. Sexually transmitted disease

      ii. Hand-to-eye inoculation of infected genital secretions

   b. Symptoms and signs

      i. Genitourinary infection (vaginal or penile discharge, dysuria, sore throat, pelvic inflammatory disease)

      ii. Nonspecific symptoms and signs of conjunctivitis (pink eye, discharge, foreign body sensation)

      iii. Persistent conjunctivitis despite multiple antibiotic courses

      iv. Unilateral more common than bilateral

   c. Diagnosis

      i. Direct immunofluorescent (DFA)

      ii. EIA

      iii. Chlamydial cultures

   d. Management

      i. Treat Chlamydial infection

        a) Oral azithromycin,

        b) Oral doxycycline

      ii. Treat for other sexually transmitted diseases

        a) Most notably Gonorrhea

      iii. Topical antibiotics are ineffective

  4. Neonatal inclusion conjunctivitis (see Pediatric chapter)

H. Hordeolum

  1. Definition

   a. **Infection** of either the eyelid margin or meibomian glands leading to an inflammatory nodule

  2. Etiology

   a. Most commonly *Staphylococcus aureus*

  3. Types

   a. Internal hordeolum: infection of meibomian gland

   b. External hordeolum (stye): infection of Zeiss or Moll glands at eyelid margins

  4. Symptoms and signs

   a. Internal hordeolum may present with localized erythema, tenderness, and swelling in the substance of the eyelid

   b. External hordeolum present with erythema and infection at the base of the eyelash

  5. Management

   a. Internal hordeolum

      i. Most resolve without drainage

        a) Warm compress

        b) Topical/oral antibiotics if concurrent cellulitis

      ii. May require incision and drainage

        a) Internal approach preferable to external scarring

        b) Large lesions should be referred to an ophthalmologist

   b. External hordeolum

      i. Warm soaks

      ii. Topical antibiotic of lid margin

      iii. Removal of single eyelash may aid resolution

I. Chalazion

  1. Definitions

   a. Deep chalazions: chronic **sterile** inflammation of the meibomian gland

   b. Superficial chalazions: chronic **sterile** inflammation of Zeiss or Moll sebaceous glands

  2. Symptoms and signs

   a. Painless

   b. Swelling and mass at either the substance of the eyelid or at its margins

   c. May be recurrent

  3. Management

   a. Topical ointments

   b. Warm compresses

   c. Defer steroid injections and surgical drainage to an ophthalmologist or plastic surgeon

J. Dacryocystitis

  1. Definition: infectious obstruction of the nasolacrimal duct

  2. Etiology: *Streptococcus pneumoniae, Haemophilus influenzae, Staphylococcus aureus, Streptococcus epidermidis*

3. Symptoms and signs
   a. Unilateral, painful, erythematous nasolacrimal duct
   b. Epiphora—an overflow of tears
   c. Digital pressure over the nasolacrimal duct may produce pus
4. Management
   a. Warm compress
   b. Topical and systemic antibiotics
   c. Ophthalmology referral

K. Periorbital (preseptal) cellulitis
   1. Definition
      a. Infection of eyelidlid, anterior to orbital septum
         i. Orbital septum: thin barrier separating the superficial eyelid from the deeper orbit
         ii. Originates from orbital periosteum and inserts into the base of the upper and lower eyelids
   2. Etiology
      a. Most commonly *Staphylococcus aureus, Streptococcus pyogenes,* and *Streptococcus pneumoniae*
   3. Symptoms and signs
      a. Acutely painful, swollen eyelid
      b. Erythema, fever
      c. Ocular motility intact
      d. No evidence of proptosis, injection, or vision change
   4. Diagnosis
      a. CT orbit (if clinical examination unequivocal)
   5. Management
      a. PO antibiotics (broad-spectrum): outpatients
         i. Amoxicillin/clavulanic acid
      b. Admit patients with more severe infection for IV antibiotics

L. Orbital (septal) cellulitis
   1. Definition
      a. Acute infection posterior to the orbital septum
   2. Etiology: same as preseptal cellulitis
   3. Symptoms and signs
      a. Red and swollen eyelid
      b. Pain, fever, and headache
      c. Increased IOP
      d. Proptosis (forward displacement of the eye)
      e. An abnormal pupil reaction afferent pupil defect
      f. Restricted or painful eye movement
   4. Diagnosis
      a. CT scan of the orbit with contrast, axial, and coronal views to rule out abscess

b. Blood culture, tissue cultures if aspirate or incision and drainage (I&D) of abscess
   5. Management
      a. Admit
      b. Immediate ophthalmology consult
      c. Parenteral antibiotics

M. Corneal ulcer
   1. Etiology
      a. Causative organisms: *Staphylococcus, Pseudomonas,* or *Streptococcus pneumoniae*
      b. *Pseudomonas* associated with contact lens usage
      c. Sleeping in contact lenses, inadequate contact lens sterilization, corneal trauma, or corneal foreign body
   2. Symptoms and signs
      a. Pain, foreign body sensation
      b. Photophobia, vision changes, eye discharge
   3. Management
      a. Ophthalmology consultation
      b. Oral or parenteral antibiotics—depends on severity
      c. Topical antibiotics—alternate aminoglycoside with a first-generation cephalosporin every 30 minutes
         i. Alternative—fluoroquinolones
      d. Addition of intravenous therapy for severe infections

N. Hypopyon
   1. Definition
      a. Leukocyte exudates (pus) in the anterior chamber
   2. Etiology
      a. Infectious (traumatic, postsurgical)
      b. Inflammatory (Behcet disease, inflammatory bowel disease)
   3. Symptoms and signs
      a. White fluid layer across inferior anterior chamber
      b. Injected conjunctiva (Figure 10–6)
   4. Management
      a. Identify and treat underlying infection

III. Inflammatory Disorders of the Eye

A. Acute anterior uveitis
   1. Definition
      a. Inflammation of the iris, ciliary body, or the choroid
   2. Etiology
      a. Autoimmune most common (rheumatoid arthritis, lupus, scleroderma, Reiter, Behcet, inflammatory bowel disease)

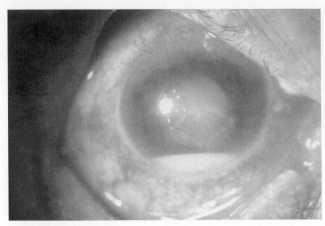

FIGURE 10–6. Hypopyon. (Reproduced, with permission, from Tintinalli JE, Kelem GD, Stapczynski JS: *Emergency Medicine A Comprehensive Study Guide,* 6th ed. Copyright © 2004, New York: McGraw-Hill.)

  b. Infectious (tuberculosis, lyme, syphilis, herpes, toxoplasmosis)
  c. Traumatic
3. Symptoms and signs
  a. Unilateral, painful red eye
  b. Vision change
  c. Photophobia
  d. Consensual photophobia (pain in affected eye when light shined into unaffected eye)
  e. Perilimbal injection (corneoscleral junction)
  f. Slit lamp: cells and flare
4. Diagnosis
  a. Clinical diagnosis
  b. Laboratory work should be directed to uncover underlying etiology
5. Management
  a. Ophthalmology consultation
  b. Prevention of synechiae (adhesion between peripheral iris and trabecular meshwork)
    i. Topical cycloplegic: block nerve impulses to the pupillary sphincter and ciliary muscles, easing pain and photophobia
    ii. Topical steroids prescribed by ophthalmologist—prednisolone 1%, 1 gtt q1 to 6 hours
  c. Evaluation of underlying systemic autoimmune and inflammatory disorder
B. Allergic
1. Etiology: IgE-mediated hypersensitivity reaction
2. Symptoms and signs
  a. Itching, tearing, redness, and mild eyelid swelling, cobblestoning
  b. Clear, watery, discharge
  c. Chemosis

3. Management
  a. Allergen avoidance
  b. Cold compresses
  c. Vasoconstrictors
  d. Antihistamine drops (levocabastine hydrochloride)
  e. Topical NSAIDs
  f. Ophthalmic mast-cell stabilizers, cromolyn sodium, or lodoxamide

C. Blepharitis
1. Definition
  a. Chronic inflammation of the eyelid near the root of the lash
2. Types
  a. Infectious
    i. Staphylococcus: scaling and crusting on eyelashes
  b. Functional
    i. Seborrheic, excess sebum production
      a) Greasy scaling along eyelashes
    ii. Meibomian gland dysfunction, excess lipid production
3. Symptoms and signs
  a. Itchy eyes, foreign body sensation
  b. Red and/or swollen eyelids
  c. Burning
  d. Crusty, flaky skin on the eyelids
  e. Dandruff
4. Management
  a. No cure
  b. Warm compresses
  c. Eyelid scrub

IV. Ophthalmologic Trauma

A. Corneal abrasion
1. Types
  a. Superficial: involves Bowman membrane
    i. Purely epithelial often heal quickly and completely without scarring
  b. Deep: penetrate Bowman membrane, but not Descemet membrane
    i. More likely to leave permanent scar
2. Symptoms and signs
  a. History of recent trauma or foreign body
  b. Acute pain, photophobia, tearing
  c. Vision change uncommon unless abrasion obstructs visual axis
  d. Foreign body sensation
  e. Foreign body revealed with eyelid eversion
  f. Conjunctival injection
3. Diagnosis
  a. Fluorescein staining detects epithelial injury
    i. Vertical abrasions indicative of foreign body lodged under lid
  b. Slit lamp examination to determine depth of injury

4. Management
   a. Topical antibiotics
   b. Contact lens abrasions: cover for *Pseudomonas*
   c. Cycloplegia for severe pain and large abrasions (atropine 1%, homatropine 5%, cyclopentolate 1%)
   d. Analgesics
   e. Ophthalmology follow-up
   f. Most corneal abrasions heal in 24 to 72 hours and rarely progress to corneal erosion or infection
   g. Update tetanus status

B. Burns
   1. Chemical (see Toxicology chapter)
      a. Acid burn
         i. Results in protein coagulation and coagulation necrosis
         ii. Limited depth of injury
      b. Alkali burn (ammonia, lye)—found in solvents, drain cleaners, detergents, cement
         i. Medical emergency
         ii. Lipophilic, penetrates more rapidly than acidic burns
         iii. Results in liquefication necrosis
         iv. Can rapidly damage cornea, iris, and lens leading to blindness
      c. Management
         i. Irrigate 2 to 5 L of saline immediately
         ii. Topical anesthesia and irrigation with ocular irrigation device
         iii. Irrigate until pH 7.4 × 2 litmus test, normal (pH is 7 to 7.4)
         iv. No corneal defect, normal anterior chamber
            a) Topical erythromycin
         v. Corneal defect or clouding of anterior chamber
            a) Topical erythromycin and cycloplegic
   2. Radiant energy and ultraviolet light- "welder" or "skier" keratitis
      a. Symptoms and signs
         i. Severe pain
         ii. Burning
         iii. Tearing
         iv. Photophobia
      b. Diagnosis
         i. Conjunctiva injected
         ii. Visual acuity decreased
         iii. Fluorescein: multiple punctate lesions
      c. Management
         i. Topical cycloplegic
         ii. Antibiotics
         iii. Oral analgesics
         iv. Ophthalmology referral

C. Hyphema
   1. Definition: blood in the anterior chamber
   2. Etiology
      a. Traumatic (most common)
         i. Contusive forces result in mechanical tearing of the fragile blood vasculature of the iris and/or ciliary body
      b. Spontaneous: associated with sickle cell disease
   3. Symptoms and signs
      a. Increased IOP caused by plugging of trabecular meshwork and Schlemm canal by RBCs
      b. Blurred vision, pain, photophobia, and tearing
   4. Diagnosis
      a. Grade 1: <33% of anterior chamber (AC)
      b. Grade 2: 33% to 50% of AC
      c. Grade 3: 50% to incomplete filling of AC
      d. Grade 4: **complete** filling of visible AC (Figure 10–7)
   5. Management
      a. Elevate head of bed
      b. Analgesics (no ASA or NSAIDS → may worsen bleed)
      c. Cycloplegics: atropine, decreases iris activity and therefore decreases chance of rebleeding
      d. Aminocaproic acid an antifibrinolytic
      e. Grade 1 can be managed outpatient; Grade 4 requires surgical intervention
      f. Admit for observation if hyphema >33% involvement or IOP >30
      g. Ophthalmology consult for disposition, secondary to high risk of complications

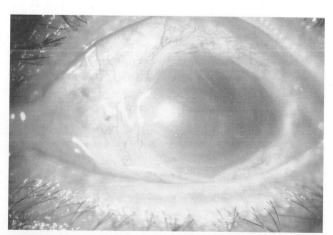

FIGURE 10–7. Hyphema. (Reproduced, with permission, from Tintinalli JE, Kelem GD, Stapczynski JS: *Emergency Medicine A Comprehensive Study Guide,* 6th ed. Copyright © 2004, New York: McGraw-Hill.)

6. Complications
   a. Rebleeding
      i. Disruption of original clot, occurs 3 to 5 days after initial bleed
      ii. Higher risk in African Americans and sickle cell patients
   b. Elevated IOP
      i. Manage with topical β-blocker, α-adrenergic agonist, and/or mannitol, acetazolamide
      ii. Sickle cell patients are at higher risk for elevated IOPs secondary to blockage caused by red blood cells that have sickled under ischemic conditions
      iii. Carbonic anhydrase inhibitors are contraindicated in sickle cell patients because they lower the pH
   c. Corneal bloodstaining and optic nerve atrophy can impair vision

D. Retrobulbar hematoma
   1. Definition
      a. Accumulation of blood behind the globe that causes a compartment syndrome of the eye
   2. Etiology
      a. Most commonly posttraumatic
   3. Pathophysiology
      a. Hematoma exerts pressure on optic nerve, globe, central retinal artery
   4. Symptoms and signs
      a. Pain
      b. Vision loss
      c. Evidence of trauma
      d. Marcus Gunn pupil
      e. Proptosis
      f. Increased IOP
      g. Ophthalmoplegia: paralysis of extraocular muscles
   5. Diagnosis
      a. CT orbits if diagnosis unclear
   6. Management
      a. Osmotic agents and carbonic anhydrase inhibitors
      b. Immediate ophthalmology consultation
      c. Emergent lateral canthotomy, to relieve rapidly rising orbital pressure which can lead to irreversible vision loss within 90 to 120 minutes of ischemia

E. Globe rupture
   1. Definition
      a. Full-thickness injury to the sclera secondary to blunt or penetrating trauma
   2. Etiology
      a. Penetrating injury (eg, hammering metal on metal)
      b. Blunt trauma (eg, closed fist injury)
   3. Symptoms and signs
      a. Subtle signs
         i. Subconjunctival hemorrhage
         ii. Uvea with dark pigmentation
         iii. Altered red reflex
         iv. Conjunctival laceration
      b. Strong signs
         i. "8-ball" or "black ball" appearance from severe conjunctival hemorrhage covering 360 degrees of the globe
         ii. Teardrop-shaped pupil
         iii. Flat anterior chamber
         iv. Iris at wound edges
      c. External evidence of globe rupture may not be visible with blunt trauma as areas of weakness occur at muscle insertion points
   4. Diagnosis
      a. CT orbit
      b. Seidel test: aqueous flow on fluorescein testing (Figure 10–8)
   5. Management
      a. Eye shield
      b. Do not manipulate or put pressure on eye
      c. IOP measurement contraindicated
      d. Elevate head of bed
      e. Antiemetics to prevent valsalva stress on eyes
      f. Tetanus
      g. Antibiotics
      h. Immediate ophthalmology consult for surgical intervention

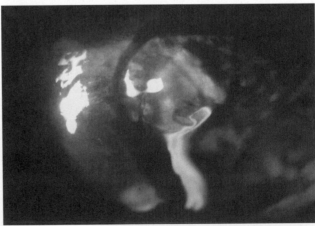

FIGURE 10–8. Seidel sign. (Reproduced, with permission, from Tintinalli JE, Kelem GD, Stapczynski JS: *Emergency Medicine A Comprehensive Study Guide*, 6th ed. Copyright © 2004, New York: McGraw-Hill.)

Chapter 11
DENTAL, EAR, NOSE, AND THROAT EMERGENCIES

Behdad Jamshahi and Anand Swaminathan

I. Oral Emergencies

A. General considerations
  1. Anatomy (Figure 11–1)
    a. Pulp
      i. Center of tooth
      ii. Provides sensation, produces dentin
    b. Crown portion
      i. Visible tooth in the oral cavity
      ii. Covered with enamel
    c. Root
      i. Part not visible
      ii. Covered with cementum
    d. Sensory innervation
      i. Maxillary teeth: anterior, middle, and posterior superior alveolar nerves (branch from cranial nerve V_2)
      ii. Mandibular teeth: inferior alveolar nerve (branch from cranial nerve V_3)
  2. Nomenclature (Figure 11–2)
    a. Numbered clockwise from maxillary third molar to bottom mandibular molars

B. Trauma
  1. Tooth avulsion (Figure 11–3)
    a. Critical to differentiate primary from secondary dentition
    b. Management
      i. Primary tooth
        a) No treatment required
        b) Do not reimplant
          i) Reimplantation may lead to fusion with underlying alveolar bone and facial deformity
      ii. Secondary tooth
        a) Reimplant immediately
          i) Preferably within first 20 minutes
          ii) Periodontal ligaments die >60 minutes

        b) Rinse gently with water, milk, or Hank solution if available (do not scrub as this may remove ligaments and fibers essential to success of reimplantation)
        c) Grasp tooth by crown and insert into socket
        d) Brace or stabilize teeth with zinc oxide paste (Coe-Pak)
        e) Antibiotics: penicillin VK, or erythromycin
          i) Tetanus if indicated
  2. Fracture of anterior teeth: Ellis classification (Figure 11–4)
    a. Class I
      i. Enamel injury
      ii. Painless
      iii. Treatment: smooth any rough edges
    b. Class II
      i. Dentin and enamel injury
      ii. May have hot or cold sensitivity
      iii. Yellow dentin exposed on exam
      iv. Management
        a) Cover with calcium hydroxide or foil
        b) Urgent oral surgery (OMFS) and dental referral
        c) Consider antibiotics
    c. Class III
      i. Enamel, dentin, and pulp injury
      ii. Severe pain, or painless if neurovascular supply is disrupted
      iii. Pink tinge visible indicating exposed pulp
      iv. Management
        a) **Immediate and emergent** OMFS and dental referral
        b) Calcium hydroxide paste or moist cotton to cover exposed pulp
        c) Oral analgesics
        d) Antibiotics: penicillin VK

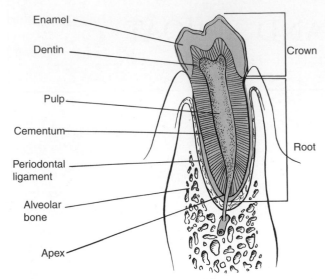

FIGURE 11–1. Tooth anatomy. (Reproduced, with permission, from Tintinalli JE, Kelen GD, Stapczynski JS: *Tintinalli's Emergency Medicine: A Comprehensive Study Guide,* 6th ed. Copyright © 2004, New York: McGraw-Hill.)

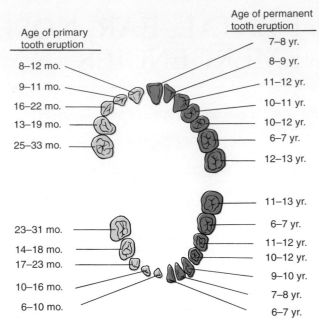

FIGURE 11–3. Timeline of tooth eruption. (Reproduced, with permission, from Tintinalli JE, Kelen GD, Stapczynski JS: *Tintinalli's Emergency Medicine: A Comprehensive Study Guide,* 6th ed. Copyright © 2004, New York: McGraw-Hill.)

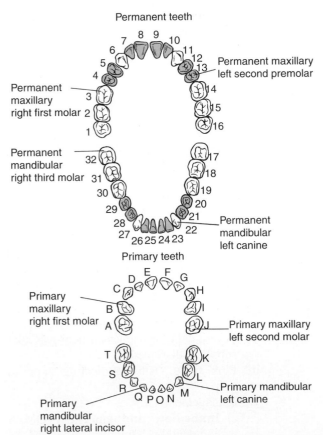

FIGURE 11–2. Tooth locations. (Reproduced, with permission, from Tintinalli JE, Kelen GD, Stapczynski JS: *Tintinalli's Emergency Medicine: A Comprehensive Study Guide,* 6th ed. Copyright © 2004, New York: McGraw-Hill.)

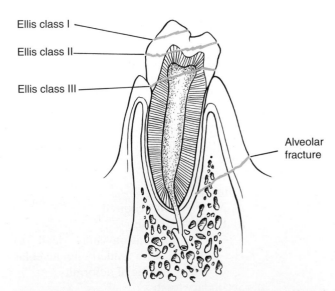

FIGURE 11–4. Ellis classification system. (Reproduced, with permission, from Tintinalli JE, Kelen GD, Stapczynski JS: *Tintinalli's Emergency Medicine: A Comprehensive Study Guide,* 6th ed. Copyright © 2004, McGraw-Hill.)

d. Complications
  i. Tooth pulp prone to infection (pulpitis)
  ii. Dentin is porous and susceptible to bacterial infiltration
3. Tooth subluxation (loose tooth)
  a. Definition: injury to the attachment apparatus of the tooth without radiographic evidence of dislodgement
  b. Management: realign tooth, oral analgesics, soft diet
    i. OMFS and dental follow-up
4. Temporomandibular joint (TMJ) dislocation
  a. Etiology: trauma, extreme opening of mouth during yawning, laughing, dystonic reactions
  b. Mechanism: Anterior movement of mandibular condyle with spasm of masseter, pterygoid, and temporalis muscles
    i. Jaw deviates to opposite side of dislocation if unilateral
  c. Diagnosis: x-ray and CT before relocation if fracture suspected
  d. Management
    i. Reduction
      a) Under procedural sedation
        i) Relax masseter spasm
      b) Gloved thumbs rest posterior to molars, fingers wrap around the outside of the jaw. Thumbs should be wrapped in gauze for protection
      c) Downward pressure applied initially, then mandible directed posteriorly and superiorly back into temporal fossae
    ii. Disposition
      a) Soft diet, warm compresses, avoidance of extreme mouth opening, soft bandage
      b) OMFS follow-up
      c) Referral for interdental fixation may be required in patients with repeated dislocation
5. Lip lacerations
  a. Management
    i. External laceration
      a) **Maintain vermilion border**
        i) Misalignment of as little as 1 mm can result in a cosmetic deformity
        ii) Mark before injection of anesthetic
        iii) Antibiotics not routinely required
    ii. Through-and-through lacerations
      a) Always approximate vermillion border first
      b) Search and remove foreign body
      c) Work from mucosa outward
      d) Mucosal and deep sutures with absorbable material

e) Vigorous irrigation after mucosa closed
f) Prophylactic antibiotics: Penicillin VK or erythromycin
    iii. Isolated intraoral mucosal lacerations
      a) Heals well due to vascularity
      b) Most heal well without suturing
        i) Consider suturing with absorbable material if larger than 2 cm
      c) Recommend frequent rinsing
6. Tongue lacerations
  a. Repair only if
    i. Large gaping injuries as food may collect
    ii. Complete anterior laceration to prevent "fork" tongue
  b. Use black silk (less irritating)
  c. Gargle after eating
7. Perioral electrical burns
  a. Epidemiology: commonly young children who bite or lick electrical cords
  b. Symptoms and signs: full-thickness burn at lip commissure
    i. May appear deceptively benign on initial presentation
    ii. Delayed bleeding from labial artery 5 to 21 days postinjury
      a) Instruct parents to anticipate bleeding
      b) Demonstrate digital compression to control bleeding
  c. Management
    i. Controversial because of possibility of delayed bleeding
    ii. Ranges from early surgical reconstruction to delayed excision
    iii. Early involvement of ENT and plastic surgery
8. Cheek lacerations
  a. Symptoms and signs: check for involvement of salivary ducts and injury to facial nerve
    i. Parotid (Stensen) and submandibular (Wharton) ducts most commonly injured
    ii. Evaluate integrity by milking saliva from the gland
  b. Management
    i. Simple interrupted sutures for uncomplicated lacerations
    ii. Duct injury requires ENT consultation

C. Infection
  1. Caries
    a. Definition: decalcification of enamel by acids as bacteria metabolize carbohydrates
    b. Symptoms and signs: dull pain, worse with chewing and temperature extremes; may be referred to ear, eye, neck, opposite jaw

c. Management
    i. Dental block
    ii. No antibiotics required for simple dental caries
    iii. Disposition: oral analgesics, dental referral
2. Periapical abscess
    a. Definition: Abscess resulting from infection of the root apex
        i. Usually confined to alveolar bone
        ii. Muscle involvement may result in spread to fascial planes
    b. Symptoms and signs: intense pain, worse if tooth manipulated; facial edema
    c. Management: antibiotics: Penicillin VK or clindamycin, OMFS and dental referral, +/– incision and drainage in ED
    d. Complications: canine space abscess (spreads through alveolar bone), Ludwig angina, cavernous sinus thrombosis, airway compromise
3. Acute necrotizing ulcerative gingivitis (ANUG): Otherwise known as Vincent angina or trench mouth (Figure 11–5)
    a. Definition: overgrowth of normally present bacteria which invade nonnecrotic tissue
        i. *Bacteriodes, Fusobacteria*, and spirochetes
        ii. Seen in immunocompromised individuals and smokers
    b. Symptoms and signs
        i. Pain, foul breath, pseudomembrane formation, metallic taste, fever, lymphadenopathy
        ii. Gingiva is fiery red, papillae between teeth are covered by grey pseudomembrane that bleeds if removed

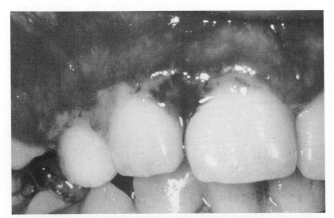

FIGURE 11–5. Necrotizing ulcerative gingivitis. (Reproduced, with permission, from Tintinalli JE, Kelen GD, Stapczynski JS: *Tintinalli's Emergency Medicine: A Comprehensive Study Guide,* 6th ed. Copyright © 2004, McGraw-Hill.)

c. Management
    i. Antibiotics: penicillin VK, clindamycin erythromycin, doxycycline
    ii. Irrigation and oral hygiene
    iii. Analgesics: viscous lidocaine, NSAIDs
    iv. Disposition: OMFS and dental follow-up a must as can result in destruction of underlying alveolar bone

D. Tooth pain
    1. Periosteitis
        a. Definition: pain and bone inflammation within 24 hours of extraction
        b. Management: oral analgesics; NSAIDs (discontinue if bleeding)
    2. Alveolar osteitis (dry socket)
        a. Definition: sudden excruciating pain 3 to 4 days after extraction
        b. Etiology: displacement of blood clot from the socket and local bone infection
        c. Symptoms and signs: pain and foul odor
        d. Management
            i. Pack socket with iodoform gauze saturated with medicated dental paste (Euginol)
            ii. Oral analgesics, OMFS, and dental follow-up
            iii. Antibiotics usually not required

E. Miscellaneous causes of oral pain
    1. Trigeminal neuralgia (tic douloureux)
        a. Etiology: idiopathic, possibly caused by vascular compression of the trigeminal nerve
        b. Symptoms and signs
            i. Excruciating, paroxysmal pain
                a) Precipitated by tapping nerve, eating, or movement
        c. Management
            i. High rate of spontaneous remission
            ii. Carbamazepine most commonly used
                a) Other options: phenytoin, baclofen, gabapentin, surgical treatment (relief of vascular compression)
            iii. Disposition: OMFS and neurologic follow-up
    2. Temporomandibular (TMJ) syndrome
        a. Caused by anatomic malalignment of joint, aggravated by trauma, clenching of teeth, bruxism (tooth grinding)
        b. Symptoms and signs
            i. Pain around area of TMJ, worse in PM
            ii. Inability to open mouth fully
            iii. Clicking of jaw
        c. Management
            i. Heat, soft diet, NSAIDs, benzodiazepines
            ii. OMFS and dental follow-up

F. Oral manifestations of systemic disease
1. Toxic and metabolic
    a. Heavy metal poisoning
        i. Lead poisoning: gingival "lead line"
        ii. Silver poisoning: blue-to-bronze discoloration of oral mucosa (argyria)
        iii. Management: depends on the heavy metal in question (see toxicology section for specific treatment)
    b. Phenytoin
        i. Epidemiology: 40% of patients develop gingival hyperplasia
        ii. Management
            a) Good dental hygiene
            b) Surgical removal of overgrowth
            c) Discontinue medication
2. Collagen vascular diseases
    a. Lupus, Reiter, Wegener, Bechet
        i. Intraoral ulcerated lesions, painful, commonly infected
    b. Sjogren
        i. Diminished secretions of salivary, lacrimal glands
        ii. Gritty sensation of eyes, diminished taste, dry mouth
3. Pyogenic granuloma (Figure 11–6)

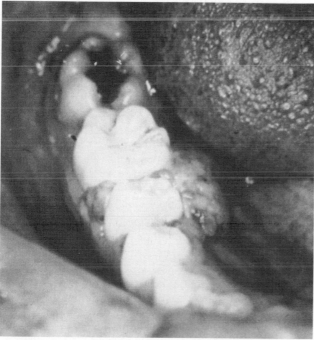

FIGURE 11–6. Pyogenic Granuloma. (Reproduced, with permission, from Tintinalli JE, Kelen GD, Stapczynski JS: *Tintinalli's Emergency Medicine: A Comprehensive Study Guide,* 6th ed. Copyright (c) 2004, New York: McGraw-Hill.)

a. Warty-like proliferation of vascular tissue in response to irritant
b. Common in pregnancy, usually resolve spontaneously 2 to 3 months postpartum
4. Blood dyscrasias
    a. Thrombocytopenia
        i. Spontaneous gingival bleeding
        ii. Soft palate petechiae
    b. Acute leukemia
        i. Edematous, bluish red gingiva
5. Aphthous stomatitis
    a. Symptoms and signs: 2 to 3 mm oral mucosal ulcers with white center often recurrent, tender and exacerbated by stress, malnutrition, oral trauma
    b. Management: hydrogen peroxide rinse, steroid ointment (Triamcinolone topical), 50:50 mix of diphenhydramine and Maalox rinse
6. Viral infections
    a. Herpes simplex virus (HSV)
        i. Gingivostomatitis
            a) Epidemiology: common presentation of primary HSV-1 infection in children <5 years
            b) Symptom and signs
                i) Fever, pharyngeal edema, erythema, cervical adenopathy
                ii) Small vesicles that ulcerate and multiply
                iii) Duration of illness: 10 to 14 days
            c) Management
                i) Topical analgesics
                    a. Viscous lidocaine
                    b. Benzocaine
                ii) Oral opioids in severe cases
                iii) Antiviral: acyclovir, valacyclovir, famcyclovir
                iv) Severe cases may require admission for pain control and dehydration
    b. Coxsackie
        i. Hand-foot-mouth syndrome
            a) Signs and symptoms
                i) Fever
                ii) Vesicles on the buccal mucosa and tongue
                iii) Peripherally distributed tender lesions on the buttock, hands, and feet
            b) Management: self-limited illness
    c. Human immunodeficiency virus (HIV)
        i. Oropharyngeal candidiasis (thrush)
            a) Symptoms and signs
                i) Curd-like plaques easily removed with tongue blade

ii) Also seen in diabetics, patients on antibiotics or steroids

b) Management: clotrimazole troches for oral lesions, systemic antifungals are required for esophageal extension and resistant lesions

ii. Hairy leukoplakia

a) Etiology: Epstein-Barr virus (EBV)

b) Symptoms and signs

i) White patches on side of tongue

ii) Cannot be removed with tongue blade

c) Management: self-limited; acyclovir, ganciclovir, foscarnet

iii. Kaposi sarcoma

a) Definition: malignant cancer of the lymphatic endothelium

b) Etiology: Human herpes virus 8 (HHV8)

i) AIDS defining illness

c) Symptoms and signs: Bluish-red lesions most commonly found on hard palate

II. Ear

A. Infection

1. Acute otitis media

a. Etiology

i. Viral > bacterial

ii. *S. pneumonia > H. influenza > M. catarrhalis > S. aureus >* Group A *Streptococci*

b. Symptoms and signs

i. More common in children <36 months

ii. Acute onset

iii. Middle ear effusion

a) Limited or absent mobility of tympanic membrane (TM) with pneumatic otoscopy (most sensitive test)

b) Bulging TM

c) Air-fluid level behind TM

iv. Middle ear inflammation

a) Erythema (though may be caused by crying, fever)

b) Pain (especially with pneumatic otoscopy)

c. Management

i. American Academy of Pediatrics Guidelines, 2004

a) Guideline based on age, certainty of diagnosis, and severity

b) Infants <6 months:, treat even if diagnosis uncertain

c) Children 6 months to 2 years: observe if unsure of diagnosis and patient has good follow-up

d) Children >2 years: treat only if certain of diagnosis, and illness is severe

ii. Antibiotics

a) Amoxicillin (80 to 90 mg/kg/day × 10 days)

i) Reevaluate those without improvement in 2 to 3 days

b) Treatment failure warrants second course of antibiotics: 3 days of amoxicillin/clavulanate or cefuroxime PO

iii. Pain management: Acetaminophen, NSAIDs

iv. No proven benefit of antihistamines, decongestants, steroids

v. Myringotomy and placement of tympanostomy tubes for persistent cases

d. Complications

i. Tympanic membrane perforation

ii. Decreased hearing

iii. Cholesteotoma

a) Accumulation of keratin-producing squamous epithelium in middle ear

b) Treatment is surgical

iv. Labyrinthitis

v. Mastoiditis

vi. Intracranial infections-meningitis, brain abscess

2. Otitis externa (swimmer's ear)

a. Definition: inflammation of the external auditory canal

b. Etiology: maceration of canal epithelium from prolonged moisture, local trauma (eg, foreign body insertion)

i. Causative orgnanisms

a) *Pseudomonas aeruginosa* (most common bacterial etiology)

b) Fungal (Aspergillus, Candida)

c. Symptoms and signs

i. Pain with pinna and auricle movement

ii. Pruritis

iii. Discharge

d. Management

i. Clean external canal of debris by means of suction, irrigation, curettage

ii. Keep canal dry (acetic acid solution may be used)

iii. Antibiotics

a) Fluoroquinolone solutions are first-line

b) Use suspension formulation if tympanic membrane perforation suspected

c) Aminoglycoside (eg, neomycin) solutions are used less frequently because of ototoxicity

d) Systemic antibiotics added for severe cases

   iv. Steroids: topical hydrocortisone reduces the duration of symptoms but not time to clinical resolution

   v. Cotton wick may be placed for better delivery of antibiotics

   vi. Pain management

   vii. Disposition

    a) Follow-up with primary care physician

    b) ENT surgery referral

 3. Necrotizing (malignant) otitis externa

  a. Definition: progression of otitis externa through the periauricular tissue and into the temporal bone

   i. Occurs in immunocompromised/diabetics patients

  b. Etiology: *P. aeruginosa*

  c. Symptoms and signs

   i. Excruciating pain

    a) Persistent, interferes with sleep, continues even after topical treatment and apparent resolution of external canal edema

   ii. Fever

   iii. Erythema of periauricular tissues

   iv. Facial and vagal nerve palsy

  d. Diagnosis

   i. CT or bone scan

  e. Management

   i. Systemic antibiotics

    a) Antipseudomonal double coverage (penicillin-based and aminoglycoside)

    b) Alternative: ciprofloxacin

   ii. Surgical debridement may be necessary if no improvement

   iii. Disposition

    a) Up to 50% mortality if untreated

    b) Admission to ENT

 4. Herpes zoster oticus (Ramsey-Hunt syndrome)

  a. Symptoms and signs

   i. Triad: ear pain, vesicles in the auricle and auditory canal, and ipsilateral facial paralysis

   ii. Multiple cranial nerve involvement (CN V, VII, IX, and X)

  b. Management

   i. Acyclovir, oral analgesics

   ii. ENT referral

 5. Bullous myringitis

  a. Etiology

   i. Predominately viral

   ii. May be caused by *Mycoplasma* infection

  b. Symptoms and signs: Hemorrhagic or clear blisters on TM, pain, mild hearing loss

  c. Management: macrolide antibiotics, heat, analgesia

B. Trauma

 1. Subperichondral hematoma

  a. Etiology: blunt trauma

  b. Management

   i. Aspiration versus incision and drainage

   ii. Postprocedure pressure × 48 to 72 hours to prevent reaccumulation

   iii. Disposition: ENT follow-up

  c. Complications: cauliflower ear may result if not promptly treated

 2. Ear laceration

  a. Anatomy

   i. Auricular skin is highly vascular

   ii. Underlying cartilage is avascular and relies on overlying skin for nourishment

   iii. Cartilage and skin are tightly adherent and difficult to separate

  b. Management

   i. All exposed cartilage **must** be completely covered with skin

   ii. Remove excess cartilage to meet above goal

    a) Consult plastic surgeon if >5 mm trimmed

   iii. Approximate edges by suturing through skin and perichondrium with 6-0 nylon

   iv. Treat and prevent subperichondral hematoma

   v. ENT follow-up

 3. TM perforation

  a. Etiology

   i. Cotton swab or foreign body

   ii. Otitis media

   iii. Barotrauma

   iv. Explosion, lightning, or high-voltage electrocution

  b. Symptoms and signs

   i. Pain

   ii. Decreased hearing (may or may not be significant)

   iii. Bleeding

  c. Management

   i. Often none required other than keeping ear dry

   ii. Analgesics

   iii. Immediate ENT referral if complete hearing loss, vertigo, facial palsy, which suggests ossicle or temporal bone injury

C. Hearing Loss (see Neurology chapter)

D. Vertigo (see Neurology chapter)

III. Nose

A. Infection
1. Sinusitis (Table 11–1)
   a. Etiology
      i. Viral infection most common
      ii. Allergic: associated with sneezing, itchy eyes
      iii. Bacterial
         a) Worsening of symptoms after 5 days or persistent symptoms after 10 days
         b) Chronic sinusitis complicated by mixed flora including anaerobes and Gram-negative organisms
   b. Symptoms and signs
      i. Headache
      ii. Unilateral facial pain
      iii. Purulent rhinorrhea
      iv. Fever
   c. Acute versus chronic
      i. Acute
         a) Develops over 5 to 7 days
         b) Associated with the classic symptoms listed above in symptoms and signs of sinusitis
         c) Difficult to differentiate viral from bacterial (bacterial worsens after 5 days)
      ii. Chronic
         a) Slow in onset and prolonged in duration (>12 weeks)
         b) Recurrent episodes
         c) Symptoms may include chronic cough, fetid breath, laryngitis, bronchitis
   d. Diagnosis
      i. Primarily a clinical diagnosis
      ii. Imaging: CT preferred to plain radiographs
         a) Air fluid levels, sinus opacification, 4 mm of sinus wall thickening
   e. Management
      i. Most resolve spontaneously
      ii. For patients with unilateral maxillary tenderness, purulent discharge, or symptoms for >1 week
         a) Amoxicillin or amoxicillin/clavulanate initially for 7 to 10 days
         b) Shorter course azithromycin for 3 days or a fluoroquinolone
      iii. Antihistamines or decongestants
         a) No good evidence supports its use
         b) Use for 3 to 5 days only
         c) Rebound vasodilation, nasal obstruction
      iv. Complications
         a) Frontal bone osteomyelitis (Pott puffy tumor)
         b) Orbital cellulitis
         c) Acute sphenoid sinusitis
2. Acute sphenoid sinusitis
   a. Anatomy
      i. Most posterior of sinuses
      ii. Sinus floor: nasopharynx
      iii. Clivus located posterior to sinus
      iv. Pituitary located superior to sinus
      v. Optic nerve passes anterolateral to sinus
      vi. Cavernous sinuses located lateral to this sinus
         a) Contains internal carotid arteries, CN II, III, IV, V_3, and VI
   b. Management
      i. Antibiotics: broad-spectrum IV antibiotics
      ii. Nasal decongestants
      iii. Surgical drainage indicated if
         a) No improvement within 24 hours with medical management
         b) Neurologic deficits
   c. Complications: Related to infection of neighboring structures
      i. Meningits, diplopia, cavernous sinus thrombosis

B. Trauma
1. Nasal fracture
   a. Clinical diagnosis
      i. X-rays not required
   b. Management
      i. Ice
      ii. Analgesia

TABLE 11–1. Acute Sinusitis Pathogens

VIRAL	BACTERIAL (COMMUNITY-ACQUIRED)	BACTERIAL (NOSOCOMIAL)	FUNGAL
Rhinovirus	S. pneumoniae	S. aureus	Aspergillus species
Parainfluenza virus	H. influenzae	Streptococcal species	P. boydii
Influenza virus	M. catarrhalis	Pseudomonal species	S. schenckii
Coronavirus	S. aureus	E. coli	Homobasidiomycetes
Respiratory vyncytial virus	Other streptococcal species	Klebsiella species	
Adenovirus	Anaerobes		

      iii. Antihistamines or decongestants

      iv. Disposition: ENT follow-up 7 to 10 days

  2. Septal hematomas

    a. Dark purple or bluish mass against the septum

    b. Management: drainage followed by anterior packing to prevent necrosis

    c. Complication: saddle nose deformity if not drained

  3. Epistaxis (see Procedure chapter)

C. Foreign body

  1. Epidemiology: Children <3 years

  2. Symptoms and signs: foul-smelling unilateral rhinorrhea or epistaxis

  3. Management: removal

    a. Positive pressure

    b. Suction catheter

    c. Forceps, wire loops

IV. Oral and Upper Airway

A. Sialadenitis and sialolithiasis

  1. Definitions

    a. Sialadenitis: inflammation of salivary glands (parotid, submandibular, sublingual)

    b. Sialolithiasis: stone formation in the salivary gland

    c. Submandibular sialadenitis and sialolithiasis most common

  2. Etiology

    a. Infectious

      i. Viral

        a) Mumps, HIV

      ii. Bacterial

        a) Most commonly *Staphylococcus aureus*

      iii. Infection and inflammation secondary to sialolithiasis

    b. Autoimmune

      i. Sjogren syndrome, systemic lupus

    c. Miscellaneous

      i. Radiation, tuberculosis, sarcoidosis, cancer, hypothyroidism, cirrhosis, diabetes

  3. Symptoms and signs

    a. Acute or chronic pain

      i. Acute inflammation painful

      ii. Less painful or even painless with chronic form

    b. Colicky postprandial pain with sialolithiasis

    c. Fever, erythema, tenderness over gland

    d. Pus from Wharton duct (submandibular) or Stenson duct (parotid)

  4. Diagnosis

    a. Clinical examination

    b. CT scanning

    c. Ultrasound may be helpful in identifying abscesses or differentiating solid versus cystic structures and may occasionally identify calcium stones

  5. Management

    a. Treat underlying pathology

    b. Acute sialadenitis

      i. Warm compress

      ii. Gland massage

      iii. Hydration

      iv. Antibiotics

      v. Sialogogues (sour candy)

      vi. Consider surgery or drainage if large abscess

    c. Simple sialolithiasis

      i. Warm compress, gland massage, hydration, and sialogogues

        a) Antibiotics if infected

    d. Disposition

      i. Admit if septic or danger of Ludwig angina

B. Ludwig angina

  1. Definition

    a. Potentially airway threatening cellulitis of the oral floor

  2. Etiology

    a. Most commonly caused by dental or salivary gland pathology

    b. Polymicrobial; *Staphylococcus, Streptococcus, Bacteroides*

  3. Symptoms and signs

    a. Pain, drooling, dysphonia

    b. Brawny edema of neck, tense edema of floor of mouth, bilateral submandibular swelling, elevation and protrusion of tongue

  4. Diagnosis

    a. Maintain high clinical suspicion

    b. Neck x-ray or CT may reveal gas collections

  5. Treatment

    a. Emergent ENT or oral maxillofacial consultation

    b. Consider prophylactic intubation as airway compromise may occur rapidly

    c. Surgical airway if endotracheal intubation not possible

    d. Broad-spectrum antibiotics

  6. Complications include internal jugular thrombosis, intracranial extension, mediastinitis

C. Retropharyngeal and prevertebral space abscesses

  1. Epidemiology: most common in children <6 years

  2. Deep neck space infection

    a. Anatomy

      i. Posterior to pharynx

      ii. Anterior to vertebral bodies

    iii. Bounded laterally by carotid sheaths
    iv. Bounded superiorly by skull base
    v. Bounded inferiorly by mediastinum

  b. Less common in adults as retropharyngeal lymph nodes regress in adulthood

3. Etiology
  a. Anaerobes: predominate in infections originating from the oral cavity
    i. *Fusobacterium, Bacteriodes*
  b. Aerobes: predominate in infections originating from the pharyngeal cavity
    i. *S. pyogenes, Staphylococcus, pseudomonal* species

4. Symptoms and signs
  a. Drooling, muffled voice, neck stiffness, fever
  b. Duck "quack" (cri du canard)
  c. Holds neck extended
  d. Trismus
  e. Stridor
  f. Tenderness on moving larynx from side to side
  g. Pain may radiate to back of neck, shoulder blades

5. Diagnosis
  a. Soft tissue neck x-rays
  b. Prevertebral soft tissue swelling
    i. Film should be obtained with neck fully extended
    ii. Film during inspiration
    iii. Prevertebral tissue space should be no wider than the vertebral body
  c. CT scan of neck
  d. Chest x-ray may indicate mediastinitis

6. Management
  a. Airway management if necessary
  b. IV antibiotics +/– surgical incision and drainage in OR
  c. Admission

7. Complications
  a. Airway compromise
  b. Mediastinitis
  c. Aspiration pneumonia
  d. Cranial nerve palsies
  e. Septic jugular thrombophlebitis
  f. Atlantoaxial separation caused by involvement of atlas transverse ligament

D. Peritonsillar abscess (Figure 11–7)
1. Polymicrobial abscess within the peritonsilar space
2. Symptoms and signs
  a. Fever
  b. Trismus
  c. Hot potato voice
  d. Contralateral uvular deviation

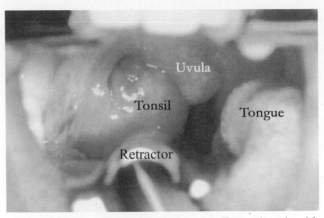

FIGURE 11–7. Peritonsillar Abscess. (Reproduced, with permission, from Tintinalli JE, Kelen GD, Stapczynski JS: *Tintinalli's Emergency Medicine: A Comprehensive Study Guide,* 6th ed. Copyright © 2004, McGraw-Hill.)

3. Management (see also Procedures section)
  a. Treatment options include antibiotics plus either needle aspiration or incision and drainage
  b. As the name indicates, the abscess is **peri**tonsillar and therefore, the needle is not placed into the tonsil
  c. Avoid internal carotid artery, which is located ~2.5 cm inferior laterally to tonsil
  d. 25% false-negative tap rate
  e. Admit patients with negative aspirations if the examination and history strongly suggest PTA
  f. Antibiotics: penicillin VK or clindamycin

4. Complications
  a. Airway obstruction
  b. Abscess rupture, aspiration
  c. Deep space, intracranial extension
  d. Inadvertent carotid artery injury during drainage

E. Pharyngitis (Table 11-2)
1. Etiology
  a. Viral
    i. Cause 50% to 60%
    ii. Enterovirus: major etiology from late spring through autumn
    iii. Adenovirus
      a) 50% associated with unilateral conjunctivitis
    iv. Ebstein-Barr virus
  b. Bacterial
    i. Group A β-hemolytic *Streptoccocus*
      a) Epidemiology: rare in children <3 years
      b) Classic symptoms and signs
        i) Tonsillar exudate
        ii) Fever

TABLE 11–2. Viral and Bacterial Causes of Pharyngitis

PATHOGEN	SYNDROME OR DISEASE	SIGNS AND SYMPTOMS	PERCENT (%)
Viral			
Rhinovirus and coronavirus	Common cold	Nonexudative; mild-to-moderate pharyngeal pain; rhinorrhea; odynophagia, fever, myalgia and malaise uncommon	25
Adenovirus	Pharyngoconjunctival fever	More common in summer; fever; malaise; HA; dizziness; conjunctivitis	5
Herpes simplex virus	Gingivitis, stomatitis	Vesicles and shallow ulcers of the palate; tender cervical adenopathy	4
Parainfluenza virus	Common cold, croup	Otitis media; cough	2
Influenza virus	Influenza	Abrupt onset; fever; chills; myalgia; HA; anorexia; severe pharyngeal pain	2
Coxsackie virus A	Herpangina	Soft palate and tonsillar pillar vesicles; fever; severe pharyngeal pain	<1
Epstein-Barr virus	Infectious mononucleosis	Fever; tender cervical adenopathy; HA; malaise; splenomegaly	<1
Cytomegalovirus	Infectious mononucleosis	Pharyngitis less severe than with EBV	<1
HIV 1	Acute retroviral syndrome	Similar to mononucleosis; nonexudative pharyngitis; truncal exanthem; aseptic meningitis	<1
Bacterial			
Streptococcus pyogenes (GABHS)	Pharyngitis and tonsillitis, scarlet fever	Fever; fiery red pharynx with patchy grey or yellow exudate; uvula edema; tender cervical adenopathy; rhinorrhea and cough uncommon	5–15
Group C β-hemolytic streptococcus	Pharyngitis and tonsillitis	Similar to GABHS, but usually less severe	5–10
Mixed anaerobic infection	Pharyngitis (Vincent angina)	Halitosis; purulent exudate	<1
Neisseria gonorrhoeae	Pharyngitis	Mild pharyngitis; usually concurrent genital infection	<1
Corynebacterium diphtheriae	Diphtheria	Slow onset; mild pharyngeal pain; firmly adherent grey tonsillar or pharyngeal membrane	<1
Arcanobacterium haemolyticum	Pharyngitis, scarlatiniform rash	Exudative pharyngitis; extremity and trunk erythematous maculopapular rash	<1
Yersinia enterocolitica	Pharyngitis, enterocolitis	Exudative pharyngitis; fever; cervical adenapathy; abdominal pain ± diarrhea; high mortality	<1
Treponema pallidum	Secondary syphilis	Silvery gray, superficial OP/OC erosions with erythematous base; other typical signs and symptoms; highly contagious	<1
Unknown			**>30**

KEY. EBV, Epstein-Barr virus; GABHS, group A β-hemolytic streptococcus; HA, headache; HIV, human immunodeficiency virus; OP/OC, oropharynx and oral cavity. Reprinted, with permission, from Tintinalli JE, Kelen GD, Stapczynski JS. *Tintinalli's Emergency Medicine: A Comprehensive Study Guide.* 6th ed. New York: McGraw-Hill, 2004 as modified, with permission, from Mandell GL, Bennett JE, Dolin R(eds): Principles and Practice of Infectious Diseases, 5th ed. Philadelphia, Chulchill Livingstone, 2000.

        iii) Tender cervical lymphadenopathy (usually anterior)
        iv) Absence of cough
    c) Diagnosis
        i) Clinical
            a. Presence of all four of the above clinical symptoms and signs give 55% probablitity of *Streptococcal* etiology
        ii) Rapid strep test (RST)
            a. 70% to >95% specificity
            b. 30% to >95% sensitivity
        iii) Culture: 90% to 95% sensitivity

2. Management of group A β-hemolytic *Streptoccocus*
    a. Treatment within 9 days to prevent rheumatic fever
        i. Glomerulonephritis not prevented by antibiotic administration
    b. Benzathine penicillin or penicillin VK
        i. Erythromycin if penicillin-allergic
    c. Corticosteroids may be indicated for patients with tonsillar hypertrophy
3. Complications
    a. Airway compromise
    b. Abscess formation

c. Rheumatic fever (0.3% to 3% of patients)
d. Poststreptococcal glomerulonephritis

F. Epiglottitis
1. Epidemiology
a. Adult incidence >children since the introduction of *H. influenza* vaccination
b. Vaccination efficacy decreases with age
c. Immigrant and unimmunized populations at increased risk
d. Diagnosis may be initially missed in up to 33% of patients
2. Etiology
a. *H. influenzae*
b. *S. pneumoniae*
c. *S. aureus*
d. Toxic fumes, superheated steam
3. Symptoms and signs
a. Toxic-appearing
b. Pain disproportionate to clinical findings
c. Dysphagia, dysphonia, muffled voice, drooling, retraction, stridor
d. Hyoid tenderness when moving larynx from side to side
e. Patient sitting in sniffing position, "tripod" position: sign of impending airway obstruction
4. Diagnosis
a. Lateral neck x-ray if stable (Figure 11–8)
i. May be negative
ii. Thumb-shaped epiglottis, obliteration of vallecula, swelling of retropharyngeal tissues
iii. Direct laryngoscopy
5. Management
a. Keep child calm as excitement may exacerbate airway compromise
b. Emergent airway management
i. Aggressive management in pediatric cases
a) Manage in OR
b) Smaller airway
c) Patients may have sudden airway compromise
ii. Airway compromise less common in adults
a) Increased ratio of trachea diameter to epiglottis
b) In rare cases, airway compromise can be sudden and catastrophic
c. Antibiotics: ceftriaxone

G. Bacterial tracheitis
1. Definition
a. Acute upper airway obstruction secondary to laryngeal, tracheal, and bronchial inflammation

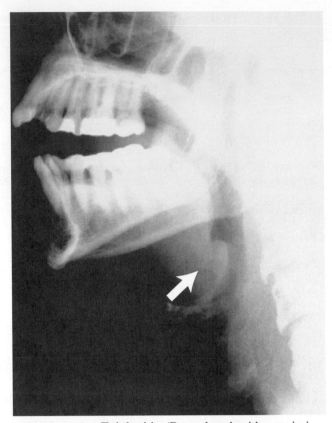

FIGURE 11–8. Epiglottitis. (Reproduced, with permission, from Tintinalli JE, Kelen GD, Stapczynski JS: *Tintinalli's Emergency Medicine: A Comprehensive Study Guide,* 6th ed. Copyright © 2004, New York: McGraw-Hill.)

2. Etiology
a. Most commonly *Staphylococcal*
b. Peak incidence in children 3 to 4 years
3. Symptoms and signs
a. Prodrome of fever, barky cough, inspiratory/expiratory stridor
b. Abrupt progression to airway obstruction
c. Difficult to differentiate from croup and epiglottitis
i. Often preceded with a viral coup-like illness
ii. Unlike croup, patients with tracheitis are toxic-appearing
iii. Unlike croup or epiglottis, patients with tracheitis may have mucopurulent cough and sputum
4. Diagnostics: x-rays may show subglottic narrowing, hazy density within the trachea
5. Management
a. Management similar to that of epiglottitis
b. Aggressive airway management in the OR

c. Bronchoscopy may be diagnostic and therapeutic
d. IV fluids
e. Broad-spectrum antibiotics

H. Croup (laryngeotracheobronchitis)
   1. Definition: Inflammation of larynx, trachea, and/or bronchial passages
   2. Epidemiology
      a. Most common cause of upper respiratory obstruction in childhood
      b. Most cases occur in late fall and early winter
      c. Peak incidence: 2 years
      d. 50% caused by *Parainfluenza* virus type 1
   3. Symptoms and signs
      a. Barking cough, hoarse voice, high-pitched inspiratory stridor

TABLE 11–3. Wesley Croup Score

CLINICAL INDICATORS	SCORE
Inspiratory stridor	
None	0
At rest, with stethoscope	1
At rest, no stethoscope required to hear	2
Level of consciousness	
Normal	0
Altered	5
Air entry	
Normal	0
Decreased	1
Severely decreased	2
Cyanosis	
None	0
Agitated	4
Resting	5
Retractions	
None	0
Mild	1
Moderate	2
Severe	3
	Total =

Reprinted, with permission, from Tintinalli JE, Kelen GD, Stapczynski JS. *Tintinalli's Emergency Medicine: A Comprehensive Study Guide,* 6th ed. New York: McGraw-Hill, 2004 as adapted, with permission, from Super DM, Cartelli NA, Brooks LJ, et al.: A prospective randomized double-blind study to evaluate the effect of dexamethasone in acute laryngotracheitis. *J Pediatr* 115:323,1989.

b. Wesley croup score (Table 11–3)
   i. Mild croup: ≤2 points
   ii. Moderate croup: 2 to 7 points
   iii. Severe croup: ≥8 points
4. Diagnosis: x-rays not helpful for management but may see steepling of subglottic trachea
5. Management
   a. Cool mist
   b. Racemic epinephrine
      i. Observe for 4 to 6 hours for rebound effect
   c. Steroids (controversial)
      i. Decreases incidence of rebound effect
      ii. Oral or intravenous dexamethasone at 0.15 to 0.3 mg/kg
   d. Admission criteria
      i. Persistence of respiratory distress, stridor at rest
      ii. Hypoxia
      iii. <6 months of age
      iv. Unreliable parents

BIBLIOGRAPHY

Adour K: Otological complications of herpes zoster. *Ann Neurol.* 1994;35(Suppl):62-64.

Amsterdam JT. Oral Medicine. In: Marx JA, ed. *Rosen's Emergency Medicine: Concepts and Clinical Practice.* 6th ed. Philadelphia, PA: Elsevier; 2006:1026.

Hickner JM, Bartlett JG, Besser RE, et al: Principles of appropriate antibiotic use for acute rhinosinusitis in adults: Background. *Ann Intern Med.* 2001;134:498.

Lew D, Southwick FS, Montgomery WW: Spenoid sinusitis. a review of 30 cases. *N Engl J Med.* 1983 Nov 10;309(19):1149.

McKay MP: Facial Trauma. In Marx JA, ed. *Rosen's Emergency Medicine Concepts and Clinical Practice.* 6th ed. Philadelphia, PA: Elsevier; 2006:382.

Pfaff JA, Moore GP: Otolaryngology. In: Marx JA, ed. *Rosen's Emergency Medicine Concepts and Clinical Practice.* 6th ed. Philadelphia, PA: Elsevier; 2006:1066.

Strupp M, Zingler VC, Arbusow V, et al: Methylprednisolone, valacyclovir, or the combination for vestibular neuritis. *N Engl J Med.* 2004 Jul 22;351(4):354-61.

Villalobos T, et al: Antibiotic prophylaxis after basilar skull fractures: a meta-analysis. *Clin Infect Dis.* 1998;27:364.

Wurman LH, et al: The Management of Epistaxis. *Am J Otolaryngol.* 1992;13:193.

Chapter 12

NEUROLOGIC EMERGENCIES

Carl A. Mealie and Mohamed A. Peera

I. Stroke

A. Definition: loss in brain function resulting from an ischemic or hemorrhagic disturbance in blood supply

B. Types
1. Ischemic
    a. Transient ischemic attack (TIA)
        i. Stroke symptoms with resolution within 24 hours
            a) Most resolve within 5 minutes
        ii. Epidemiology
            a) 10% of patients with a TIA will have a stroke within 3 months
            b) ~5% of the above patients have a stroke within 48 hours of TIA
        iii. Risk factors for early stroke after TIA
            a) Age >60 years
            b) Diabetes
            c) Symptom duration >10 minutes
            d) Motor deficit
            e) Speech deficit
    b. Thrombotic
        i. Etiology
            a) Large vessel
                i) Carotid artery system
                ii) Men >woman
                iii) Whites >African Americans
            b) Small vessel
                i) Intracerebral arteries (eg, middle cerebral artery)
                ii) African Americans >whites
                iii) Hypertensive patients
                iv) Diabetic patients
                v) Sickle cell, protein C deficiency, polycythemia vera
    c. Cardioembolic
        i. Etiology
            a) Atrial fibrillation
            b) Carotid stenosis with plaque
            c) Mural thrombi secondary to myocardial infarction (MI)
2. Hemorrhagic strokes (20% of all strokes)
    a. Intracerebral hemorrhage (ICH)
        i. Epidemiology
            a) Comprises about 66% of hemorrhagic strokes
            b) 30-day mortality approaches 50%
            c) Men >Women
    b. Subarachnoid hemorrhage (SAH)
        i. Epidemiology: 33% of hemorrhagic strokes
        ii. Etiology
            a) Associated with rupture of saccular (berry) aneurysms
            b) Associated with **polycystic kidney disease**, Marfan syndrome, coarctation of aorta, and fibromuscular dysplasia
        iii. Symptoms and signs: classic "thunderclap" headache with meningeal signs

C. Location
1. Anterior circulation (supplies 80% of the cerebral circulation)
    a. Anterior cerebral artery stroke: frontal lobe dysfunction
        i. Symptoms and signs
            a) Altered mentation, impaired judgment
            b) Contralateral extremity paralysis and numbness: lower extremity weakness >upper extremity weakness
            c) Apraxia (inability to perform learned purposeful movements) and gait ataxia
    b. Middle cerebral artery stroke
        i. Symptoms and signs
            a) Contralateral paralysis or weakness: upper >lower extremity
            b) Numbness and weakness is on the same side of the body
            c) Ipsilateral hemianopsia (blindness in 50% of visual field)

d) Aphasia or agnosia (inability to recognize objects, persons, shapes, or smells) if the lesion is on the dominant (usually left) hemisphere

e) Neglect or inattention if lesion on non-dominant hemisphere

2. Posterior circulation (supplies 20% of the cerebral circulation)

   a. Posterior cerebral artery stroke and vertebral basilar insufficiency: affect the brainstem, cranial nerves, cerebellum, and reticular activating system (RAS)

      i. Symptoms and signs

         a) Loss of consciousness by affecting the RAS

         b) Nausea and vomiting

         c) Visual agnosia and alexia: inability to recognize an object or to understand a written word by (damage to the occipital lobe)

         d) Various cranial nerve dysfunctions: diplopia, nystagmus, dysarthria, dysphagia, homonymous hemianopsia

         e) Ataxia and spasticity from cerebellar dysfunction

D. Diagnosis

  1. Noncontrast computed tomography (CT)

   a. Will diagnose 99% of ICH >1 cm and 95% of SAH

      i. Early signs of ischemic infarct found in 33% of stroke patients within 3 hours

         a) Loss of grey-white interface

         b) Acute hypodensity

         c) Hyperdensity within the artery from a thrombus

E. Management

  1. TIAs

   a. Neurology consultation

   b. Consider admitting secondary to high risk of impending stroke

   c. Repeat CT as ischemic changes may not be apparent until >24 hours

   d. Carotid Doppler

   e. Echocardiogram (if indicated)

  2. Ischemic stroke

   a. Thrombolytics to appropriate candidates (Table 12–1)

      i. Fingerstick for glucose as hypoglycemia may present with focal deficits

      ii. CT head to exclude hemorrhagic stroke

   b. Blood pressure (BP) control (Table 12–2)

   c. No aspirin in the first 24 hours if given thrombolytic therapy

TABLE 12–1. Thrombolytic Therapy for Acute Ischemic Stroke

Thrombolytic candidates: presenting within 3 hours of symptom onset

Inclusion Criteria

1. Age ≥18 years
2. Clinical diagnosis of ischemic stroke causing a measurable neurologic deficit
3. Time of symptom onset <180 minutes before treatment begins

Exclusion Criteria

1. Intracranial hemorrhage (ICH) on head CT
2. Minor or rapidly improving stroke symptoms
3. High suspicion for subarachnoid hemorrhage
4. Active internal bleeding (eg, gastrointestinal bleed or urinary bleeding within last 21 days)
5. Bleeding diathesis including but not limited to:
   Platelet <100,000 mm^3
   Heparin administration within 48 hours and elevated PTT
   Recent coumadin use and PT >15 seconds
6. History of head trauma, intracranial surgery or previous CVA within 3 months
7. Major surgery or trauma within 14 days
8. Recent arterial puncture at noncompressible site
9. Lumbar puncture within 7 days
10. History of ICH, AVM, or aneurysm
11. Witnessed seizure at stroke onset
12. Recent acute myocardial infarction
13. SBP >185 or DBP >110 at time of drug administration or requiring aggressive treatment to maintain BP below that

(Reproduced, with permission from Marx JA, Hockberger RS: *Rosen's Emergency Medicine Concepts and Clinical Practice*, 6th ed. Philadelphia, PA: Mosby Elsevier: 1615.)

3. Hemorrhagic stroke

   a. Hypertension management: maintain mean arterial pressure (MAP) at approximately 110 mm Hg

   b. Neurosurgical consultation

   c. Seizure prophylaxis: phenytoin 18 to 20 mg/kg (seizures will occur in 10% of patients in a neurosurgic ICU with ICH)

II. Seizures

A. Definition: temporary abnormal synchronization of electro-neural activity

  1. In seizures, eye movement is away from the side of the pathology. Mnemonic: "see a stroke, shake away from a seizure"

B. Types

  1. Generalized seizures: involves both hemispheres that result in mental status change

TABLE 12–2.   Emergency BP Management for Acute Ischemic Strokes

Nonthrombolytic Candidates	Treatment
SBP >220, DBP >120, or MAP >130	Labetolol IV or nicardipine drip for a 10 to 20 decrease in MAP
SBP <220, DBP <120, or MAP <130	Defer treatment unless concomitant aortic dissection, acute MI, severe CHF, or hypertensive encephalopathy
Thrombolytic Candidates Pretreatment	
SBP >185 or DBP >110	Labetalol 10 to 20 mg IV over 1 to 2 minutes, may repeat once, or Nitropaste 1 to 2 inches, or Nicardipine drip 5 mg/h titrate up to 15 mg/h and then reduce to 3 mg/h after target BP met
During and after Thrombolytic Therapy	
DBP >140	Sodium nitroprusside drip
SBP >230 or DBP 121 to 140	Labetalol IV ± labetalol drip, if BP is not controlled use nitroprusside drip
SBP 180 to 230 or DBP 105 to 120	Labetalol IV ± Labetalol drip

(Modified with permission from Marx JA, Hockberger RS: *Rosen's Emergency Medicine Concepts and Clinical Practice*, 6th ed. Philadelphia, PA: Mosby Elsevier: 1614.)

a. Absence (petit mal): brief mental status change without aura, postictal state, or loss of postural tone
b. Tonic: tensing of muscles that cause either flexion or extension of muscle groups
c. Clonic: repetitive, rhythmic contraction and relaxation of muscle and muscle groups
d. Tonic-clonic (grand mal): tonic phase followed by clonic ictal phase
e. Myoclonic: brief arrhythmic contraction that occurs in clusters <1 second each
f. Atonic: (drop attack) sudden, brief loss of postural tone

2. Partial (focal) seizures
   a. Simple partial
      i. Seizures with preserved consciousness
   b. Complex partial (eg, temporal lobe epilepsy)
      i. Partial alteration in consciousness, although patient can still react to surroundings
      ii. Associated with automatisms such as lip smacking
      iii. Can be preceded by olfactory aura
   c. Secondary generalized partial seizure: simple or complex seizure that progresses to a generalized seizure

3. Status epilepticus
   a. Traditionally defined as prolonged seizure activity >30 minutes or ≥2 seizures without return to consciousness
   b. Some advocates redefine status as continuous seizures >5 minutes
   c. May be the presenting seizure in 10% to 30% of patients

4. Pseudoseizures
   a. Usually female patient with history of physical or sexual abuse

b. Generalized seizure without loss of consciousness
c. No postictal phase
d. Occurs only when witnesses are present
e. Patient retains ability to protect self from noxious stimuli
f. Characterized by variable activity, side-to-side head movement, pelvic thrusting, alternating extremity movement

C. Management
   1. Rule out treatable causes of seizures
      a. Bedside glucose determination (finger stick dextrose)
      b. Rule out pregnancy and eclampsia
      c. **Lindane** use in pediatric for the treatment of head lice
      d. Check electrolytes and thyroid function
      e. Consider head CT to rule out mass or bleeding
      f. Consider lumbar puncture to rule out infection
      g. Toxins
         i. Sympathomimetics (cocaine, PCP)
         ii. Anticholinergic (jimson weed, organophosphates)
         iii. Withdrawal states (alcohol, benzodiazepines)
         iv. Tricyclic overdose, **isoniazid**, theophylline, lidocaine, lindane
      h. Cardiogenic syncope may mimic seizures
         i. Depending on the study, anywhere from 40% to 90% of patients with cardiogenic syncope had seizure-like activity
   2. Medications
      a. First-line drugs: benzodiazepines (diazepam, lorazepam, or midazolam)

b. Second-line drugs: phenytoin (or phosphenytoin)
  i. Phenytoin ineffective in drug-induced seizures
  ii. For drug-induced seizures use phenobarbital, if benzodiazepines fail
  iii. Phenytoin is contraindicated in tricyclic antidepressant (TCA) overdose as it is arrythmogenic in animal models and of limited efficacy in toxin-induced seizures
c. Third-line drugs: no consensus exists for best third-line therapy
  i. Barbiturates
    a) Phenobarbital
    b) Pentobarbital
      i) Use only when other options fail
      ii) Pentobarbital coma requires intubation
  ii. Valproate
  iii. Propofol
  iv. Isoflurane
d. Vitamin B_6 (pyridoxine) for INH-related seizures or refractory seizures in the neonate
3. EEG monitoring may be required if persistent seizure activity suspected despite lack of or inability to monitor visible seizure activity

III. Headache

A. Primary headaches: benign
  1. Tension headaches
    a. Epidemiology
      i. Most common headache syndrome
        a) Affects >75% of population
      ii. Women >men
    b. Symptoms and signs
      i. Gradual onset
      ii. Bilateral tight, band-like pain radiating from neck around head to forehead
      iii. Lasts 4 to 13 hours
      iv. Less severe in morning and worsens after work
      v. Nausea, vomiting, and photophobia uncommon
    c. Management
      i. NSAIDs and acetaminophen
  2. Migraine headaches
    a. Epidemiology
      i. Second most common headache syndrome
      ii. First episode usually <30 years (onset >50 years rare)
      iii. Frequency of attacks decrease with age
      iv. Women >men (3:1)
    b. Symptoms and signs

      i. Migraine without aura or common migraine (80%)
        a) Worsening unilateral or bilateral throbbing headache associated with nausea and vomiting, photophobia, and phonophobia
      ii. Migraine with aura or classic migraine
        a) Sudden onset sensory auras
          i) Visual auras such as scotomas occur in central field as a bright and expanding "C" or herringbone pattern
      iii. Ophthalmoplegic migraine
        a) Rare headache associated with paresis or plegia of extraocular muscles
        b) May last from days to weeks
      iv. Hemiplegic migraine
        a) Migraine associated with temporary paralysis
      v. Basilar artery migraine (Bickerstaff migraine)
        a) Abrupt onset of total blindness
        b) Usually in adolescent girls
        c) Vertigo, ataxia, nausea, vomiting lasting 30 minutes followed by occipital throbbing headache
    c. Management
      i. Rule out life-threatening causes of headache (subarachnoid hemorrhage, mass)
      ii. Avoid triggers: alcohol, foods (chocolate, monosodium glutamate), hunger, sleep deprivation, prolonged exertion
      iii. Medication
        a) Mild migraine
          i) NSAID,
          ii) Oral 5-HT agonist (sumatriptan)
            (a) Contraindicated with basilar migraine, cardiovascular disease, ischemic cerebrovascular disease, and peripheral vascular disease
        b) Moderate migraine: oral, nasal, subcutaneous 5-HT agonist, or dopamine antagonist (prochlorperazine or metoclopramide)
        c) Severe migraine: 5-HT agonist IM, IV or SC, dopamine antagonist IM or IV and prophylactic medication (β-blockers, calcium channel blockers, valproic acid, TCA, and monoamine oxidase inhibitors)
  3. Cluster headaches
    a. Epidemiology
      i. **Men >** women (8:1)
      ii. 20 to 50 years

b. Symptoms and signs
  i. Sudden onset, explosive unilateral peri-orbital pain
  ii. Lasts 30 minutes to 2 hours
  iii. Lacrimation, coryza, injected eye on the side of pain
  iv. 85% have an attack occuring at the same time each day
c. Management
  i. Avoid alcohol, which triggers attacks in 70% of patients
  ii. High-flow oxygen
  iii. Medications
    a) Oxygen
    b) 5-HT agonist (triptans)
    c) Lithium 600 to 900 mg daily
    d) Prednisone 60 mg/day for 10 days
    e) Sublingual ergotamine
    f) Nasal anesthetic: lidocaine

B. Secondary headaches—dangerous
  1. Epidural hematoma: blood between the skull and dura
    a. Epidemiology
      i. Uncommon in the elderly and in children <2 years because of close attachment of the skull to the dura
      ii. Present in 0.5% of all head-injured patients and in 1% of all head-injured patients presenting with coma
    b. Pathophysiology
      i. Usually associated with skull fractures across the **middle meningeal artery** (temporoparietal region)
      ii. Arterial bleeding in 66% and the remainder venous
      iii. Usually rapid bleeding
      iv. Usually unilateral, 20% of the time associated with other intracranial lesions (eg, contusions or subdural hematomas)
    c. Symptoms and signs
      i. Severe headache, drowsiness, nausea, and vomiting
      ii. Classically associated with **lucid interval** just prior to rapid deterioration (present <30% of epidural bleeds)
      iii. Evidence of trauma most commonly at temporoparietal region
    d. Diagnosis
      i. CT shows hyperdense, biconvex, or lenticular-shaped hematoma usually in the temporal region
      ii. The hematoma is sharply defined

      iii. Does not cross suture lines, may cross midline
    e. Management
      i. Burr hole placement if herniation present
        a) Place next to but not on skull fracture
        b) Place ipsilateral to dilated pupil if CT scan unavailable
      ii. Neurosurgical consult for hematoma evacuation
      iii. Good prognosis if promptly treated and patient is not in coma
  2. Subdural hematoma—blood collection between the dura and arachnoid mater
    a. Epidemiology
      i. More common in individuals with brain atrophy (alcoholics and elderly)
      ii. More common than epidural hematomas
    b. Pathophysiology
      i. Rupture of the **bridging veins** from movement of the brain relative to the skull (eg, acceleration-deceleration injury)
      ii. Blood fills the potential space between dura and arachnoid
      iii. Usually slow venous bleeding
    c. Symptoms and signs
      i. Acute
        a) Typically after trauma
        b) Headache, mental status change, seizures, focal deficits
      ii. Subacute and chronic
        a) No history of trauma in 50%
        b) Headache, mental status change, seizures, focal deficits
        c) Personality change (depression, psychosis)
    d. Diagnosis
      i. CT findings: hyperdense crescent-shaped hematoma (if acute), isodense (if subacute) or hypodense (if chronic)
      ii. Can cross suture lines, but does not cross midline
    e. Management
      i. Neurosurgical consultation for possible surgical evacuation
      ii. Very small subdural hematoma may be observed closely with plans to repeat emergent CT if any signs of deterioration
      iii. Burr holes are temporary non-curative measures
        a) Burr hole ipsilateral to dilated pupil if CT scan not available in a timely fashion
      iv. Indications for immediate surgery
        a) Neurologic deterioration
        b) >5 mm midline shift

3. Spontaneous subarachnoid hemorrhage (SAH)
    a. Definition
        i. Blood between arachnoid and pia mater
        ii. Entity distinct from traumatic SAH (see Trauma chapter)
    b. Epidemiology
        i. 1% of all patients presenting with headache
        ii. 10% of all strokes
        iii. Peak 40 to 60 years
    c. Etiology
        i. Saccular (berry) aneurysm (80%)
        ii. Arteriovenous malformation, cavernous angiomas, and mycotic aneurysms
    d. Symptoms and signs
        i. Sudden **thunderclap headache**
            a) Reaches maximum intensity within 1 hour
        ii. Worst headache of life
        iii. Migrating headache down spine
        iv. Nausea and vomiting
        v. Meningismus
        vi. Hunt and Hess grading scale (Table 12–3)
            a) Scale applies to non-traumatic SAH
            b) Grades IV and V have dismal outcomes
            c) Grades I to III have good outcomes in 50% to 90%
    e. Diagnosis
        i. CT Scan (Figure 12–1)
            a) 95% sensitivity within first 24 hours
            b) Sensitivity 50% after first week
        ii. Lumbar puncture: to detect xanthochromia
            a) 6 to 12 hours required for xanthochromia to form
            b) Peaks at 48 hours
            c) May last 1 to 4 weeks
            d) False positives with hyperbilirubinemia and hypercarotenemia
    f. Management
        i. Surgical clipping
        ii. Interventional radiology coil placement
            a) Thrombosis of platinum coil stops bleeding

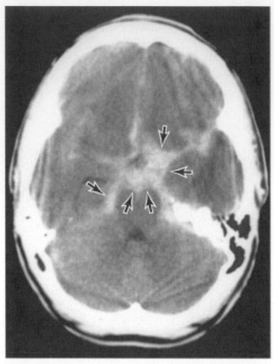

FIGURE 12–1. Subarachnoid hemorrhage. The star sign. (Reproduced, with permission, from Aminoff MJ, Greenberg DA, Simon RP: *Clinical Neurology*, 6th ed. Copyright © 2005, New York: McGraw-Hill.)

            b) Higher re-bleed rate compared to clipping
        iii. Nimodipine PO
            a) Prevents cerebral vasospasm
    g. Complications: hydrocephalus in 15% to 20%
        i. Require ventricular shunt
4. Cerebral sinus vein thrombosis
    a. Etiology
        i. Infectious/septic thrombosis **or**
        ii. Hypercoagulable state (see Hematology/oncology chapter)
    b. Symptoms and signs
        i. Varies with location (cavernous sinus, sagittal sinus)
        ii. Difficult diagnosis
        iii. Nonspecific headache
        iv. May present similarly to meningitis or stroke
        v. Fever if septic thrombosis
        vi. Diploplia
    c. Diagnosis
        i. Head CT poor sensitivity
            a) May see hyperdense thrombosis on CT
        ii. Magnetic resonance venography (MRV) has best sensitivity and specificity

TABLE 12–3. Hunt and Hess Classification for Subarachnoid Hemorrhage

0	Unruptured aneurysm
1	Minimal symptoms, mild headache or nuchal rigidity
2	Moderate to severe headache or nuchal rigidity and/or isolated oculomotor palsy
3	Lethargy, confusion and/or mild neurologic deficit(s)
4	Stupor with moderate to severe focal neurologic deficit(s)
5	Deep coma, decerebrate posturing

iii. Spinal fluid may show white cells with septic thrombosis

iv. Spinal fluid may reveal high opening pressures

d. Management

  i. Neurosurgical consultation

  ii. Anticoagulation with heparin and warfarin

  iii. Consider thrombolytics with severe symptoms refractory to treatment

  iv. Increased intracranial pressure may require shunt placement

  v. Antibiotics if septic thrombosis suspected

5. Giant cell (temporal) arteritis

a. Epidemiology

  i. <50 years rare

  ii. Higher incidence in Scandinavian population

  iii. Women >men

b. Pathophysiology

  i. Vasculitis of large and medium size arteries

c. Symptoms and signs

  i. Temporal headache

  ii. Jaw claudication

  iii. Loss of vision

d. Diagnosis

  i. Clinical diagnosis

  ii. Elevated ESR

    a) Often >100 mm/h

    b) 10% to 25% have a normal level

  iii. Mild-to-moderate anemia

  iv. Temporal artery biopsy

    a) Best done within 48 to 72 hours of treatment onset since responds rapidly to steroids

e. Management

  i. High-dose, tapered steroids for up to 72 months

6. Carotid and vertebral artery dissection

a. Epidemiology

  i. Most occur in fifth decade

  ii. Common cause of ischemic stroke in patients aged 25 to 45

b. Risk factors

  i. Underlying ateriopathy due to underlying connective tissue disease

    a) Fibromuscular dysplasia, Marfan' syndrome, type IV Ehler-Danlos syndrome

  ii. May be triggered by minor truama

    a) Neck rotation injuries, minor fall, chiropractic manipulation

c. Symptoms and signs

  i. Carotid artery dissection

    a) Severe neck, facial, or retroorbital pain

    b) Pulsatile tinnitus

    c) Visual disturbance from ophthalmic artery occlusion (amaurosis fugax)

    d) Ipsilateral **partial** Horner syndrome

      i) Miosis, ptosis

      ii) Anhydrosis **not** present (unlike typical Horner syndrome)

    e) Contralateral hemiparesis, neglect, or frontal lobe findings

  ii. Vertebral artery dissection

    a) Occipital and/or posterior neck pain

    b) Progressive brain stem and cerebellar findings such as severe ataxia, vertigo, vomiting, cranial nerve dysfunction with diplopia, dysarthria, and dysphagia

d. Diagnosis

  i. CT scan with contrast

  ii. Ultrasound

  iii. Magnetic resonance arteriography (MRA)

e. Management

  i. Anticoagulation after ruling out intracranial bleeding

    a) Morbidity caused by clotting and consequent stroke

7. Idiopathic intracranial hypertension (pseudotumor cerebri)

a. Risk factors

  i. Young, obese, females

  ii. Vitamin A toxicity

  iii. Vitamin A derivative

    a) All-trans-retinoic acid: treatment of promyelocytic leukemia

    b) Isotretinoin: treatment of acne

  iv. Oral contraception

  v. Steroids

  vi. Tetracycline

b. Pathophysiology

  i. Impaired cerebrospinal fluid (CSF) absorption by arachnoid villi

c. Symptoms and signs

  i. Morning headaches

  ii. Worse with coughing and straining

  iii. Pulsatile tinnitus

  iv. Papilledema

  v. Diploplia with lateral gaze: cranial nerve (CN) VI palsy

  vi. Loss of peripheral visual fields

  vii. Central visual loss may become permanent

d. Diagnosis

  i. Normal head CT or slit-like ventricles

  ii. Elevated (>20 cm Hg) opening pressure on lumbar puncture

e. Management

  i. Weight loss

  ii. Carbonic anhydrase inhibitor: acetazolamide

iii. Serial lumbar puncture to decrease pressure
iv. Surgical intervention if above measures fail
   a) Neurosurgical shunt placement, or
   b) Optic nerve sheath fenestration: window cut into the dura of the optic nerve sheath to relieve papilledema and prevent loss of optic nerve fibers

8. Lumbar puncture and postprocedural headache
  a. Epidemiology
    i. Occurs in 10% to 30% of lumbar punctures
  b. Pathophysiology
    i. Traction on brain structures caused by persistent CSF leak
  c. Symptoms and signs
    i. Bilateral headache typically 48 hours after procedure
    ii. Worse with standing or sitting
    iii. Relieved by abdominal compression
    iv. Symptoms resolve over several days to weeks
  d. Management
    i. Best treatment is prevention
      a) Use small caliber needle (23 or 25)
      b) Use blunt needle
      c) Adopt bevel orientation that minimizes damage to dural fibers
      d) Stylet replacement before needle removal
    ii. Only anecdotal evidence to support caffeine sodium benzoate
    iii. Epidural blood patch using 15 mL autologous blood

IV. Vertigo

A. Definition
  1. The illusion of motion
  2. Often described as whirling, spinning, rotating, rocking, falling etc.

B. Symptoms and signs
  1. Various degrees of ear pain and hearing disturbance depending on etiology
  2. Nausea and vomiting
  3. Horizontal or rotary nystagmus

C. Etiology: central versus peripheral (Table 12–4)
  1. Central vertigo
    a. Stroke
    b. Multiple sclerosis
    c. Infection
      i. Meningitis, mastoiditis, syphilis
  2. Peripheral vertigo
    a. Benign paroxysmal positional vertigo (BPPV)
      i. Most common cause of vertigo
      ii. Instigated by position change
      iii. Caused by obstructing otoliths in semicircular canals
    b. Meniere disease
      i. **Recurrent** triad of vertigo, tinnitus, and hearing loss
      ii. Caused by endolymphatic hydrops or excess fluid in inner ear
    c. Labyrinthitis
      i. Inner ear inflammation (cochlea, semicircular canals, utricle)
      ii. Sudden, severe vertigo and hearing loss
      iii. May be confused with Meniere disease but **rarely** recurrent
      iv. Usually viral (serous), less commonly bacterial (suppurative)
    d. Vestibular neuritis
      i. By strict definition, a process distinct from labyrinthitis
      ii. Vestibular nerve inflammation: 1 of 2 branches of CN VIII (vestibulocochlear nerve)
        a) Vestibular nerve transmits information from semicircular canals to the brain

TABLE 12–4. Central Vertigo versus Peripheral Vertigo

CENTRAL VERTIGO	PERIPHERAL VERTIGO
Long duration, continuous in nature	Short duration, intermittent in nature
Not worsening with change in position	Worsens with change in position
Mild intensity	Severe intensity
Can be associated with central symptoms, but not associated with hearing loss	Not associated with central symptoms, but can involve hearing loss and tinnitus
Gradual onset	Sudden onset
Non-fatigable nystagmus (persists despite head kept still)	Fatigable nystagmus
Multidirectional nystagmus	Nystagmus is unidirectional (never vertical)
Nystagmus persists despite fixation of focus on stationary target (non-inhibited)	Nystagmus can be inhibited

iii. Does **not** involve hearing loss as cochlea not affected

iv. Viral etiology most common

    a) Ramsay-Hunt syndrome: reactivation of the herpes zoster virus in the geniculate ganglion of the facial nerve

    b) Symptoms and signs

        i) Dermatologic: painful, vesicular rash of external auditory canal, tongue and/or hard palate

        ii) Facial nerve: Bell palsy

        iii) Vestibulocochlear nerve (effected due to close proximity): tinnitus, hearing loss, vertigo

e. Acoustic neuroma (vestibular schwannoma)

    i. Tumor of myelin cells of the cochlear branch of CN VIII

    ii. Gradual hearing loss and tinnitus

    iii. CN V and VII most commonly involved as tumor enlarges

    iv. May present with truncal ataxia and diminished corneal reflex

f. Medications

    i. May cause both vestibular neuritis and labyrinthitis

    ii. NSAIDs, antiepileptic medications, loop diuretics, aminoglycosides

g. Peri-lymphatic fistula

    i. Opening in round window that allows transmission of pressures from middle to inner ear

    ii. Most commonly posttraumatic

3. Diagnosis

a. Head CT

    i. Helps to rule out mastoiditis

    ii. Assessment for stroke or bleeding in high-risk patients

    iii. Contrast enhanced study will detect most large acoustic neuromas

b. Magnetic resonance imaging (MRI)

    i. Assess for presence of even small acoustic neuromas

    ii. Enhanced uptake with contrast in vestibular organs may make the diagnosis of labyrinthitis

c. Dix-Hallpike maneuver (or Nylen-Barany)

    i. Evaluates benign paroxysmal positional vertigo

    ii. Dix-Hallpike maneuver: patient is moved quickly from an upright-seated position to supine position with the patient's head rotated 45 degrees to one side and extended 30 degrees. If no nystagmus is observed, the test is repeated in the other direction

    iii. Horizontal or rotary nystagmus reproducing symptoms indicate a positive test

4. Management

a. General management

    i. Treat underlying cause and rule out life-threatening processes

    ii. Antihistamines and/or anticholinergics (meclizine, diphenhydramine, scopolamine)

    iii. Prochlorperazine or metoclopramide may be required for control of nausea and vomiting

    iv. Diazepam

b. Specific management

    i. BPPV may benefit from the Epley maneuver

        a) Relieves vertigo by dumping otoliths from canals into utricle

        b) Patient positioned supine with head extended 30 degrees and rotated 45 degrees to more affected side (as determined by slow phase of nystagmus incuced by the Dix-Hallpike maneuver)

        c) Rotate head 90 degrees to opposite side

        d) Rotate patient onto shoulder effectively turning patient 180 degrees from original position

        e) Sit patient up with chin to chest and slowly look up

        f) Each position should be held until nystagmus fatigues

            i) May require a few minutes

    ii. Meniere disease may benefit from a low sodium diet, smoking and alcohol cessation, and correction of hypokalemia

    iii. Antiviral medication may be beneficial with Ramsay-Hunt syndrome

    iv. Bacterial (suppurative) labyrinthitis may require admission for intravenous antibiotics

    v. Surgery may be indicated for acoustic neuromas and repair of perilymphatic fistula

V. Mental Status Change

A. Differentiate psychiatric from organic etiologies

B. Organic versus psychiatric (Table 12–5)

C. Delirium: disturbance of consciousness

1. Waxing and waning

2. Acute onset with diurnal fluctuations

3. Usually caused by a medical condition (eg, metabolic, toxic, drugs, infection)

4. Management: treat underlying medical condition

TABLE 12–5. Organic versus Psychiatric Causes of Mental Status Change

ORGANIC	PSYCHIATRIC
Gradual onset	Sudden onset
Waxing and waning	Progressive
Visual hallucinations	Auditory hallucination
Medical illness, fever	Family history, drug abuse

D. Dementia: cognitive impairment without disturbance of consciousness
   1. Gradual onset with memory impairment
   2. Usually from physiologic changes from general medical condition
   3. Reversible causes (20%) include normal pressure hydrocephalus, Wilson disease, and nutritional deficiencies
   4. Irreversible causes dementia (80%) include Alzheimer disease, multiinfarct dementia, and Creutzfeldt-Jakob disease

VI. Central Nervous System Infections

A. Meningitis (see Infectious Diseases chapter)
   1. Epidemiology
      a. Bacterial meningitis: more common in late winter and early spring
      b. Viral meningitis: more common in summer, caused by enterovirus
   2. Etiology
      a. *Streptococcus pneumoniae* (most common)
      b. *Neisseria meningitides*
      c. *Haemophilus influenza* type B
      d. Fungal meningitis: immunocompromised individuals
      e. Tuberculosis
      f. Herpes simplex

g. HIV: more likely to develop community-acquired bacterial and viral meningitis
   i. Early: aseptic meningitis related to HIV-1 virus
   ii. Late: AIDS defining fungal infections (cryptooccosis, coccidioidomycosis, histoplasmosis), CMV, *Listeria monocytogenes*, and other opportunistic infections
   3. Diagnosis
      a. Clinical: start antibiotics empirically
      b. Head CT prior to lumbar puncture if
         i. ≥60 years
         ii. History of CNS disease
            a) Immunocompromised
            b) CVA
            c) Mass: tumor or abscess
            d) Trauma
            e) Seizure within the last 7 days
         iii. Neurologic deficits or altered mental status
            a) Inability to answer 2 consecutive questions correctly or follow 2 consecutive commands
            b) Arm or leg drift
      c. CSF interpretation (Table 12–6)
   4. Management
      a. Do not delay antibiotic administration while awaiting CSF analysis
         i. Increased morbidity and mortality with antibiotic delay
      b. Antibiotic therapy is based on most common organisms
         i. Cefotaxime or ceftriaxone, plus vancomycin (if penicillin or cephalosporin allergy use chloromphenicol plus vancomycin)
         ii. Ampicillin in the neonates and elderly to cover *Listeria*
         iii. Infectious disease consultation if tuberculosis or fungal meningitis suspected

TABLE 12–6. CSF Interpretations in Meningitis

	BACTERIAL	VIRAL	FUNGAL
WBC	>1000	<1000	<500
% PMN	>80%	1% to 50%	1% to 50%
Glucose	<40 mg/dL	>40 mg/dL	<40 mg/dL
Protein	>200 mg/dL	<200 mg/dL	>200 mg/dL
Gram stain	Organism identified 80% of the time	No organism	Negative
Lactic acid	>35 mg/dL in bacterial and TB	<35 mg/dL	<35 mg/dL
Bacterial antigen test	>95% specific for organism tested; up to 50% false-negative rate	Negative	Negative

c. Steroids: dexamethasone 10 mg IV every 6 hours should be given **before** or **with** the first dose of antibiotics to improve outcome
d. Prophylaxis of close contacts
   i. *N. meningitidis* and *H. influenzae* have increased risk of transmission hence prophylaxis of houschold contacts
   ii. Prophylaxis **not** required for pneumococcal meningitis
   iii. Prophylaxis for *N. meningitidis* in adults
     a) Rifampin 600 mg PO every 12 hours × 4 doses or
     b) Cipro 500 mg × 1 or
     c) Ceftriaxone 250 mg IM × 1 or
     d) If pregnant single dose of azithromycin 500 mg PO or Ceftriaxone 250 mg IM × 1
   iv. Prophylaxis for *H. influenzae* meningitidis in adults
     a) Rifampin 600 mg PO every 12 hours × 4 days

B. Encephalitis
1. Epidemiology
  a. Only 10% of the incidence of bacterial meningitis
2. Etiology
  a. Most common causes: West Nile, Eastern and Western equine, St. Louis, and California encephalitis
  b. Other causes: CMV, varicella, Lyme, syphilis, Epstein-Barr, mumps, and measles
  c. Herpesviridae
   i. Herpes simplex type 1: older children and adults
   ii. Herpes simplex type 2: neonates, with devastating outcome
   iii. Affects the temporal lobe
   iv. 70% mortality without treatment
   v. 30% mortality when treated with acyclovir
3. Symptoms and signs
  a. Fever, headache, and altered mental status
  b. Hallucination and change in personality
  c. May mimic psychiatric illness
  d. Bizarre behavior usually precedes neurologic manifestations by several days, progressing to confusion lethargy and coma
4. Diagnosis
  a. MRI: modality of choice
   i. Herpes simplex virus: hyperintensity corresponding to edematous changes, commonly in the temporal horns
  b. CT
   i. Herpes simplex virus: hypodensity in the in the temporal horns

c. EEG: almost always abnormal in encephalitis and normal in meningitis
   i. Pathognomonic in HSV with episodic asymmetric spikes
d. LP: CSF lymphocytic pleocytosis (5 to 500 cells/mm^3), elevated protein, normal glucose
5. Management
  a. HSV: acyclovir
  b. CMV: gancyclovir
  c. Lyme disease: ceftriaxone
  d. Syphilis: ceftriaxone

VII. CNS Disorders: Brain and Cranial Nerves

A. Multiple sclerosis
1. Definition
  a. An auto-immune disease in which the immune system responds against the myelin proteins of the CNS (white matter) resulting in a triad of inflammatory changes, demyelination, and scarring (gliosis)
2. Epidemiology
  a. 2:1 female to male ratio
  b. 20 to 30 years old. May occur later in men
  c. Increasing incidence closer to the equator
3. Symptoms and signs: may be triggered by infection, fever, or stress
  a. Sensory loss, optic neuritis, weakness, paresthesia, diplopia, ataxia, bladder dysfunction, and depression
  b. Lhermitte sign: electric shock sensation down back with neck flexion
  c. Diploplia with lateral gaze (intranuclear ophthalmoplegia)
  d. Acute transverse myelitis (see "transverse myelitis" below)
4. Diagnosis
  a. Consider multiple sclerosis if one is unable to account for multiple symptoms and neurologic findings with a single anatomic lesion
   i. Symptoms occurring in different parts of the body at least 3 months apart. Mnemonic: "separated by time and space"
  b. Multiple plaques visible on MRI in 95%
  c. Lumbar puncture
   i. CSF pleocytosis
   ii. Elevation of CSF proteins such as immunoglobulin G (IgG)
   iii. Immunoglobulin G (IgG) oligoclonal band pattern on electrophoresis of CSF proteins
5. Prognosis
  a. 15 years after diagnosis 50% of patients will develop secondary symptoms
  b. 25 years after diagnosis >80% of patients develop secondary symptoms

6. Management
   a. Glucocorticoids
   b. Plasma exchange
   c. Disease-modifying therapies
      i. Interferon β-1a (Avonex)
      ii. Interferon β-1b (Betaserone)

B. Cranial nerve palsies (Table 12–7)
   1. Trigeminal neuralgia
      a. Symptoms and signs
         i. Sudden, lancing paroxysm of pain in chin, gums, cheek, or temporal forehead
         ii. Triggered by chewing, swallowing, brushing teeth, touching face, or exposure to hot or cold

   b. Diagnosis
      i. Clinical: rule out temporomandibular disorder, sinus infection, dental infection, tumor, or AVM
   c. Management
      i. Carbamazepine
      ii. Surgical management for refractory cases
2. CN VII (Bell palsy)
   a. Etiology
      i. Idiopathic most common
      ii. Viral
         a) HSV-1
         b) Herpes Zoster: Ramsay-Hunt syndrome
      iii. Bilateral Bell palsy may result from **Lyme disease** or **mononucleosis**

TABLE 12–7. Cranial Nerve Palsies

CN	FINDINGS	COMMON CAUSES
I Olfactory nerve	Anostomia: loss of smell	Traumatic transection of nerve Compression from frontal lobe mass
II Optic nerve	Unilateral vision loss	Traumatic optic neuropathy Compression from lesion Optic neuritis (multiple sclerosis) Ischemic optic neuropathy
III Oculomotor nerve	Ptosis, diplopia Eye deviated laterally and down Dilated, nonreactive pupil Loss of accommodation	Transtentorial herniation of the temporal lobe Ischemic injury (as in diabetes) Intracranial aneurysms Myasthenia gravis
IV Trochlear nerve	Inability to move eye downward, and laterally Diplopia	Trauma
V Trigeminal nerve	Partial facial anesthesia Trigeminal neuralgia	Facial bone fracture Tic douloureux
VI Abducens nerve	Inability to move affected eye laterally Diplopia on lateral gaze	Tumor in the cerebellopontine angle Compression from lesion in the cavernous sinus Elevated intracranial pressure
VII Facial nerve	Lower motor neuron lesion: entire side of face paralyzed Upper motor neuron lesion: spares forehead Abnormal taste Intolerance to sudden loud noises	Lower motor neuron: viral infection (Bell palsy), Lyme disease, bacterial infection (otitis media) Upper motor neuron: stroke, tumor
VIII Vestibulocochlear nerve	Unilateral hearing loss Tinnitus Vertigo	Trauma Infection Acoustic neuroma
IX Glossopharyngeal nerve	Painful paroxysms radiating from the throat down the side of the neck	Brainstem lesion Glossopharyngeal neuralgia
X Vagus nerve	Unilateral loss of palatal elevation Unilateral vocal cord paralysis Hoarse voice	Brainstem lesion Injury to the recurrent laryngeal nerve during surgery
XI Spinal accessory nerve	Downward and lateral rotation of the scapula and shoulder drop	Trauma
XII Hypoglossal nerve	Upper motor neuron lesion: tongue deviates contralaterally Lower motor neuron lesion: ipsilateral tongue deviation	Upper motor neuron: stroke or tumor Amyotrophic lateral sclerosis (ALS) can cause bilateral lower motor neuron lesions

iv. Malignant otitis externa secondary to pseudomonas infection in the immunocompromised

v. Tumor

b. Symptoms and signs

    i. Facial droop of ipsilateral upper and lower face

    ii. Unable to close ipsilateral eye

    iii. Taste disturbance in anterior two-thirds of tongue

    iv. 50% have postauricular pain

c. Diagnosis of exclusion

    i. Differentiate from central causes of facial weakness where the upper one-third of the face is spared due to dual innervation of the forehead (orbicularis and frontalis muscles)

    ii. Pseudo-Bell: CN VI stroke may masquerade as a peripheral lesion, check for lateral gaze

d. Management

    i. Prednisone 1 mg/kg/day for 7 to 10 days (controversial)

    ii. Acyclovir 400 to 800 mg orally five times daily for 10 days (controversial)

    iii. Eye protection

        a) Artificial tears

        b) Tape eye shut during sleep

VIII. Peripheral Nervous System Disorders

A. Guillain-Barre syndrome

1. Etiology

  a. Usually follows a upper respiratory or a gastrointestinal (GI) illness

  b. Associated with antecedent *Campylobacter jejuni* infection

2. Symptoms and signs

  a. Progressive, symmetrical weakness

  b. Lower extremities weakness >upper extremities

  c. Weakness causes ascending paralysis, which may affect respiratory muscles

    i. Miller Fisher variant results in descending paralysis

  d. Variable sensory findings

  e. Diminution or loss of deep tendon reflexes

  f. Anal sphincter tone **sparing**

3. Diagnosis

  a. Electrophysiologic testing

  b. CSF analysis reveals elevated proteins with mild pleocytosis

4. Management

  a. Neurologic consultation and hospital admission

b. Plasma exchange or intravenous immunoglobulin

c. Avoid steroids

d. Follow vital capacity (normally >15 cc L/kg)

    i. Prophylactic intubation if signs of weakness, CO_2 retention, or early ventilatory failure

5. Prognosis

  a. ~33% require intubation and ventilatory support

  b. Mortality and recurrence rate ~3%

IX. Spinal Cord Lesions (myelopathy)

A. Classification of spinal cord syndromes by function

1. Anatomy

  a. Corticospinal tract (efferent motor): ipsilateral deficits

  b. Spinothalamic tract (afferent pain/temp): contralateral deficits

  c. Dorsal column (afferent fine touch, vibration, proprioception): ipsilateral deficits

2. Complete spinal cord syndrome

  a. Etiology

    i. Acute: trauma, infarction, and hemorrhage

    ii. Subacute: multiple sclerosis, transverse myelitis, syringmyelia, and primary lateral sclerosis

  b. Symptoms and signs: complete loss of all sensory, motor and autonomic activities distal to the level of injury

3. Incomplete spinal cord syndromes

  a. Central cord syndrome

    i. Epidemiology: most common incomplete spinal cord syndrome

    ii. Etiology: hyperextension injury

    iii. Symptoms and signs: Bilateral motor weakness

        a) Upper >lower extremity weakness

        b) Upper >lower extremity sensory loss

  b. Anterior cord syndrome

    i. Etiology: disruption of blood supply to the anterior cord

        a) Aortic surgery, hypotension, and myocardial infarction

    ii. Symptoms and signs

        a) Bilateral loss of pain and touch

        b) Bilateral weakness or paralysis below the lesion

        c) Loss of sphincter control

        d) Vibration and position in the posterior columns are preserved

    iii. Poor prognosis—only 10% to 20% of patients regain some strength

c. Brown-Sequard syndrome
   i. Eiology: commonly penetrating injury, but can occur from compressive lesions such as tumors or hemorrhage
   ii. Symptoms and signs
      a) Ipsilateral motor, position and vibration loss
      b) Contralateral pain and temperature loss
      c) ± Bladder and sphincter weakness
      d) Mnemonic: Brown Bear Sequard Syndrome
         i) Half of your spine/lower extremity is bitten off by a bear, and in order to escape, you hop away barefoot on the other leg
         ii) On the injured side, there is pain but no strength because the leg is gone
         iii) In order to hop, proprioception must be intact contralaterally
         iv) Furthermore, since one is hopping away barefoot, pain and sensation must be lost contralaterally
d. Conus medullaris syndrome
   i. Symptoms and signs (terminal cord and therefore central)
      a) Saddle anesthesia
      b) Loss of bladder control, impotence
      c) Upper motor symptoms
         i) **Spasticity** of lower extremities
         ii) Usually bilateral
e. Cauda equina syndrome (peripheral nerve)
   i. Etiology: compression of cauda equina by herniated disc, tumor, or abscess
   ii. Symptoms and signs
      a) Urinary retention most common symptom
         i) Post-void residual urine volume >100 cc
      b) Saddle anesthesia
      c) Loss of bladder control, impotence
      d) Lower motor symptoms with increased **flaccidity** of lower extremities
         i) Usually unilateral
   iii. Better prognosis than conus medullaris syndrome (Table 12–8)

B. Classification of spinal cord syndromes by location
   1. Intrinsic cord lesions
      a. Transverse myelitis
         i. Etiology: inflammatory process of spinal cord causing axon demylination
            a) Associated with infections, vaccinations, and multiple sclerosis

TABLE 12–8. Upper Versus Lower Neuron Signs

	UPPER MOTOR NEURON SIGNS	LOWER MOTOR NEURON SIGNS
Reflexes	Increased	Decreased
Tone	Increased	Decreased
Atrophy	Absent	Present
Babinski	Present	Absent
Fasciculations	Absent	Present

      ii. Symptoms and signs: motor and sensory deficits with sphincter function compromise
      iii. Diagnosis:
         a) MRI
         b) Lumbar puncture
            i) Elevated protein in CSF
   b. Spinal subarachnoid hemorrhage
      i. Etiology: AVM, tumors, or anticoagulation
      ii. Symptoms and signs
         a) Sudden onset of severe back pain at level of hemorrhage
         b) Meningismus may develop if blood migrates cephalad
         c) Extremity sensory loss and weakness
      iii. Diagnosis
         a) MRI
      iv. Management
         a) Neurosurgical consult
            i) Clot evacuation if causing compression
            ii) Angiography if cause is believed to be from an AVM
   c. Amyotrophic lateral sclerosis (Lou Gehrig disease)
      i. Most common motor neuron disease
      ii. Definition: neurodegenerative disease resulting in lesions of anterior horn cells giving pure motor symptoms
         a) **Sensory intact**
      iii. Symptoms and signs
         a) Upper and lower motor neuron signs
            i) Early: spasticity, hyperreflexia, weakness, dysphagia
            ii) Late: intercostal muscle weakness, decreased forced vital capacity
      iv. Management is supportive
   2. Extrinsic cord lesions
      a. Epidural spinal hematoma
         i. Risk factors: lumbar puncture, epidural anesthesia, spinal AVM, and anticoagulation
         ii. Symptoms and signs: sudden radicular pain aggravated by straining or coughing

    iii. Diagnosis: MRI
    iv. Management: emergent surgical decompressive laminectomy
  b. Epidural spinal abscess
    i. Anatomy: most frequently located in the thoracic and lumbar spine
    ii. Etiology
      a) Hematogenous seeding in 25% to 50%
      b) *S. aureus* most common organism
    iii. Risk factors include diabetes, alcoholism, intravenous drug use, and renal failure
    iv. Symptoms and signs: back pain with fever, followed by radicular neurologic symptoms
    v. Diagnosis: MRI
      a) Lumbar puncture **contraindicated**
    vii. Management
      b) Antibiotics
      c) Surgical consult
    vi. Neurologic deficit rarely improves if treated >36 hours from initial symptoms
      a) Mortality rate 20%
  c. Diskitis
    i. Etiology: primary infection of the nucleus pulposus with extension to the cartilaginous end-plate
      a) May occur after surgical procedures
        i) Can occur spontaneously in children
          (a) Mean childhood age is 7 years
    ii. Symptoms and signs: localized radicular pain worsened by movement
      a) Lumbar spine is the most common site
    iii. Diagnosis: MRI
      a) Plain films may show destruction of disc space after 2 to 4 weeks of disease
    iv. Management: parenteral antibiotics
  d. Neoplasm (see Hematology/oncology chapter)
    i. Spinal cord tumors <10% of all CNS tumors
    ii. Metastatic from lung, breast, and lymphoma
    iii. Thoracic spine most commonly affected
    iv. Nighttime pain is characteristic
    v. 70% to 85% of plain films will be abnormal
    vi. Diagnosed by MRI
    vii. Cord compression is an oncologic emergency → Rx high-dose steroids and radiotherapy (Tables 12-9, 12-10, and 12-11)

X. Neuromuscular Disorders

A. Anatomy: the neuromuscular unit is composed of the anterior horn cell in the spinal cord, the peripheral nerve, the neuromuscular junction, and the muscle

TABLE 12–9. Sensory Levels (Dermatome)

LEVEL	SENSATION
C2	Occiput
C3	Exposed neck corresponding to turtle neck of shirt
C4	Suprasternal notch
C5	Below lateral clavicle
C6	Thumb
C7	Index and middle finger
C8	Ring and pinky finger
T4	Nipple line
T6-T7	Xiphoid process
T10	Umbilicus
L1	Inguinal ligament
L2-L3	Medial thigh
L4	Patella
L5	Lateral calf
S1	Lateral foot
S2-S4	Perianal region

TABLE 12–10. Motor Levels (Myotomes)

LEVEL	FUNCTION
C4	Spontaneous breathing
C5	Shoulder shrug
C6	Elbow flexion (biceps)
C7	Elbow extension (triceps)
C8-T1	Hand grasp
T2-T7	Chest muscles
T9-T12	Abdominal muscles
L2	Hip flexion
L3	Knee extension
L4	Ankle dorsiflexion
L5	Great toe extension
S1-S2	Foot plantar flexion
S2-S4	Voluntary rectal tone

TABLE 12–11. Reflexes

LEVEL	REFLEX
C6	Biceps
C7	Triceps
L4	Patellar
S1	Achilles

B. Disorders at the neuromuscular junction
  1. Myasthenia gravis (MG)
    a. Epidemiology
      i. 1 case in 100,000
      ii. Bimodal onset: women aged 20 to 30 years >men; men aged 60 to 70 years >women
    b. Pathophysiology
      i. Autoimmune destruction of acetylcholine receptors (AChR) on the **postsynaptic** membrane

c. Symptoms and signs
  i. Muscle weakness with repeated stimulation
    a) Autoimmune destruction of postsynaptic receptors leaves a limited number or receptor. A greater percent of these limited receptors are in refractory phase with repetitive depolarization
  ii. Facial and bulbar weakness
    a) Ptosis worse in the evening
    b) Blurred vision and diplopia
    c) Dysphagia
  iii. Weakness of respiratory muscles
d. Differential diagnosis: Eaton-Lambert syndrome (ELS)
  i. Autoimmune antibodies against **presynaptic** acetylcholine
  ii. Repeated stimulation **increases** muscle strength with ELS in contrast to myasthenia
  iii. Diagnosis
  iv. Serum for AChR antibody testing
    a) 80% to 90% of patients will test positive
    b) Unlikely to be helpful in ED
  v. Tensilon (edrophonium test: short-acting acetylcholinesterase inhibitor)
    a) Used to help diagnose MG and to differentiate MG exacerbations from cholinergic crisis
      i) 2 mg test dose given to identify patient with adverse reaction
        (a) Severe bradycardia: keep atropine at bedside
        (b) Exacerbation of asthma and COPD
        (c) Acute or chronic overdose of cholinesterase inhibitors may present similar to a MG exacerbation
          (i) Tensilon test will worsen symptoms
      ii) If no adverse reaction or improvement occurs within 90 seconds, give additional 3 mg IV
      iii) If still no improvement within 90 seconds, give the final dose of 5 mg IV
    b) Improvement measured by increased distance between the lower and upper eyelids
  vi. Ice test
    a) Apply ice pack to patient's eye for 2 minutes

b) A positive test is defined as improvement in the measured distance between the lower and upper eyelids
c) 80% of patients with MG will improve
e. Management
  i. Intubation if vital capacity <1 L (15 mL/kg)
    a) Rapid sequence intubation
      i) May require higher doses of succinylcholine since fewer AChR
      ii) Smaller doses of non-depolarizing paralytics preferred in these patients
  ii. Cholinesterase inhibitors
    a) Pyridostigmine (60 to 120 mg every 4 to 6 hours) or
    b) Neostigmine (15 to 30mg every 4 to 6 hours)
  iii. Immunomodulatory therapy
    a) Plasmapheresis 3 times a week to remove AChR antibodies
    b) IVIG
  iv. Thymectomy: can cause remission or improvement in 50% of patients <60 years
  v. Check prior to administering medications that can exacerbate symptoms
    a) Aminoglycosides, ciprofloxacin, erythromycin
    b) Penicillamine
    c) β-blockers
2. Botulism (see Infectious Disease chapter)
  a. Three forms exist
    i. Food-borne botulism
      a) Occurs 6 to 8 hours after toxin ingestion
      b) Symptoms and signs
        i) Abdominal pain, nausea/vomiting
        ii) **Descending** flaccid paralysis
        iii) Bulbar symptoms: diplopia, ptosis, dysphagia, and dysarthria
        iv) May lead to respiratory failure
    ii. Wound botulism
      a) Spores of *Clostridium botulinum* contaminate an open wound (cesarean section) or are injected (black-tar heroin)
      b) Symptoms similar to food-borne botulism without the GI symptoms
    iii. Infant botulism
      a) Spores are ingested and toxins produced most commonly after unprocessed honey ingestion
  b. Pathophysiology
    i. Toxin **irreversibly** binds to presynaptic membrane that prevents acetylcholine release

c. Diagnosis
   i. Toxin assays in serum and stool
d. Management
   i. Supportive
   ii. Bivalent (A, B) and a monovalent (E) horse-based antitoxin may shorten illness duration
   iii. Erythromycin
3. Tick paralysis (see Infectious Diseases chapter)
  a. Pathophysiology
    i. Ixovotoxin in tick saliva
    ii. **Reversible** binding at presynaptic membrane that prevents acetylcholine release
  b. Etiology
    i. 40 known tick species capable of producing ixovotoxin
    ii. Dermacentor andersoni (wood tick)
    iii. Dermacentor veriabilis (dog tick)
  c. Symptoms and signs
    i. **Ascending** flaccid paralysis
    ii. Symmetric paralysis
    iii. Occurs 5 to 6 days after female tick feeding
  d. Management
    i. Locate and remove tick
    ii. Patient symptoms resolve 1 to 24 hours after tick removal

C. Disorders of the muscle (myopathies)
1. Painful inflammatory diseases: affect 1 in 100,000
  a. Types
    i. Polymyositis: gradually increasing multiple myalgias
    ii. Dermatomyositis: similar presentation to polymyositis but with dermatologic features
     a) Periorbital heliotrope rash of a blue-purple discoloration of the upper eyelids with swelling
     b) Grotton papules: bilateral, erythematous, scaly rash over the MCP's and interphalangeal joints,
    iii. Inclusion body myositis: often misdiagnosed as polymyositis
     a) Definition: inflammatory muscle disease in which autoimmune and degenerative destruction of muscle cells occur in parallel
     b) Symptoms and signs: proximal and distal muscle weakness with eventual pharyngeal muscle weakness
     c) Does not respond well to treatment
  b. Symptoms and signs
    i. Proximal >distal weakness
    ii. Pain
    iii. Symmetrically decreased reflexes

c. Diagnosis
   i. Elevated creatinine phosphokinase (CPK) with predominance of skeletal muscle isoform
   ii. CPK-muscle type (MM): has limited sensitivity and specificity, neuropathies will also increase CPK
    a) Electromyography and muscle biopsy confirms the diagnosis
d. Management
   i. Prednisone 1 to 2 mg/kg/day
   ii. Add methotrexate if steroids ineffective
2. Painless generalized weakness
  a. Metabolic and electrolyte abnormalities
    i. Hypo- and hypercalcemia
    ii. Hypo- and hyperkalemia
    iii. Hypophosphatemia
    iv. Hypomagnesemia
  b. Familial periodic paralysis
    i. Definition: intermittent episodes of weakness associated with either hyper- or hypokalemia
    ii. Etiology: genetic predisposition: males >females, more common in Asians especially Japanese
    iii. Usually a history of similar events in other family members
    iv. Management: supportive. Hyper- or hypokalemia may need to be treated, but most often it is caused by transient transmembrane shifts rather than changes in total body stores
    v. Precipitating factors: can occur on awakening from sleep after a high-carbohydrate meal the previous night
  c. Thyrotoxic periodic paralysis
    i. Epidemiology: higher incidence in hyperthyroid patient of Asian ancestry
    ii. Etiology: genetic predisposition
    iii. Management: evidence that potassium does improve weakness until symptoms of hyperthyroidism treated

XI. Neurology Physical Exam Pearls

A. Weber and Rinne test
1. Tests complement one another
2. Sensorineural hearing loss is caused by problems with the inner ear, CN VIII, or the brain
3. Conductive hearing loss is secondary to problems with the outer ear, tympanic membrane, or the middle ear
4. Weber test
  a. Place tuning fork in middle of head
  b. Sound will localize to ear of conductive loss and opposite that of sensorineural hearing loss

5. Rinne test
   a. Tests for conductive hearing loss
   b. Air conduction (AC) is normally twice as long as bone conduction (BC)
   c. Tuning fork is placed on mastoid (bone conduction) and the moment the vibration is no longer heard, the tuning fork is placed next to the auditory meatus (air conduction)
   d. Patient should continue to hear vibration. If not, there is conduction loss on that side

6. Examples
   a. Weber test lateralizes to left ear. One now has to determine if a conductive loss on the left exists or if testing indicates sensorineural hearing loss on the right. The Rinne test is performed next and it is determined that air conduction is greater than bone conduction on both ears (which is normal). One can then conclude that there is a sensorineural impairment of the right ear
   b. Weber test lateralizes to left ear. BC > AC in left ear and AC > BC in right ear. One can then conclude that conductive hearing loss exists on the left
   c. Weber test lateralizes to left ear. BC > AC in left ear and BC > AC in right ear. Now what? A combined hearing loss is likely

B. Romberg sign
   1. Indications
      a. Used primarily to diagnose sensory ataxia
      b. Is not a test of cerebellar function as commonly misunderstood
      c. Tests for vestibular system and dorsal column dysfunction
   2. Testing technique
      a. Patient stands with feet together and eyes open initially
      b. Patient subsequently closes his/her eyes
         i. Cerebellum provides stability via input from 3 sensory modes
            a) Proprioceptive: dorsal column and peripheral nerves
            b) Visual: eyes and CN II
            c) Vestibular: inner ear and CN VIII
         ii. The Romberg test removes visual input
         iii. Patient with intact vestibular apparatus and proprioception remains stable
   3. Test interpretation
      a. Test is positive if **both** criteria met
         i. Patient stable with eyes open **and**
         ii. Unsteady when eyes shut
      b. Patients with cerebellar disease sway with eyes open or closed, which does **not** constitute a positive test

   c. Positive test indicative of
      i. Bilateral vestibular dysfunction
      ii. Proprioceptive dysfunction
         a) Dorsal column pathology such as tabes dorsalis
         b) Peripheral sensory nerve disease such as in chronic inflammatory demyelinating polyradiculoneuropathy (CIDP), which is the chromic form of Guillain-Barré syndrome

C. Oculovestibular reflex (cold calorics)
   1. Indications
      a. Assess brainstem, cortical function, and brain death
      b. Identify malingering patients
   2. Testing technique
      a. Position patient supine with head at 30 degrees elevation
      b. Instill 10 to 30 mL of ice cold water into the ear canal
      c. Normal response is transient conjugate slow deviation of gaze **ipsilateral** to the cold water stimulus (brainstem mediated)
      d. This is followed by rapid corrective motion (nystagmus) to bring the eyes back to midline (cortically mediated)
      e. Direction of nystagmus is indicated by the direction of the rapid component
   3. Test interpretation
      a. Presence of horizontal nystagmus, with quick component away from irrigated ear implies normal response in a patient who is not comatose (ie, there is cortical correction to the brainstem-mediated response)
      b. Presence of only slow ipsilateral eye deviation towards the stimulated ear implies a comatose patient (ie, brainstem-mediated response occurs but there is no cortically medicate corrective response)
      c. If no eye movement is noted upon testing, it implies that patient is comatose with brainstem dysfunction (ie, there is no brainstem-mediated gaze towards stimulated ear)
      d. Normal response in a "comatose appearing" patient implies malingering

D. Oculomotor kinetics
   1. Used to determine malingerers feigning blindness
   2. If nystagmus is exhibited by spinning of optokinetic drum, this provides evidence of vision and suggests malingering
   3. Passing a tape measure back and forth in front of the patient can be used as an alternative to the optokinetic drum

BIBLIOGRAPHY

Adams JHP, et al: Guidelines for the management of patients with acute ischemic stroke. *Stroke.* 1994;25:1901.

American Heart Association: *Heart and Stroke Facts*, Dallas, TX: American Heart Association; 2003.

American Heart Association: *Heart Disease and Stroke Statistics—2004 Update.* Dallas, TX: American Heart Association; 2003.

American Psychiatric Association Practice Guidelines: Practice guidelines for the treatment of patients with delirium. *Am J Psychiatry.* 1999;156(Suppl):5.

American Psychiatric Association: *Diagnostic and Statistical Manual of Mental Disorders: DSM-IV-TR, text revision*, Chicago, IL: American Psychiatric Association, 2000.

Bartt R: *Autoimmune and inflammatory disorders.* In: Goetz CG, (ed). *Goetz Textbook of Clinical Neurology*, Philadelphia: WB Saunders; 1999.

Boon PA, Williamson PD: The diagnosis of pseudoseizure. *Clin Neurol Neurosurg.* 1993;95:1.

Broderick JP, et al: Guidelines for the management of spontaneous intracerebral hemorrhage: a statement for healthcare professionals from a special writing group of the Stroke Council, American Heart Association. *Stroke.* 1999;30:905.

Brott T. The National Institute for Neurological Disorders and Stroke rt-PA Study Group, et al: Hypertension and its treatment in the NINDS rt-PA Stroke Trial. *Stroke.* 1998;29:1504.

Commission on Classification and Terminology of the International League Against Epilepsy: Proposal for revised clinical and electroencephalographic classification of epileptic seizures. *Epilepsia.*1989;30:389.

deGans J, van de Beek D: Dexamethasone in adults with bacterial meningitis. *N Eng J Med.* Nov 2002;347:1549.

Drachman DB: Myasthenia gravis. *N Engl J Med.* 1994;330:1797.

Edmeads J: Emergency management of headache. *Headache.* 1988;28:675.

Giovannoni G, Miller D: Multiple sclerosis and its treatment. *J R Coll Physicians Lond.* 1999;33:315.

Goadsby PJ, Lipton RB, Ferrari MD: Migraine—Current understanding and treatment. *N Engl J Med.* 2002;346:257.

Goetz CG, ed: *Goetz Textbook of Clinical Neurology*, Philadelphia: WB Saunders; 1999.

Goldman B. Vertigo and dizziness. In: Tintinalli JE, et al (eds): *Emergency Medicine, A Comprehensive Study Guide,* 6th ed. 2004;1400. (Note: The content of this reading also relates to Content Area 12, Nervous System Disorders. This reference has been updated from the 5th edition of this text, 3/30/2005.)

Hasbun R, Abrahams J, Jekel J, et al: Computed tomography of the head before lumbar puncture in adults with suspected meningitis. *N Engl J Med.* Dec 2001;345:1727.

Hauser WA, Hesdorffer DC: *Epilepsy: Frequency, Causes and Consequences*, New York: Demos; 1990.

Hogenkamp WE, et al: The epidemiology of multiple sclerosis. *Mayo Clin Proc.* 1997;72:871.

Hohl CM, et al: Polypharmacy, adverse drug-related events, and potential adverse drug interactions in elderly patients presenting to an emergency department. *Ann Emerg Med.* 2001; 38:661.

Hunt WE, Hess RM: Surgical risk as related to time intervention in the repair of intracranial aneurysm. *J Neurosurg.* 1968;28:14.

Kaniecki R: Headache assessment and management. *JAMA.* 2003;289:1430.

Kasper DL, Braunwald E, Fauci AS, et al: *Harrison's Principals of Internal Medicine.* 16th ed. New York: McGraw-Hill; 2004.

Kidwell CS, Chalela JA, Saver JL, et al: Comparison of MRI and CT for detection of acute intracerebral hemorrhage. *JAMA.* Oct 2004;292(15):1823.

Lempert T, Bauer M, Schmidt D: Syncope: a videometric analysis of 56 episodes of transient cerebral hypoxia. *Ann Neurol.* 1994;36:233.

Lewandowski C, Barsan W: Treatment of acute ischemic stroke. *Ann Emerg Med.* Feb. 2001; 37:202.

Marx JA, Hockberger RS, Walls RM, et al, eds: *Rosen's Emergency Medicine Concepts and Clinical Practice*, 6th ed. Philadelphia, PA: Elsevier; 2006.

Petersen LR, Marfin AA, Gubler DJ: West Nile virus. *JAMA.* July 2003; 290:524.

Pollack CV, et al: Case conference: two crack cocaine body stuffers. *Ann Emerg Med.*1992;21:1370.

Rothrock SG: *Tarascon Adult Emergency Pocketbook*, 2nd ed. 2002; 96.

Rothrock SG: *Tarascon Adult Emergency Pocketbook*, 2nd ed. 2002; 93.

Rowland LP: Familial periodic paralysis. In: Rowland LP, ed. *Merritt's Textbook of Neurology*, 9th ed. Philadelphia: Williams & Wilkins; 1995.

Saper JR: Headache disorders. *Med Clin North Am.* 1999;83:663.

The National Institute of Neurological Disorders t-PA Stroke Study Group: Generalized efficacy of t-PA for acute stroke: Subgroup analysis of the NINDS t-PA Stroke Trial. *Stroke.* 1997;28:2119.

The NINDS rt-PA Stroke Study Group: Tissue plasminogen activator for acute ischemic stroke. *N Engl J Med.* 1995;333:1581.

Thomas PK: Clinical features and investigation of diabetic somatic peripheral neuropathy. *Neuroscience.* 1997;4:341.

Tintinalli JE, Ruiz E, Krome RL, et al eds: *Emergency Medicine. A Comprehensive Study.* 6th ed. New York: McGraw-Hill; 2006.

Warden CR, Zibulewsky J, Mace S, et al: Evaluation and management of febrile seizures in the out-of-hospital and emergency department settings. *Ann Emerg Med.* Feb 2003; 41:215-222.

Watanabe K, et al: Characteristics of cranial nerve palsies in diabetic patients. *Diabetes Res Clin Pract.* 1990;10:19.

Working Group on Status Epilepticus: Treatment of convulsive status epilepticus. *JAMA.* 1993;270:854.

Chapter 13
ENDOCRINE AND METABOLIC EMERGENCIES

Gary Mazer, Nicole Kriss, and Leo Pritsiolas

I. Acid-Base Disorders

A. General principles

1. Acidosis = pH <7.40. Can result from a respiratory (PCO_2 >40) or a metabolic disorder (HCO_3 <24)

2. Alkalosis = pH >7.40. Can result from a respiratory (PCO_2 <40) or a metabolic disorder (HCO_3 >24)

3. Can have only 1 primary pulmonary disturbance but up to 2 separate primary metabolic disorders (triple acid-base disorder)

   a. Therefore, nephrologists claims to be smarter than pulmonologists

4. Respiratory compensation occurs immediately

5. Metabolic compensation occurs over days

   a. Therefore, pulmonologist claims that nephrologists are slow

6. Compensation never overcorrects a primary acid-base disturbance

B. Respiratory disturbances

1. Primary respiratory acidosis: pH <7.40 and CO_2 >40

   a. Acute versus chronic disorders

      i. In acute respiratory acidosis, for each 10 mm Hg increase in $PaCO_2$, pH should decrease by 0.08 units

      ii. In chronic respiratory acidosis, for each 10 mm Hg increase in $PaCO_2$, pH should decrease by 0.03 units

      iii. If the HCO_3 is above normal, it may be a chronic (compensated) process, and the pH may be low but near normal range (eg, COPD)

      iv. If the HCO_3 is normal or low, there is an acute problem, such as respiratory distress or failure (remember: metabolic compensation occurs over days)

      v. Acute respiratory acidosis may be an indicator of impending respiratory failure

   b. Etiology

      i. Central nervous system (CNS): oversedation (eg, opiates), intracranial pathology (bleed, obesity, hypoventilation)

      ii. Neurologic and neuromuscular disorders: Guillain-Barré syndrome, myasthenia gravis, botulism

      iii. Pleural diseases: large pneumothorax or pleural effusion

      iv. Lung disease: COPD, ARDS, pneumonia, pulmonary embolism

      v. Musculoskeletal disorders: kyphoscoliosis, polymyositis

2. Secondary respiratory acidosis: pH >7.40 and CO_2 >40

   a. Compensation for a primary metabolic alkalosis

3. Primary respiratory alkalosis: pH >7.40 and CO_2 <40

   a. Etiology: breathing too rapidly or increased minute ventilation

      i. Anxiety and pain

      ii. Medications: salicylates, progesterone

      iii. Liver failure

      iv. Seen normally in pregnancy caused by increased tidal volume; there may be full compensation with normal pH

      v. High altitude

   b. Treatment aimed at correcting underlying cause

4. Secondary respiratory alkalosis: pH <7.40 and CO_2 <40

   a. A compensatory process for a metabolic acidosis

   b. The pH is acidemic

   c. Treat underlying metabolic etiology in a tachypneic patient who has a normal lung examination and no lung pathology

C. Metabolic disturbances
1. Primary metabolic acidosis: pH <7.40 and HCO_3 <25 categorized as anion gap (AG) or nonanion gap acidosis (NAG)
   a. AG metabolic acidosis
      i. $AG = Na - (Cl + CO_2)$ normally between 5 to 12 mEq/L
      ii. Etiology: mnemonic **MUDPILES**: **M**ethanol, **U**remia, **D**iabetic ketoacidosis (or any ketosis), **P**araldehyde, **P**henformin, **I**ron, **I**soniazid, **L**actic acidosis (shock, seizures, cyanide, carbon monoxide), **E**thylene glycol, **S**alicylates
      iii. Use Winter formula to help determine if respiratory compensation is appropriate
         a) Winter formula: expected $PCO_2 = 1.5$ $(HCO_3) + 8 \pm 2$
            i) If measured PCO_2 equals expected PCO_2, there is appropriate compensation
            ii) If measured PCO_2 is higher than expected PCO_2, there is an additional primary respiratory acidosis
            iii) If measured PCO_2 is lower than expected PCO_2, there is an additional primary respiratory alkalosis
            iv) A quick rule of thumb in metabolic acidosis: the last 2 digits of the pH should approximate the expected PCO_2. For example, if the pH is 7.20, the PCO_2 should be approximately 20. If the measured PCO_2 is 25, there is an additional primary respiratory acidosis
      iv. Consider Delta AG-Delta HCO_3 gap (bicarbonate gap)
         a) With pure AG metabolic acidosis, there should be a 1:1 correlation between the rise in AG and the fall in HCO_3
         b) Delta anion gap – Delta HCO_3 where
            i) Delta $AG = AG - 12$ (normal gap)
            ii) Delta $HCO_3 = 25$ (normal HCO_3) – measured HCO_3
         c) If gap is very negative or very positive, a secondary metabolic disturbance is likely
            i) If >6, a concurrent metabolic alkalosis is likely since the rise in the AG is greater than the fall in HCO_3
            ii) If <6, a concurrent metabolic acidosis is likely because the fall in HCO_3 is greater than the rise in the AG
   b. NAG metabolic acidosis: HCO_3 loss with subsequent increase in chloride, thereby maintaining a normal AG (hyperchloremic acidosis)
      i. Most cases in ED are attributable to gastrointestinal (GI) loss (diarrhea) or massive saline administration
      ii. Mnemonic **HARD UP**
         a) **H**ypoaldosteronism, **H**ydration (saline)
         b) **A**cetazolamide
         c) **R**enal tubular acidosis
         d) **D**iarrhea
         e) **U**reteroenterostomy
         f) **P**ancreatic fistula
2. Metabolic alkalosis: pH >7.4 and HCO_3 >25, caused by either loss of H^+ or increase in HCO_3
   a. Generally speaking, metabolic alkalosis results from increased renin or aldosterone activity. This occurs secondary to decreased renal perfusion (saline responsive) or mineralocorticoid excess (saline unresponsive)
   b. Characterized as saline (chloride) responsive or saline resistant
      i. Saline responsive (Urine chloride <10 mEq/L)
         a) Etiology
            i) Dehydration, vomiting
            ii) Renal artery stenosis
         b) Treatment
            i) Administer IV fluids
            ii) Watch for hypokalemia
      ii. Saline resistant (urine chloride >10 mEq/L)
         a) Etiology
            i) Mineralocorticoid excess (HCO_3 is retained and H^+ is excreted)
               (a) Licorice poisoning
               (b) Exogenous steroids, hyperaldosteronism
               (c) Hypomagnesemia
         b) Treat underlying etiology

D. Acid-base pearls
1. Isopropyl alcohol causes an osmolar gap without an AG acidosis
2. If a patient presents with tinnitus, increased AG metabolic acidosis, and a primary respiratory alkalosis, consider aspirin overdose
3. A patient with an asthma exacerbation who has a normal or decreased pH and a rising CO_2 may

have impending respiratory failure. (Early asthma causes hyperventilation and respiratory alkalosis)

II. Electrolyte Disturbances

A. Hyperkalemia
  1. Etiology
    a. Pseudohyperkalemia
      i. Tourniquet use
      ii. Hemolysis (in vitro)
      iii. Leukocytosis
      iv. Thrombocytosis
    b. Intra- to extracellular shift
      i. Acidosis (eg, diabetic ketoacidosis [DKA])
      ii. Drugs: β-blockers, digitalis, succinylcholine
      iii. Cell breakdown (rhabdomyolysis, tumor lysis syndrome)
    c. Decreased excretion
      i. Renal failure and insufficiency
      ii. Drugs (ACE inhibitors, NSAIDs, potassium-sparing diuretics)
      iii. Aldosterone deficiency
      iv. Type IV RTA
  2. Symptoms and signs
    a. Neuromuscular: weakness, paresthesias, areflexia
    b. Hypotension, dysrhythmias, asystole
  3. Diagnosis
    a. Serum level
    b. ECG progression
      i. Peaked T waves
      ii. Shortened QT interval
      iii. ST depression
      iv. Bundle branch block and widened QRS
      v. Widened PR interval
      vi. Decreased P wave
      vii. Sine wave, ventricular fibrillation, and asystole
  4. Management
    a. Calcium chloride
      i. Provides membrane stabilization (1 to 3 minute onset)
      ii. Indicated with widened QRS complex
      iii. Use caution if patient is on digoxin
        a) Calcium may potentiate the effects of digoxin and its administration may lead to failure of diastolic relaxation and cardiac tetany termed "stone heart" (in animal studies only)
    b. Bicarbonate: leads to shift of potassium into cell (5 to 10 minute onset)
    c. Insulin and glucose: shifts potassium into cell (30 minute onset)
    d. Albuterol (nebulized): upregulates cAMP, shifts potassium into cell (15 to 30 minute onset)
    e. Kayexalate: GI potassium excretion (2 to 12 hour onset)
    f. Furosemide: renal potassium excretion (variable onset)
    g. Hemodialysis: removes potassium within minutes

B. Hypokalemia
  1. Etiology
    a. Transcellular shifts: alkalosis, insulin treatment, β agonists
    b. Decreased intake
    c. GI loss: vomiting, nasogastric tube suctioning, diarrhea
      i. Dehydration leads to metabolic "contraction" alkalosis and relative hyperaldosteronism with renal loss and intracellular potassium shift
    d. Renal loss: diuretics, hyperaldosteronism, type I RTA
  2. Symptoms and signs
    a. Occur when serum concentration <2.5 mEq/L
    b. Cardiovascular: hypotension, orthostatic hypotension, dysrhythmias
    c. Neuromuscular: weakness, muscle cramping, fatigue, hyporeflexia, paresthesias, periodic paralysis
    d. GI: ileus
  3. Diagnosis
    a. Serum levels
    b. ECG changes
      i. U waves, T-wave flattening, ST depression, QT prolongation
      ii. Risk for torsade de pointes
  4. Management
    a. Oral replacement in stable patient
    b. IV replacement if severely hypokalemic
    c. Consider hypomagnesemia in patients with resistant hypokalemia

C. Hypernatremia
  1. Etiology
    a. Osmotic diuresis: poorly controlled diabetes, hyperalimentation, mannitol
    b. Extrarenal water loss: fever, burns, vomiting, diarrhea
    c. Renal water loss: kidney is unable to conserve water
      i. Diabetes insipidus:
        a) Central diabetes insipidus: the kidney is unable to concentrate urine because of absent or deficient ADH

b) Nephrogenic diabetes insipidus: the kidney is unresponsive to the effects of ADH

2. Symptoms and signs
   a. Neurologic symptoms usually seen when sodium >158 mEq/L
   b. Irritability, lethargy, and weakness, and can progress to seizures and coma
   c. Intracerebral or subarachnoid hemorrhage may occur with brain shrinkage and tearing of cerebral blood vessels

3. Management
   a. Volume repletion
   b. Start with 0.9% normal saline (NS). Subsequent fluids should be hypotonic
   c. Calculate water deficit and correct over 48 hours
      i. H_2O deficit = TBW × ([Na]$_{(measured)}$ − [Na$_{(desired)}$]/[Na$_{(desired)}$]
   d. Correct no faster than 0.5 mEq/L/h
   e. Maximum 12 mEq/L/day
   f. Over correction may cause cerebral edema
   g. Treatment of diabetes insipidus
      i. Central
         a) Desmopressin: increases ADH which decreases urine output and therefore decreases further water loss
      ii. Nephrogenic
         a) Discontinue offending drug (eg, lithium)
         b) Thiazide diuretics: mild volume depletion, increasing proximal sodium and water reabsorption. Diminished water delivery to the ADH-sensitive sites in the collecting tubules reduces urine output
         c) Exogenous ADH: most patients with nephrogenic DI have partial rather than complete resistance to ADH. Supraphysiologic hormone levels may increase the renal effect of ADH
         d) NSAIDs: prostaglandins antagonize the action of ADH

D. Hyponatremia
   1. Etiology
      a. Pseudohyponatremia
         i. Check serum osmolality. With true hyponatremia, serum osmolality is low (remember serum osmolality = 2 Na + BUN/2.8 + Glucose/18)
         ii. Hypertonic pseudohyponatremia (osmolality >295)

            a) Hyperglycemia (adjust sodium up 1.6 for every 100 glucose level >100)
            b) Mannitol
         iii. Normotonic pseudohyponatremia (osmolality = 295)
            a) Severe hyperlipidemia
            b) Hyperproteinemia such as multiple myeloma
      b. True hyponatremia (osmolality <295)
         i. Determine volume status
            a) Hypovolemic hyponatremia: vomiting, diarrhea
            b) Hypervolemic hyponatremia: congestive heart failure (CHF), cirrhosis, renal failure
            c) Euvolemic hyponatremia
               i) Psychogenic polydipsia
               ii) SIADH (most common cause of euvolemic hyponatremia)
               iii) Hypoadrenalism
               iv) Hypothyroidism

   2. Symptoms and signs
      a. Depends on cause, volume status, and acuity
      b. Acute: nausea, vomiting, confusion, lethargy, stupor, seizures
      c. Chronic: milder neurologic symptoms. (patients usually asymptomatic until sodium is <120 mEq/L)

   3. Management
      a. Neurologically stable
         i. Volume status dependent
            a) Hypovolemic
               i) Replace volume with 0.9% NS
               ii) Do not correct >0.5 to 1 mEq/L/h. Maximum 12 mEq/L/24 h
               iii) Acute hyponatremia tolerates correction more safely than chronic hyponatremia
               iv) Central pontine myelinolysis may occur with excessively rapid correction
            b) Euvolemic
               i) Free water restriction (<1 L/day)
               ii) Demeclocycline for severe SIADH
            c) Hypervolemic
               i) Free water restriction
               ii) Loop diuresis
      b. Neurologically unstable (coma, seizures)
         i. 3% hypertonic saline
            a) Correct no faster than 1 to 2 mEq/L/h for 3 hours or until Na >120

b) Then switch to 0.9% NS so that the serum sodium is increased at a rate of 0.5 mEq/L/h

c) Max 8 mEq/L total in 24 h

E. Hypercalcemia
1. Pathophysiology
   a. 3 calcium states in body: protein bound (40%), bound to anions (10%), and free ionized form (50%)
      i. Only the free ionized form is biologically active
      ii. Ionized calcium levels are difficult to measure so total calcium levels are typically used as a surrogate
      iii. Hypoalbuminemia results in falsely low calcium levels but does **not** affect ionized calcium levels
      iv. Add 0.8 mg/dL to serum calcium levels for every 0.8 g/dL decrease in albumin (normal 4 g/dL)
   b. Calcium homeostasis
      i. Calcium resorption from bone regulated by parathyroid hormone (PTH) and incorporation into bone regulated by calcitonin
      ii. Vitamin D is a cofactor involved with gut absorption
2. Etiology
   a. Mnemonic **CHIMPANZEES**
      i. **C**alcium supplementation
      ii. **H**yperparathyroidism (most common outpatient etiology)
      iii. **I**atrogenic (thiazide diuretics), **I**mmobility
      iv. **M**etastases/**M**ilk alkali syndrome
      v. **P**aget disease
      vi. **A**ddison disease
      vii. **N**eoplasm (most common inpatient etiology)
      viii. **Z**ollinger-Ellison syndrome
      ix. **E**xcessive vitamin D
      x. **E**xcessive vitamin A
      xi. **S**arcoid disease
   b. Metastases to bone. Mnemonic **Pb KTL** (lead kettle)
      i. **P**rostate, **B**reast, **K**idney, **T**hyroid, **L**ung
3. Symptoms and signs
   a. Mnemonic **bones, stones, groans, psychiatric overtones**
      i. Bones (abnormal bone remodeling and fracture risk)
      ii. Renal stones
      iii. Abdominal groans (pain, nausea, ileus, and constipation)
      iv. Psychiatric disturbances (lethargy, depressed mood, psychosis, cognitive dysfunction, and coma)
4. Diagnosis
   a. Usually asymptomatic unless calcium >14 mg/dL
   b. Serum protein levels affect total calcium levels
      i. Corrected total calcium (mg/dL) = (measured total calcium mg/dL) + 0.8 (4.4 – measured albumin g/dL)
   c. ECG findings: shortened QT interval, flattened T-wave and QRS widening with very elevated values
5. Management
   a. Intravenous 0.9% NS is first step in management
   b. Loop diuretics may be added after adequate hydration (forced diuresis)
      i. Facilitates urinary excretion of calcium and prevent volume overload
   c. Bisphosphonates inhibit calcium release from bone
      i. Onset of action 2 to 4 days
      ii. Associated with jaw osteonecrosis (avascular necrosis)
   d. Steroids can be used in chronic granulomatous disease (sarcoidosis) and hematologic malignancies
   e. Calcitonin binds to osteoclasts and inhibits bone resorption
   f. Parathyroidectomy, if hyperparathyroidism is the etiology
   g. Dialysis for severe hypercalcemia

F. Hypocalcemia
1. Etiology
   a. Pseudohypocalcemia (correct for hypoalbuminemia; see Diagnosis of Hypercalcemia above)
   b. Postoperative from thyroid and parathyroid surgery
   c. Low vitamin D levels
      i. Renal failure: decreased 1, 25-$(OH)_2$ vitamin D production causes decreased intestinal absorption of calcium
   d. Malabsorption syndromes (celiac sprue, Crohn disease)
   e. Liver failure
   f. Hydrofluoric acid exposure
   g. Hyperphosphatemia: as in rhabdomyolysis and tumor lysis syndrome
      i. Phosphorus binds calcium and leads to calcium deposition in bone

h. Citrate toxicity from massive blood transfusions
i. Bicarbonate administration
j. Sepsis and surgery: high incidence in critically ill and postsurgical
k. Pancreatitis: precipitation of calcium soaps in abdominal cavity
l. Hypomagnesemia

2. Symptoms and signs
a. Reduced myocardial contractility
b. Perioral and distal extremity paresthesias
c. Tetany: repeated neuromuscular discharge after a single stimulus
   i. Chvostek sign: facial twitching caused by tapping facial nerve anterior to ear (present in 10% to 30% of normal individuals)
   ii. Trousseau sign: carpal spasm when blood pressure cuff inflated on upper arm above systolic >3 minutes (more specific than Chvostek sign)

3. Diagnosis
a. Corrected total serum calcium level
b. Serum-free ionized calcium level most accurate
c. Serum 25-(OH) and 1,25-(OH) vitamin D and PTH levels
d. ECG findings: prolonged QT interval

4. Management
a. Treat the underlying cause
b. Consider magnesium therapy with refractory hypocalcemia
c. Asymptomatic or mild hypocalcemia
   i. Oral therapy with or without vitamin D
d. Symptomatic, severe hypocalcemia
   i. IV calcium chloride (10 mL of 10% $CaCl_2$) or calcium gluconate (10 to 30 mL of 10% solution) over 10 to 20 minutes
      a) Calcium chloride has 3 times more calcium than calcium gluconate per equal volume
      b) Calcium gluconate preferred in case of accidental tissue extravasation
      c) IV calcium may cause vasoconstriction and ischemia
      d) Use caution in patients on digitalis, as it may theoretically precipitate "stone heart" (see Management of Hyperkalemia above)

G. Hypermagnesemia
1. Etiology
a. Renal failure is most common cause
b. Ingestion of vitamins, antacids, and cathartics in patients with chronic renal insufficiency
c. Iatrogenic: treatment of eclampsia and torsade de pointes

d. Tumor lysis syndrome and rhabdomyolysis
e. Rarely hypothyroidism

2. Symptoms and signs
a. Neuromuscular: muscle weakness including heart and diaphragm → CHF, lethargy, paralysis, diminished or **absent reflexes**, confusion, coma, and hypoventilation
b. Cardiovascular: arrhythmias, hypotension from vasodilation

3. Diagnosis
a. Serum magnesium level
b. ECG
   i. PR prolongation
   ii. QRS widening
   iii. Bundle branch blocks
   iv. Atrial fibrillation

4. Management
a. Supportive
b. Cessation of magnesium-containing medications (antacids)
c. Fluids
d. Furosemide
e. Intravenous **calcium**
f. Dialysis if renal failure

H. Hypomagnesemia—far more common than hypermagnesemia
1. Etiology
a. Decreased absorption from renal disease
b. Increased losses from diarrhea
c. Malnutrition
d. Alcoholism, cirrhosis (30% to 80% incidence in alcoholics)
e. Endocrine disorders: DKA, hyperaldosteronism, hyperparathyroidism
f. Pancreatitis
g. Medications: pentamidine, diuretics, aminoglycosides

2. Symptoms and signs
a. Neuromuscular: weakness, tremors, fasciculations, nystagmus, tetany, confusion, seizures, cerebellar (ataxia, nystagmus, vertigo)
b. GI: nausea, anorexia
c. Cardiovascular: hypotension, arrhythmias including torsades, PVCs, Vfib, Vtach
d. Interferes with PTH leading to hypocalcemia
e. Leads to hypokalemia with ECG changes of hypokalemia

3. Diagnosis
a. Low serum magnesium levels are reliable indicators of low body levels but may not become decreased until late. Therefore, have low threshold to administer in patients with alcohol abuse and resistant hypocalcemia and/or hypokalemia

4. Management
   a. Replete magnesium: intravenously if symptomatic
   b. Treat concurrent hypocalcemia and hypokalemia

III. Parathyroid Disorders

A. Hyperparathyroidism
   1. General considerations
      a. PTH is inversely proportional to serum calcium
      b. PTH causes an increase in serum calcium
         i. Stimulates bone reabsorption and calcium and phosphate release
         ii. Acts on the kidney to decrease calcium clearance and phosphate reabsorption
         iii. PTH increases 1,25-dihydroxyvitamin D, the active form of the vitamin, which increases gut absorption of calcium
   2. Etiology
      a. Parathyroid adenoma: 85%
      b. Hyperplasia: 15%
      c. Carcinoma: 0.5%
   3. Symptoms and signs
      a. Similar to that of hypercalcemia
   4. Diagnosis
      a. Primary hyperparathyroidism: elevated PTH levels inappropriate for elevated serum calcium
      b. Secondary hyperparathyroidism
         i. Malabsorption syndromes
         ii. Rickets
         iii. Chronic renal failure: phosphate excretion decreases with GFR. As serum phosphate levels increase, PTH increases in order to decrease renal phosphate reabsorption. Over the long-term the hyperparathyroidism is maladaptive, producing bone disease (renal osteodystrophy)
   5. Symptoms and treatment are attributed to hypercalcemia

B. Hypoparathyroidism
   1. Etiology
      a. Can be acquired after thyroid surgery (most commonly) or radiation
      b. Congenital or acquired deficiency in PTH or its receptors
      c. Infiltration of the parathyroid glands from metastatic carcinoma, hemochromatosis, Wilson disease
   2. Symptoms and signs
      a. Related to hypocalcemia (see hypocalcemia section)

3. Management
   a. Consists of calcium and vitamin D supplementation

IV. Thyroid Disorders

A. Hypothyroidism
   1. Etiology
      a. Causes of primary thyroid failure
         i. Radioactive iodine treatment for Graves disease (most common cause in United States)
         ii. Previous thyroid surgery or radiation.
         iii. Autoimmune disease, such as burnt-out Hashimoto thyroiditis
         iv. Subacute thyroiditis, postpartum thyroiditis
         v. Medications: amiodarone (also causes hyperthyroid), dopamine, lithium
      b. Causes of secondary thyroid failure
         i. Pituitary tumor, hemorrhage, or infiltrative disease
         ii. "Tertiary hypothyroid" or hypothalamic dysfunction
   2. Symptoms and signs
      a. Symptoms: fatigue, weight gain, cold intolerance, menstrual irregularities, constipation, and depression
      b. Signs: nonpitting edema, goiter, hoarseness, bradycardia, dry skin, delayed relaxation phase of deep tendon reflexes, carpal tunnel syndrome, thinning of the outer third of the eyebrows, and thyroidectomy scar
   3. Diagnosis
      i. Thyroid-stimulating hormone (TSH)
         a) Controls the synthesis and release of thyroxine (T_4) and triiodothyronine (T_3)
         b) Elevated with primary hypothyroidism
         c) May be low with secondary hypothyroidism
         d) Regulated by negative feedback from T_3 and T_4
         e) High TSH and low T_4 is diagnostic for primary hypothyroidism
      ii. T_4 or free T_4
         a) Decreased with hypothyroidism
         b) May be normal early on in disease or with subclinical disease
      iii. T_3 or free T_3
         a) More biologically active than T_4
         b) Levels may be normal early in disease
         c) T_3 levels drop later than T_4
            i) Decreased T_4 results in elevated TSH and thyroid hypertrophy

with increased T_3 secretion early in disease

  iv. Thyrotropin-releasing hormone (TRH)

    a) Produced by hypothalamus and acts on anterior pituitary to release TSH and prolactin

    b) Helps regulate TSH production

    c) Low levels with tertiary hypothyroidism (hypothalamic failure)

  4. ED management

    a. Rule out central causes of hypothyroidism (eg, pituitary mass)

    b. Initiation of therapy generally deferred to the primary care physician

    c. First-line therapy involves levothyroxine (LT_4), usually initiated at 50 to 100 mcg/day

B. Myxedema coma

  1. Definition

    a. Severe hypothyroidism resulting in a decompensated metabolic state and mental status change

    b. Myxedema refers to the thickened, nonpitting edema of skin associated with severe chronic hypothyroidism

      i. Not to be confused with pretibial myxedema which is associated with **hyper**thyroidism

  2. Precipitating factors

    a. Infection, cold exposure, stroke, or medications (amiodarone and lithium)

  3. Symptoms and signs

    a. Hypothermia: mortality proportional to severity of hypothermia

    b. Hypoventilation

    c. Cardiovascular: bradycardia, decreased contractility, cardiac output, and pericardial effusion

    d. CNS: altered mental status

  4. Diagnosis

    a. Initially made by history, physical examination, and exclusion of other causes of coma

    b. Thyroid function tests should be ordered to confirm diagnosis

    c. Laboratory findings

      i. Metabolic: hypoglycemia, hyponatremia (50%)

      ii. ABG: hypoxemia, hypercapnea

      iii. ECG: prolonged QT, low voltage, flattened or inverted T waves

      iv. CXR: pericardial effusion causing enlarged cardiac silhouette

      v. Search for precipitant

  5. Management

    a. Supportive

      i. Airway protection

      ii. Cardiac monitoring

      iii. Passive rewarming

      iv. Frequent glucose monitoring

    b. Treatment should not be delayed while awaiting laboratory results

    c. Hydrocortisone 100 mg IV every 8 hours to prevent precipitation of possible concurrent adrenal crisis

    d. Levothyroxine (T_4) 300 to 500 mcg IV initially, then 50 to 100 mcg IV daily (Some sources recommend T_3 supplementation)

C. Hyperthyroidism

  1. Etiology

    a. Graves disease

      i. Most common etiology of hyperthyroidism

      ii. Autoimmune thyroid-stimulating antibody binds to TSH receptors

      iii. These patients may display signs of hyperthyroidism, goiter, pretibial myxedema, and opthalmopathy

    b. Toxic adenoma and toxic multinodular goiter: hyperplasia of thyroid follicular cells

    c. Thyroiditis: inflammation of thyroid tissue with hyperthyroidism followed by hypothyroidism then recovery phase

      i. Includes subacute painful (de Quervain), silent subacute, radiation-induced, and postpartum

    d. Other causes: pituitary tumors, thyroid cancer, medications (iodine, lithium, amiodarone, thyroid hormone)

  2. Symptoms and signs

    a. Symptoms: heat intolerance, palpitations, weight loss, sweating, tremor, weakness and fatigue, menstrual irregularities, diarrhea, anxiety

    b. Signs: warm skin, stare and lid lag, enlarged thyroid, pain (consider thyroiditis with a tender thyroid), tachycardia with widened pulse pressure, tremor, proximal muscle weakness, atrial fibrillation

    c. Ophthalmopathy (periorbital edema, chemosis, and proptosis) is a hallmark of Graves disease

    d. Elderly may present with apathetic hyperthyroidism

      i. Rare form of thyrotoxicosis usually seen in the elderly

      ii. Paradoxically presents with lethargy, slowed mentation, goiter, weight loss, and muscle weakness; may see atrial fibrillation with CHF

3. Diagnosis
  a. Elevated free T_4, with low or undetectable TSH
  b. Pituitary adenoma: T_4 and TSH will be high
4. Management: etiology dependent
  a. Graves disease
    i. β-blockers for palpitations, anxiety, and tremulousness and peripheral $T_4 \rightarrow T_3$ conversion
    ii. Thionamides such as methimazole and propylthiouracil (PTU) prevent the release of thyroid hormone
      a) Methimazole unsafe in pregnancy (leaves a "mess")
    iii. Ablative therapy with radioiodine provides more definitive treatment and is therapy of choice in United States
  b. Toxic multinodular goiter and solitary adenomas may be treated with radioiodine
  c. Hyperthyroidism due to thyroiditis often resolves without therapy

D. Thyroid storm
1. Definition
  a. Rare, life-threatening hypermetabolic state caused by severe thyrotoxicosis
2. Precipitating factors
  a. Infection most common inciting factor)
  b. Trauma (surgery, burns)
  c. Molar and normal pregnancy (β-hCG has subunit structure identical to TSH with 1/27th of the potency)
  d. Diabetic ketoacidosis
  e. Myocardial infarction or stroke
  f. Thyroid-medication withdrawal
  g. Iodine administration
3. Symptoms and signs
  a. CNS
    i. Early: anxiety, tremulousness, emotional lability, psychosis
    ii. Late: obtundation, seizures, and coma
  b. Fever
  c. Cardiovascular: sinus or supraventricular tachycardia (out of proportion to fever), new atrial fibrillation, CHF, circulatory collapse
  d. GI: diarrhea, hyperdefecation, vomiting, hepatic failure
4. Diagnosis
  a. Clinical diagnosis
  b. Thyroid hormone levels usually no different from those with symptomatic, uncomplicated hyperthyroidism
5. Management
  a. Supportive therapy
    i. Airway protection, IV fluids, monitoring, supplemental oxygen
    ii. Diuretics for CHF
    iii. Digitalis for atrial fibrillation
    iv. Treat fever with acetaminophen
    v. Avoid salicylates which can increase T_4 and T_3 levels
  b. Adrenergic blockade: **propanolol** decreases sympathetic hyperactivity and partially blocks peripheral conversion of T_4 to T_3
  c. Antithyroid drugs: PTU and methimazole; block synthesis of thyroid hormone. PTU also decreases conversion of T_4 to T_3 and works faster than methimazole
  d. Iodide administration inhibits release of stored thyroid hormone. Administer only after synthetic pathway has been blocked by PTU or methimazole
  e. Steroids decrease peripheral conversion of T_4 to T_3 and may treat the autoimmune process in Graves disease

V. Adrenal Disorders

A. General considerations
1. The adrenal gland consists of the medulla and cortex
  a. Adrenal medulla secretes catecholamines (epinephrine and norepinephrine)
  b. The adrenal cortex produces glucocorticoids (cortisol), mineralocorticoids (aldosterone), and androgens
2. The hypothalamus releases corticotrophin-releasing factor (CRF) which stimulates the pituitary to secrete adrenocorticotropic hormone (ACTH), which stimulates the adrenal cortex to produce and secrete cortisol

B. Adrenal insufficiency
1. Etiology
  a. Primary adrenal insufficiency (Addison disease)
    i. Idiopathic (autoimmune)
    ii. Infectious: TB (most common infectious cause worldwide), fungal, meningococcemia (adrenal hemorrhage in Waterhouse-Friderichsen syndrome)
    iii. Infiltrative: sarcoid, amyloid, hemochromatosis, and cancer
    iv. Medication-induced (eg, ketoconazole)
  b. Secondary adrenal insufficiency (hypothalamic-pituitary-adrenal disturbance)
    i. Sudden withdrawal of **prolonged exogenous steroid** usage (most common cause of adrenal insufficiency)

a) Exogenous steroid suppresses ACTH release and sudden stoppage is not met with an appropriate response
  ii. Panhypopituitarism
  iii. Pituitary tumor, Sheehan syndrome (postpartum infarction)
  iv. Infiltrative: sarcoidosis, hemochromatosis
  v. Infectious: meningitis, cavernous sinus thrombosis
  vi. Head trauma
 c. Acute adrenal crisis
  i. Above conditions may be triggered by acute stressors (eg, infection, trauma, myocardial infarction, stroke)
2. Symptoms and signs
 a. General: weakness and lethargy
 b. GI: anorexia, nausea, vomiting, **abdominal pain**
 c. Dermatologic
  i. **Hyperpigmentation** caused by melanocyte-stimulating activity of high plasma ACTH concentrations (seen in primary adrenal insufficiency)
  ii. Most conspicuous in sun-exposed areas (face, neck, hands) or areas exposed to friction or pressure (elbows, knees, and waist)
 d. Cardiovascular
  i. Postural hypotension or syncope
  ii. **Hypotension resistant to fluid or vasopressor therapy**
 e. Musculoskeletal symptoms: diffuse myalgia and arthralgia
 f. Psychiatric manifestations: confusion, depression, psychosis
3. Diagnosis
 a. Serum electrolytes
  i. Hyponatremia, hyperkalemia, and hypoglycemia
  ii. NAG acidosis
 b. Serum cortisol
  i. Levels <20 mcg/dL during periods of stress or post-ACTH administration
 c. Failure of rise in cortisol after ACTH administration
  i. Usually diagnosed by admitting physician
4. Management
 a. Do not delay treatment in favor of diagnosing disease
 b. IV fluids
 c. Medications
  i. Dexamethasone or hydrocortisone
   a) Dexamethasone
    i) Does not interfere with ACTH stimulation testing

    ii) Lacks mineralocorticoid activity:— monitor electrolytes
    iii) May require addition of mineralocorticoid (fludrocortisone acetate)
   b) Hydrocortisone
    i) Possesses mineralocorticoid activity but interferes with ACTH stimulation testing
  ii. Vasopressors effective only after steroids administration
 d. Treat underlying precipitant/trigger event

C. Cushing syndrome and disease
1. Definition
 a. Cushing syndrome results from an excessive exposure to glucocorticoids
 b. Cushing disease is a specific form of Cushing syndrome due to the hypersecretion of ACTH by a pituitary tumor
2. Etiology
 a. Exogenous corticosteroids
 b. Ectopic ACTH-producing tumor (oat, small cell lung cancer)
 c. Primary adrenal tumor
3. Symptoms and signs: proximal muscle weakness, easy bruising, poor wound healing, weight gain, hirsutism, hyperpigmentation, moon facies, facial plethora, supraclavicular fat pads, buffalo hump, truncal obesity, purple striae, menstrual irregularities, osteoporosis, glucose intolerance, and hypertension
4. Diagnosis
 a. Serum chemistry
  i. Hypokalemia and hyperglycemia
  ii. Metabolic alkalosis
 b. Elevated white cell count
 c. Urine, saliva, and serum cortisol levels
 d. Overnight dexamethasone suppression test
5. Management
 a. Taper off steroids (if exogenous cause)
 b. Treat underlying disorder (eg, surgical removal of tumor with adrenalectomy or transsphenoidal surgery for Cushing disease)

D. Pheochromocytoma
1. Definition
 a. Catecholamine-secreting tumor
 b. Adrenal (90%) or extraadrenal (10%)
 c. Malignancy rate of 10%
 d. Rare: ~1/1000 of patients with hypertension
2. Symptoms and signs
 a. Episodic signs of excess catecholamine activity (palpitations, sweating, tremor, weight loss, fever, and hypertension)
 b. Headache, flushing, flank pain, and constipation

3. Diagnosis
   a. Plasma metanephrine testing
   b. 24-hour urine creatinine, catecholamines, vanillylmandelic acid, and metanephrine collection
   c. Abdominal CT scan
4. Management
   a. Surgical resection of tumor curative
   b. Hypertensive emergency
      i. Treatment similar to cocaine-induced hypertension (cocaine blocks norepinephrine reuptake and effectively mimics pheochromocytoma)
         a) α-blockade prior to β-blockade
            i) Phenoxybenzamine (α_1- and α_2-blockers)
            ii) Phentolamine (nonspecific α-blocker)

VI. Glucose Disorders

A. DKA
   1. General considerations
      a. DKA is more common in insulin-dependent diabetics
      b. Insulin deficiency causes hyperglycemia, which leads to an osmotic diuresis and dehydration
      c. Unable to metabolize glucose, ketosis occurs as the body breaks down fatty acids for calories
      d. Ketosis causes acidosis with resultant abdominal pain, vomiting, and the characteristic "fruity odor" of breath
   2. Etiology
      a. Noncompliance with insulin therapy is most common cause
      b. Stressors
         i. Most commonly infection
         ii. Myocardial infarction (MI), CVA, trauma, surgery, and pancreatitis
   3. Symptoms and signs
      a. Tachycardia and hypotension from volume loss
      b. Mental status change
      c. Tachypnea (Kussmaul respiration) as respiratory response to acidosis
      d. Low or elevated temperature may indicate infectious etiology
      e. Dry mucous membranes
      f. Abdominal pain
      g. Blurry vision
      h. Fruity odor of breath resulting from ketosis
      i. Evidence of DKA precipitant such as infections
   4. Diagnosis
      a. Hyperglycemia (usually >300)
      b. AG metabolic acidosis
         i. Vomiting may cause a metabolic alkalosis and normalize the pH
         ii. Increased AG may be the only clue
      c. Serum chemistry
         i. Pseudohyponatremia or true hyponatremia
         ii. Hyperkalemia (but total body potassium is depleted)
      d. Urine may reveal elevated specific gravity, glucosuria, and ketonuria
      e. Look for serum or urine acetone
         i. Urine may be negative for ketones as β-hydroxybutyrate not measured with most urine reagents
         ii. Paradoxically, this reverses with treatment as acetoacetate forms during clinical improvement
   5. Management
      a. Cardiac monitoring
      b. Aggressive IV hydration
         i. Titrate fluids so glucose decreases at a rate of 50 to100 mg/dL/h
      c. IV Insulin
         i. 0.1 unit/kg IV bolus (controversial)
         ii. Follow with 0.1 units/kg/h IV drip
         iii. Continue therapy until AG normalizes
         iv. Administer glucose-containing fluids once glucose <250
         v. Administer long-acting subcutaneous insulin 30 minutes prior to discontinuing IV insulin
      d. Potassium supplementation
         i. Profound hypokalemia often masked by acidosis and extracellular shift
            a) Supplement if potassium <5 mEq/L and adequate urine output
            b) Check electrolytes every 2 hours
      e. Bicarbonate therapy controversial
         i. Fluids and insulin will correct acidosis
         ii. Consider if pH <7 with impaired cardiac contractility
      f. Cerebral edema complicates DKA management primarily in the pediatric population
         i. Most common in children <5 years
         ii. Careful fluid hydration
         iii. Loading dose of IV insulin not used in pediatric population
      g. Search for underlying precipitants and triggers

B. Hyperosmolar hyperglycemic nonketotic coma
   1. Definition
      a. Characterized by hyperglycemia induced dehydration usually accompanied by mental status change
      b. Higher mortality than DKA

2. Epidemiology
   a. Associated with type 2 diabetes and insulin resistance (rather than insulin deficiency)
   b. Affects mainly the elderly, patients on psychiatric medications, and handicapped persons unable to access fluids
3. Etiology
   a. Infection is leading precipitant (pneumonia and UTI account for 30% to 50%)
   b. As with DKA, any physiologic stressor can precipitate this condition
4. Symptoms and signs
   a. Neurologic complaints (lethargy, delirium, coma)
   b. Dehydration
   c. Only 10% of patients present with coma
   d. Ketosis rarely present, and therefore fewer GI complaints
5. Diagnosis
   a. Serum glucose is usually >600
   b. Serum osmolarity is often >315
   c. Minimal to absent ketosis
   d. pH is usually >7.25
6. Management
   a. Fluids: may need 4 to 6 L NS before any insulin given
      i. Osmotic diuresis causes a more profound dehydration than in DKA
      ii. Average fluid deficit is 8 to 12 L
   b. After fluid therapy, treatment is similar to DKA
   c. Search for a precipitant

C. Alcoholic ketoacidosis
   1. Definition
      a. Severe metabolic DKA-like syndrome after binge alcohol drinking with little or no hyperglycemia
   2. Etiology
      a. Poor nutrional status secondary to chronic alcoholism
      b. Typically occurs 2 to 3 days after alcohol cessation
      c. Alcohol levels may also be absent or low unless recent ingestion
         i. No alcohol to metabolize
         ii. Decreased carbohydrate intake reduces insulin secretion
         iii. Alcohol inhibits gluconeogenesis and stimulates lipolysis
      d. All of the above contribute to ketoacid formation and a severe metabolic acidosis
   3. Symptoms and signs
      a. Dehydration, nausea, vomiting

   b. Rigid, surgical-like abdomen secondary to severe ketosis
   4. Diagnosis
      a. Clinical history of alcohol cessation after binge
      b. AG acidosis
      c. Normal or slightly elevated glucose
      d. Rapid resolution of symptoms with glucose and hydration
   5. Management
      a. Administer dextrose containing solution
         i. Dextrose increases insulin and reduces glucagon secretion
      b. Thiamine 100 mg IV prior to glucose to avoid precipitating Wernicke encephalopathy
      c. Treat underlying precipitant

D. Hypoglycemia
   1. Etiology
      a. Insulin or oral hypoglycemic medication (particularly sulfonylureas)
      b. Renal failure or insufficiency (insulin and sulfonylureas are metabolized by the kidneys)
      c. Liver disease, insulinoma, adrenal insufficiency, hypothyroidism
      d. Malingering
         i. Consider in health-care worker or relative of a diabetic
         ii. Low C-peptide levels in patients self-administering insulin
         iii. Send urine or serum for presence of sulfonylureas
            a) Urine only detects presence of first generation sulfonylureas
   2. Symptoms and signs
      a. Usually with glucose level <60
      b. Symptoms may be masked by β-blockers
      c. Mental status change (confusion, agitation, unresponsiveness)
      d. Tachycardia, diaphoresis, and tremulousness
      e. Focal neurologic deficit (can be mistaken for CVA) or seizure
   3. Management
      a. Feed patient if symptoms mild
         i. A sandwich that contains protein, carbohydrate, and fat will provide sustained increase in serum glucose (orange juice and D50 only transiently increases serum glucose)
      b. IV dextrose with altered mental status
      c. For patients on long-acting oral hypoglycemic or insulin, follow ampule of D50 with D10 NS by continuous infusion, or a meal

d. IM Glucagon 1 mg if IV access unattainable
  i. Ineffective in patients with low glycogen stores (alcoholism, cirrhosis)
e. Glucose gel on buccal mucosa
f. Octreotide for sulfonylurea overdose
  i. Octreotide inhibits insulin release
g. Admission criteria
  i. Patients on long-acting insulin or oral hypoglycemics
  ii. Those without an obvious etiology
  iii. Continued or recurrent hypoglycemia during ED stay
  iv. Intentional overdose for medical and psychiatric care

VII. Nutritional Disorders

A. Thiamine (B_1) deficiency
  1. General considerations
    a. Found in wheat germ, seeds, nuts, and most vegetables
    b. Thiamine necessary for glucose utilization
    c. Deficiency may occur either by insufficient ingestion or by excessive demand/metabolism (hyperthyroid, pregnancy, and lactation)
    d. Stored in muscle and depleted >1 month without repletion
      i. Fad diets often do not contain enough thiamine
  2. Symptoms and signs
    a. Symptoms may occur in as little as 1 week without thiamine ingestion
    b. Two distinct clinical presentations
      i. Dry beriberi
        a) Nervous system involvement
        b) Sensory and motor deficits especially in lower extremities
        c) Wernicke-Korsakoff syndrome
          i) Medical emergency
          ii) Wernicke syndrome consists of triad of ophthalmoplegia, ataxia, and acute confusion
          iii) Korsakoff syndrome is the persistent and irreversible memory and learning disturbance from chronic thiamine deficiency
      ii. Wet beriberi (3 stages)
        a) Vasodilation leads to high cardiac output
        b) Salt retention leads to systemic edema exacerbating fluid overload
        c) Structural cardiac changes occur that lead to frank CHF
  3. Management
    a. Thiamine 100 mg IM/IV prior to glucose to avoid theoretical precipitation of Wernicke encephalopathy

B. Niacin (B_3) deficiency
  1. General considerations
    a. Found in poultry, meat, fish, and yeast
    b. Deficiency is rare in industrialized countries, but may be seen in alcoholics and patients on long-term isoniazid
  2. Symptoms and signs
    a. Involve skin, CNS, and GI tract
    b. Pellagra is the end result (3 Ds of niacin deficiency)
      i. Dermatitis: pellagra means "raw skin." A photosensitive pigmented dermatitis typically affecting sun-exposed areas
      ii. Diarrhea
      iii. Dementia
  3. Management
    a. Treat with niacin
    b. Treat concurrent deficiencies

C. Pyridoxine (B_6) deficiency
  1. General considerations
    a. Associated with extreme malnourishment and medications that increase metabolism of or bind B_6
      i. Penicillamine
      ii. Isoniazid (INH): binds to the active form of pyridoxine
  2. Symptoms and signs
    a. Nausea and vomiting
    b. Intractable seizures
    c. Fever
    d. Tachycardia
  3. Management
    a. Pyridoxine 5 g IV over 30 minutes, or 1 g of pyridoxine for every gram of isoniazid consumed
    b. Consider in patients with intractable seizures and a history of tuberculosis
    c. Consider in the newborn or infants <18 months with intractable seizures

D. Cyanocobalamin (B_{12}) deficiency
  1. General consideration
    a. Found in meats, cheese, milk, eggs, and fish
    b. Absorption requires gastric acidity and gastric intrinsic factor (IF) to cleave and bind B_{12} prior to absorption in terminal ileum
    c. Etiology of deficiency

    i. Decreased intake
       a) Strict vegetarians
       b) Alcoholics
    ii. Impaired absorption
       a) Gastric abnormalities: pernicious anemia (autoimmune attack on gastric intrinsic factor), gastrectomy, and achlorhydria (antacids)
       b) Disease of terminal ileum (Crohn disease and celiac sprue)

2. Symptoms and signs
  a. Classic triad of weakness, sore tongue, and paresthesias
  b. Multiple nonspecific neurologic symptoms
  c. Subacute combined degeneration: spinal cord disease involving posterior and lateral spinal columns. Characterized early on by paresthesias, ataxia, loss of vibration and position sense, it can progress to severe weakness, spasticity, paraplegia, and bowel and bladder incontinence
    i. Patient may exhibit positive Romberg testing
  d. Macrocytic anemia (red blood cell mean corpuscular volume (MCV) >100 fL, hypersegmented neutrophils on peripheral smear
  e. Patients with symptoms may have normal or low normal B_{12} levels
3. Management
  a. Oral B_{12}
  b. Intramuscular or subcutaneous route if malabsorptive process exists

BIBLIOGRAPHY

Brady W, Harrigan R: Hypoglycemia. In: Tintinalli JE, ed. *Emergency Medicine: A Comprehensive Study Guide,* 6th ed. New York: McGraw-Hill; 2004:1283.

Braen GR: Vitamins and herbals. In: Tintanelli JE, ed. *Emergency Medicine: A Comprehensive Study Guide,* 6th ed. New York: McGraw-Hill; 2004:1160.

Chansky ME, Lubkin CL: Diabetic ketoacidosis. In: Tintinalli JE, ed. *Emergency Medicine: A Comprehensive Study Guide,* 6th ed. New York: McGraw-Hill; 2004:1287.

Graffeo CS: Hyperosmolar hyperglycemic state. In: Tintinalli JE, ed. *Emergency Medicine: A Comprehensive Study Guide,* 6th ed. New York: McGraw-Hill; 2004:1307.

Kelen GD, Gabor D, Nicolau DD: Acid-base disorders. In: Tintinalli JE, ed. *Emergency Medicine: A Comprehensive Study Guide,* 6th ed. New York: McGraw-Hill; 2004:154.

Liang HK: Hyperthyroidism and thyroid storm. In: Tintinalli JE, ed. *Emergency Medicine: A Comprehensive Study Guide,* 6th ed. New York: McGraw-Hill; 2004:1311.

Liang HK: Hypothyroidism and myxedema coma. In: Tintinalli JE, ed. *Emergency Medicine: a Comprehensive Study Guid,* 6th ed. New York: McGraw-Hill; 2004:1313.

Lodner M, Hammer D, Gabor D: Fluid and electrolyte problems. In: Tintinalli JE, ed. *Emergency Medicine: A Comprehensive Study Guide,* 6th ed. New York: McGraw-Hill; 2004:167.

Shoenfeld CN: Adrenal insufficiency and adrenal crisis. In: Tintinalli JE, ed. *Emergency Medicine: A Comprehensive Study Guide,* 6th ed. New York: McGraw-Hill; 2004:1315.

Woods WA, Perina DG: Alcoholic ketoacidosis. In: Tintinalli JE, ed. *Emergency Medicine: A Comprehensive Study Guide,* 6th ed. New York: McGraw-Hill; 2004:1304.

Chapter 14
GASTROINTESTINAL EMERGENCIES

Gar Chan and Wayne Ramcharitar

I. Esophagus

A. Dysphagia
   1. Etiology
      a. Difficulty with solids usually indicates mechanical obstruction
      b. Difficulty with liquids and solids may indicate motility dysfunction (neurologic or muscular coordination)
   2. Phases of swallowing
      a. Physiology and pathology
         i. Oral phase
            a) Dysfunction usually obvious
               i) Poor dentition
               ii) Unable to keep lip closed (CVA, Bell palsy)
               iii) Tongue pathology
               iv) CN V, CN VII, and CN XII
         ii. Pharyngeal phase
            a) Reflexive (gag reflex)
            b) CN IX and CN X
            c) Neurological dysfunction
               i) Neuromuscular junction disease (eg, myasthenia, botulism)
                  (a) Bulbar symptoms (difficulty initiating swallow, nasal voice)
               ii) Motor dysfunction
                  (a) CVA and brainstem lesions, cranial nerve palsies, ALS
            d) Mechanical dysfunction
               i) Zenker diverticula, mass, or obstruction (pharyngeal webs, cancers)
         iii. Esophageal phase
            a) Under influence of medulla
            b) Sensation of sticking as food passes
            c) Upper third of esophagus localizes well
            d) Distal esophageal discomfort difficult to differentiate cardiac chest pain
            e) Motility disorder
               i) Brainstem and medulla pathology
               ii) Peristalsis pathology: achalasia
               iii) Esophageal sphincter dysfunction
               iv) Scleroderma
            f) Mechanical obstruction
               i) Mass, webs, or rings
               ii) History of caustic ingestion (see Toxicologic Emergencies chapter)
   3. Diagnosis
      a. Endoscopy
      b. Esophagram
      c. Esophageal motility studies

B. Swallowed foreign body (FB)
   1. Site of obstruction (in order of frequency)
      a. C6 most common: cricopharyngeal muscle
      b. T4: aortic arch
      c. T11: gastroesophageal junction
      d. T6: tracheal bifurcation
      e. T1: thoracic inlet
   2. Diagnosis
      a. Plain radiography may or may not reveal FB
         i. Soda can tabs may not show on x-ray
         ii. Coins
            a) AP soft-tissue neck radiograph
               i) In esophagus, will show "en face" or in coronal plane
               ii) In trachea, will appear "on edge" or in sagital plane
      b. Endoscopy or direct laryngoscopy
   3. Management
      a. Most FBs pass spontaneously if they pass the pylorus
      b. Observe esophageal FB for 24 hours unless contraindicated (see "exceptions and contraindications" below)
      c. 10% to 20% require endoscopic assistance and 1% require surgery
      d. Most objects <2 cm by 5 cm will usually pass
      e. Exceptions and contraindications

　　　i. Button battery
　　　　　a) If in esophagus, needs to be **removed** endoscopically
　　　　　b) If in stomach, observe to see if battery clears the pylorus within 48 hours
　　　ii. Sharp object (eg, open safety pins, needles, nails)
　　　　　a) Remove endoscopically or surgically **prior** to transit through pylorus
　　　　　b) Surgical consultation for any sharp object past pylorus
　　　　　c) May cause perforation at ileocecal junction

C. Food impaction
　1. Etiology: esophageal dysfunction
　　a. Esophageal narrowing: Schatzki rings, peptic stricture, webs, cancer
　　b. Esophageal dysmotility
　　　i. Achalasia: inability of esophageal sphincter to relax
　2. Symptoms and signs
　　a. Dysphagia, chest pain, regurgitation
　　　i. Upper third of esophagus localizes pain well
　3. Management
　　a. Medical
　　　i. Glucagon reduces lower esophageal sphincter tone. Useful if symptoms <24 hours
　　　ii. Nifedipine lowers esophageal tone
　　　iii. Sublingual nitroglycerin
　　　iv. Carbonated or gas-forming agents
　　b. Interventional
　　　i. Endoscopy
　　　ii. Surgical intervention rarely required

D. Boerhaave syndrome—esophageal rupture
　1. Definition
　　a. Full-thickness esophageal rupture after forceful emesis
　2. Epidemiology
　　a. 50 to 70 years of age
　　b. Men >women
　3. Etiology
　　a. Retching and vomiting (alcohol binge, bulimia)
　　b. Occurs most commonly at distal posterolateral esophagus
　4. Symptoms and signs
　　a. Does **not** typically present with bleeding (in contrast to Mallory-Weiss)
　　b. Chest pain, may be pleuritic (caused by esophageal-pleural communication)
　　c. Back pain
　　d. Dysphagia

　　e. Subcutaneous emphysema
　　f. Hamman crunch (auscultation of mediastinal air disturbed by the beating heart)
　5. Diagnosis
　　a. Chest x-ray (CXR) is initial study
　　　i. Subcutaneous emphysema
　　　ii. Pleural effusion (left > right)
　　　iii. Widened mediastinum
　　b. Esophogram
　　　i. Identifies leak site
　　　ii. Contrast material
　　　　a) Use water-soluble first
　　　　b) Barium if water-soluble contrast study negative but clinical suspicion remains high
　6. Management
　　a. Surgical consultation
　　b. Antibiotics to cover oral and gastrointestinal (GI) flora
　　c. 35% mortality even with treatment

II. Upper GI Bleed (UGIB)—bleeding proximal to the ligament of Treitz

A. Peptic ulcer disease
　1. Definition: mucosal erosion in an area of the GI tract, most commonly in the duodenum, stomach or esophagus
　2. Epidemiology
　　a. Most common cause of UGIB (15% to 40%)
　　b. Duodenal >gastric
　3. Etiology
　　a. Smoking, *H. pylori* infection (80%), NSAIDS, aspirin, steroids, and alcohol use, Dieulafoy lesion (superficial, large caliber gastric arteriole)
　4. Symptoms and signs
　　a. Duodenal ulcers
　　　i. Awakens patient at night
　　　ii. Pain relieved by food
　　　　a) Postprandial pain (1 to 2 hours delay)
　　b. Gastric ulcers
　　　i. Early satiety
　　　ii. Pain immediately after meals
　5. Management
　　a. Active bleeding
　　　i. Consider airway protection if active bleeding
　　　ii. IV hydration and blood transfusion if hemodynamically unstable or myocardial ischemia
　　　iii. Proton pump inhibitor[4]
　　　　a) Alkalinization of gastric content allows clot stabilization

b) May decrease blood transfusion requirements

iv. Immediate GI consultation for endoscopy (sclerotherapy, injection, cauterization)

6. Complications of peptic ulcer disease
   a. Perforation
      i. Upright CXR best for free air
      ii. Free air more visible under right hemidiaphragm
      iii. May not see free air if the perforation is in posterior duodenum (retroperitoneal)
         a) Retroperitoneal perforations have been estimated ≥30%
      iv. Surgical management
   b. Gastric outlet syndrome
      i. May develop after ulcer causes scarring that blocks gastric outlet and pylorus
      ii. Presents with weight loss, abdominal pain, and vomiting 20 to 30 minutes after eating
      iii. Abdominal x-ray reveals dilated stomach
      iv. Management
         a) Nasogastric decompression
         b) Fluid and electrolyte management
         c) Surgical consultation

B. Esophageal varices
   1. Definition
      a. Dilated esophageal veins caused by portal hypertension that can lead to life-threatening bleeding
   2. Symptoms and signs
      a. Evidence of cirrhosis
         i. Jaundice, dark urine, abdominal ascites, pruritis, easy bruising and bleeding
         ii. Enlarged parotid glands signify poor nutrition and alcohol abuse
         iii. Fetor hepaticus: musty sweet odor caused by inability of liver to metabolize mercaptans produced by bacteria
         iv. Gynecomastia, telangiectasias, testicular atrophy, caput medusae (dilated umbilical veins)
      b. Evidence of portal hypertension
         i. Splenomegaly
   3. Diagnosis
      a. Laboratory
         i. Complete blood count (CBC)
         ii. Abnormal liver function tests and hepatitis panels
         iii. Prolonged prothrombin time
      b. Endoscopy
   4. Management
      a. ABCs: aggressive airway management

   b. GI consultation for banding or sclerotherapy
   c. Balloon tamponade with Sengstaken-Blakemore or Minnesota tubes are temporary measures
   d. Medical management
      i. Antibiotics (third-generation cephalosporin)
      ii. Somatostatin or octreotide[2]
      iii. Vasopressin less frequently used (complications include chest pain, myocardial infarction (MI), arrhythmias)
      iv. Consider fresh frozen plasma and platelets
      v. Blood transfusion
      vi. Consider vitamin K (may be ineffective with cirrhosis)
      vii. β-blockers and nitrates have **no** role in the acute management of variceal bleeding (useful for prophylaxis of recurrent bleeding)

C. Mallory-Weiss syndrome
   1. Definition
      a. **Partial** thickness longitudinal mucosal tear of distal esophagus
   2. Risk factors
      a. Alcohol binge
      b. Hiatal hernia
   3. Symptoms and signs
      a. Hematemesis after retching
      b. Chest, epigastric, and upper abdominal pain
   4. Management
      a. Usually self-limiting
      b. Blood transfusion if necessary
      c. Endoscopy if necessary
      d. Surgery and Sengstaken Blakemore tube rarely indicated

III. Lower GI Bleed (LGIB)—bleeding distal to the ligament of Treitz

A. General considerations
   1. Epidemiology: 10% to 15% of bright red blood per rectum (BRBPR) has an upper GI source[1]
   2. Etiology
      a. Traditionally taught the most common cause of lower GI bleeds is upper GI bleed
         i. May not apply in the post-proton pump inhibitor, H_2-blocker era[3]
      b. Diverticulosis, hemorrhoids, angiodysplasia
      c. Less common: malignancy, polyps, arteriovenous malformation, aortoenteric fistula, inflammatory bowel disease, infectious colitis
      d. Hematochezia may be imitated by certain foods such as beets

3. Diagnosis
   a. Negative nasogastric lavage with presence of bile
      i. Bilious return frequently not demonstrated
      ii. False negatives
         a) Intermittent bleeding
         b) Pyloric edema
   b. Controversy surrounds the order or preference of nuclear scintigraphy, angiography, and colonoscopy
      i. Nuclear scan
         a) Sensitive to bleeding of 0.1 mL/min
         b) Does not localize site of bleeding well
         c) Taken up by liver and spleen confounding localization
      ii. Angiogram
         a) Not as sensitive to bleeding: 0.5 to 2.0 mL/min
         b) Better at pinpointing location of bleeding
         c) Angiographic embolization is an option although ischemic colitis is a complication
      iii. Colonoscopy can be both therapeutic and diagnostic

B. Diverticulosis
   1. Definition
      a. Diverticula are mucosal lined pockets that protrude through weaknesses in the lumen of the large intestine (rarely small bowel)
   2. Epidemiology
      a. Most common cause of LGIB
      b. Found in 10% of patients >40 years
      c. Found in >50% of patients >60 years
   3. Etiology
      a. Low-fiber diets are associated with smaller stool bulk that requires more pressure to remove or excrete
      b. Diverticula form in lumen wall weakened by vessel entrance
      c. Artery weakened by adjacent diverticula and bleed
      d. Most common in sigmoid colon
   4. Symptoms and signs
      a. Often asymptomatic
      b. May have minimal bloating and/or crampy abdominal pain
      c. Painless rectal bleeding
   5. Diagnosis
      a. CT scan
      b. Colonoscopy
      c. Nuclear scan or angiogram

6. Management of acute bleeding
   a. Fluids and blood transfusion as necessary
   b. Most patients stop bleeding spontaneously
   c. Surgery for persistent bleeding

C. Mesenteric ischemia
   1. Definition
      a. **Small** bowel ischemia
   2. Etiology
      a. Venous obstruction
         i. Least common form of mesenteric ischemia
         ii. Risk factors: hypercoagulable state
      b. Arterial
         i. Low flow (aka non-occlusive)
            a) Risk factors[11,12]: advanced CHF, cardiogenic shock, dysrhythmias
         ii. Thrombotic (more chronic)
            a) Risk factors: HTN, DM, CAD, hypercholesterolemia, vasculopathic disease (PVD)
         iii. Embolism
            a) Superior mesenteric artery most likely involved
            b) Risk factors
               1) Atrial fibrillation
               2) Digoxin use
   3. Symptoms and signs
      a. Pain out of proportion to examination
      b. Varying patterns of pain pattern progression
         i. Embolic: sudden onset of severe abdominal pain, +/- gut emptying (vomiting and/or diarrhea) with possible history of atrial fibrillation
         ii. Thrombotic: usually history of progressing abdominal pain during/after eating, +/- anorexia (limited appetite), +/- history of weight loss
      c. Rectal bleeding
         i. May be frank or heme (+) stool
      d. Shock from bowel gangrene
   4. Diagnosis
      a. Laboratory
         i. Leukocytosis may be present but insensitive
         ii. Lactic acidosis is a late finding
         iii. Elevated phosphorus level has low sensitivity
      b. Imaging
         i. Radiographic: CXR and abdominal series (supine and upright) to rule out bowel obstruction or perforation
         ii. CT scan with IV contrast
            a) Some studies find CT scan to be as sensitive as angiography

b) May demonstrate edema of bowel wall and mesentery, ascites, intramural gas, and rarely direct evidence of mesenteric venous thrombus

    iii. **Angiography** is the gold standard

  c. Management

    i. Immediate surgical consultation

    ii. Intra-arterial papavarine is a temporarizing measure employed during angiography

    iii. Antibiotics (Gram-negative and anaerobic coverage)

    iv. Mortality rate 80% to 90% with late diagnosis

D. Ischemic colitis

  1. Definition

    a. **Large bowel** ischemia

    b. Frequently confused with mesenteric ischemia

    c. Two unique diseases with separate treatment options that happen to share the same organ system

    d. Multiple blood supplies makes the colon more resistant to ischemia. Therefore, ischemic colitis is a global low flow state rather than an embolic phenomenon

  2. Etiology

    a. Hypotension of various etiology

      i. CHF

      ii. Myocardial infarction

      iii. Sepsis

      iv. **Hemorrhage**

  3. Symptoms and signs

    a. Pain out of proportion to examination

    b. Abdominal distension

    c. Bloody stools or diarrhea

  4. Diagnosis

    a. Clinical suspicion in hypotensive patient with low flow to splanchic vessels

      i. For example, CHF patient with abdominal pain and distension

      ii. Difficult to differentiate from mesenteric ischemia

    b. Often diagnosed on CT scan

      i. Nonspecific edema, colitis

      ii. Often involves splenic flexure or "watershed region"

      iii. Difficult to differentiate from infectious colitis

  5. Management

    a. Treating underlying etiology of hypoperfusion reverses ischemia in 66% of patients

    b. Rebound tenderness, acidosis, and worsening clinical status may signal full-thickness involvement and perforation

c. Antibiotics and surgery/surgical consultation may be required in patients with progression of symptoms

E. Aortoenteric fistula

  1. Definition

    a. Communication between the aorta and bowel lumen

  2. Risk factors

    a. History of abdominal aortic aneurysm (primary)

    b. History of aortic repair or aortic graft placement (secondary)

  3. Symptoms and signs

    a. Hematemesis, melena, or hematochezia

    b. Minor bleeding (herald bleed) may precede catastrophic rectal bleeding

    c. Abdominal auscultation may reveal harsh machinelike bruit

  4. Management

    a. CT scan with IV contrast to diagnose

    b. IV crystalloid and blood product transfusion

    c. Immediate surgical consultation

F. Anal fissure

  1. Symptoms and signs

    a. Minor rectal bleeding

    b. Sharp pain with defecation

    c. May lead to constipation secondary to pain

    d. Posterior midline location in 90%

      i. Non-posterior midline fissures should raise concern for Crohn disease, ulcerative colitis, sexual abuse, syphilis, tuberculosis, and cancer

  2. Management

    a. Sitz baths 3 times a day

    b. Topical anesthetic and steroid preparation may retard healing

    c. Pain medication

    d. Stool softeners

G. Hemorrhoids

  1. Definition

    a. Internal hemorrhoids

      i. Defined as proximal to dentate line (series of anal crypts)

      ii. Visible only if protruding externally

      iii. **Painless** bleeding

    b. External hemorrhoids

      i. Below dentate line

      ii. Visible

      iii. Thrombosed clot appears blue beneath hemorrhoid and causes severe pain

  2. Management

    a. Sitz baths 3 times a day

    b. Stool softener

c. Thrombosed external hemorrhoid may benefit from excision with "fishmouth" incision

IV. Abdominal Hernias

A. Definitions
1. Reducible: hernia able to be put back into native cavity
2. Incarcerated: irreducible hernia
3. Strangulated: ischemic incarcerated hernia

B. Types
1. Inguinal
   a. Direct
      i. Definition: hernia secondary to defect in Hesselbach triangle (inguinal ligament, inferior epigastric vessel laterally, lateral border of rectus abdominus medially)
         a) Strangulation uncommon
      ii. Physical examination: feel hernia on "pad" of finger tip with valsalva
   b. Indirect
      i. Definition: hernia secondary to failure of embryonic closure of the internal inguinal ring
      ii. Epidemiology
         a) Most common cause of groin hernia
         b) More common on right
         c) More common than direct inguinal hernias
         d) Higher risk of strangulation since contents pass through internal and external inguinal ring
      iii. Physical examination: during testicular examination, feel hernia on "tip" of finger with valsalva or cough
         a) May bulge in scrotal sac
   c. Pantaloon
      i. Concurrent direct and indirect inguinal hernias
2. Femoral
   a. Hernia below inguinal ligament
   b. Difficult to diagnose
   c. More common in women than men
3. Obturator
   a. Definition: hernia into the obturator foramen (hole created by the pubis and ishium bones)
   b. Epidemiology: "little old ladies" hernia
      i. Thin elderly women have less fat to prevent passage of hernia through obturator canal
      ii. Women have larger obturator canals than men
   c. Symptoms and signs
      i. Pain may radiate to inner thigh

ii. More commonly on right side since left partially protected by sigmoid colon
iii. Howship-Romberg sign
   a) Pain secondary pressure on obturator nerve with hip extension, adduction, and external rotation
4. Umbilical hernia
   a. Rarely strangulates
   b. Delay surgery until child 4 years of age
   c. Most close spontaneously
5. Richter hernia: hernia of 1 wall of a hollow viscus

C. Management
1. Reduction (see Procedures chapter)
2. Surgical consult
3. Complications
   a. Reduction of ischemic gut into peritoneal cavity
      i. Do **not** reduce hernia if patient febrile or exhibits leukocytosis or acidosis

V. Bowel Obstruction

A. Types
1. Small bowel obstruction (SBO)
   a. More common than large bowel obstruction
   b. Most common etiology is adhesions followed by inguinal hernias
   c. Less common causes include lymphoma, polyps, cancer, and gallstone ileus
2. Large bowel obstruction (LBO)
   a. Most commonly associated with neoplasms followed by diverticulitis, volvulus, and strictures formed from chronic inflammation
   b. Rarely caused by adhesions or hernias
3. Adynamic ileus
   a. Gut activity slows or stops in response to systemic illness, shock, toxins and drug reaction, or abdominal surgery and injury
4. Ogilvie or pseudo-obstruction
   a. Massive dilatation of the colon through to the cecum in the absence of mechanical obstruction
   b. Risk factors
      i. Elderly in nursing home
      ii. Bed bound
      iii. Anticholinergic medication
      iv. Frequently associated with large vacuous rectal vault

B. Symptoms and signs
1. Especially rapid progression of symptoms with closed loop obstruction
2. Pain

a. Intermittent crampy pain
  i. May be less pronounced with adynamic ileus and Ogilvie syndrome
3. Vomiting
  a. Bilious vomiting if proximal obstruction
  b. Feculent vomitus with distal ileal obstruction
4. Constipation and obstipation
  a. May not be present with partial bowel obstruction
  b. Partial obstruction may present with diarrhea
5. Fever with bowel perforation, gangrene
6. Abdominal distention
7. High-pitched or hyperactive bowel sounds in 50%[5]

C. Diagnosis
  1. Plain abdominal radiography
    a. General considerations
      i. Diagnostic in 50%
      ii. Completely normal in 20%
    b. SBO
      i. Dilated small bowel with paucity of distal colonic air
      ii. Air fluid levels
      iii. "Stack of coins" appearance of small bowel
    c. LBO
      i. Dilated large bowel
      ii. Small bowel distension may also be seen if ileocecal valve incompetent
      iii. Bird beak pattern with sigmoid or cecal volvulus
    d. Adynamic ileus
      i. Dilated small and large bowel
    e. Ogilvie syndrome
      i. Typically very dilated distal colon
      ii. Difficult to differentiate from LBO with incompetent ileocecal valve
  2. Abdominal CT
    a. May aid surgeons by identifying point of obstruction
  3. Sigmoidoscopy/colonoscopy
    a. Test of choice for suspected volvulus
    b. Diagnostic and therapeutic
  4. Barium enema
    a. Useful diagnosis site of LBO
    b. May be useful to diagnose cecal volvulus
    c. Avoid use in Ogilvie syndrome as patient unable to evacuate barium

D. Management
  1. General considerations
    a. Increased mortality if obstruction >24 hours
    b. Fluid and electrolyte maintenance

  c. **Closed loop** obstruction requires immediate surgery
  d. Preoperative antibiotics often indicated
2. SBO
  a. Nasogastric tube decompression
  b. Surgical consultation
3. LBO
  a. Rectal tube or sigmoidoscopy
  b. Nasogastric tube decompression if iliocecal valve incompetent
  c. Surgical consultation
4. Adynamic ileus
  a. Diagnosis of exclusion
  b. Nasogastric decompression
  c. Manage conservatively if patient tolerates
5. Management of Ogilvie syndrome
  a. Diagnosis of exclusion
  b. Mortality related to perforation and sepsis
  c. May require colonoscopy
  d. **Rectal tube** and sigmoidoscopy
  e. Nasogastric tube if iliocecal valve incompetent
  f. Neostigmine of possible benefit
  g. Surgery rarely helpful, often harmful

E. Volvulus
  1. Sigmoid: most common site of volvulus
    a. Risk factors
      i. Nursing home patients
      ii. Elderly
      iii. Bed bound
      iv. Chronic constipation
    b. Symptoms and signs
      i. May present insidiously with chronic abdominal pain or distension in the elderly
    c. Diagnosis
      i. Abdominal x-ray (Figure 14–1)
        a) Diagnostic 50% to 80%
        b) Inverted U-shaped dilated sigmoid
        c) Limbs of sigmoid colon directed toward pelvis
        d) Coffee bean sign
      ii. Barium enema may reveal bird beak deformity at site of torsion
    d. Management
      i. Sigmoidoscopy to decompress volvulus
      ii. Surgical resection in patients suspected of perforation or gangrenous bowel
      iii. Antibiotics if indicated
  2. Cecal: second most common site of volvulus
    a. Risk factors
      i. Age: relatively younger than sigmoid volvulous (early 50's)
      ii. Associated with marathon runners

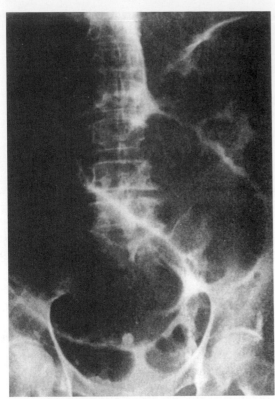

Figure 14–1. Sigmoid volvulus. (Reproduced with permission from Tintinalli JE, Kelen GD, Stapczynski JS: *Tintinalli's Emergency Medicine. A Comprehensive Study Guide,* 6th ed. Copyright © 2004, New York: McGraw-Hill.)

    b. Abdominal x-ray
      i. Kidney-shaped loop pointing left
    c. Management
      i. Surgery
      ii. Antibiotics if perforation

VI. Inflammatory Bowel Disease

A. Crohn disease
  1. Epidemiology
    a. Bimodal age of onset: 15 to 25 years, 55 to 60 years
    b. Whites >Blacks or Asians
    c. Jewish ancestry highest incidence
  2. Symptoms and signs
    a. Presents with chronic abdominal pain, diarrhea +/– fever
    b. Bloody diarrhea uncommon
    c. Perianal fistulas, fissures, abscesses
    d. Complications include
      i. Perianal abscess
      ii. Fistulas
      iii. Thromboembolic disease

      iv. Threefold to fivefold increase in GI malignancy
      v. Extraintestinal manifestations (see "extraintestinal manifestations of inflammatory bowel disease" below)
  3. Diagnosis: dependent on site of involvement
    a. Upper GI: upper GI Series (show segmental narrowing of small intestine, fistulae, mucosal destruction)
    b. Lower GI: colonoscopy permits biopsy
    c. CT scan of abdomen and pelvis: useful in exacerbations to identify abscesses, fistulae, obstruction, or toxic megacolon
  4. Management
    a. Diarrhea
      i. Cholestyramine may benefit terminal ileitis-related diarrhea (unable to absorb bile salts)
    b. Cramping pain
      i. Relieved by dicyclomine or hyoscyamine
    c. Large intestine inflammation
      i. Sulfasalazine metabolized into 5-aminosalicylic acid by gut bacteria (5-ASA)
    d. Small and large intestine inflammation
      i. Mesalamine metabolized into 5-ASA in distal small bowel
    e. Steroid for severe symptoms after abscess ruled out
    f. Antibiotics with coexistent infection
    g. Immune modulating medications

B. Ulcerative colitis
  1. Definition
    a. Chronic idiopathic inflammation of the colon and rectum
      i. Inflammation usually begins in the rectum and extends proximally through the colon
      ii. Small intestines not involved
      iii. Usually spares the perianal area, mild disease may occur (fissures, hemorrhoids)
        a) Extensive perianal lesions suggest Crohn disease
  2. Epidemiology
    a. Peak incidence 15 to 28 years
    b. Whites >Blacks or Asians
    c. Jewish ancestry highest incidence
  3. Symptoms and signs
    a. Bloody diarrhea and abdominal pain
    b. Tenesmus
    c. Weight loss
  4. Diagnosis
    a. Colonoscopy for definitive diagnosis

5. Management
   a. Colectomy is curative
   b. Sulfasalazine and mesalamine deliver local 5-ASA
   c. Steroids for severe disease and flares
   d. Immune modulating medications for refractory cases
6. Complications
   a. Associated with primary sclerosing cholangitis
   b. Colon cancer risk is ~8%
7. Extraintestinal manifestations (see "extraintestinal manifestations of inflammatory bowel disease" below)

C. Extraintestinal manifestation of inflammatory bowel disease
   1. Toxic megacolon
      a. Definition
         i. Transmural inflammation of the colon resulting in atony and distension
      b. Etiology
         i. Ulcerative colitis
         ii. Crohn disease
         iii. *Clostridium difficile* colitis
      c. Symptoms and signs
         i. Toxic appearance
         ii. Abdominal pain and distension
         iii. Colon perforation and Gram-negative sepsis
         iv. Rectal bleeding
      d. Diagnosis
         i. Kidneys and upper bladder (KUB) or CT scan
            a) Continuous loop with diameter >6 cm colon dilation is abnormal
            b) Transverse colon most commonly involved
            c) "Thumb-printing" of bowel wall may be seen (bowel wall edema)
      e. Management
         i. Immediate decompression with nasogastric tube (+/– rectal tube)
         ii. Broad-spectrum antibiotics (anaerobic, Gram-negative, enteric flora; consider ciprofloxacin and metronidazole, or ampicillin and clindamycin, cefotetan/cefoxitin)
         iii. Immediate surgical consultation
         iv. Surgery if no resolution within 24 to 48 hours
         v. 50% mortality if perforation occurs
   2. Kidney stones and gallstones (Crohn >UC)
   3. Arthritis and arthralgias
   4. Ankylosing spondylitis
   5. Iritis and conjunctivitis
   6. Erythema nodosum (see Dermatology chapter)
   7. Pyoderma gangrenosum: pretibial ulcerative lesion with necrotic center

VII. Infectious Bowel Disease

A. Appendicitis
   1. Epidemiology
      a. Lifetime incidence 7%
      b. Incidence peak in teen years
      c. Prevalence higher in countries with poor fiber intake
   2. Symptoms and signs
      a. Anorexia, nausea, abdominal pain are common symptoms
      b. Classic pain pattern begins periumbilical and migrates to right lower quadrant (occurs in only 50%)
      c. Symptoms vary with contact point of inflamed appendix
         i. UTI symptoms occur if bladder irritated by inflamed appendix
         ii. Watery profuse diarrhea may occur with inflammation of large intestine by inflamed appendix
         iii. Back pain may occur with a retrocecal appendix
         iv. Obturator sign: pain with internal rotation of a flexed hip secondary to contact of the inflames appendix with the obturator internus muscle
         v. Psoas sign: pain with hyperextension of right leg secondary to contact of the inflames appendix with the iliopsoas muscle
      d. Rovsing sign: LLQ palpation elicits RLQ pain
      e. Children may present with scrotal swelling much like testicular torsion
   3. Diagnosis
      a. Clinical diagnosis
      b. Laboratory values insensitive and nonspecific
         i. Up to 30% may have normal WBC
         ii. Up to 48% may be afebrile
      c. Urinalysis
         i. Sterile pyuria (presence of leukocytes caused by bladder irritation by an inflamed appendix, but absence of bacteria distinguishes this from a urinary tract infection)
         ii. Hematuria
      d. KUB may reveal an appendicolith (calcified deposit within the appendix)

e. Ultrasound: may see dilated segment (not compressible is positive)
   i. 75% to 93% sensitivity
f. CT scan if diagnosis unclear
4. Management
   a. Surgical consultation
   b. Consider broad-spectrum antibiotics if strong suspicion of perforation or abscess while awaiting **or**
      i. Antibiotics should cover anaerobes, Gram-negatives (cefoxitin/cefotaxime, ciprofloxacin + metronidazole)

B. Diverticulitis
1. Definition
   a. Inflammation of diverticula occluded by food or feces, with or without microperforation
2. Symptoms and signs
   a. Left lower quadrant pain most common
      i. Sigmoid diverticulosis most common
   b. Fever
   c. Constipation more common than diarrhea
   d. Complications
      i. Colovesicular fistulas in men
      ii. Colovaginal fistulas in women as the uterus lies between the colon and bladder
      iii. Abscess formation
3. Diagnosis
   a. Clinical diagnosis
   b. CT scan
   c. Colonoscopy
4. Management
   a. Outpatient for mild disease
      i. Ciprofloxacin and metronidazole
      ii. Alternative
         a) Moxifloxacin monotherapy
         b) Amoxicillin/clavulonic acid monotherapy
   b. Inpatient for severe disease (systemic signs of infection, peritonitis, outpatient treatment failure or inability to tolerate oral hydration)
      i. Clear liquids
      ii. Metronidazole and third-generation cephalosporin or fluoroquinolone
         a) Alternative
            i) Tigecycline (monotherapy in severe penicillin allergy)
            ii) Imipenem (immune compromised)
   c. Colonoscopy after acute episode to rule out malignancy

C. Rectal abscess
1. Types (Figure 14–2)
   a. Perianal, intersphinteric, ischiorectal, supralevator
2. Risk factor
   a. Diabetes, immunosuppression, inflammatory bowel disease

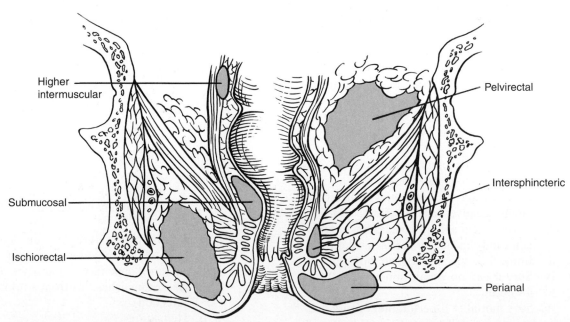

Figure 14–2. Rectal abscess types. (Reproduced with permission from Tintinalli JE, Kelen GD, Stapczynski JS: *Tintinalli's Emergency Medicine. A Comprehensive Study Guide,* 6th ed. Copyright © 2004, New York: McGraw-Hill.)

3. Symptoms and signs
   a. Pain with sitting, coughing, or defecation
   b. May be afebrile
   c. Pus in rectum
   d. Tender rectal mass
   e. Erythema over buttock if ischiorectal abscess
   f. Deep ischiorectal and supralevator abscesses may not have any external manifestation
   g. Rectal examination often requires anesthesia
4. Diagnosis
   a. Exploration in operating room
   b. CT scan
5. Management
   a. Only perianal abscesses should be drained in ED
   b. Surgical or interventional drainage

VIII. Diarrhea

A. General considerations
   1. Viruses >50%
   2. Antibiotics can shorten course of disease by 24 hours
      a. Cipro 500 mg PO bid × 5 days
      b. Bactrim if fluoroquinolone allergy
      c. Fear of prolonging salmonella carrier state unfounded
   3. Diphenoxylate and atropine (lomotil) safe
      a. No increase in fatal shigellosis

B. Invasive (bloody or occult bloody stool) diarrhea
   1. *Campylobacter jejuni*
      a. Most common bacterial diarrhea
      b. Associated with Guillan-Barre syndrome
   2. *Salmonella*
      a. Contaminated eggs and poultry products
      b. Associated with imported turtles
      c. Sickle cell patients susceptible
         i. More prone to osteomyelitis
   3. *Shigella*
      a. Associated with febrile seizures in children
   4. *Vibrio parahaemolyticus*
      a. Raw seafood
      b. Most common cause of bacterial diarrheal illness in Japan
   5. *Yersinia*
      a. Undercooked pork
      b. May mimic appendicitis
   6. *E. coli* (0157:H7)
      a. Verotoxin (shiga-like toxin) may lead to hemolytic uremic syndrome
         i. Children at greatest risk
         ii. Antibiotic treatment may increase toxin production

C. Noninvasive diarrhea
   1. Enterotoxigenic *E. coli*
      a. Traveler diarrhea
      b. Toxin similar to cholera toxin
      c. Onset from 17 to 72 hours
   2. *Staphylococcus aureus*
      a. Toxin-mediated
      b. Onset to illness 1 to 6 hours
   3. *Bacillus cereus*
      a. Old fried rice
      b. Onset 8 to 16 hours
   4. Cholera
      a. Rice water stools
   5. *Clostridium difficile*
      a. Epidemiology
         i. Up to 25% mortality in ill elderly
      b. Etiology
         i. Spore-forming Gram-positive anaerobe bacillus
      c. Risk factors
         i. Surgery or other GI instrumentation
         ii. Advanced age
            a) Antibiotic use
            b) Historically J-strain type predominant
               i) Resistance to clindamycin (so patients symptomatic after a course of clindamycin)
            c) Recently, NAP1/B2/027 strain identified
               i) Greater fluoroquinolone resistance
               ii) Much more virulent toxin
      d. Symptoms and signs
         i. Typically within 1 to 2 weeks of antibiotic discontinuation
         ii. Suspect if diarrhea >3 days after hospitalization
         iii. Frequent watery stools
         iv. Crampy abdominal pain
         v. Spectrum of presentation from well appearing to deathly ill
         vi. Increasing mortality rate with resistant strains
      e. Diagnosis
         i. Colonoscopy reveals pseudomembrane (yellowish plaques)
         ii. Stool culture
            a) High sensitivity but low specificity
         iii. Toxin detection
            a) Stool cytotoxin test is best but most expensive
            b) ELISA most commonly used
               i) Sensitivity 63% to 94%
               ii) Specificity 75% to 100%[6]
            c) Latex agglutination has poor sensitivity

f. Management
  i. If possible, stop antibiotics
  ii. Mild to moderate disease
    a) Metronidazole 250 mg PO qid
  iii. Severe disease or failure of metronidazole
    a) Vancomycin 125 mg to 250 mg PO qid
  iv. Complications: toxic megacolon and perforation

6. Scombroid: most common fish-borne toxin
  a. Etiology
    i. Histaminic toxin found in poorly kept dark-fleshed fish
    ii. Tuna, mackerel, and mahi mahi
    iii. Fish is said to have peppery taste
    iv. Toxin is **not** deactivated by heat
  b. Symptoms and signs
    i. Onset within 30 minutes of ingestion
    ii. Histamine-release type symptoms
      a) Flushing, diarrhea, nausea, vomiting, palpitations, and headache
      b) Hypotension, wheezing, tachycardia, and diffuse erythema
  c. Management
    i. Supportive
    ii. Self-limited illness
    iii. Antihistamines

7. Ciguatera: second most common fish-borne toxin
  a. Etiology
    i. Ciguatoxin concentrated in larger fish that ingest smaller fish
      a) Barracuda, grouper, and red snapper
    ii. Small fish feed on coral reef dinoflagellates that form the toxin
      a) Toxin is odorless, colorless, and tasteless
      b) Toxin is not deactivated by heat
    iii. Tropical warm weather fish is exported around the world causing disease
  b. Symptoms and signs
    i. Variable from 2 hours to 30 hours
    ii. Mortality uncommon but severe morbidity
    iii. Abdominal pain, vomiting, and diarrhea
    iv. Unique neurologic symptoms
      a) Hot-cold reversal
      b) Sensation of tooth looseness
    v. Ataxia and coma
    vi. Bradycardia, hypotension, and pulmonary edema
  c. Management
    i. Supportive care
      a) Antiemetics
      b) IV fluids for hypotension
      c) Atropine if bradyarrhythmia

  ii. Mannitol to prevent or alleviate neurologic morbidity

D. Parasitic diarrheal illnesses
  1. *Giardia lamblia*
    a. Most common parasitic diarrhea
    b. Explosive profuse diarrhea
    c. Drinking contaminated lake water
    d. Anal-oral sexual exposure
  2. *Cryptosporidium*
    a. HIV patients susceptible
    b. Untreated contaminated water
    c. Swimming in contaminated lake
  3. *Entamoeba histolytica*
    a. Amebiasis and liver abscess
    b. Fecal-oral route
    c. Homosexual men

E. Noninfectious causes of diarrhea
  1. Colchicine
  2. Theophylline (diarrhea and seizures)
  3. Cholinergics
  4. Ischemic colitis
  5. Inflammatory bowel disease
  6. Carcinoid tumor or VIPomas

IX. Hepatobilliary

A. Hepatocellular versus cholestatic disease
  1. Hepatocellular necrosis presents with nonspecific symptoms including nausea, vomiting, fever, weight loss, and anorexia
  2. Cholestatic (biliary obstructive) processes present with jaundice, dark urine, and clay-colored stools

B. Liver function tests
  1. Transaminases
    a. Elevated in both hepatocellular and cholestatic diseases
    b. Mild elevations occur with chronic disease such as viral hepatitis
    c. Severe elevations indicate hepatic necrosis as found in acetaminophen overdose
    d. Aspartate aminotransferase (AST)
      i. Nonspecific: also found in heart, smooth muscle, kidney, and brain
      ii. Elevated with alcohol, acetaminophen, NSAIDs, ACE inhibitor, isoniazid, erythromycin, and many antifungal medication usage
    e. Alanine aminotransferase (ALT)
      i. More specific to liver than AST
        a) AST:ALT ratio >2 may indicate alcohol abuse

b) AST:ALT >1 in the absence of alcohol use may indicate cirrhosis

c) AST:ALT ratio <1 with acute or chronic hepatocellular necrosis

2. Alkaline phosphatase
   a. Elevated in both hepatocellular or cholestatic diseases
   b. Significant elevations >fourfold indicate cholestatic disease as opposed to hepatocellular necrosis
   c. Alkaline phosphatase also found in bone, placenta, intestine, kidneys, and WBCs
   d. May be twofold and threefold elevated in healthy children and pregnant women

3. Gamma-glutamyl transpeptidase (GGT)
   a. Concurrent elevation with alkaline phosphatase indicative of cholestasis
   b. GGT also elevated with alcohol, phenobarbital, and warfarin use
   c. GGT can be elevated with pancreatitis, myocardial infarction, uremia, chronic obstructive pulmonary disease (COPD), rheumatoid arthritis, and diabetes

4. Bilirubin
   a. Breakdown product of heme containing proteins such as hemoglobin and myoglobin
   b. Circulating unconjugated (indirect) bilirubin is transformed by liver to conjugated (direct) bilirubin
   c. Indirect bilirubin normally 70% of total bilirubin
      i. Accumulates with increased production
         a) Hemolysis
      ii. Accumulates with decreased conjugation
         a) Gilbert syndrome
   d. Conjugated (direct) bilirubin
      i. Accumulates in diseases that slow secretion of bilirubin into bile or bile into the intestine
      ii. Usually shows a mixed hyperbilirubinemia due to reflux of conjugated bilirubin back to the plasma

5. Prothrombin time
   a. Hepatocellular disease with decreased protein synthesis of factors II, VII, IX, and X causes PT prolongation

C. Viral hepatitis
   1. Hepatitis A
      a. Transmission
         i. Fecal-oral route
         ii. Rarely blood borne
         iii. Ingesting shellfish from infected water
      b. Symptoms and signs
         i. Most infections in the United States result in jaundice and impressive transient hepatitis
         ii. Nausea, vomiting, fever, abdominal distension
         iii. Jaundice, dark urine, clay-colored stool
         iv. Hepatomegaly
         v. Splenomegaly (10% to 20%)
      c. Complications
         i. Relatively benign course in most patients other than acute illness
         ii. 1% risk of fulminant hepatitis
         iii. No chronic stage exists
         iv. Infection confers long-term immunity
      d. Diagnosis
         i. Anti-HAV = antibody to hepatitis A virus
            a) IgM = acute infection or
            b) IgG = prior infection (IgG- think "G" for "GONE")
         ii. AST and ALT elevated (4-100 times normal)
         iii. Elevated bilirubin (usually below 10 mg/dL)
      e. Management
         i. Supportive
         ii. Immunoglobulin prophylaxis within 2 weeks of exposure

   2. Hepatitis B
      a. Transmission
         i. Blood-borne
         ii. Sexually transmitted
         iii. Vertical maternal-fetal transmission
         iv. 30% have no identifiable source
      b. Symptoms and signs
         i. As with hepatitis A
      c. Complications
         i. Adult infection
            a) Asymptomatic infection (60% to 65%) without long-term sequelae
            b) Symptomatic hepatitis (25%) that resolves without long-term sequelae
            c) Chronic carrier (5% to 10%) who is asymptomatic but remains infectious
            d) Fulminant hepatitis (<0.5%)
               i) Acute liver failure secondary to acute hepatic necrosis
                  (a) Results in encephalopathy and decreased protein synthesis
                  (b) Often requires transplant
            e) Chronic hepatitis (5%)
         ii. Newborns and children have much more difficulty fending off virus
            a) 90% of infected babies will develop either chronic carrier or hepatitis status

    iii. Cirrhosis

    iv. Hepatocellular carcinoma

  d. Diagnosis

    i. HB_sAg = surface antigen of HBV indicates acute or chronic infection

      a) First detectable antigen

      b) May not be detectable during phase in which patient is clearing antigen

      c) Positive for >6 months indicates carrier or chronic hepatitis B

    ii. HB_cAb-IgM = core IgM antibody indicates acute infection

      a) Only serological evidence of disease during "window" in which patient is clearing virus but is still infected

    iii. HB_eAg = hepatitis B "e" antigen indicates active infection and high infectivity (think "e" antigen is evil)

    iv. HB_eAb = antibody to "e" antigen indicates decreased infectivity

    v. HB_sAb-IgG = antibody to hepatitis B surface antigen

      a) Acute or prior infection, or immunity

      b) Appears just after "disappearance" of HB_sAg

  e. Post-exposure prophylaxis from known carrier (see Infectious Disease chapter)

3. Hepatitis C

  a. Transmission

    i. Blood-borne (needle stick, injection drug use, blood product transfusion)

    ii. Vertical transmission mother to fetus not as efficient as hepatitis B

    iii. Uncommonly sexually transmitted

  b. Symptoms and signs

    i. Most patients with acute infection are asymptomatic

    ii. Affected individuals may present with nonspecific signs of hepatitis as above

  c. Complications

    i. Chronic infection occurs in 70% to 80%

    ii. Chronic infection progresses to cirrhosis in 20% within 20 years

    iii. Increased rate of hepatocellular carcinoma

  d. Diagnosis

    i. Difficult diagnosis because acute and chronic infections are typically asymptomatic

    ii. Anti-HCV antibodies

      a) Generated about 15 weeks after exposure

      b) May indicate acute or prior hepatitis C infection

      c) Must be followed by PCR testing for the virus itself

  e. Treatment: immunoglobulin against hepatitis C has not yet been developed

4. Hepatitis D

  a. Endemic to Mediterranean, Middle East, and South America (consider in travelers)

  b. Transmission: parenteral (blood product transfusion, needle stick or injection drug user)

  c. Requires **hepatitis B coinfection** synergy

5. Hepatitis E

  a. Seen in epidemics in India, Southeast Asia, Africa, and Mexico

  b. Transmission: fecal-oral

  c. Similar transmission and progression pattern as hepatitis A

  d. High fatality rate among **pregnant** women

6. General management for acute hepatitis

  a. Supportive (fluid intake, avoid hepatotoxic intake, alcohol, tylenol)

  b. Immunoglobulin passive immunity exist for hepatitis A and B

  c. Hospital admission criteria

    i. Altered mental status, encephalopathy

    ii. INR >1.5 (could progress to fulminant hepatitis)

    iii. Bilirubin >20

    iv. Dehydration, refractory emesis

    v. Significant electrolyte imbalance, hypoglycemia

    vi. Significant comorbid conditions

  d. Antiviral therapy (interferon alpha, ribavirin) for hepatitis B and C coordinated by infectious disease specialist or gastroenterologist

  e. Consider liver transplantation for fulminant hepatitis

D. Hepatic encephalopathy

  1. Definition

    a. Reversible mental status change in the setting of liver failure, acute or chronic (cirrhosis), secondary to neurotoxins including ammonia that cross leaky blood brain barrier

  2. Etiology

    a. Occurs in patients with advanced cirrhosis and portal hypertension

  3. Risk factors in the presence of cirrhosis

    a. Infection most common

    b. GI bleeding

    c. Constipation

    d. High-protein diet

    e. Zinc deficiency—needed to metabolize nitrogen

    f. Medications: benzodiazepines

    g. "TIPS" procedure (transjugular intrahepatic portosystemic shunt)

4. Diagnosis
   a. Ammonia level correlates poorly with symptoms
      i. Compare level to baseline
      ii. Serial level monitoring aids management in the individual
5. Management
   a. Uncover and treat exacerbating condition(s)
   b. Increase nitrogen elimination with lactulose
   c. Decrease ammonia-producing flora with metronidazole (neomycin formerly recommended but may lead to renal failure)
   d. Protein restriction
   e. Zinc replacement with zinc acetate or sulfate
   f. Flumazenil may give short-term benefit

E. Spontaneous bacterial peritonitis (SBP)
   1. Etiology
      a. Bowel edema caused by portal hypertension (liver disease) will result in bacterial migration from the GI tract
      b. The majority of organisms involved are Gram-negative (eg, *E. coli* and *Klebsiella)*
   2. Symptoms and signs
      a. Asymptomatic (30%)
      b. Fever and chills (80%)
      c. Abdominal pain (70%)
   3. Diagnosis
      a. Peritoneal fluid analysis
         i. WBC >1000 mm^3
         ii. PMN >250 mm^3
         iii. pH <7.34
         iv. Cultures poorly sensitive
         v. Repeat paracentesis >48 hours to monitor treatment response
   4. Management
      a. Antibiotics (third-generation cephalosporin, ampicillin/sulbactam, piperacillin/tazobactam, or ampicillin/aminoglycoside)

F. Biliary colic and cholecystitis
   1. Etiology
      a. Obstructing gallstone
      b. Acalculous cholecystitis occurs in up to 10%
         i. Due to bile stasis resulting from coexisting, serious illness (sepsis)
         ii. Associated with more rapid and malignant disease
   2. Risk factors
      a. Increased age, female sex, multiparity, pregnancy, obesity, diabetes, hypertriglyceridemia
      b. Profound weight loss, prolonged fasting state
      c. Chronic intravascular hemolysis
         i. Sickle cell disease
         ii. Hereditary spherocytosis

   d. Medications: oral contraceptives, estrogens/progesterones, clofibrate, ceftriaxone
   3. Symptoms and signs
      a. Most patients present with epigastric discomfort with or without radiation to right or left shoulder
      b. Circadian rhythm of symptoms
         i. Peaks at midnight
         ii. Usually between 9 p.m. and 4 a.m. (or whenever ultrasound becomes unavailable at your institution)
      c. No temporal relationship with food in up to 40%
      d. Traditionally taught that pain relieved within 6 hours is biliary colic, and to consider cholecystitis if pain persists longer
      e. Positive Murphy sign: inspiratory arrest during deep RUQ palpation
      f. Afebrile cholecystitis in 59% to 90%[7,8]
   4. Diagnosis
      a. Laboratory
         i. CBC
            a) 27% to 40% of gangrenous cholecystitis lack leukocytosis[7,8]
            b) 16% of gangrenous cholecystitis lack both fever and leukocytosis[7]
         ii. Liver function tests
            a) Normal tests do not rule out cholecystitis or biliary colic
         iii. Elevated lipase suggests gallstone pancreatitis
      b. Plain films
         i. Usually unhelpful as most stones are radiolucent (cholesterol and pigment)
      c. Abdominal CT
         i. Detection of acute cholecystitis
            a) Thickened gallbladder wall
            b) Pericholecystic stranding/fluid
            c) Dilated intrahepatic and extrahepatic ducts
            d) Unlikely to visualize stone
         ii. May be unable to detect up to 20% of gallstones (pigment stones) as it may be the same density as bile[9]
      d. Ultrasound
         i. Findings as with CT, but more likely to visualize stone
         ii. Sensitivity of 94% to 98% and specificity of 75% to 78%[10]
      e. Nuclear with technetium-iminoacetic acid analogues (HIDA)
         i. Sensitivity of 97% and specificity of 90%
         ii. Normal scan will outline cystic duct and gallbladder within 1 hour
         iii. May be inaccurate in patients with bilirubin levels >5

5. Management
   a. Biliary colic
      i. Symptomatic management
         a) Antiemetics
         b) Analgesia
      ii. Outpatient surgical referral
      iii. Consider admission if intractable emesis or pain
   b. Acute cholecystitis
      i. IV fluids (NPO)
      ii. Antibiotics (broad-spectrum to cover anaerobes, Gram-positives and Gram-negatives)
      iii. Surgical consultation

G. Cholangitis
   1. Definition
      a. Obstruction of common bile duct (usually stone) with superimposed retrograde ascending bacterial infection
   2. Symptoms and signs
      a. Charcot triad: fever, RUQ pain, jaundice
      b. Reynold pentad: Charcot triad with hypotension and altered mental status
      c. Dark urine, clay-colored light stools
   3. Diagnosis
      a. Laboratory
         i. Leukocytosis
         ii. Elevated direct bilirubin
         iii. Elevated alkaline phosphatase and GGT
      b. Radiologic imaging
         i. Ultrasound, CT scan, or HIDA
         ii. Reveals obstruction or dilation of common bile duct
            a) Fluid may represent pus
   4. Management
      a. Broad-spectrum antibiotics (Gram +/– and anaerobic)
      b. Endoscopic retrograde cholangiopancreatography (ERCP) followed by cholecystectomy if necessary
      c. Surgical consult (for percutaneous or surgical decompression)
      d. ICU admission

X. Pancreatitis

A. Definition(s)
   1. Pancreatitis: inflammation and auto-digestion of the pancreas
   2. Necrotizing pancreatitis: severe inflammation resulting in cell death and devitalized pancreatic tissue (gangrene)
   3. Acute fluid collection: fluid-filled thin-walled sac which results from pancreatic edema
   4. Pseudocyst: localized fluid collection of digestive enzymes contained in a fibrous, non-epithelialized capsule
      a. Forms 4 to 5 weeks after acute episode of pancreatitis

B. Epidemiology
   1. Women more likely to have gallstone pancreatitis
   2. Men more likely to have alcohol pancreatitis

C. Etiology
   1. Gall stones (45%)
   2. Ethanol (35%)
   3. Others include medications (corticosteroids, pentamidine), scorpion envenomation, hypertriglyceridemia, trauma, complication of ERCP

D. Symptoms and signs
   1. Epigastric pain radiating to back
   2. Grey Turner sign: flank ecchymosis caused by retroperitoneal hemorrhage
   3. Cullen sign: periumbilical ecchymosis caused by subcutaneous intraperitoneal hemorrhage

E. Diagnosis
   1. Laboratory
      a. CBC and metabolic panel
      b. Liver function testing
      c. Amylase >3 times normal (75% to 90% sensitivity and 20% to 60% specificity)
      d. Elevated lipase is the preferred laboratory marker (86% to 100% sensitivity and 50% to 95% specificity)
      e. Values help estimate mortality using Ranson criteria (Table 14–1)
         i. Note: neither amylase or lipase are part of Ranson criteria

TABLE 14–1 Ranson Criteria

AT ADMISSION	WITH 48 HOURS
Age >55 years	HCT decline >10%
WBC >16,000	BUN rise >5 mg dL
Glucose >200 mg dL	Calcium <8 mg dL
LDH >350 IU L	PaO$_2$ <60 mm Hg
AST >250	Base deficit >4 mEq L
	Fluid balance – 6 L

TOTAL SIGNS	MORTALITY
0 to 3	1%
3 to 4	15%
5 to 6	40%
>7	100%

2. Plain radiography
   a. May reveal calcifications in epigastrium particularly with chronic pancreatitis
   b. Sentinel loop may reveal focal small bowel ileus
3. Ultrasound
   a. May help determine gallstone etiology of pain
   b. May identify pseudocysts and abscesses
4. CT scan
   a. Rarely useful in acute pancreatitis
      i. Helpful to diagnosis pancreatic necrosis, abscesses, and pseudocysts

F. Management
   1. Fluid resuscitation
   2. NPO
   3. β-lactam antibiotics may improve mortality and prevent pancreatic necrosis (controversial)
      a. Imipenem with best pancreatic penetration if suspect necrosis secondary to bacterial infection

G. Complications
   1. Pancreatic pseudocyst
      a. Occurs, generally >4 weeks after acute inflammation
      b. Scarred pancreatic exocrine ducts lead to spillage of digestive enzymes and formation of pseudocysts
      c. Fluid-filled structures associated with acute pancreatitis are called acute fluid collections until 4 weeks
         i. Acute fluid collections have low concentrations of caustic pancreatic enzymes and more transudative fluid and therefore are not dangerous if ruptured
         ii. 50% of acute fluid collections become pseudocysts.
      d. Pseudocysts filled with digestive enzymes can be deadly when ruptured
      e. Pseudocysts are generally drained if they persist >6 weeks or are larger than 5 to 6 cm in diameter

2. Diabetes
3. Chronic pancreatitis

REFERENCES

1. Wilcox CM, Alexander LN, Cotsonis G: A prospective characterization of upper gastrointestinal hemorrhage presenting with hematochezia. *Am J Gastroenterol.* 1997;92:231.
2. Jenkins SA, Shields R, Davies M, et al: A multicenter randomized trial comparing Octreotide and injection sclerotherapy in the management and outcome of acute variceal hemorrhage. *Gut.* 1997;41:526.
3. Collins R, Langman M: Treatment with histamine H_2 antagonists in acute upper gastrointestinal hemorrhage: implications of randomized trials. *N Engl J Med.* 1985;313:660.
4. Khuroo MS, Yattoo GN, Javid G, et al: A comparison of omeprazole and placebo for bleeding peptic ulcer. *N Engl J Med.* 1997;336:1054.
5. Staniland JR, Ditchburn J, de Dombal FT: Clinical presentation of the acute abdomen: study of 600 patients. *BMJ.* 1972;3:393.
6. Gerding DN, Johnson S, Peterson LR, et al: Clostridium difficile associated diarrhea and colitis. *Infect Control Hosp Epidemiol.* 1995;16:459.
7. Gruber PJ, Silverman RA, Gottesfeld S, et al: Presence of fever and leukocytosis in acute cholecystitis. *Ann Emerg Med.* 1996;28(3):273.
8. Singer AJ, McCracken G, Henry MC, et al: Correlation among clinical, laboratory, and hepatobiliary scanning findings in patients with suspected acute cholecystitis. *Ann Emerg Med.* 1996;28(3):267.
9. Fidler J, Paulson EK, Layfield L: CT evaluation of acute cholecystitis: findings and usefulness in diagnosis. *AJR.* 1996;166:1085.
10. Shea JA, Berlin JA, Escarce JJ, et al: Revised estimates of diagnostic test sensitivity and specificity in suspected biliary tract disease. *Arch Intern Med.* 1994;154.
11. Marx JA, Hockberger RS, Walls RM, eds: *Rosen's Emergency Medicine: Concepts and Clinical Practice.* 6th ed. St. Louis, MO: Mosby; 2006.
12. Tintinalli JE, Kelen GD, Stapczynski JS, eds: *Emergency Medicine: A Comprehensive Study Guide.* 6th ed. New York: McGraw-Hill; 2003.

Chapter 15
INFECTIOUS EMERGENCIES

Howard A. Greller

SEXUALLY TRANSMITTED DISEASES

I. Ulcerative Sexually Transmitted Diseases (Table 15–1)

A. Genital herpes
  1. Epidemiology
      a. Most common ulcerative sexually transmitted disease (STD) in United States
      b. 1 in 5 sexually active adults infected[1]
      c. 45 million affected in United States with 1 million new cases per year
  2. Etiology: herpes simplex virus (HSV)
      a. HSV-2 more commonly causes genital infection and transmission is by sexual contact
      b. HSV-1 more commonly causes oropharyngeal infection and transmission is by nongenital personal contact
      c. Both forms can cause either genital or oropharyngeal infection
  3. Symptoms and signs
      a. Incubation period 2 to 7 days
      b. Transmission via direct contact with secretion
      c. Multiple, **painful**, shallow ulcers which may coalesce (Figure 15–1)
      d. Systemic symptoms of fever, myalgias, headache
      e. Bilateral, tender adenopathy develops during second to third week of disease
      f. Lesions heal by 2 to 4 weeks
      g. Shedding lasts up to 3 weeks and may occur in asymptomatic patients
      h. Recurrence in 60% to 90% of patients
          i. Virus latent in spinal cord ganglia for life
          ii. Recurrent episodes milder and shorter in duration
          iii. Risk factors include immunosuppression, stress, ultraviolet light, birth control, and fever
          iv. Prodrome of paresthesias, burning, and itching at site of lesions

      i. Transmission
          i. Highest viral load and transmitability during primary infection
          ii. May be contagious during reactivation even before lesions become visible
  4. Diagnosis
      a. Clinical diagnosis if vesicles intact
      b. Viral culture from vesicles (test of choice) for confirmation of clinical diagnosis
          i. False negatives common secondary to improper collection, storage, or transport
      c. Direct antigen testing; immunofluorescent testing; polymerase chain reaction (PCR) testing
          i. Low sensitivity
          ii. Cannot distinguish between HSV-1 and HSV-2
      d. Serologic testing
          i. May take 6 to 8 weeks to become positive and false-negative results may occur early in infection
          ii. Positive results do not differentiate present from past infection
      e. Tzanck smear
          i. Multinucleated giant cell
          ii. No longer recommended because of lack of sensitivity
  5. Management
      a. Treat primary infection for 7 to 10 days
          i. Acyclovir 200 mg 5 times daily, or 400 mg 3 times daily
          ii. Famciclovir 250 mg 3 times daily (enhanced absorption)
          iii. Valacyclovir 1 g twice daily (high oral bioavailability)
          iv. Does not eradicate latent infection
      b. Treatment of recurrence: effective if initiated during prodrome or within 1 day of lesion onset
          i. Acyclovir 200 mg 5 times daily × 5 days
          ii. Famciclovir 125 mg twice daily × 5 days
          iii. Valacyclovir 500 mg twice daily × 5 days

TABLE 15–1.   Ulcerative Sexually Transmitted Diseases

NAME	ORGANISM	PRESENTATION	DIAGNOSIS	TREATMENT
Genital Herpes	*Herpes simplex*	Clusters of vesicles with an erythematous base	Clinical, viral culture or tzank smear	Acyclovir Valacyclovir Famciclovir
Syphilis	*Treponema pallidum*	Painless chancre (1°), diffuse rash, condyloma lata (2°), thoracic aneurysm, dementia, tabes dorsalis (3°)	VDRL, RPR, FTA-ABS	Benzathine PCN Doxycycline Tetracycline Erythromycin
LGV	*Chlamydia trachomatis*	Small ulcer, tender inguinal lymphadenopathy, Proctocolitis	PCR or culture	Doxycycline Azithromycin Erythromycin
Chancroid	*Haemophilus ducreyi*	Painful chancres	Gram stain	Ceftriaxone Azithromycin Ciprofloxacin Erythromycin
Granuloma Inguinale	*Calymmatobacterium granulomatis*	Painless papule, vesicle, or nodular lesion of the genitalia, red ulcers with a rolled border	Biopsy showing Donovan bodies in monocytes	Trimethoprim-sulfamethoxazole Doxycycline Ciprofloxacin Erythromycin

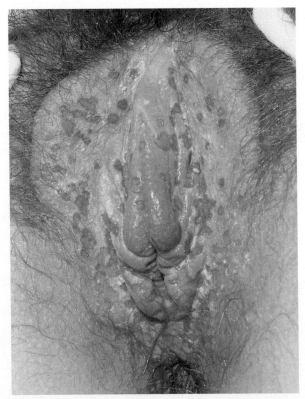

FIGURE 15–1. Genital herpes. Multiple, painful, shallow ulcers. (Reproduced, with permission, from Wolff K, Johnson RA, Suurmond D: *Fitzpatrick's Color Atlas and Synopsis of Clinical Dermatology,* 5th ed. Copyright © 2005, New York: McGraw-Hill.)

    c. Suppressive therapy recommended for >6 episodes per year
    d. Suppressive therapy during pregnancy
      i. Safety not definitively established
      ii. No increased risk of major birth defects with acyclovir use during the first trimester according to available data
      iii. Acyclovir treatment late in pregnancy reduces frequency of C-section by decreasing recurrences at term

B. Syphilis
  1. Epidemiology
    a. Known as the "great imitator" because its signs and symptoms are often indistinguishable from other diseases
    b. 7000 new cases in United States each year—increasing rates
  2. Etiology
    a. Organism: spirochete *Treponema pallidum*
    b. Transmitted by
      i. Sexual direct contact with infected lesion
      ii. Maternal-fetal transmission
  3. Symptoms and signs
    a. Primary syphilis
      i. Incubation 9 to 90 days
      ii. Chancre: begins as papule then ulcerates
      iii. **Painless,** clean-based, sharply defined, circular ulcer
      iv. Usually solitary (Figure 15–2)

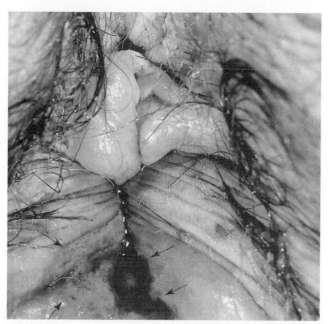

FIGURE 15–2. Primary chancre. Large painless ulcer. (Reproduced, with permission, from Wolff K, Johnson RA, Suurmond D: *Fitzpatrick's Color Atlas and Synopsis of Clinical Dermatology,* 5th ed. Copyright © 2005, New York: McGraw-Hill.)

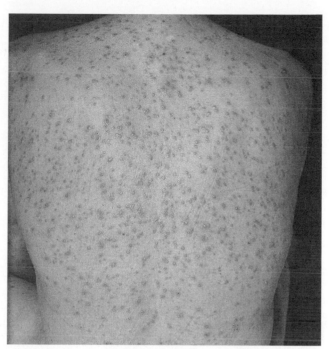

FIGURE 15–3. Secondary syphilis. Disseminated eruption. (Reproduced, with permission, from Wolff K, Johnson RA, Suurmond D: *Fitzpatrick's Color Atlas and Synopsis of Clinical Dermatology,* 5th ed. Copyright © 2005, New York: McGraw-Hill.)

     v. Occurs at site of inoculation
    vi. Resolves spontaneously after 2 to 6 weeks
   vii. May have bilateral, painless, nonfluctuant, inguinal adenopathy

  b. Secondary syphilis
    i. Occurs 5 to 8 weeks after resolution of primary syphilis
    ii. Rash
      a) Initially maculopapular, copper-colored, becomes papulosquamous
      b) May resemble pityriasis rosea
      c) Starts on trunk, spreads outward, may involve **palms** and **soles** (Figure 15–3)
   iii. Condyloma lata
      a) Broad-based papules with flat, moist tops, occurring in the perineal region (Figure 15–4)
   iv. Constitutional symptoms: fever, malaise, and arthralgias
    v. Resolves spontaneously in 1 to 2 months if untreated
   vi. 25% will have relapse of secondary syphilis (usually within 1 year)

  c. Latent syphilis
    i. Asymptomatic period

  d. Tertiary syphilis
    i. Occurs after latent period of 3 to 4 years (up to 20 years later)

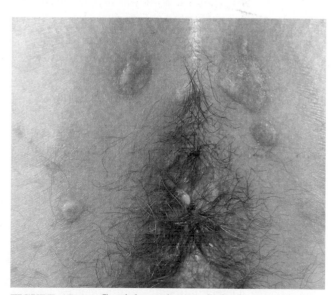

FIGURE 15–4. Condyloma latum. Soft, flat-topped, pink papules on perineum. (Reproduced, with permission, from Wolff K, Johnson RA, Suurmond D: *Fitzpatrick's Color Atlas and Synopsis of Clinical Dermatology,* 5th ed. Copyright © 2005, New York: McGraw-Hill.)

ii. Gumma: benign granulomatous lesion that causes local destruction in any organ system, most commonly skin, mucous membranes, and bone

iii. Neurosyphilis

  a) Asymptomatic neurosyphilis: lacks symptoms but has cerebrospinal fluid (CSF) evidence of syphilis, including pleocytosis, elevated protein, decreased glucose or have reactive CSF VDRL (Venereal Disease Research Laboratory test for syphilis)

  b) Meningeal syphilis (meningitis): <1 year after infection

  c) Meningovascular syphilis: 5 to 10 years after infection; manifests as stroke syndrome caused by endarteritis

  d) General paresis (dementia paralytica): 20 years after infection, changes in personality, affect, intellect that result from progressive frontotemporal meningoencephalitis

  e) *Tabes doralis* (peripheral neuropathy): 25 to 30 years after infection, loss of pain/vibration/position sensation, ataxia, that result from progressive degeneration of posterior columns, positive Romberg test

iv. Cardiovascular

  a) Classification of tertiary syphilis that occurs anytime during tertiary stage

  b) Thoracic aortic aneurysms caused by obliterative endarteritis of vaso vasorum

4. Diagnosis

  a. Darkfield microscopy of scrapings from primary and secondary lesions with 80% sensitivity

  b. Nontreponemal tests :VDRL and rapid plasma Reagin (RPR)

    i. Measure nonspecific antibodies 100% sensitive in secondary syphilis

    ii. Titers correlate with disease progression and activity

    iii. Positive 2 weeks after appearance of primary chancre

    iv. Used to follow treatment response; become nonreactive after treatment or reactive at lower titers

  c. Treponemal tests: MHA-TP and FTA-ABS

    i. Detect antibodies to treponemes

    ii. Used as confirmation for positive nontreponemal tests

    iii. Titers do not correlate with treatment response; often reactive after therapy

    iv. Not helpful testing in patients with previously treated syphilis

    v. Positive tests must be reported to the public health department

5. Management

  a. Primary, secondary, and early latent syphilis (<1 year)

    i. Benzathine penicillin (PCN) G 2.4 million units IM (treatment of choice)

    ii. Doxycycline 100 mg oral, twice daily × 14 days

    iii. Tetracycline or erythromycin 500 mg oral, 4 times daily × 14 days

  b. Tertiary syphilis

    i. Cardiovascular syphilis or late latent syphilis (>1 year)

      a) Benzathine PCN G 2.4 million units IM weekly × 3 weeks

      b) Doxycycline 100 mg oral twice daily × 4 weeks

      c) Tetracycline 500 mg oral 4 times daily × 4 weeks

      d) Pregnant women allergic to PCN should be desensitized and treated with PCN

    ii. Neurosyphilis

      a) Aqueous PCN G 3 to 4 million units IV every 4 hours × 10 to 14 days

      b) Procaine PCN G 2.4 million units IM daily plus probenecid 500 mg × 10 to 14 days

  c. Jarisch-Herxheimer reaction associated with treatment

    i. Caused by inflammatory reaction secondary to release of endotoxins from death of spirochetes

    ii. 1 to 2 hours after antibiotic therapy

    iii. Fever, headache, myalgia, worsening rash

    iv. Usually self-limited, supportive therapy

C. Lymphogranuloma venereum (LGV)

1. Epidemiology: prevalent in tropical countries, rare in United States

2. Etiology: *Chlamydia trachomatis*

  a. Gram-negative, aerobic, intracellular

  b. Serotypes L1 to L3 responsible for LGV

3. Symptoms and signs

  a. Primary stage

    i. Incubation 3 to 21 days

    ii. Small, painless, transient genital ulcers

  b. Secondary stage

    i. Occurs 7 to 30 days after primary lesions resolves

    ii. Regional lymphadenitis

a) Buboes: unilateral, **painful**, firm adenopathy

b) Groove sign: adenopathy above and below pouparts ligament

4. Diagnosis
   a. Clinical diagnosis
   b. Serology (complement fixation)
   c. Aspiration and culture of bubo
5. Management
   a. Doxycycline 100 mg oral twice daily × 3 weeks (treatment of choice)
   b. Erythromycin 500 mg oral 4 times daily × 3 weeks

D. Chancroid
   1. Epidemiology: common in developing countries, rare in United States
   2. Etiology: *Haemophilus ducreyi*, Gram-negative bacillus
   3. Symptoms and signs
      a. Incubation period <1 week
      b. Initially small pustules at site of inoculation
      c. Progresses to multiple, **painful** ulcerations with sharp, purulent bases, distinguishing it from syphilitic chancre (Figure 15–5)
      d. Associated with **painful** inguinal lymphadenopathy which may become suppurative
         i. Bubo: unilateral, large, painful, fluctuant, inguinal lymph node
      e. Dysuria with chancre contact
   4. Diagnosis
      a. Gram stain aspirate from bubo that demonstrates Gram-negative bacilli in linear or parallel formation
      b. Culture
      c. Often clinical diagnosis once herpes and syphilis excluded
   5. Management
      a. Azithromycin 1 g PO × 1
      b. Ceftriaxone 250 mg IM × 1
      c. Ciprofloxacin 500 mg oral twice daily × 3 days
      d. Erythromycin 500 mg oral 4 times daily × 7 days

E. Condyloma acuminatum
   1. Etiology
      a. Human papilloma virus types 6, 11
   2. Symptoms and signs
      a. Single or multiple, broad-based, pedunculated or pigmented warts (Figure 15–6)
         i. Can be painful, friable, or pruritic
         ii. Biopsy indurated, fixed, ulcerated, darkly pigmented warts to rule out carcinoma

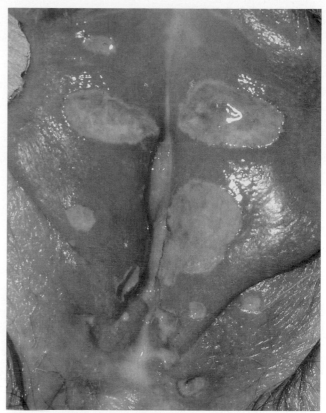

FIGURE 15–5. Chancroid. Multiple, painful ulcers. (Reproduced, with permission, from Wolff K, Johnson RA, Suurmond D: *Fitzpatrick's Color Atlas and Synopsis of Clinical Dermatology,* 5th ed. Copyright © 2005, New York: McGraw-Hill.)

   3. Diagnosis
      a. Clinical
      b. Biopsy
      c. Rule out syphilis (condyloma latum)
   4. Management
      a. If untreated may
         i. Resolve spontaneously
         ii. Remain unchanged
         iii. Increase in number
      b. Removal
         i. Topical (Podofilox, Imiquimod)
         ii. Cryotherapy
         iii. Surgical removal
   5. Recurrence
      a. Can occur in >50% of patients
      b. Repeat infection
      c. Immunosuppression
      d. Missed lesions on first treatment

F. Granuloma inguinale (donovanosis)
   1. Etiology: *Calymmatobacterium granulomatis*, Gram-negative, pleomorphic bacillus

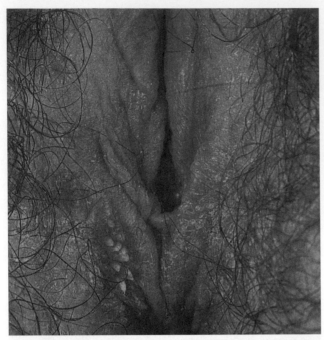

FIGURE 15–6. Condyloma acuminatum. Verrucous lesions. (Reproduced, with permission, from Handsfield HH. *Atlas of Sexually Transmitted Diseases*. Copyright © 2005, New York: McGraw-Hill, 1992.)

2. Symptoms and signs
    a. Incubation period 1 to 12 weeks
    b. **Painless** papule, vesicle, or nodular lesion of genitalia
    c. Red ulcers with a rolled border
3. Diagnosis: biopsy with Donovan bodies (safety pin-shaped intracellular organisms in monocytes)
4. Management
    a. Trimethoprim-sulfamethoxazole 1 DS tablet twice daily × 3 weeks
    b. Doxycycline 100 mg oral twice daily × 3 weeks
    c. Ciprofloxacin 750 mg oral twice daily × 3 weeks
    d. Erythromycin 500 mg oral 4 times daily × 3 weeks

II. Nonulcerative Sexually Transmitted Diseases (Table 15–2)

A. *Chlamydia*
    1. Epidemiology: most common bacterial STD in the United States
    2. Etiology: *Chlamydia trachomatis*
        a. Obligate intracellular Gram-negative organism
        b. Serotypes D to K
    3. Symptoms and signs
        a. Incubation period of 1 to 3 weeks
        b. Female: 80% of infected females are initially asymptomatic
            i. Mucopurulent cervicitis
            ii. Pelvic inflammatory disease (PID): 40% of untreated females
            iii. 5% to 10% will go on to have perihepatitis (ie, Fitz-Hugh-Curtis syndrome)
            iv. Urethritis
        c. Male: 50% of infected males are asymptomatic
            i. Epididymitis, most common cause in males <35 years
        d. Male and female
            i. Dysuria
            ii. Yellow mucopurulent discharge from the urethra
            iii. Mucopurulent rectal discharge (from anal intercourse)
            iv. LGV: serovars L1 to L3 (see description above)
        e. Neonatal conjunctivitis (see Common Infections in Pediatrics chapter)
        f. Reiter syndrome
            i. A reactive arthritis associated with immune response to enteric or genitourinary organisms, frequently *Chlamydia*
            ii. Results in conjunctivitis, urethritis, asymmetric polyarthritis (mnemonic Can't see, pee, or climb a tree)
            iii. Associated with HLA-B27

TABLE 15–2. Nonulcerating Sexually Transmitted Diseases

Chlamydia	*Chlamydia trachomatis*	Urethritis, epididymitis, dysuria, discharge, mucopurulent cervicitis PID	LGV fixation test	Doxycycline Azithromycin Erythromycin
Gonorrhea	*Neisseria gonorrhea*	Urethritis, discharge, or PID	Gram stain, PCR	Ceftriaxone Cefixime
Trichomoniasis	*Trichomonas vaginalis*	Vaginal (frothy) discharge, itchy, fishy odor, mucosa and cervix with erosions, "strawberry" appearance	Wet mount-shaped organism with flagella	Metronidazole Tinidazole

4. Diagnosis
   a. Cell culture
      i. Labor intensive
      ii. Sensitivity 60% to 80%, specificity 99%
      iii. No longer routinely done
   b. Urine for nucleic acid amplification tests (NAATs), including PCR and ligase chain reaction (LCR) tests
      i. Gold standard
      ii. Sensitivity >90%, specificity 99%
      iii. Males
         a) No difference in urine specimen versus genital specimen
      iv. Females
         a) May be less sensitive than genital swab for females
      v. May treat presumptively in high-risk populations with poor follow-up
5. Management
   a. Empiric therapy prior to definitive diagnosis
   b. Antibiotics
      i. Azithromycin 1 g PO
      ii. Doxycycline 100 mg PO twice daily × 7 days
      iii. Erythromycin 500 mg 4 times daily × 7 days
      iv. Fluoroquinolones inferior to macrolides and doxycycline and are not recommended[2]
   c. Antibiotics safe in pregnancy
      i. Azithromycin
      ii. Erythromycin
   d. Sexual abstinence for 7 days after completion of treatment
   e. Treat for coinfection with gonorrhea
   f. Test and treat partner

B. Gonorrhea
   1. Epidemiology: second most frequently reported STD
   2. Etiology: *Neisseria gonorrhea*, Gram-negative diplococcus
   3. Symptoms and signs
      a. Incubation period 7 to 14 days
      b. Female
         i. Often asymptomatic but may present with nonspecific lower abdominal discomfort
         ii. Vaginal discharge or urethritis
         iii. PID: 20% of untreated females
      c. Male
         i. Urethritis (purulent discharge)
         ii. Epididymitis-orchitis
         iii. Proctitis should be considered in those with rectal discharge

   d. Male and female
      i. Can affect oropharynx and anorectal area
      ii. Conjunctivitis
      iii. Neonatal conjunctivitis (see Pediatrics chapter)
      iv. Disseminated gonococcal infection (DGI)
         a) More common in young, sexually active females
         b) Bacteremia, fevers, or chills
            i) May progress to endocarditis, meningitis, or sepsis
         c) Oligoarticular arthritis or arthralgias
            i) Knees most commonly involved
            ii) Erythematous, warm joint
            iii) Asymmetrical arthralgia, tenosynovitis
            iv) Septic arthritis or migratory polyarthritis
         d) Rash
            i) Petechial or pustular acral skin lesions
            ii) Result from septic emboli to small vessels (Figure 15–7)
         e) Tenosynovitis
         f) Diagnosis of DGI made on clinical suspicion and with isolation of gonococci from blood, synovium, or skin
4. Diagnosis
   a. Gram stain and culture required for diagnosis from oropharynx, synovium, anorectum, and CSF
   b. NAATs for diagnosis of cervical or urethral gonorrhea only
   c. Clinical suspicion

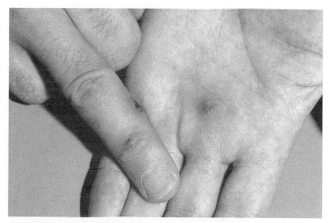

FIGURE 15–7. Disseminated gonococcal infection. Hemorrhagic painful pustules on erythematous base. (Reproduced, with permission, from Wolff K, Johnson RA, Suurmond D: *Fitzpatrick's Color Atlas and Synopsis of Clinical Dermatology,* 5th ed. Copyright © 2005, New York: McGraw-Hill.)

5. Management
   a. Empiric therapy prior to definitive diagnosis
   b. Coinfection with *Chlamydia* in 45%; treat for both
   c. Test for syphilis because of increased risk for other STDs
   d. Test and treat sexual partner
   e. Treatment for uncomplicated gonococcal infection
      i. Ceftriaxone 125 mg IM (for uncomplicated infections)
      ii. Cefixime 400 mg PO
      iii. Ceftizoxime 500 mg IM; cefoxitin 2 g IM, administered with probenecid 1 g PO; or cefotaxime 500 mg IM
      iv. Azithromycin 2 g as a single oral dose is highly efficacious but not recommended secondary to expense and gastrointestinal (GI) distress[3]
      v. Spectinomycin 2 g IM
      vi. Fluoroquinolones no longer recommended for treatment of gonorrhea secondary to increased resistance[4]
   f. Antibiotics safe in pregnancy: ceftriaxone, cefixime spectinomycin, azithromycin, erythromycin
   g. Treatment of gonococcal arthritis
      i. Ceftriaxone 1 g IM or IV every 24 hours, continue for 24 to 48 hours after improvement begins
      ii. Follow by an oral regimen to complete at least 1 week of treatment
         a) Cefixime 400 mg PO twice daily × 7 days
   h. Treatment of DGI
      i. Admit for IV antibiotics

C. PID
   1. Epidemiology
      a. The most common severe infection of reproductive-aged women
   2. Etiology
      a. Ascending infection from asymptomatic cervicitis
      b. Polymicrobial infection
         i. *Gonorrhea* and *Chlamydia* most common
         ii. *Mycoplasma* and endogenous vaginal flora also implicated
   3. Risk factors
      a. Young age
      b. Multiple partners
      c. Smoking
      d. Menses, secondary to breakdown of natural barriers
   4. Symptoms and signs
      a. Lower abdominal pain, vaginal bleeding or discharge, cervical motion tenderness, fever

   b. Adnexal mass with tuboovarian abscess
   c. Fitz-Hugh-Curtis syndrome
      i. Inflammation of hepatic capsule and diaphragm: perihepatitis
      ii. Can present without signs and symptoms of PID
      iii. **Violin string** sign during laparotomy: adhesions between liver and abdominal wall
   d. Complications
      i. **Infertility**
      ii. **Ectopic pregnancies**
      iii. Chronic pelvic pain
5. Diagnosis
   a. Clinical diagnosis
   b. Empiric therapy in patients at risk for STDs with pelvic and lower abdominal pain after other causes excluded and at least one of the following minimum criteria is present[5]
      i. Uterine tenderness
      ii. Adnexal tenderness
      iii. Cervical motion tenderness
   c. Other criteria to increase specificity include
      i. Fever
      ii. Abnormal discharge
      iii. WBCs in vaginal secretions
      iv. Elevated C-reactive protein
      v. Elevated erythrocyte sedimentation rate
      vi. Laboratory documentation of gonococcal or chlamydial cervical infection (negative results do not rule out infection)
   d. Ultrasound useful for detecting tuboovarian abscess or pyosalpinx
   e. Computed tomography (CT) scan to rule out other possible causes of lower abdominal pain
   f. Laparoscopy definitive
6. Management
   a. Admission criteria
      i. Peritonitis
      ii. Pregnancy
      iii. Failure of outpatient therapy
      iv. Unable to tolerate PO
      v. Uncertain diagnosis
      vi. Tuboovarian abscess
      vii. Presence of IUD
   b. Outpatient treatment[4]
      i. Ceftriaxone + doxycycline with or without metronidazole **or**
      ii. Cefoxitin, probenecid + doxycycline with or without metronidazole
      iii. Treat partners
   c. Inpatient treatment
      i. Cefotetan **or** cefoxitin plus doxycycline **or**
      ii. Clindamycin + gentamycin

D. Trichomoniasis
  1. Etiology: *Trichomonas vaginalis,* flagellated protozoan
  2. Symptoms and signs
     a. Incubation period 4 to 28 days
     b. Female
        i. 50% of females asymptomatic
        ii. Vaginal discharge (itchy, fishy odor)
        iii. Vaginal pH > 4.5
        iv. Nonspecific lower abdominal pain
        v. Vaginal mucosa and cervix with erosions, "strawberry" appearance
     c. Males: usually asymptomatic
  3. Diagnosis
     a. Wet mount
        i. Direct visualization of pear-shaped, flagellated organisms
        ii. 60% to 70% sensitivity
     b. Culture not routinely done
     c. PCR
  4. Management[5]
     a. Metronidazole 2- g PO × 1, or 500 mg PO × 7 days
        i. Disulfiram: reaction with alcohol up to 72 hours after last dose
        ii. Safe in pregnancy
        iii. Topical metronidazole less efficacious
     b. Tinidazole 2-g single dose, may use in metronidazole-resistant trichomonas
     c. Treat all symptomatic pregnant women to decrease risk of
        i. Premature rupture of membranes
        ii. Premature labor
        iii. Low birth weight
        iv. Posthysterectomy infection
     d. Treat partners

BACTERIAL ILLNESS

I. Anthrax (*Bacillus anthracis*)

A. Etiology
  1. Spore-forming Gram-positive rods
  2. Spores can persist indefinitely
  3. Generally, a disease of grazing animals (cows, sheep, goats, horses)
  4. No human-to-human spread
  5. Potential weapon of mass destruction

B. Symptoms and signs (3 distinct clinical presentations)
  1. Intestinal and oropharyngeal
     a. Rarest of clinical presentations
     b. Ingestion of contaminated meat
     c. Abdominal pain or dysphagia and oropharyngeal edema
     d. Dysentery like presentation
     e. 20% to 60% mortality
  2. Cutaneous anthrax
     a. Black eschar that begins as a papule or vesicle
     b. Pruritic but rarely painful
     c. Painful lymphadenopathy
     d. Associated with animal fluid, hair, wool, or hide exposure
     e. Most cases are mild and resolve with antibiotics

  3. Pulmonary
     d. Woolsorter disease
     e. Contracted from inhaled spores
     f. Incubation period up to 1 week
     g. Presentation
        i. Nonspecific flu-like symptoms
        ii. Hypoxia and dyspnea
        iii. Chest pain
        iv. Worst prognosis of anthrax types
        v. 100% mortality if not treated within 24 hours

C. Diagnosis
  1. Blood cultures
     a. Useful in disseminated septicemia
     b. High sensitivity if patient not on antibiotics
  2. Cutaneous anthrax: tissue and ulcer exudate culture
  3. Intestinal anthrax is difficult to differentiate from dysentery
  4. Pulmonary anthrax: chest x-ray (CXR) and CT scan
     a. **Widened mediastinum**
        i. Lymphadenopathy
        ii. Hemorrhagic mediastinitis
     b. Hemorrhagic pleural effusion
     c. **Absence** of pulmonary infiltrates

D. Management
   1. Prevention
      a. Household bleach solution to decontaminate victims
      b. Iodine or hypochlorite to destroy spores on equipment
      c. Vaccine administered to soldiers
      d. Postexposure chemoprophylaxis with ciprofloxacin
   2. Uncomplicated cutaneous anthrax
      a. Outpatient doxycycline
   3. Suspected inhalation, intestinal, or complicated cutaneous anthrax
      a. Admission
      b. Antibiotics: fluoroquinolones
      c. Supportive care

II. Botulism[6] (*Clostridium botulinum*)

A. Epidemiology
   1. <100 cases annually in United States
   2. Almost two-thirds of cases are infant botulism

B. Etiology
   1. Anaerobic, Gram-positive, rod-shaped
   2. Spores germinate under anaerobic environment
   3. Infant botulism
      a. Ingestion of honey or corn syrup contaminated with spores
   4. Food-borne botulism
      a. Inadequately preserved or undercooked foods
      b. Home canning
      c. Ingestion of preformed toxin
   5. Wound botulism
      a. Wounds contaminated by spores
      b. Increased during 1990s because of popularity of "black tar" heroin
      c. Iatrogenic or inadvertent from cosmetic or therapeutic injection

C. Pathophysiology
   1. Most potent biologic toxin in the world
      a. Doses as small as 0.05 to 0.1 mcg can be fatal
      b. Toxins resistant to digestive enzymes
      c. Spores are highly heat-resistant
   2. Neurotoxin inhibits acetylcholine release by blocking presynaptic receptors

D. Symptoms and signs
   1. Infant botulism
      a. Constipation
      b. Weak suck, feeble cry, poor gag reflex, and pooled secretions
      c. Generalized weakness and hypotonia with loss of head control
      d. Cranial nerve involvement follows
   2. Food-borne and wound botulism have similar presentation
      a. Nonspecific flu-like symptoms
         i. Usually afebrile
      b. Postural hypotension
      c. Cranial nerves affected first
         i. Diplopia, blurred vision, ptosis, pupillary dilation
         ii. Dysphonia, dysphagia, dysarthria, decreased gag reflex
      d. Parasympathetic blockade
         i. Decreased salivation, dry mouth
         ii. GI ileus
         iii. Urinary retention
      e. **Descending, flaccid paralysis**
         i. Symmetric descending muscular weakness
            a) Upper extremity more than lower extremity
         ii. Muscles of respiration often affected
            a) Tachypnea and respiratory failure
         iii. DTR may be decreased
         iv. Normal sensory examination

E. Diagnosis
   1. Initial diagnosis is clinical
   2. Electromyography to differentiate from other paralytic illness
   3. Confirmation is through detection of toxin in blood, wound, gastric contents, stool or food source

F. Differential
   1. Guillain-Barré (ascending weakness)
   2. Tick paralysis (ascending weakness)
   3. Miller-Fisher variant of Guillain-Barré (descending paralysis)
   4. Diphtheria (descending weakness)
   5. Myasthenia gravis
   6. Poliomyelitis
   7. Eaton-Lambert syndrome

G. Management
   1. Contact CDC if infection suspected
   2. Supportive care
      a. Respiratory monitoring
         i. Frequent vital capacity evaluation
         ii. Consider intubation if vital capacity <15 mL/ kg, or a negative inspiratory force is < −20 cm H_2O
      b. GI and GU decompression
   3. Antitoxin administration

a. Botulism equine trivalent antitoxin (CDC)
   i. Does not decrease mortality
   ii. May decrease length of disease
   iii. **Not** for infant botulism
4. Antibiotics for secondary infections
   a. No utility for botulism disease itself
   b. Also consider wound debridement for wound botulism

III. Diphtheria[6] (*Corynebacterium diphtheriae*)

A. Etiology
   1. Gram-positive bacillus
   2. Produces exotoxin
   3. Person-to-person contact
   4. Nasopharyngeal secretions
   5. Humans only known reservoir

B. Symptoms and signs[7,8]
   1. Weakness, dysphagia, voice change, anorexia
      a. Descending weakness with decreased or absent reflexes
   2. Diphtheritic membrane
      a. Necrosis caused by exotoxin
      b. Edema and cervical adenitis
      c. Adherent, bleeds if scraped
      d. Pharyngeal membrane severity correlates with disease severity
   3. "Bull-neck": cervical lymphadenopathy and edema
   4. "Malignant" diphtheria: 25% mortality
      a. High fever, severe weakness, vomiting, diarrhea, delirium
      b. Death from respiratory failure or myocarditis
   5. Complications
      a. **Airway obstruction** (membrane)
      b. Respiratory failure from neuromuscular compromise
      c. Congestive heart failure (CHF), myocarditis, conduction disturbance
      d. Paralysis

C. Diagnosis
   1. **Not** identified on "routine" cultures
   2. Membrane swabs on tellurite media with immunofluorescent stain
   3. PCR testing
   4. Leukocytosis, thrombocytopenia

D. Management
   1. Airway management
   2. Hospitalization and isolation
   3. Equine serum diphtheria antitoxin
      a. Dose based on size and location of membrane, duration of illness, and degree of toxicity
   4. Antibiotics: PCN or erythromycin
   5. Immunize close contacts
      a. Previously unimmunized or unknown should receive antibiotic therapy and immunization

IV. Endocarditis[6]

A. Risk factors
   1. Rheumatic heart disease
   2. Congenital or acquired valvular disease
   3. Intravenous drug use
   4. Cardiac procedures
   5. Indwelling venous catheters

B. Classification
   1. Acute versus subacute endocarditis
      a. Acute
         i. Predilection for normal valves
         ii. Young patients affected
         iii. Embolic stroke and acute heart failure more common
         iv. Sicker appearing than subacute form
      b. Subacute
         i. Predilection for abnormal valves
         ii. Older patients affected
         iii. Anemia common
         iv. Right-sided endocarditis less likely
         v. Organisms
            a) HACEK Gram-negative organisms *Haemophilus, Actinobacillus, Cardiobacterium, Eikinella, Kingella*
         vi. Intermittent fever and nonspecific constitutional complaints often missed on presentation
   2. Left- versus right-sided
      a. Left-sided
         i. Aortic and mitral valve
         ii. More common than right-sided endocarditis
         iii. Organisms
            a) *S. viridans*
            b) *S. aureus*
            c) *Enterococcus*
            d) Fungal
         iv. Complications
            a) CHF
            b) Stroke
            c) Systemic infarcts from septic emboli
            d) Atrioventricular block
      b. Right-sided
         i. Pulmonic and tricuspid valve
         ii. Usually in intravenous drug users

iii. Organisms
   a) *S. aureus*
   b) *S. pneumonia*
   c) Gram-negative bacteria
   d) Fungal

C. Symptoms and signs
  1. Left-sided endocarditis
    a. Septic-appearing
    b. Cardiac
      i. Acute CHF
      ii. Heart block
      iii. Chest pain
    c. Neurologic
      i. Stroke, aseptic meningoencephalitis, hemiplegia, and monocular blindness
    d. Dermatologic manifestation
      i. Roth spots (retinal hemorrhages with central clearing): immunologic vasculitis
      ii. Osler nodes (painful nodes on toes and fingers): immunologic vasculitis
      iii. Janeway lesions (painless plaques on palms and soles): infectious vasculitis most likely from *S. aureus*
      iv. Embolic splinter hemorrhages on nails
      v. Petechiae
    e. Murmurs are often indicative of aortic or mitral valve infection
  2. Right sided endocarditis
    a. Subacute illness unlikely
    b. Acute presentation of fever with respiratory symptoms
      i. Cough
      ii. Chest pain
      iii. Hemoptysis
      iv. Dyspnea
    c. Often misdiagnosed as pneumonia
    d. Murmurs less prominent

D. Diagnosis
  1. Maintain high clinical suspicion
    a. Treat empirically
  2. Echocardiography
    a. Preferably transesophageal
  3. Blood cultures
  4. Diagnostic criteria requires 2 major or 1 major and 3 minor, or 5 minor
    a. Major criteria
      i. 2 positive blood cultures
        a) At least 3 sets sent 1 hour apart
        b) Cultures of organisms common to infectious endocarditis
        c) Persistence of cultures >12 hours

      ii. Abnormal echocardiography
        a) Prior prosthetic valve dehiscence
        b) New valvular regurgitation
        c) Myocardial abscess
        d) Visible vegetation
    b. Minor criteria
      i. Predisposing risk factors or IV drug use
      ii. Fever
      iii. Vascular events such as septic emboli and Janeway lesions
      iv. Immunologic events such as Osler nodes, Roth spots, and glomerulonephritis
      v. Echo findings consistent with endocarditis not meeting major criteria
      vi. Positive blood cultures otherwise not meeting major criteria

E. Management
  1. Antibiotics
    a. Add vancomycin if high resistance area or patient already on antibiotics
    b. Special considerations
      i. Prosthetic valves: cover *S. epidermidis* with vancomycin
      ii. IVDA: cover *Pseudomonas aeruginosa* and *Serratia marcescens*
  2. Admit pending cultures particularly if history of IV drug abuse
  3. Surgical evaluation for suspected valve rupture

V. Meningococcemia[6] (*Neisseria meningitides*)

A. Epidemiology
  1. Spring and fall
  2. Military recruits and children <5 years
  3. Mortality of meningococcal disease
    a. Meningitis alone ~5%
    b. **Septicemia** without meningitis >20%

B. Etiology
  1. Aerobic, Gram-negative diplococcus
  2. Nasopharynx is the portal of entry

C. Symptoms and signs
  1. Rash
    a. May be papular, macular, or maculopapular
    b. Petechiae present in 50% to 60%
      i. Appears within 24 hours
      ii. Can involve mucous membranes
      iii. Most common on trunk and extremities
    c. Severe cases can include purpura fulminans
      i. Rapidly spreading ecchymosis
      ii. Gangrene of extremities
      iii. Associated with DIC

2. Waterhouse-Friderichsen syndrome
   a. Bilateral adrenal hemorrhage
   b. Fulminant meningococcemia
   c. Endotoxin mediated
   d. Diffuse petechial and extensive intercutaneous hemorrhage
   e. Myocarditis
   f. DIC
   g. Renal failure

D. Diagnosis
   1. Clinical diagnosis
   2. Blood and lesion culture and Gram stain
   3. Lumbar puncture for suspected meningitis

E. Management
   1. Immediate antibiotics
   2. Antibiotic prophylaxis for close contacts, health-care workers
      a. Rifampin
      b. Ceftriaxone
      c. Ciprofloxacin
   3. Quadrivalent vaccination
      a. Recommended for
         i. Military personnel
         ii. Functional asplenia
      b. Vaccination is short-lasting (<3 years)

VI. Pertussis[6-8] (*Bordetella pertussis*)

A. Etiology
   1. Highly contagious respiratory droplets
   2. Toxin production
   3. Vaccination and natural immunity do **not** confer lifelong immunity

B. Symptoms and signs
   1. Three clinical phases
      a. Catarrhal phase (1 to 2 weeks)
         i. Upper respiratory infection-like symptoms
         ii. Cough, low grade fever, rhinitis, anorexia
         iii. Highest infectivity
      b. Paroxysmal phase (2 to 6 weeks)
         i. Cough increases, fever subsides
         ii. Paroxysms of coughing (50 times per day)
      c. Convalescent phase
         i. Residual cough lasting weeks to months
         ii. Paroxysms may be triggered by URI or irritants
   2. Atypical presentations often misdiagnosed as bronchitis
      a. Occur in young infant and adults as immunity wanes

3. Complications
   a. Central nervous system (CNS)
      i. Seizures
      ii. Encephalopathy
      iii. Hemorrhage
   b. Bradycardia, hypotension, and cardiac arrest
      i. Primarily neonates and young infants
      ii. This group requires ICU admission

C. Diagnosis
   1. Often missed (atypical presentations, over-reliance on vaccination)
   2. **Lymphocytosis**
   3. CXR: peribronchial thickening, atelectasis, or consolidation
   4. Nasopharyngeal culture
      a. Bordet-Gengou medium for 7 days
      b. PCR

D. Management
   1. Medical
      a. Antibiotics: erythromycin (limited utility after catarrhal phase)
      b. Corticosteroids
      c. β-adrenergic agonists
      d. Prophylactic antibiotics for close contacts
         i. Immunity wanes >10 years
         ii. Acellular pertussis vaccine recommended for high-risk exposures. Routine booster not recommended
   2. Supportive
      a. Oxygenation and pulmonary toilet
      b. Severely ill and children <1 year require hospitalization
      c. Neonates require ICU admission
      d. Respiratory isolation

VII. Pneumococcemia[6] (*Streptococcus pneumoniae*)

A. Etiology
   1. Encapsulated, **lancet-shaped** Gram-positive coccus in pairs (diplococcus)

B. Symptoms and signs
   1. Pneumonia
      a. Severe rigors
      b. Rusty sputum
   2. Meningitis
   3. Septicemia
   4. Endocarditis

C. Diagnosis
   1. CBC
      a. Low WBC count prognostic of more serious disease

2. Blood and urine cultures
3. CXR
4. LP if meningitis suspected

D. Management
  1. Prompt antibiotic therapy
     a. Ideally based on local resistance patterns
     b. PCN, cephalosporins, macrolide, vancomycin, chloramphenicol
     c. Empiric therapy for meningitis with ceftriaxone
  2. Adult vaccination indicated for:
     a. Immunocompetent adults with chronic illness
     b. Age >65 years
     c. Immunocompromised adults
     d. Asymptomatic HIV infection
     e. Anatomic or functional asplenia

VIII. Tetanus[8] (*Clostridium tetani*)

A. Etiology
  1. Anaerobic, motile, spore forming Gram-positive rod-shaped ("drumstick")
  2. Found in soil, dust, and feces
  3. Ubiquitous spores are hearty and resistant to heat and chemicals
  4. >70% from wound (postoperative infection common)

B. Symptoms and signs
  1. Incubation is generally 3 days to 2 weeks
  2. No mental status change
  3. Weakness, myalgias, dysphagia, hydrophobia, and drooling
  4. Trismus ("Lockjaw")
  5. Risus sardonicus (facial muscle involvement)
  6. Generalized tetanus
     a. Full skeletal muscle hypertonicity
     b. Severe spasms are spontaneous or triggered by external stimuli
     c. Opisthotonos (severe spasm with arching of the back and head and heels bent backwards)
     d. Laryngeal and respiratory spasm can cause respiratory failure
     e. Autonomic dysfunction

C. Diagnosis
  1. Clinical diagnosis
  2. Wound cultures rarely helpful
  3. Rule out strychnine poisoning

D. Management
  1. Supportive care
     a. Benzodiazepines
     b. Narcotics
     c. Nondepolarizing neuromuscular blockade
     d. Continuous spinal anesthesia
     e. Consider ICU care
  2. Gentle handling
     a. Keep quiet environment
     b. Minimize unnecessary procedures and movements
  3. Elimination of toxin production
     a. Wound cleaning and debridement
     b. Metronidazole (flagyl) preferable to PCN
  4. Tetanus immunoglobulin (TIG)
     a. May shorten course and severity of disease
     b. Administer on opposite arm of tetanus booster
     c. Safe in pregnancy
  5. Td booster: every 5 to 10 years
     a. Safe in pregnancy
     b. Infection **does not** confer lifelong immunity

E. Tetanus immunization and wound care
  1. TIG not indicated if primary series completed (3 or more tetanus toxoid received)
  2. If required, administer TIG to separate site from Td
  3. If dirty wound, administer Td if >5 years since last booster
  4. If clean wound, administer Td if >10 years since last booster
  5. Administer TIG if Td allergic and consider prophylactic antibiotics

IX. Tuberculosis (*Mycobacterium tuberculosis*)

A. Epidemiology
  1. Present throughout recorded history
     a. Global emergency
     b. Leading infectious cause of death worldwide
     c. One-third of world population infected by TB
  2. Increased resurgence and emergence of drug resistant strains through 1980s
     a. Elderly harboring dormant infection reactivated by illness or immunosenescence
     b. Immigration from endemic countries
     c. Homelessness
     d. Pandemic of HIV-related TB

B. Etiology
  1. *M. tuberculosis*
     a. Humans are sole reservoir
     b. Intracellular, aerobic, nonmotile, nonspore-forming
  2. Transmitted through respiratory route
     a. Airborne particles (see Infection Control below)
     b. Only few respiratory droplets necessary for infection
  3. TB can remain dormant for years in granulomas(s)

C. Risk factors
  1. Immunocompromised (HIV, malignancy, DM, extremes of age)

2. Close contacts or occupational exposures
3. Foreign-born: Asia, Africa, and Latin America
4. Medically underserved, low-income populations
   a. Elderly
   b. Residents of long-term care facilities (nursing home, prison, shelter, etc.)
   c. Intravenous drug abuse

D. Symptoms and signs
1. Primary tuberculosis
   a. Only 10% of exposed individuals develop primary tuberculosis
      i. Positive PPD and Ghon complex may identify asymptomatic individuals
      ii. Remaining 90% of healthy asymptomatic patients with latent tuberculosis are noninfectious
   b. Constitutional symptoms
      i. Cough
         a) Most common symptom of pulmonary TB
         b) Initially nonproductive or nonspecific sputum
         c) Hemoptysis may be presenting complaint
      ii. Pleuritic chest pain
         a) Parenchymal irritation of pleural surface
         b) May represent spontaneous pneumothorax
      iii. Night sweats
         a) Fever, defervesces while sleeping
      iv. Weight loss, cachexia, and failure to thrive
   c. "Classic" presentation uncommon
      i. Fever of unknown origin may represent TB
      ii. Atypical presentations common
         a) Infants: hilar lymphadenopathy and bronchial obstruction
         b) Elderly: chronic cough and failure to thrive
   d. Physical examination findings
      i. Abnormal chest auscultation
      ii. Lymphadenopathy
      iii. Hypersensitivity reaction to tuberculosis
         a) Erythema nodosum
         b) Phlyctenular keratoconjunctivitis (severe unilateral eye inflammation)
2. Postprimary tuberculosis (reactivation TB)
   a. Lifetime risk
      i. In immunocompetent individual is 10% to 15%
      ii. In HIV-positive patients
         a) 37% with disease in 6 months
         b) 10% incidence of disease per year
   b. Signs and symptoms similar to primary tuberculosis

3. Extrapulmonary tuberculosis (EPTB)[6,9]
   a. Lymphadenitis (scrofula)
      i. Most common EPTB
      ii. Enlarging, painless, erythematous firm mass near cervical nodes
      iii. **Do not I&D**
   b. Pleural effusion
      i. Small and unilateral
      ii. Diagnosis through pleurocentesis
         a) Acid-fast bacilli (AFB) smears rarely positive
   c. Bone and joint infection
      i. Pott's disease (spinal)
         a) Spinal cord injury possible
         b) Lumbar infection may lead to psoas abscess
   d. Acute disseminated
      i. Generalized systemic illness
      ii. Typically in elderly and HIV patients
      iii. Clinical presentation varies widely
         a) Fever, weight loss, anorexia, weakness
         b) SIADH is common, often associated with meningitis
   e. CNS
      i. 6% of cases, peak in newborn to 4 years
      ii. SIADH
      iii. Tuberculous meningitis
         a) Subependymal tubercle rupture into subarachnoid space
         b) Malaise, nausea, headache, low-grade fever
         c) Focal neurologic signs, confusion, meningismus
         d) Diplopia in 70%
         e) CSF analysis
            i) **Lowest glucose** CSF levels of any meningitis
            ii) Opening pressure slightly elevated or normal
            iii) Pleocytosis: initially polymorphs then lymphocytes
            iv) Elevated protein
            v) Positive AFB culture
4. Complications
   a. Pneumothorax (<5%)
   b. Empyema (1% to 4%)
      i. Rupture of cavity is catastrophic
   c. Superinfection
      i. Healing of extensive TB leaves open cavities and bronchiectasis
      ii. *Aspergillus fumigatus* superinfection ("fungus ball")
         a) May lead to massive, fatal hemoptysis

d. Hemoptysis
   i. Mild hemoptysis is a common complication
   ii. Massive bleeding from rupture of parenchymal vessels
   iii. Rasmussen aneurysm (rare)
      a) Erosion into pulmonary artery, leading to pseudoaneurysm formation
e. Primary tuberculosis pericarditis

E. Diagnosis
   1. Tuberculin skin testing
      a. Read 48 to 72 hours later, induration not erythema
         i. 15 mm in low-risk, immunocompetent patients
         ii. 10 mm in high-risk, health-care workers, foreign born, IVDU, homeless
         iii. 5 mm in HIV, close contacts infectious TB, abnormal CXR, immunocompromised from steroids
      b. May need to repeat PPD testing in 1 to 3 weeks in the elderly (see below "booster effect")
      c. False-negative result
         i. 20% false negative in active disease
         ii. Booster effect
            a) Remote tuberculosis exposure in distant past may lead to a false-negative PPD
            b) A second PPD placement 1 to 3 weeks after the first may help detect those with waning skin reactivity (aka the "booster effect")
            c) No evidence that repeated PPD testing causes skin reactions in and of itself
      d. False-positive result
         i. Infection with nontuberculous mycobacteria (eg, leprosy)
      e. BCG (bacilli Calmette-Guérin) vaccination should not alter interpretation of PPD reading
   2. CXR
      a. Negative CXR has high negative predictive value
         i. False-negative rate 1% in immunocompetent
         ii. False-negative rate 15% in HIV-positive
      b. Primary tuberculosis
         i. Infiltrate difficult to differentiate from typical pneumonia
            a) More common in primary than reactivation tuberculosis
            b) Homogeneous, involves single lobe
         ii. Hilar and mediastinal lymphadenopathy common in primary disease and uncommon with reactivation tuberculosis
            iii. Miliary TB: multiple basilar prominent non-calcified nodules bilaterally
            iv. Tuberculoma
               a) Present in primary and reactivation disease
               b) Round nodules that harbor slow-growing bacilli
      c. Reactivation (postprimary) tuberculosis
         i. Cavitation without lymphadenopathy
            a) High infectivity
            b) Ill-defined wall suggests active lesion
         ii. Fibrosis
            a) Irregular, angular lesions with multiple calcifications
            b) Distortion of normal structures secondary to contraction
               i) Severe fibrosis with upward hilar displacement
         iii. Pleural effusion more common in reactivation disease in comparison with primary tuberculosis
   3. Microbiology
      a. Sputum sample
         i. Fiberoptic bronchoscopy or BAL may be needed
         ii. Early morning sputum collection × 3 (not recommended in the ED)
      b. AFB sputum smear
         i. Stained and looked under microscope
         ii. Results available within hours
         iii. Many false negatives and false positives
            a) Only 30% to 60% sensitivity even with 3 early morning samples
            b) Cannot differentiate between *M. tuberculosis* and nontuberculous mycobacterium
         iv. Positive sputum smear may indicate higher bacilli burden and infectivity
      c. AFB Culture
         i. Gold standard for microbiologic testing
         ii. Only 87% sensitive ("Culture negative tuberculosis")
         iii. All sputum samples regardless of smear results should be cultured
         iv. Slow-growing organism requiring 2 to 8 weeks for results
         v. Newer growth media may yield results in 4 to 8 days
         vi. Drug susceptibility testing
            a) Emergence of multidrug-resistant TB
            b) Check susceptibility to isoniazid, rifampin, ethambutol
      d. New PCR testing may provide results within hours to days

i. High specificity

ii. High sensitivity if AFB smear positive

iii. Poor sensitivity if AFB smear negative

F. Management

1. Exchanging contaminated air is essential

a. Negative pressure isolation

b. Ultraviolet radiation destroys organism

c. 3 negative smears necessary to remove from isolation (debated)

2. Massive hemoptysis

a. Defined as 600 mL of blood in 24 hours

b. Airway management with largest endotracheal tube possible

i. Patient with bleeding lung in dependent position (unlike pulmonary contusion where the **good** lung goes down)

ii. Consider selective main stem intubation

c. Emergent consultation for bronchoscopy, surgery, or angiography

3. Medical therapy

a. General considerations

i. Latent tuberculosis: infections without active disease (eg, asymptomatic individual with positive PPD)

a) Chemoprophylaxis with isoniazid for 9 months

ii. Active tuberculosis

a) Treated for 6 months

b) 4 drugs until resistance pattern determined

c) After 2 months, may discontinue pyrazinamide if TB isolates do not demonstrate resistance

iii. Extrapulmonary tuberculosis: treat for 6 months

a) CNS infection (tuberculous meningitis) is the exception, requires 9 to 12 months of treatment

iv. Consider steroids for CNS and pericardial tuberculosis

b. First-line agents

i. Isoniazid (INH)

a) 8% resistance rate

b) Prevent INH-related seizures: supplement with pyridoxine (B_6)

c) Hepatitis risk increases >35 years

d) Peripheral neuropathy

ii. Rifampin (RIF)

a) Orange discoloration of bodily fluids

b) Oral contraception failure

iii. Pyrazinamide (PZA)

a) Hepatotoxicity

b) Polyarthralgias

iv. Ethambutol (ETH)

a) Prevents emergence of RIF resistance

b) Retrobulbar neuritis

i) Decreased visual acuity or red-green color blindness

c. Multidrug-resistant TB (MDRTB)

i. Resistance to 2 or more first-line agents

ii. Most commonly from suboptimal treatment, or adding a single drug to a failed regimen

iii. Resistance spreads faster in areas of high HIV prevalence

d. Pregnancy

i. INH, RIF, ETH cross placenta and are safe

4. Noncompliant patients

a. Uncooperative and potentially infectious patients may be compelled to comply

i. Court-ordered directly-observed therapy (DOT)

ii. House arrest with DOT

iii. Incarceration as last resort

b. Example

i. Schizophrenic homeless man with symptoms and radiographs suspicious for tuberculosis may be held against his will to protect society

X. *Yersinia pestis* (the plague)

A. Etiology

1. Intracellular Gram-negative bacillus

2. Potentially devastating biological weapon

3. Traditional reservoirs were infected rats

a. More recent reservoirs include squirrels and cats

b. Vector is the rat flea *Xenopsylla cheopis*

4. Transmission

a. Bite of vector the rat flea, ticks, and human lice

b. Close contact with infected body tissue and fluids

c. Direct inhalation

B. Symptoms and signs

1. Nonspecific systemic symptoms such as fever and myalgias

a. Susceptible populations (veterinarians, animal handlers, etc.)

2. Three distinct clinical syndromes

a. Bubonic: bubos form on skin with eventual invasion of lymphoid tissue and vasculature. Generalized painful lymphadenopathy

b. Septicemic: direct invasion of vasculature without formation of bubos

c. Pneumonic: most aggressive form; severe pneumonia, sepsis, and death

3. Black plague refers to the deep cyanosis and gangrene of disseminated disease
4. Rose-colored purpura ("ring around the rosy")
5. Advanced disease leads to DIC, shock, and death ("Ashes, ashes, we all fall down")

C. Diagnosis
1. Gram stain of bubo aspirate
2. Blood, sputum, and bubo cultures

3. CXR: may reveal infiltrate or hilar lymphadenopathy with pneumonic plague

D. Management
1. Respiratory isolation if respiratory symptoms exist
2. Contact precautions until bubos dried out
3. Antibiotics: streptomycin or doxycycline
4. Supportive care as most patients present with some degree of shock

VIRAL ILLNESS

I. *Herpesviridae*[6]

A. Herpes simplex virus
1. Genital herpes (see Ulcerative Sexually Transmitted Diseases above)
2. Ocular involvement
   a. Branching dendritic ulcers
   b. Conjunctivitis, blepharitis, corneal epithelial opacities
   c. Emergent ophthalmology consultation
   d. Do not administer topical steroids
   e. Administer topical antiviral drops and oral acyclovir
3. Herpetic whitlow
   a. Herpetic finger infection (HSV-1 in medical and dental personnel, HSV-2 in general population)
   b. Intense pain and pruritis
   c. Resolves in 2 to 3 weeks
   d. Do not I&D
4. Neonatal herpes
   a. Transmission at time of delivery
      i. Requires cesarean section for delivery
   a. Presents days to weeks after birth
   b. Vesicles, conjunctivitis
   c. Neurologic involvement is common
   d. Untreated disseminated or CNS involvement high mortality
2. Herpes encephalitis (see Neurology chapter)
   a. Most common cause of encephalitis in United States
   b. Fever and bizarre behavior
   c. May be confused for psychiatric illness
   d. CSF fluid analysis may show many red blood cells (RBCs)

   e. Early initiation of IV acyclovir if clinically suspected

B. Varicella-zoster virus (VZV)[6]
1. Chickenpox
   a. Acute, generalized viral illness
   b. Fever, malaise
   c. Initially maculopapular, then vesiculated
      i. Lesions occur in crops, multiple stages present
      ii. Lesions everywhere on skin and mucous membranes
      iii. Palms and soles spared
   d. Severe disease
      i. Children with acute leukemia
      ii. Neonates <10 days
      iii. Pneumonia development in adults
2. Herpes zoster (shingles)
   a. Reactivation infection of VZV latent in dorsal root ganglion
   b. Multiple vesicles on an erythematous base
      i. Preceded by tingling or hyperesthesia
      ii. Appears along paths of single/grouped sensory nerves
      iii. Usually unilateral and dermatomal
   c. Postherpetic neuralgia: persistent pain >3 months
   d. Check for corneal involvement with lesions of the ophthalmic branch of the trigeminal nerve
      i. Suspect with lesions of ophthalmic branch of trigeminal nerve: Hutchinson sign (lcsion on tip of nose)
   e. Ramsey Hunt syndrome
      i. Facial paralysis (Bell palsy) with herpetic blisters in the auditory canal or pinna

3. Management
  a. Chickenpox
    i. Incubation period is ~2 weeks
      a) Transmits 5 days before to 5 days after vesicles
    ii. Acyclovir is safe but only modestly effective
      a) Famciclovir, valacyclovir
      b) **No aspirin in children**—Reye syndrome association
    iii. Pneumonitis or severe disease
      a) IV acyclovir
      b) Varicella-zoster immunoglobulin (VZIG)
    iv. Vaccine
      a) Live, attenuated (immunocompetent only)
      b) Primary prevention
      c) Postexposure prophylaxis (PEP) of nonimmune host
  b. Herpes zoster
    i. Pain control
    ii. Acyclovir, famciclovir, valacyclovir for simple disease, within 48 to 72 hours of eruption
    iii. IV acyclovir for disseminated disease, multidermatomal or ophthalmic involvement
    iv. Consider comorbid immunocompromise
      a) HIV testing
      b) Diabetic testing
  c. Postherpetic neuralgia
    i. Tricyclic antidepressants
    ii. Opioids
    iii. Gabapentoids
    iv. Lidocaine and capsaicin patches

C. Epstein-Barr virus (EBV)
  1. Symptoms and signs
    a. Fever
    b. Exudative pharyngotonsilitis (kissing tonsils)
    c. Peripheral lymphocytosis with atypical lymphocytes
    d. Posterior cervical lymphadenopathy
    e. Hepatosplenomegaly in 50%
    f. Evanescent rash
    g. Resolves 1 to 3 weeks although fatigue and malaise may persist
    h. Complications
      i. Splenic rupture (traumatic and atraumatic)
      ii. Tonsilar swelling that causes respiratory compromise
      iii. Characteristic rash after treatment with ampicillin

  2. Management
    a. Supportive
    b. Steroids for severe tonsilar edema
    c. Restrict from contact sport

II. Human Immunodeficiency Virus (HIV)

A. Epidemiology[6-9]
  1. Over 37 million adults and 2 million children in 2003
  2. 95% of HIV-infected individuals in developing world
  3. In United States, highest concentration in urban centers
    a. Disproportionate rate in minority groups
    b. Females account for 26% of cases

B. Etiology
  1. HIV is cytopathic human retrovirus of the lentivirus subfamily
    a. HIV-1 (most common), HIV-2 (Western Africa)
    b. Very labile, easily neutralized by heat and disinfectants
  2. Transmitted through semen, vaginal secretion, blood, breast milk
  3. Attacks primarily T 4 helper cells
  4. Viral load corresponds with clinical outcome

C. Risk factors
  1. IV drug use
  2. Unprotected sexual contact
  3. Blood transfusion prior to 1985
  4. Vertical or horizontal maternal-neonatal transmission

D. Diagnosis
  1. Serology
    a. Enzyme-linked immunoassay (EIA) and Western blot (WB) assay
    b. Positive EIA confirmed with positive WB
    c. Sensitivity and specificity is >99.9%
    d. False-negative tests occur during "window" period
      i. After viral transmission
      ii. Prior to appearance of antibodies
      iii. 95% of false-negative tests become positive in 3 months, 98% in 6 months
    e. False-positive results rare
      i. Blood transfusion containing HIV-antibody (not virus)
      ii. Children <6 months with transplacental-acquired antibody

2. Case definition of AIDS (in addition to positive HIV serology)
   a. CD4 <200 cells/mm^3
   b. AIDS-defining illness
      i. Coccidiodomycosis, cryptococcus (extrapulmonary), cryptosporidiosis (diarrhea >1 month), CMV (any system other than liver, spleen, or lymph nodes), HSV (ulcer >1 month, pneumonitis, esophagitis), histoplasmosis (extrapulmonary), isosporiasis (diarrhea >1 month), TB (pulmonary or disseminated), PCP, recurrent bacterial pneumonia, *Salmonella* septicemia, toxoplasmosis
   c. Oncologic
      i. Cervical cancer
      ii. Kaposi sarcoma (KS)
      iii. Lymphoma (<60 years)
   d. Other
      i. HIV-associated dementia
      ii. HIV-wasting syndrome
      iii. Progressive multifocal leukoencephalopathy

E. Complications (selected diseases)[8-11]
   1. Primary HIV infection (acute seroconversion syndrome)
      a. Follows primary exposure by 2 to 6 weeks
         i. Present 1 to 3 weeks
      b. Nonspecific viral syndrome
         i. Fever, fatigue, adenopathy
         ii. Pharyngitis, diarrhea, weight loss, rash
   2. Tuberculosis
      a. Dramatic increase in HIV-infected patients (50- to 200-fold)
      b. May present atypically in patients with CD4 <200 cells/mm^3
      c. Extrapulmonary disease is more common (>75% of patients)
      d. False-negative PPD common
      e. Frequent-false negative CXR
   3. Pneumonia
      a. Most common reason for ED presentation
      b. CD4 >500 cells/mm^3: encapsulated bacteria, TB, malignancy
      c. CD4 <500 cells/mm^3: PCP, atypical mycobacteria, fungal, CMV, lymphoma, KS, lymphoproliferative disorders
   4. PCP (*Pneumocystic carinii*, now known as *Pneumocystis jiroveci*)
      a. More than 80% AIDS patients acquire PCP
      b. CXR
         i. Diffuse interstitial infiltrate. "Bat-wing" configuration
         ii. May be normal

   c. Gallium scanning
      i. False positive more than 50%
   d. Bronchoscopy or induced sputum
      i. Monoclonal antibody staining of sputum
5. Cytomegalovirus (CMV)
   a. Disseminated disease is common
   b. Most common cause of retinitis in HIV-infected patients
   c. Colitis and esophagitis may also result
6. Cryptococcus neoformans
   a. 10% of patients with HIV
   b. Most commonly with CD4 <100
   c. Mortality up to 30%
   d. Sudden clinical deterioration from cerebral herniation common
   e. Fever and headache, nausea and vomiting
      i. Less common: visual changes, cranial nerve, seizures
   f. Head CT may be normal. IV contrast aids little
   g. Lumbar puncture
      i. Elevated opening pressure
      ii. Mononuclear pleocytosis
      iii. CSF studies
         a) Cryptococcal antigen in CSF (100% sensitive and specific)
         b) Fungal culture (95% sensitive)
         c) India ink staining (80% sensitive)
7. Toxoplasma gondii
   a. Most common cause of focal intracranial mass lesion (~4%)
   b. Headache, fever, altered mental status and seizure
   c. Focal neurologic deficits common (80%)
      i. Serologic testing not useful
   d. CT scan
      i. Noncontrast initial study
      ii. Contrast adds little to normal scan
         a) If clinically suspicion is high, perform contrast scan
         b) Multiple subcortical lesions
         c) With contrast, ring enhancing with surrounding edema
      iii. MRI more sensitive
8. Primary CNS lymphoma
   a. CD4 <100 cells/mm^3
   b. Altered mental status is most common clinical finding
   c. Hyper or iso-dense multiple round enhancing lesions on CT
   d. Poor prognosis, median survival <1 month
9. GI involvement
   a. Diarrhea
      i. Most common GI complaint in AIDS patients (50% to 90%)

    ii. Cryptosporidium and isospora
      a) Prolonged watery diarrhea
      b) Acid-fast stain of stool, monoclonal antibodies
    iii. CMV, adenovirus, rotavirus, others
  b. Oropharyngeal
    i. Oral candidiasis *(Candida albicans)*
      a) >80% of AIDS patients
      b) Whitish, lacy plaques easily scraped off erythematous base
      c) Indicator of HIV disease progression
    ii. Hairy leukoplakia
      a) Associated with EBV infection
      b) White, corrugated, or filiform-thickened lesions on tongue (not easy to scrape away)
      c) Often asymptomatic
      d) An indicator of HIV disease progression
  c. Esophagus
    i. Complaints of dysphagia, odynophagia, or chest pain
    ii. *Candida*, HSV, CMV, KS, MAI, or gastroesophageal reflux disease (GERD)

10. Cutaneous
  a. Preexisting dermatologic conditions can be exacerbated
  b. Kaposi sarcoma
    i. Second most common manifestation of AIDS
    ii. Widely disseminated with mucous membrane lesions
      a) Pink, red, or purple papules, plaques, nodules, and tumors
  c. Varicella-zoster
    i. Multidermatomal involvement very common
    ii. 17 times more likely than general population
  d. HSV infection
    i. Very common
    ii. Atypical presentation
    iii. May be difficult to distinguish from varicella-zoster

11. Ophthalmologic
  a. Cotton wool spots on retina are common
  b. CMV retinitis: most common cause of blindness in AIDS patients

B. Management[6-9]
  1. PCP
    a. TMP-SMX
    b. Steroids if PaO_2 <70 mm Hg
    c. Prophylaxis with TMP-SMX, dapsone or aerosolized pentamidine for CD4 <200 cells/m^3
  2. Cryptococcal meningitis

    a. IV amphotericin B: watch for nephrotoxicity
    b. Chronic fluconazole to prevent high relapse rate
  3. Toxoplasmosis
    a. Pyrimethamine
    b. Sulfadiazine PO with folinic acid
    c. Steroids if edema or mass effect
    d. Chronic therapy indicated because of high relapse rate
      i. Pyrimethamine, sulfadiazine, and folinic acid
      ii. TMP-SMX or dapsone plus folinic acid
  4. Primary CNS lymphoma
    a. Whole brain irradiation
    b. Corticosteroids
    c. Chemotherapy (methotrexate and zidovudine)
  5. Candidiasis
    a. Oral
      i. Clotrimazole troches
      ii. Nystatin
      iii. Systemic therapy (fluconazole, itraconazole) for resistant lesions
    b. Esophageal
      i. Presumptive treatment based on symptoms
      ii. Fluconazole or ketoconazole daily × 3 weeks
      iii. IV amphotericin B for refractory cases
  6. *Cryptosporidium* and *Isospora* diarrhea
    a. Symptomatic with dietary modification and loperamide
    b. Azithromycin (*Cryptosporidium*)
    c. TMP-SMX (*Isospora*)
  7. CMV retinitis
    a. Ganciclovir or foscarnet
      i. Ganciclovir intravitreal implants reduce risk of retinal detachment
    b. Intravitreal injection of fomivirsen
  8. Chemoprophylaxis
    a. Prevent initial and subsequent opportunistic infections
    b. Initiation based on CD4 count
    c. Works best against PCP, toxoplasmosis, TB, MAI

III. Marburg and Ebola Viruses

A. Epidemiology
  1. Mortality of 25% (Marburg) and 90% (Ebola)

B. Symptoms and signs
  1. 7 to 10 days after exposure
  2. Hemorrhagic fever
    a. Headache, fever, myalgias, arthralgias, lethargy

   b. Thrombocytopenia
   c. Hemorrhage (particularly GI)

C. Management
   1. Supportive

IV. Rabies[6]

A. Epidemiology
   1. Over 40,000 deaths per year worldwide
   2. ~3 cases per year in the United States
   3. Dogs and bats most important reservoir worldwide

B. Etiology
   1. Neurotropic rhabdovirus: Lyssa virus
   2. Transmitted through saliva into bite wounds or mucous membranes
   3. Virus replicates in muscle cells near bite site
      a. Stays at inoculation site for incubation period (30 to 90 days)
         i. Bite on head and neck with shorter incubation period than extremity or trunk
      b. Rapidly ascends along peripheral nerves to CNS
         i. Predilection for brainstem and medulla
      c. Enters salivary glands after replication

C. Symptoms and signs
   1. Viral prodrome
      a. Headache, fever, rhinorrhea, sore throat, myalgias, GI distress
      b. Back pain and muscle spasm common
   2. "Furious" rabies (encephalitic)
      a. Agitation and extreme irritability
      b. May be mistaken for psychiatric illness
      c. Hallucinations, ataxia, weakness, seizures can occur
      d. Aerophobia: fear of air in motion
      e. Hydrophobia
         i. Exaggerated protective airway gag reflex
         ii. Violent diaphragmatic contraction while drinking
   3. Coma after 1 week, death within days soon after
      a. Only 6 reported recoveries from clinical rabies

D. Diagnosis
   1. History of bite or exposure to animal
      a. Animal should be observed for 10 days
      b. Vaccination status should be obtained
   2. History of travel to endemic region

3. Antemortem diagnosis involves isolation of virus from brain biopsy

E. Management
   1. No specific or effective treatment for clinical rabies exists
   2. Mainstay of management is PEP
      a. PEP indicated for:
         i. Mucous membrane or open wound contact with saliva
         ii. High-risk animal bites
            a) Raccoon, skunk, fox, bats, and coyote (U.S.)
            b) Carnivores in endemic areas
         iii. PEP recommended for seemingly insignificant exposure to bats in endemic regions
            a) Sleeping in room where bat was found
            b) Unattended child
            c) Unable to obtain history from patient (ie, dementia)
      b. PEP not indicated for:
         i. Petting animal
         ii. Contact with blood, urine, or feces
         iii. Skunk spray
         iv. Domestic animals generally low risk
         v. Small rodents and lagomorphs (rabbits, hares) low risk
            a) Groundhogs and woodchucks in endemic areas are high risk
            b) Small animals die when bitten by rabid animals
   3. PEP involves 3 steps[6,9]
      a. Wound care
         i. **Scrubbing** with soap within 3 hours nearly 100% protective
         ii. Benzalkonium chloride, povidone-iodine recommended
      b. Passive immunization
         i. Human rabies immunoglobulin (HRIG) 20 IU/kg
            a) As much of dose into and around wound
            b) Remaining volume injected IM at distant site
      c. Active immunization
         i. Human diploid cell vaccine (HDCV)
         ii. If not previously vaccinated
            a) 1 mL IM (deltoid) on days 0, 3, 7, 14, 28
         iii. If previously vaccinated
            a) 1 mL IM (deltoid) on days 0, 3
      d. HRIG and HDCV must be given in different anatomic sites

V. Variola (Smallpox)

A. Epidemiology
   1. Eradicated disease as declared by WHO in 1980
   2. Last naturally occurring disease in 1977, Somalia
   3. United States vaccination program against small-pox ended in 1972
      a. Estimated protection from vaccine <10 years
   4. Untreated mortality rate of 30%

B. Etiology
   1. Airborne pathogen
   2. Potential devastating biologic weapon

C. Symptoms and signs
   1. Prodrome with fever, myalgias, back pain, and malaise
   2. Rash
      a. Easily **confused with varicella**
      b. Macules and papules that progress to classic pustules
         i. Deep-seated, firm, and well circumscribed
         ii. Lesions progress slowly as each stage lasting 1 to 2 days
         iii. Unlike varicella, the rash of variola present uniformly in the same stage
      c. Centrifugal distribution
         i. Face and limbs involvement >trunk involvement
         ii. Often forms first on oral mucosa and face

D. Diagnosis
   1. Suspect clinically
   2. Viral swab of oral mucosa or open pustule

E. Management
   1. Immediate contact and droplet isolation
   2. Isolate family members and contacts
   3. Contact authorities as terrorist attack likely
   4. Vaccination and immunoglobulin during first few days of exposure may attenuate disease severity
   5. Supportive care once rash appears

PARASITIC ILLNESS

I. Malaria[6]

A. Etiology
   1. *Plasmodium falciparum, ovale, vivax,* and *malariae*
      a. *Falciparum* is deadliest
   2. Transmitted by the female *Anopheles* mosquito
   3. Transmission by IV drug use, perinatal, organ transplant, airport malaria (airport with "stowaway" mosquitoes on board)

B. Symptoms and signs
   1. Consider in anyone with fever and travel
   2. Irregular fevers are hallmark of malaria
   3. Hepatosplenomegaly may be present in chronic cases
   4. Anemia may be present with evidence of hemolysis
      a. "Blackwater" fever: hemoglobinuria caused by severe hemolysis

C. Complications
   1. Cerebral malaria
      a. *P. falciparum* infection
      b. Fever, altered mental status, seizure, coma
      c. Mortality is high, especially children (>30%)
   2. Anemia
      a. Acute: massive hemolysis
         i. Immune destruction of RBCs from cell-surface antibodies
         ii. Thrombocytopenia
         iii. Consider G6PD-deficiency in patients treated with primaquine (therapeutic complication)
   3. Pulmonary
      a. *P. falciparum* may present with fever and cough
      b. May develop noncardiogenic pulmonary edema or ARDS

D. Differential considerations[6-9]
   1. Babesiosis
   2. American trypanosomiasis (Chagas disease)
      a. Transmitted by Reduviid bug
      b. Cardiomyopathy from parasitization of myocardium

E. Diagnosis
   1. Thick and thin blood smears are gold standard for diagnosis
   2. Thrombocytopenia common
   3. False positive VDRL

F. Management
   1. Uncomplicated malarial infection
      a. Chloroquine phosphate was treatment of choice
         i. Resistance has been increasing
      b. Only useful for areas with continued sensitivity (Haiti, Dominican Republic, Central America, areas of Middle East)
   2. Chloroquine-resistant uncomplicated malarial infection
      a. Quinine and doxycycline
   3. Complicated malarial infection *P. falciparum*
      a. Intravenous quinine or quinidine
         i. Can cause profound hypoglycemia, cardiac dysrhythmia
   4. Cerebral malaria
      a. IV quinine, quinidine or artemisinin (Primaquine)
      b. Supportive care and mechanical ventilation
      c. Anticonvulsant therapy
      d. Corticosteroids **not** beneficial
   5. Primaquine
      a. Expunge hepatic phases of *P. ovale* and *P. vivax*
      b. Must test patient for G6PD

II. Sporotrichosis[6]

A. Etiology
   1. Fungal infection by *Sporothrix schenckii*
      a. Mold on plants and roses
      b. Cats and armadillos
   2. Inoculation into skin (classically rose thorn) or inhalation
   3. Farmers, gardeners, and forestry workers at risk

B. Symptoms and signs
   1. Often painless red papule
   2. Delayed lesions form up to one month after exposure
   3. Lymphocutaneous spread
   4. Indolent form may persist intermittently for years if untreated
   5. Constitutional symptoms if spread
      a. Osteoarticular: joint pain, tenosynovitis, osteomyelitis
      b. Pulmonary involvement with cough, fever, and weight loss
      c. CNS involvement uncommon

C. Diagnosis
   1. Detection of organism in tissue or body fluids
      a. Skin biopsy
      b. Blood, sputum, joint fluid cultures

D. Management
   1. Cutaneous involvement only
      a. Antifungal azoles such as itraconazole
      b. Treatment may take months
   2. Disseminated infection
      a. Itraconazole for well appearing patients
      b. Amphotericin B for ill patients

TICK-BORNE ILLNESS

I. Babesiosis

A. Epidemiology
   1. Northeastern United States
   2. "Malaria of the Northeast"

B. Etiology
   1. Malaria-like parasite
      a. Protozoan *Babesia*
      b. Multiplies in RBCs resulting in hemolysis
      c. Causes sludging and stasis of microvasculature

2. Transmission vectors
   a. *Ixodes dammini*
      i. Concurrent infection with Lyme disease possible
   b. *Ixodes scapularis*
   c. *Ixodes pacificus*
3. Primary reservoir is the white-footed mouse

C. Symptoms and signs
   1. Spiking fevers, myalgias, dark urine, headache, fatigue
   2. Hepatosplenomegaly
   3. Hemolysis
      a. Anemia, thrombocytopenia, elevated LFTs, elevated LDH

D. Diagnosis
   1. Giemsa and Wright stain of thin blood smears reveals rings of *Babesia*
   2. "Tetrad" forms are pathognomonic

E. Management
   1. Remits spontaneously in most healthy adults
   2. Can be deadly in **splenectomized** patients
   3. Treat with quinine and clindamycin if ill-appearing

II. Colorado Tick Fever[6]

A. Epidemiology
   1. Western United States, Germany
   2. Late spring through summer

B. Etiology
   1. Orbivirus
   2. *Dermacentor andersoni* (wood tick)
      a. Concurrent Rocky Mountain spotted fever (RMSF) possible

C. Symptoms and signs
   1. Incubation of 3 to 6 days after tick bite
   2. Fever is biphasic
      a. Acute chills, lethargy, headache, ocular pain, photophobia, abdominal pain, severe myalgias
      b. Fever breaks after 2 or 3 days
      c. Recurs for another 3 days

D. Management
   1. Supportive

III. Ehrlichiosis[6]

A. Epidemiology
   1. Nicknamed "Spotless RMSF"
   2. South Central, South Atlantic
   3. Peak incidence between June and August

B. Etiology
   1. Gram-negative, obligate intracellular rickettsia-like coccobacilli
   2. Transmission through tick bite
      a. *Ixodes scapularis*
      b. Organism reside in circulating leukocytes

C. Symptoms and signs
   1. Onset ~9 days after discovery of tick (90% report bite)
   2. Abrupt onset fever, headache, myalgias, and shaking chills
      a. Less frequent nausea, vomiting, diarrhea, abdominal pain
   3. Rash in one-third of patients
   4. Complications
      a. Optic neuritis
      b. ARDS
      c. Meningitis
      d. Pericarditis
      e. Renal failure
      f. DIC

D. Diagnosis
   1. Leukopenia, thrombocytopenia, and elevated LFT in 50% to 90%
   2. Peripheral smear shows **morulae** (intracellular mulberry like clusters)

E. Management
   1. Doxycycline or tetracycline for 7 to 14 days
   2. Rifampin
   3. Most recover without residual problems

IV. Lyme Disease[6]

A. Epidemiology
   1. Most common vector-borne disease in United States (95%)
      a. Endemic in Northeastern coastal, mid-Atlantic, north central
   2. Found on every continent except Antarctica

B. Etiology
   1. Spirochete *Borrelia burgdorferi*
   2. Transmission occurs 2 days after tick attachment

a. Tick *Ixodes dammini*
b. Nymph is responsible for transmission of disease
3. Primary reservoir is the field mouse

C. Symptoms and signs—3 stages
1. Early Lyme disease
a. Erythema migrans (EM)
i. Most characteristic clinical manifestation (>60%)
ii. Well demarcated, flat-bordered, blanching erythematous oval patch
iii. Hematogenous spread leads to secondary lesions (spares palms and soles)
b. Nonspecific constitutional symptoms
c. Meningeal irritation
d. GI
i. Hepatitis
ii. Pharyngitis
2. Acute disseminated infection
a. Neurologic manifestations
i. ~4 weeks after onset of EMC
ii. Clinical triad
a) Meningoencephalitis
b) Cranial neuropathy (most commonly Bell palsy)
i) 50% with Lyme meningitis
ii) Bilateral Bell palsy in one-third of patients
c) Radiculopathy
i) Weakness, pain, and dysesthesia
ii) Extremity involvement often asymmetric
b. Cardiac manifestations
i. ~3 to 5 weeks from EMC
ii. AV block is most common with gradual resolution and favorable prognosis
c. Arthritis
i. Weeks to months after initial illness
ii. Monoarticular or oligoarticular arthritis of large joints
iii. Nondiagnostic arthrocentesis
3. Late Lyme disease
a. >1 year
b. 10% develop chronic arthritis
c. Neurologic
i. Fatigue syndromes
ii. Chronic encephalopathy is most common
a) Mild-to-moderate memory impairment
b) Hypersomnolence
c) Mild psychiatric disturbances

D. Diagnosis
1. History of tick bite in only <50%
2. EM is diagnostic

3. Serologic testing
a. Must be cautiously interpreted in context of clinical picture
b. False-negative and false-positive results are common
c. IgM
i. Peak titers 3 to 6 weeks after onset of illness
ii. Returns to nondiagnostic levels 4 to 6 weeks after peak
d. IgG
i. Detectable 2 months after exposure
ii. Peaks at 12 months
e. Early antibiotic therapy blunts the antibody response
f. ELISA, Western blot, and PCR confirmation of diagnosis
4. Lumbar puncture if neuro Lyme suspected

E. Management[6,9]
1. Vaccination
a. Considered for high-risk areas and frequent exposures
b. Efficacy of 76%
2. Prophylaxis (questionable efficacy)
a. Doxycycline 200 mg single dose PO if
i. Endemic area
ii. 72 hours after discovery of an **engorged** deer tick
iii. Tick was attached for >72 hours
b. Not recommended
i. Not engorged therefore not feeding
ii. Attached <36 hours
3. Early Lyme disease
a. Doxycycline 100 mg PO twice a day for 3 weeks
i. Amoxicillin in children or pregnant women
b. Jarish-Herxheimer reaction may occur in first 24 hours
i. Fever, myalgias, headache, tachycardia, tachypnea
ii. Rest and aspirin are therapeutic
4. Early disseminated infection
a. Neurologic disease
i. Doxycycline or amoxicillin for mild symptoms
a) Antibiotics for 1 month
b) Prednisone for facial palsy **not** recommended
ii. Meningitis, encephalitis, cranial neuritis, CSF spirochetes
a) Intravenous ceftriaxone or PCN
b. Cardiac disease
i. Mild disease (first degree AV block, PR <0.30 seconds)
a) Doxycycline or amoxicillin for 21 to 30 days

ii. High-degree block
a) Admit for telemetry monitoring
b) Intravenous ceftriaxone or PCN
5. Late Lyme disease
a. Arthritis
i. Doxycycline or amoxicillin for 30 days
ii. If arthralgias recur or persist
a) Second 4-week course of oral antibiotics
b) 2- to 4-week course of IV ceftriaxone
b. Neurologic
i. Ceftriaxone 2 g IV daily for 2 to 4 weeks
ii. Response is slow, and often incomplete

V. Rocky Mountain Spotted Fever[6]

A. Epidemiology
1. Only rickettsial illness still associated with significant mortality
a. Case fatality rate of ~5%
b. ~40 deaths in United States per year
2. Despite its name, disease is rare in Rocky Mountain states
a. Endemic in 48 contiguous states (except Maine)
b. Most prevalent in southeastern United States

B. Etiology
1. *Rickettsia rickettsii*
a. Obligate Gram-negative intracellular coccobacillus
2. Ticks that carry feed on any warm-blooded animal
a. *Demacentor andersoni* (wood tick)
b. *Dermacentor variabilis* (dog tick)
c. Dogs can become symptomatic

C. Pathophysiology
1. Organism multiplies in vascular endothelium and smooth muscle
a. Causes tPA and von Willebrand factor release
i. Microhemorrhage
ii. Microthrombus formation
iii. Increased vascular permeability
b. Type III immune response (antibody antigen activation of complement)

D. Symptoms and signs
1. Symptoms are myriad and the disease has aptly been called the "great imitator" (along with syphilis)
2. Tick bite history in most patients
3. Abrupt onset of symptoms
4. Headache, myalgias, nausea, and vomiting
a. Myositis of abdominal wall

5. Calf tenderness
6. Rumpel-Leede phenomenon
a. Petechiae formation after blood pressure cuff inflation
7. Cutaneous
a. Centripetal rash
i. Initial blanching pink or red pruritic discrete macules
ii. Initial lesions ankles and wrists and goes to the trunk
iii. Lesions may involve the palms and soles
8. Complications
a. Gangrene can occur from small-vessel occlusion
b. Cardiopulmonary
i. **Myocarditis** and decreased left ventricular contractility is usually the cause of death
ii. Interstitial pneumonitis and acute respiratory distress syndrome (ARDs)
c. Neurologic
i. Rickettsial encephalitis
ii. Meningismus
iii. Focal neurologic deficits
iv. Seizures
v. Coma
d. Renal: acute renal failure and hypovolemic shock

E. Diagnosis
1. Clinical diagnosis
2. Serology
a. Serology results are not back in a clinically timely manner
b. Indirect immunofluorescence assay (IFA)
3. Laboratory testing
a. Thrombocytopenia and hyponatremia are the most common laboratory abnormality, both occurring in ≥50%
b. Anemia, azotemia, hyperbilirubinemia, and other liver function test abnormalities occur in a minority of patients
4. Electrocardiogram (ECG) may reveal conduction abnormalities

F. Management
1. Empirically treat with antibiotics if diagnosis suspected
a. Doxycycline 100 mg PO/IV twice a day
b. Chloramphenicol 50 mg/kg/day PO/IV (max 1 g IV)
2. Supportive care
a. ARDS, DIC, CHF, shock should be anticipated
3. Steroids

a. Not routinely recommended
b. Recommended for severe RMSF with
   i. Extensive vasculitis
   ii. Encephalitis
   iii. Cerebral edema

VI. Tick Paralysis[6]

A. Epidemiology
   1. Reported worldwide, but most common in southeast and northwest United States
   2. Spring and summer

B. Etiology
   1. Most cases caused by *Dermacentor* species
   2. Toxin secreted by salivary glands during blood meal
   3. Poorly understood mechanism
      a. Conduction block in peripheral branches of motor fibers
      b. Acetylcholine release inhibited at neuromuscular junction

C. Symptoms and signs
   1. Restlessness and irritability 4 to 7 days after tick attachment
   2. Followed by ascending flaccid paralysis +/– acute ataxia
      a. Loss of deep tendon reflexes
      b. Bulbar involvement
      c. Respiratory paralysis
   3. May present with ataxia without muscular weakness ("tick ataxia")
   4. Systemic symptoms such as fever are unusual
   5. Complications
      a. Respiratory failure

D. Differential considerations
   1. Guillain-Barré (ascending weakness)
   2. Eaton-Lambert
   3. Myasthenia gravis
   4. Poliomyelitis
   5. Botulism (descending weakness)
   6. Diphtheritic polyneuropathy (descending weakness)

E. Management
   1. Find and remove tick
   2. Improvement in few hours, recovery within 48 hours

VII. Tularemia[6]

A. Epidemiology
   1. Roughly 200 cases per year in the United States
   2. Most common in southwest central

3. Untreated mortality ranges from 5% to 30%
4. Treated mortality <1%

B. Etiology
   1. *Francisella tularensis*
      a. Gram-negative pleomorphic bacillus
   2. Wide range of animal reservoirs
      a. White cottontail rabbit
      b. Domestic cat
      c. Tick
         i. *Amblyomma americanum* (Lone Star tick) and *Dermacentor variabilis* (dog tick)
   3. Mode of transmission dictates illness form (see below)
      a. Direct contact, ingestion, inhalation

C. Symptoms and signs
   1. Clinical presentations depends on entry site
      a. Ulceroglandular tularemia
         i. Most common form (80%)
         ii. Ulceration of erythematous papule 2 days after inoculation
      b. Glandular tularemia
         i. Second most common form
         ii. Lymphadenopathy without ulceration
      c. Oculoglandular in 1% to 2 %
         i. Unilateral conjunctivitis with regional preauricular adenopathy
      d. Typhoidal tularemia
         i. Systemic disease without identified entry site
         ii. Fever, chills, abdominal pain, weight loss
      e. Pulmonary tularemia
         i. Similar to bacterial pneumonia
         ii. Direct inhalation or bacteremic spread
         iii. Concern for use as biologic warfare agent
      f. Oropharyngeal
         i. Least common form
         ii. Ingestion of undercooked infected rabbit meat
         iii. Nonspecific GI symptoms that may progress to bleeding

D. Diagnosis
   1. Clinical history and physical examination findings (bubos)
   2. Serologic testing
   3. Aspiration of lymph nodes **not** recommended
      a. Risk of transmission to health-care practitioner or laboratory worker

E. Management
   1. Isolation not required
   2. Streptomycin
   3. Prophylaxis
      a. Doxycycline 100 mg PO twice a day for 14 days

MISCELLANEOUS

I. Infection Control

A. Standard precautions
  1. Apply to all patients
  2. Hand washing after secretions, excretions, and other body fluid handling
     a. Wash regardless whether or not gloves were used
     b. Plain soap and water acceptable
  3. Nonsterile gloves adequate when touching patient body and fluids
  4. Clean gown/coat to be worn by health-care provider

B. Airborne-spread
  1. Applies to infectious particles <5 microns
  2. Particles remained suspended in air
  3. Patients need to be in negative pressure isolation
  4. Door needs to remain closed
  5. Limit patient movement
  6. Health-care workers need respiratory protection when entering room
  7. Applicable infections include
     a. Rubeola (measles)
     b. Varicella (including disseminated zoster)
     c. Tuberculosis

C. Droplet spread
  1. Particles >5 microns
  2. Particles formed during talking, sneezing, or coughing
  3. Negative pressure **not** required
  4. Patients should be placed in private rooms
  5. Doors may remain open
  6. At least 3 feet between patients and health-care providers if private rooms unavailable
  7. Health-care providers should observe standard precautions and wear face mask when within 3 feet of patient
  8. Applicable infections include
     a. Meningitis (*Haemophilus, Neisseria*)
     b. Diphtheria, pertussis, plague, mycoplasma, streptococcal pharyngitis, bacterial pneumonia, and scarlet fever
     c. Adenovirus, influenza, rubella (German measles), mumps, and parvovirus

D. Contact precautions
  1. Nonsterile gown in addition to gown worn with standard precaution
  2. External gown removed prior to leaving examination room
  3. Such infections include
     a. *Clostridium difficile, E. coli* 0157:H7, *Shigella,* hepatitis A, and rotavirus
     b. Skin infections including herpes simplex, impetigo, cellulitis, scabies, lice, and herpes zoster
     c. Hemorrhagic conjunctivitis
     d. Ebola, Lassa, Marburg viruses

II. Occupational Infectious Exposure

A. Needle stick risks
  1. Higher risk with the following
     a. Deeper depth of injury
     b. Larger amount of blood/fluids involved
     c. Hollow needle higher risk than solid needle
     d. Greater viral load of source patient
  2. Hepatitis B
     a. If patient HBV positive
        i. 20% to 30% transmission risk if HBsAg and HBeAg positive
     b. Management[10]
        i. Prior immunization with antibody level ≥10 mIU/mL 3 months after third dose
           a) Consider booster immunization if >10 years since last (Controversial).
           b) HBIG not indicated
        ii. Prior immunization but non-responder
           a) 2 treatment options
              i) HBIG and vaccine concurrently
              ii) HBIG at time of injury and again 1 month later
        iii. Prior immunization but unknown titer
           a) Draw titers and treat depending on results
           b) If laboratory results delayed >48 hours, treat as if nonresponder
        iv. If no prior immunization
           a) Administer HBIG and hepatitis vaccination
           b) Administer second dose of HBIG 1e month later unless source patient HbsAg negative
  3. Hepatitis C
     a. Transmission risk is approximately 2% to 7% if source patient HCV positive
     b. No treatment or vaccination yet exists

4. HIV[11]
   a. Risk from all percutaneous exposure is 0.3% if source is HIV positive
   b. Viral load of source patient is an important variable
   c. Mucous membrane exposure with infected blood is ~0.1%
   d. PEP
      i. Recommend only for high risk exposures
         a) Source patient has advanced AIDS plus mucous membrane or skin integrity compromised
         b) Patients with symptomatic HIV
         c) Acute seroconversion
         d) High viral load >1500 copies/mL
      ii. Basic regimen includes zidovudine and lamivudine × 1 month
      iii. Administer as soon as possible
      iv. May be ineffective if started >24 hours

REFERENCES

1. Fleming DT, McQuillan GM, Johnson RE, et al: Herpes simplex virus type 2 in the United States, 1976 to 1994. *N Engl J Med.* 1997;337:1105.

2. Di Carlo RP, Martin DH: Use of quinolones in sexually transmitted disease. In: Andriole VT, ed. *The Quinolones.* 3rd ed. San Diego: Academic Press; 2000:227.

3. Gruber F, Brajac I, Jonijic A, et al: Comparative trial of azithromycin and ciprofloxacin in the treatment of gonorrhea. *J. Chemother.* 1997 Aug;9(4):263.

4. Centers for Disease Control and Prevention: Updated recommended treatment regimens for gonococcal infections and associated conditions, April 2007. Available at: http://www.cdc.gov/std/Treatment/.

5. Workowski KA, Berman SM: Sexually transmitted diseases treatment guidelines, 2006. *MMWR.* 2006;55(RR11):1.

6. Marx JA, Hockberger RS, Walls RM, eds: *Rosen's Emergency Medicine: Concepts and Clinical Practice.* 6th ed. Mosby; 2006.

7. Aghababian RV, Allison EJJ, Boyer EW, et al., eds.: *Essentials of Emergency Medicine.* Boston: Jones and Bartlett; 2006.

8. Rivers C: *Preparing for the Written Board Exam in Emergency Medicine.* 5th ed. Milford, OH: Emergency Medicine Educational Enterprises, Inc.; 2006.

9. Tintinalli JE, Kelen GD, Stapczynski JS, eds: *Emergency Medicine: A Comprehensive Study Guide.* 6th ed. McGraw-Hill; 2003.

10. Kubba AK, Taylor P, Graneek B, Strobel S: Non-responders to hepatitis B vaccination: a review. *Commun Dis Public Health.* 2003;6:106.

11. www.cdc.gov/mmwr/preview/mmwrhtml/r5011a1.html

Chapter 16

EMERGENCY PROCEDURES

Gino Farina and Kyle Vanstone

I. Abdominal Procedures

A. Diagnostic peritoneal lavage
  1. Indications
    a. Used to determine the presence of internal bleeding in patients after trauma
  2. Procedure
    a. Prepare patient
      i. Foley and nasogastric lavage to decompress organs
      ii. Patient supine
      iii. Sterile preparation
    b. Site of entry
      i. Typically infraumbilical and midline
        a) Fewer vessels
        b) Less fat to obscure anatomy
      ii. Suprauterine fully open technique preferred in second and third trimester pregnancy
      iii. Supraumbilical fully open technique preferred in pelvic trauma
    c. Open and semi-open versus closed technique
      i. Open and semi-open
        a) Use #15 blade to cut down and through linea alba
        b) Lift both rectus fascia away with towel clips to allow passage of catheter or trocar
        c) Semi-open technique utilizes catheter over trocar to penetrate peritoneum
        d) Fully open technique involves cutting through peritoneum after exposing linea alba
          i) Open technique difficult in obese patients secondary to heavy bleeding that results in false-positive lavage
      ii. Closed
        a) Infraumbilical midline entrance of needle
        b) Seldinger technique
          i) Place guide wire through finder needle
          ii) Remove needle
          iii) Pass catheter over guide wire into cavity
    d. Aspiration and lavage: 2 distinct components of procedure
      i. Aspiration
        a) 15 mL of blood (positive)
        b) Bile, feces, urine, or food aspirated (positive)
      ii. Lavage
        a) 1 L of normal saline infused in adults
        b) Gently shake or mix fluid in abdomen
        c) 700 mL of return fluid adequate for evaluation
      iii. Interpretation of aspirate fluid
        a) Positive with >100,000 RBC/mm^3, >500 WBC, or presence of amylase, in blunt trauma
  3. Contraindications
    a. Multiple abdominal surgeries
    b. Unstable patient who obviously requires laparotomy

B. Paracentesis
  1. Indications
    a. Diagnostic evaluation of ascites fluid
    b. Therapeutic relief of cardiovascular and respiratory compromise secondary to abdominal distension
  2. Technique
    a. Preparation
      i. Foley catheter to decompress bladder
      ii. Patient supine
      iii. Sterile prep
    b. Site of entry
      i. Infraumbilical midline entry: relatively avascular
        a) 2 cm below umbilicus where the rectus abdominal fasciae join to form linea alba

ii) Left lower quadrant entry- no bowel resides there

    a) 4 or 5 cm above and medial to anterior superior iliac spine

    b) Keep lateral of rectus sheath to avoid vessels

    c) Lateral decubitus positioning of patient

c. Enter with metal needle or spinal needle in obese patients

    i. Advance needle slowly to avoid perforation of intestines

    ii. Free-floating intestine will move away from needle if advanced slowly

    iii. Avoid continuous suction as it may attract bowel walls to sharp needle

d. Send fluid for cell count, total protein, cultures and Gram stain, bilirubin, albumin, LDH, amylase, glucose, triglycerides, and cytology dependent upon clinical picture

C. Gastric lavage for toxic ingestion

  1. General considerations

    a. Benefits are questionable >1 hour after ingestion

    b. No evidence that lavage improves final outcome

    c. Lavage may force duodenal passage of toxin

    d. Procedural time often exceeds 30 minutes

  2. Relative indications

    a. Ingestion within 1 to 2 hours

    b. Poison not absorbed by activated charcoal

      i. Small molecules: metals (iron, lithium), the alcohols, strong acids and alkalis, sodium, chloride, etc

    c. No adequate antidote exists

    d. Ileus-promoting toxins

    e. Formations of concretions possible (aspirin, enteric-coated medications, iron, meprobamate)

    f. Sustained-release medications

  3. Contraindications

    a. Caustic ingestions

    b. Large foreign bodies or sharp objects

    c. Inability to protect the airway (or no endotracheal tube)

    d. When drug is no longer considered to be accessible in the stomach

  4. Procedure

    a. IV and monitor

    b. Suction prepared

    c. Mild sedation if necessary

    d. Left lateral decubitus position

      i. Keeps contents in stomach rather than passage into duodenum

      ii. Decreases risk and volume of aspiration

e. Orogastric tube most commonly used

    i. Bite block of oral airway inserted

    ii. 36 to 40 Fr in adults

    iii. 24 to 28 Fr in children

    iv. Visually approximate passage distance

f. Orogastric tube gently passed

    i. Never force tube

    ii. Chin to chest may aid passage

    iii. Auscultation of stomach during air injection to confirm placement

g. Lavage with 200 to 300 mL of tap water at a time

    i. Avoid large volumes to lower aspiration risk

    ii. Substitute lavage fluid with normal saline in children to prevent electrolyte shifts

    iii. Lavage until fluid clears or no more pill fragments return

h. Administer activated charcoal after lavage

  5. Complications

    a. Aspiration

    b. Esophageal and gastric perforation

    c. Dysrhythmias

    d. Laryngospasm

    e. Hypothermia

    f. Inability to remove tube

      i. Perform fluoroscopy to exclude tube kinking

        a) Lower esophageal sphincter spasm: administer glucagon

        b) Surgical removal if kinking or knotting of tube

D. Hernia reduction

  1. General consideration

    a. Reducible hernia: contents of the hernia can be reduced back into the abdominal cavity either spontaneously or manually

      i. Nontender mass

    b. Incarcerated hernias: contents of the hernia out of the abdominal cavity enough to cause pain or symptoms of obstruction but does not compromise the blood supply to the bowel; not easily reducible

      i. Tender mass

      ii. Nausea and vomiting possible

    c. Strangulated hernias are typically incarcerated ischemic hernias whose blood supply has been compromised—do **not** reduce

      i. Tender mass

      ii. Peritoneal signs

      iii. Fever, chills, and leukocytosis

      iv. Nausea and vomiting

      v. Overlying erythema

2. Procedure
   a. Preparation
      i. Trendelenburg for inguinal hernias
      ii. Supine for abdominal hernias
   b. After optimal positioning
      i. Wrapped ice or ice water over area
      ii. Attempt to identify the edge of abdominal weakness or hernia
      iii. Firm, gentle pressure until hernia reduced
3. Complications
   a. Reduction of ischemic strangulated bowel can lead to bowel perforation and peritonitis

E. Anoscopy
   1. General considerations
      a. Useful in examination of the anus and distal rectum
      b. Anus measures ~3 to 4 cm distal to the pectinate line
      c. Rectum is ~10 to 15 cm in length and extends from the rectosigmoid junction to the pectinate line
   2. Indications
      a. Performed to locate source of rectal pain or bleeding (internal hemorrhoids, fissures, anorectal masses, or foreign bodies)
   3. Procedure
      a. Perform digital examination first to assess for pain, bleeding, or obstructing mass
      b. Place patient in lateral decubitus position
      c. Advance well lubricated anoscope with thumb firmly holding obturator in place
      d. Remove obturator and inspect 360 degrees
   4. Complications
      a. Irritation to anal mucosa, mild bleeding

II. Airway Procedures

A. Rapid sequence intubation (RSI)
   1. General considerations
      a. Used to minimize risk of aspiration and facilitate rapid intubation
      b. Results in fewer complications and higher successful rates
   2. Procedure
      a. Place patient on monitor and place IV
      b. Prepare and check equipment
      c. Pre-oxygenate with 100% oxygen for a minimum of 2 or 3 minutes
         i. Oxygen displaces alveolar nitrogen and increases reserve
         ii. 3 minutes of pre-oxygenation maintains systemic oxygen saturation for 8 minutes in healthy adults

   d. Premedicate
      i. Lidocaine (1.5 to 2.0 mg/kg over 1 minute)
         a) Used in patients with head trauma, intracranial hemorrhage
            i) Theoretically attenuates increased intracranial pressure (ICP)
            ii) Prevent vasopressor response: increase in blood pressure (BP) and heart rate secondary to airway manipulation
      ii. Fentanyl (2 to 3 mcg/kg)
         a) Also may be used when ICP elevations are a concern
            i) Helps prevent pressor response
               (a) Hypertension/tachycardia from increased circulating catecholamine associated with laryngoscopy
      iii. Atropine (0.01 mg/kg, minimum 0.1 mg)
         a) Attenuates vagal response in children and infants during laryngeal manipulation
   e. Administer sedative induction agents
      i. Etomidate (0.3 mg/kg)
         a) Advantages
            i) Does not decrease blood pressure
            ii) Quick onset and short acting
            iii) Decreases intraocular pressure (IOP)
            iv) Decreases ICP
         b) Disadvantages
            i) Theoretical risk of adrenal insufficiency even after 1 dose
            ii) May cause transient myoclonus
            iii) May lower seizure threshold
            iv) May cause nausea and vomiting
      ii. Ketamine (1 to 2 mg/kg)
         a) Advantages
            i) Bronchodilator, may be useful in asthmatics and COPD patients
            ii) Positive chronotrope and inotrope and useful in hypotensive patients
         b) Disadvantages
            i) Positive chronotrope and inotrope: use care in elderly with cardiac disease
            ii) Increases ICP
            iii) Patient may become combative with "emergence phenomenon"
      iii. Midazolam (0.1 mg/kg)
         a) Advantages
            i) Amnesic
            ii) Anticonvulsant
         b) Disadvantages
            i) Hypotension
            ii) Highly variable effective dose

iv. Thiopental (3 to 5 mg/kg)
   a) Short-acting barbiturate
   b) Advantages
      i) Onset within 1 minute
      ii) May prevent seizures
   c) Disadvantages
      i) Can last up to 30 minutes
      ii) Hypotension
         (a) Venodilation
         (b) Cardiac suppression
      iii) Laryngospasm
      iv) Trismus reported with rapid administration
v. Propofol (2 mg/kg)
   a) Advantages
      i) More rapid onset than etomidate
      ii) Extremely short half-life
      iii) Anticonvulsant properties
      iv) Antiemetic properties
   b) Disadvantages
      i) Hypotension
vi. Fentanyl (3 to 8 mcg/kg)
   a) Advantages
      i) Rapid onset within 1 to 2 minutes
      ii) Analgesia reversible with naloxone
      iii) No histamine release, does not induce hypotension
   b) Disadvantages
      i) Highly variable effective dose
      ii) Theoretical risk of chest wall rigidity ("wooden chest syndrome")
f. Administer paralytic
   i. Depolarizing agents: combines with cholinergic receptor to produce persistent depolarization
      a) Succinylcholine (1.5 mg/kg)
         i) Advantages
            (a) Extremely rapid onset <1 minute
            (b) Short duration 5 or 6 minutes
         ii) Disadvantages
            (a) Fasiculations
            (b) Increases ICP and IOP
            (c) Increased intragastric pressure predisposing to aspiration
            (d) Transiently raises serum potassium by 0.5 meq/L
            (e) Avoid in patients with severe burns and crush injuries
            (f) Malignant hyperthermia
               (i) Genetic predisposition
               (ii) Treated with **dantrolene**
         iii) Consider pretreat with one-tenth the dose of the following nondepolarizing paralytics prior to succinylcholine use to prevent the above complications
   ii. Nondepolarizing agents: competitive neuromuscular blockade
      a) Used when succinylcholine contraindicated and for prolonged paralysis
      b) Generally have a longer time to onset (1 to 5 minutes) and longer duration (10 to 120 minutes) in comparison with succinylcholine
      c) Vecuronium (0.1 to 0.25 mg/kg)
         i) Advantages
            (a) Hypersensitivity rare
            (b) Doses minimally cumulative
            (c) Generally does not alter BP or heart rate
         ii) Disadvantages
            (a) Prolonged recovery time in obese and elderly or those with hepatorenal dysfunction
      d) Atracurium (0.5 mg/kg)
         i) Advantages
            (a) OK in hepatic or renal failure
            (b) Short half-life
         ii) Disadvantages
            (a) Histamine release that causes hypotension and laryngospasm
      e) Mivacurium (0.15 mg/kg)
         i) Advantages
            (a) Shortest duration of action (5 to 10 minute half-life)
         ii) Disadvantages
            (a) Hypotension, histamine release, bronchospasm
      f) Rocuronium (1 mg/kg)
         i) Advantages
            (a) Fastest onset of action
         ii) Disadvantages
            (a) May cause histamine release
            (b) Tachycardia

B. Orotracheal intubation
   1. Laryngoscope
      a. Curved (Macintosh)
         i. Pros
            a) Less likely to touch larynx directly
               i) Less trauma
               ii) Less likely to stimulate airway reflex
            b) Provides more room for direct visualization
         ii. Cons
            a) Difficult to see vocal cords with floppy epiglottis or anterior airway

      iii. Preferred in uncomplicated adult intubation

      iv. Use size 3 blade for most adults

  b. Straight (Miller)

    i. Pros

      a) May be better in young children

        i) Miller size 0 for premature infants

        ii) Size 1 for normal infants

        iii) Size 2 for older children

      b) Better with anterior airway

      c) Better with floppy epiglottis

    ii. Cons

      a) May have higher rates of laryngospasm

      b) More difficult with large upper teeth

      c) Requires more forearm strength

2. Tracheal tubes

  a. Males

    i. Use 8 or 9 mm tube

  b. Females

    i. Use 7 to 8.5 mm tube

    ii. May need to use smaller tubes in pregnant females secondary to laryngeal edema

  c. Nasal intubation: choose a size 1 mm smaller

  d. Pediatric

    i. Traditionally use uncuffed tubes in children <8 years

      a) May use cuffed tubes without inflation

    ii. Tube size

      a) Diameter of pinky finger

      b) Age (years)/4 + 4

3. Procedure

  a. Equipment check

    i. Suction

    ii. Endotracheal tube with stylet

      a) Stylet should not jut out of tube as it may cause injury

      b) Check proper inflation of balloon at end of endotracheal tube

    iii. Laryngoscope with adequate light source

  b. Patient preparation

    i. Keep height of stretcher comfortable for practitioner

    ii. Check for and remove dentures (dentures may allow for easier bag valve mask administration)

    iii. Place patient's head forward in "sniffing" position with towel under occiput (not shoulders)

    iv. Extend neck once in "sniffing" position

  c. Employ RSI and Sellick maneuver

    i. Pressure on cricoid cartilage (not thyroid)

      a) Cricoid is fully circumferential and anterior pressure transmitted to posterior esophagus

  d. Insert blade

    i. Macintosh blades

      a) Insert from right to left, sweeping the tongue

      b) Place tip of blade firmly in valecula to bring cords into view

    ii. Miller blades are inserted midline and repositioned until under the epiglottis

    iii. Tips

      a) Novices often pass blade too deeply into pharynx

        i) Mucosa of the posterior esophagus is smooth. Pull blade back until transverse mucosal folds of larynx seen

      b) Vocal cord is attached to thyroid cartilage. Thyroid (not cricoid) cartilage manipulation with free hand may aid vocal cord visualization

  e. Lift blade in direction of handle (direct toward ceiling corner of opposite wall)

    i. Do not pull back on upper teeth as fulcrum

  f. Gently pass endotracheal tube through true vocal cords

  g. Placement depth

    i. Generally 21 cm deep in females and 23 cm in males measured mouth corner

    ii. Children, tube depth: age (years)/2 + 12

4. Placement confirmation

  a. Direct visualization

  b. End tidal CO_2 device

    i. Most commonly used device

    ii. Changes color (purple and yellow)

    iii. May be unreliable in

      a) Cardiac arrest. Ventilate at least 6 breaths prior to reading

      b) Recent carbonated drink

      c) Does not rule out glottic positioning (tip of ET tube above vocal cords that causes false-positive CO_2 change detection)

  c. Esophageal detection

    i. If proper tracheal placement, syringe plunger will pull back without resistance or bulb will reinflate. Tracheal cartilage prevents collapse

    ii. Esophageal intubation results in resistance or failure of bulb reinflation. Pliable walls of esophagus collapse

    iii. May be unreliable in obese or pregnant patients because of lower esophageal incompetence that causes false filling of syringe or bulb

5. Chest x-ray (CXR) confirmation
   a. Not definitive
   b. ~5 cm above carina
   c. If carina not visualized, tip of ET tube should align with T3 or T4 vertebra

C. Nasal intubation
   1. Advantages
      a. Minimizes neck movement
      b. Patient cannot open mouth, although emesis and aspiration can be complication
      c. Patient can be in sitting position
      d. Cannot bite tube and easier to care for
      e. More comfortable for patient
   2. Disadvantages
      a. Blind placement
      b. **Requires spontaneous respirations**
   3. Contraindications
      a. Apnea
      b. Severe facial fractures
      c. Coagulopathy is a relative contraindication
      d. Nasal intubation may be impossible with severe septal deviation
   4. Procedure
      a. Sniffing position
      b. Topical anesthetic and local vasoconstriction essential
      c. Dilate with nasal trumpet if time allows
      d. Use endotracheal tube one size smaller
      e. Direct lubricated endotracheal tube parallel to floor of nostril with bevel facing nasal septum
      f. Rotate tube when pharynx reached
      g. Advance tube decisively during inspiration at point where breath sounds are most clearly heard (above the glottis)
   5. Tips
      a. Patient will cough briefly with successful passage
      b. Slightly tilt head laterally to side of intubated nostril
         i. Turning head 30 degrees toward intubated nostril may aid passage

D. Cricothyoidotomy
   1. Indicated when endotracheal intubation cannot be performed or is contraindicated
   2. Contraindications
      a. Absolute
         i. Complete tracheal disruption
         ii. Fractured larynx
      b. Relative
         i. Age <12 years

3. Procedure
   a. Hyperextend neck if no contraindications
   b. Locate membrane below laryngeal prominence
      i. Alternative: 4 fingers above suprasternal notch
   c. Horizontal or vertical skin incision controversial
      i. Horizontal incision when membrane easily palpated
      ii. Vertical incision if palpation difficult
   d. Locate membrane and stab membrane with scalpel horizontally so that only the tip enters
   e. Incision along the inferior portion of the cricothyroid membrane will avoid heavy bleeding
   f. Dilate opening with trousseau dilator, taking care never to leave the membrane opening unattended. In other words, keep something in the "hole" at all times
   g. Insert ET tube or size 4 or 5 tracheostomy tube
4. Complications
   a. Hemorrhage
   b. Vocal cord injury
   c. Laryngeal fracture
   d. Subglottic stenosis

E. Percutaneous trans-laryngeal jet ventilation
   1. General considerations
      a. Temporary oxygenation, poor ventilation
      b. Can be used in infants and children
      c. Requires high-pressure oxygen source (50 psi)
   2. Indications same as for cricothyroidotomy
   3. Procedure
      a. Large bore IV catheter used to puncture cricothyroid membrane. Aim catheter caudally
      b. Attach 3-mL syringe to aspirate air in order to confirm placement
      c. Remove syringe plunger and attach standard endotracheal tube connector
      d. Attach high-pressure oxygen source
      e. 20 bursts per minute of 100% oxygen ~1 second each. (1 second for inspiration. 2 seconds for expiration)
   4. Complications are the same as for cricothyroidotomy

III. Arthrocentesis

A. Indications
   1. Diagnostic
      a. Septic joint
         i. Culture and sensitivity of organism
      b. Diagnosis of crystalline disease

c. Diagnosis of fractures/tendon/meniscus with aspiration of blood or fat particles

d. Determine open fractures or penetration of joint by projectile

   i. Inject with methylene blue

2. Therapeutic

   a. Aspiration of tense effusion or hemarthrosis

   b. May replace fluid with lidocaine, bupivacaine, morphine, and/or corticosteroids

B. Contraindications

1. Overlying cellulitis

   a. Do not puncture infected skin and enter joint space

2. Coagulopathy is a relative contraindication

C. Fluid interpretation (see Immunology and Rheumatology chapter)

1. Normal joint fluid

   a. Clear enough to read newsprint

   b. Straw colored

   c. Normal fluid will not clot

      i. However, mixed with 4 parts 2% acetic acid will form a good clot when normal

      ii. Infected fluid will have poor clotting with acetic acid

   d. Positive "string sign"

      i. Dropped fluid from a syringe will form a string 5 to 10 cm long

      ii. Poor string sign indicates decreased viscosity and possible infection

2. Abnormal fluid

   a. Gram stain is positive in only 65% of patients with septic arthritis which depends on organism

D. Shoulder

1. Anterior approach

   a. Insert needle inferior and lateral to coracoid process toward the glenoid

2. Posterior approach

   a. From behind patient, "walk" fingers laterally along scapular ridge

   b. Insert needle 1 finger breadth below the scapular ridge into the depression felt prior to the bend of the scapular ridge into the acromion

E. Elbow (Figure 16–1)

1. Lateral approach

   a. Position elbow flexed to 90 degrees

   b. Identify the lateral epicondyle and radial head (lateral to the olecranon)

      i. Radial head can be easily identified with protonation and supination of the forearm while palpating the elbow

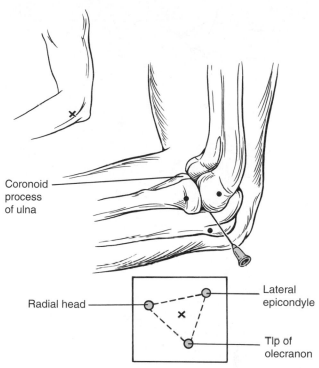

FIGURE 16–1. Arthrocentesis of elbow. (Reproduced, with permission, from Tintinalli JE, Kelen GD, Stapczynski JS: *Tintinalli's Emergency Medicine: A Comprehensive Study Guide*, 6th ed. Copyright © 2004, New York: McGraw-Hill.)

   c. Insert needle in the "trisection" of radial head, lateral epicondyle, and olecranon

2. **Avoid medial approach** as vessel and ulnar nerve may be damaged

F. Wrist (Figure 16–2)

1. Position 20 degrees flexion and slight ulnar deviation

2. Identify Listers tubercle

   a. Located in the center of the dorsal aspect of the distal end of the radius

3. Insert needle in depression slightly distal and ulnar to Lister tubercle

G. Knee

1. Approach medially or laterally

2. Keep leg flexed slightly at 20 to 30 degrees and have quadriceps muscles relaxed for easier access

3. Insert needle at midpoint or upper portion of patella directed beneath the posterior surface of patella into joint

4. May distract patella off intercondylar notch for assistance

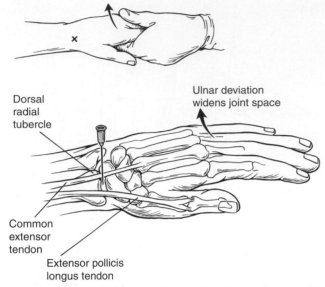

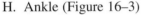

FIGURE 16–2. Arthrocentesis of wrist. (Reproduced, with permission, from Tintinalli JE, Kelen GD, Stapczynski JS: *Tintinalli's Emergency Medicine: A Comprehensive Study Guide*, 6th ed. Copyright © 2004, New York: McGraw-Hill.)

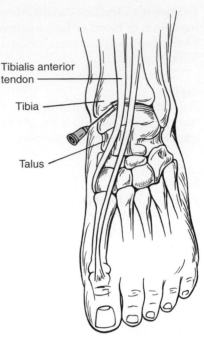

FIGURE 16–3. Arthrocentesis of ankle. (Reproduced, with permission, from Tintinalli JE, Kelen GD, Stapczynski JS: *Tintinalli's Emergency Medicine: A Comprehensive Study Guide*, 6th ed. Copyright © 2004, New York: McGraw-Hill.)

H. Ankle (Figure 16–3)
 1. Keep foot plantar flexed
 2. Insert needle medial to anterior tibial tendon
 3. Direct needle to the anterior edge of medial malleolus

IV. Cardiothoracic Procedures

A. Carotid sinus massage
 1. Indications
  a. Differentiating supraventricular tachycardia (SVT) with aberrancy versus ventricular tachycardia etiology of a wide complex tachycardia
  b. Evaluation of narrow complex tachycardia where p waves are not visible
  c. Aborting SVT
 2. Procedure
  a. General considerations
   i. Affects both SA node and AV node
  b. Contraindications
   i. Carotid bruit present
   ii. Do not perform simultaneous bilateral carotid massage
   iii. Avoid in patients with recent MI
  c. Procedure
   i. Monitoring and pacing/defibrillator equipment
   ii. Atropine and amiodarone and lidocaine at bedside

   iii. Slight reverse trendelenburg to distend carotid bulb
   iv. The carotid bulb is located midway between the angle of the mandible superiorly and the superior pole of the thyroid cartilage inferiorly
   v. Apply pressure for 5 seconds
    a) Preferentially massage right carotid to prevent stroke on dominant left hemisphere
   vi. Repeat in 1 minute if necessary

B. Cardiac Pacing
 1. Indications
  a. Symptomatic sinus disease
   i. Bradycardia
  b. Myocardial infarction associated with
   i. New left bundle branch block (LBBB) if symptomatic
   ii. Right bundle branch block (RBBB) with left anterior fascicle block if symptomatic
   iii. Alternating RBBB and LBBB block
   iv. Mobitz II second degree heart block
  c. Third-degree heart block
  d. Asystoli
  e. Overdrive pacing for tachycardia

2. Transcutaneous pacing
   a. Rapid and easy to apply
   b. May not capture
   c. Uncomfortable for patient
3. Transvenous
   a. Right internal jugular and left subclavian veins most commonly used although femoral access also feasible
   b. Electrocardiographic guidance if patient has cardiac activity (does not show up on ECG unless native cardiac activity present)
      i. Attach V lead to **negative** electrode (distal terminal) of the pacer wire
         a) Any V lead may be used
      ii. Attach limb leads to patient
      iii. Monitor QRS complex of attached V lead for location of wire
         a) Large, biphasic P waves indicate wire in right atrium
         b) Successful placement in right ventricle results in ST segment elevation (current of injury)
4. Threshold
   a. Good positioning of transvenous pacemaker leads indicated by capture with <1 mA
   b. Typical transcutaneous capture requires 54 mA
   c. Start mA high and decrease until you lose capture
      i. This is the threshold
         a) Usually between 0.3 and 0.7 mA
      ii. Set mA 1.5 to 2 times threshold for safety
5. Complications
   a. Same as for internal jugular, subclavian vein central line placement

C. Pericardiocentesis
1. General considerations
   a. 100 to 150 of **acute** fluid accumulation can be symptomatic
   b. Small amounts of fluid removal can lead to significant amelioration of symptoms
   c. Ultrasound or fluoroscopic guidance for all nonemergent situations
2. Procedure
   a. IV line and monitoring
   b. Premedication with atropine may prevent bradycardia
   c. Head of bed to 45 degrees to bring heart closer to chest wall
   d. Nasogastric decompression if distended abdomen
   e. Landmarks are controversial
      i. Subxiphoid approach
         a) Needle inserted at 30 to 45 degree angle towards the left shoulder (controversial)
            i) Directing towards right shoulder may lead to injury of thin-walled right atria
         b) Angle to skin >45 degrees may injure abdominal organs
         c) Usually about 6 to 8 cm to pericardial fluid
      ii. Apical subcostal approach may be best visualized by ultrasound
      iii. Parasternal approach
         a) 3 or 4 cm lateral to sternal border to avoid internal mammary artery in fifth intercostal space
         b) Higher incidence or pneumothorax
   f. Electrocardiographic assistance
      i. Attach needle to V lead with alligator clips
      ii. A current of injury pattern indicates contact with epicardium. Withdraw needle a few mm until current of injury disappears
   g. Guidewire can be advanced and catheter placed into pericardial space via seldinger technique
3. Complications
   a. Myocardial or coronary vessel laceration with beating heart
      i. Left anterior descending artery particularly at risk
   b. Dysrhythmias
   c. Pneumothorax
   d. Air embolism

D. Resuscitative thoracotomy
1. Indications
   a. Time of injury <30 minutes prior to arrival
   b. <5 minutes CPR in nonintubated patients, <10 minutes CPR in intubated patients
   c. Mechanisms of injury
      i. Blunt trauma, vital signs in field, electrical activity on monitor
      ii. Penetrating trauma with organized electrical activity
2. Contraindications
   a. Must consider limited patient survival to injury risk for health-care provider
   b. American College of Surgeons recommend **not** performing emergency thoracotomy for blunt trauma patients who arrest prior to ED arrival (controversial)
3. Procedure (Figure 16–4)
   a. Intubate patient and pass nasogastric tube to help differentiate esophagus from aorta. Perform simultaneously with thoracotomy
   b. Anterolateral incision traditionally used over fifth intercostal space when site of injury is unclear

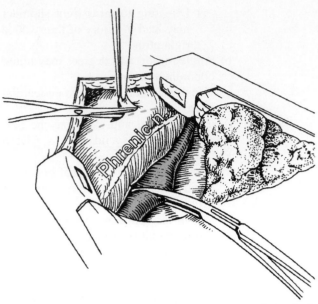

FIGURE 16–4. Thoracotomy. Phrenic nerve parallel to incision. (Reproduced, with permission, from Brunicardi FC, Andersen DK, Billiar TR, et al: *Schwartz's Principles of Surgery,* 8th ed. Copyright © 2005, New York: McGraw-Hill.)

c. Extend incision across sternum to right if necessary

d. Start 2 or 3 cm lateral to sternum to avoid injury to internal mammary artery

e. Hold ventilation momentarily and allow lung to collapse prior to entering pleura

f. Pericardiotomy

   i. Open pericardial sac if cardiac injury suspected

   ii. Start incision near diaphragm and up vertically anterior and medial to the phrenic nerve

   iii. Direct cardiac compression

      a) Avoid using fingertips. Use palm or entire palmer surface of fingers

      b) Keep heart as close to anatomical position to avoid kinking of vessels

      c) Compress perpendicular to septum (landmark—left anterior descending artery is located over the interventricular septum)

   iv. Cardiac lacerations

      a) May use Foley catheter for temporary control of bleeding as suture or stapling takes place

        i) Insert Foley into defect

        ii) Inflate balloon

        iii) Pull back to occlude

      b) Avoid suturing and occluding coronary vessels

g. Aortic cross-clamping

   i. Identify aorta

      a) Aorta lies directly anterior to vertebrae

      b) Esophagus lies anterior and medial to aorta but sometimes difficult to differentiate. Palpation of nasogastric tube in esophagus may aid differentiation

   ii. Apply DeBakey aortic clamp

      a) Temporary occlusion of descending aorta to maintain cerebral and myocardial perfusion >70 mm Hg

      b) Adjust and loosen aortic occlusion to keep brachial pulse ~120 mm Hg

E. Thoracentesis

1. Indications

  a. Generally nonemergent

  b. Diagnostic

    i. Transudate versus exudates (see Pulmonary chapter)

    ii. Diagnosis of empyema requiring chest tube (thick pus, glucose <60, pH <20)

  c. Therapeutic

    i. Severe dyspnea secondary to effusion

2. Relative contraindications

  a. Overlying cellulitis or herpes zoster

  b. Mechanical ventilation

  c. Coagulopathy

3. Landmarks

  a. Position

    i. Preferred position is with patient upright, arms resting forward on a table

  b. Identify the midscapular line

  c. Percuss dullness or decreased fremitus to localize fluid level

  d. Avoid puncture below eighth intercostal space

    i. At or just below the inferior angle of the scapula

4. Procedure

  a. Anesthesize generously using anesthetic needle to locate pleural fluid

    i. Hold needle perpendicular entering above the lower rib

  b. Enter using needle, over-the-needle catheter or through-the-needle catheter (most common) apparatus

    i. All require 3-way stopcock to allow fluid removal with minimal manipulation of needle or catheter

    ii. At all times during procedure care should be taken to place slight negative pressure on needle entering the thorax and at no

time should an uncovered needle hub be in the pleural space
   - a) This will prevent communication of air with the pleural space and pneumothorax
5. Complications
   a. Pneumothorax
   b. Hemothorax
   c. Localized organ puncture (spleen, liver)

F. Tube thoracostomy
1. Indications
   a. Tension pneumothorax
   b. Empyema
   c. Hemothorax and trauma
   d. Pneumothorax with positive pressure ventilation
2. Relative contraindications
   a. Multiple pleural adhesions
   b. Multiple emphysematous blebs
3. Procedure
   a. Skin incision
      i. Location: fourth or fifth intercostal space
         a) Nipple line
      ii. Midaxillary line
      iii. Above the lower rib
         a) To avoid neurovascular structures that run below the rib
   b. Blunt dissection with large Kelly clamp above the lower rib
   c. Push through parietal pleura. A "pop" may be felt and gush of air released
   d. **Finger sweep** for lung adhesions and assurance of safe passage
   e. Advance tube superiorly, posterior and medially toward lung apex
   f. Check to see all holes inserted into chest cavity
   g. Prophylactic antibiotics controversial
4. Complications
   a. Infection
   b. Lung laceration
   c. Re-expansion pulmonary edema
      i. Rare and unpredictable
      ii. Higher incidence in subacute pneumothorax
      iii. May have unilateral pulmonary edema
      iv. Recommend slow re-expansion of pneumothorax. Avoid wall suction

V. Head and Neck Procedures

A. Peritonsilar abscess (PTA)
1. General considerations
   a. Treatment options include antibiotics plus either needle aspiration or incision and drainage
   b. As the name indicates, the abscess is **peri**tonsillar and therefore, the needle is not placed into tonsil
   c. Avoid internal carotid artery, which is located ~2.5 cm inferior laterally to tonsil
   d. 25% false-negative tap rate
   e. Admit patients with negative aspirations if the examination and history strongly suggest PTA
2. Procedure
   a. Premedicate with an opioid and an **intramucosal** local anesthetic
   b. Use finger to sweep anterior to posterior across palate to peritonsilar area mimicking the path of food. This will reduce gag and minimize chances of the patient's biting, and enables you to check for area of greatest fluctuance
   c. Insert 18- or 20-gauge needle into area of greatest fluctuance
   d. If no obvious fluctuance is appreciated, the superior pole of the peritonsilar space should be aspirated first as most PTAs arise there
   e. If a dry tap occurs, the second and third attempts should be made in the middle then inferior pole of the peritonsilar space
   f. Do not aspirate a depth >1 cm to avoid hitting the internal carotid artery. Great depths can be avoided by cutting off the distal 1 cm of the plastic needle cover and placing it back on the needle as a guard

B. Epistaxis control
1. General consideration: epistaxis characterized by location
   a. Anterior epistaxis most common
      i. **Kiesselbach plexus**, located at the anterior portion of the nasal septum, is the most common source of anterior bleeds
   b. Posterior epistaxis
      i. **Sphenopalatine artery**, located at the posterior aspect of middle turbinate, is the most common source of posterior bleeds
      ii. Patients complain of bleeding from both nostrils
      iii. Oropharyngeal inspection may reveal profuse bleeding
2. Inspection
   a. Have patient blow nose or suction blood
   b. If bleeding profuse, apply cotton soaked in topical anesthetic/vasoconstrictor, for 5 minutes. Options include
      i. 1% tetracaine + 0.05% oxymetazoline (Afrin) solution
      ii. 2% lidocaine with 1:100,000 epinephrine
      iii. 4% cocaine solution
   c. Once localized can attempt to treat

3. Management of anterior epistaxis
   a. Cautery and hemostatic gels
      i. Cautery
         a) Silver nitrate stick: apply in circular motion outside-in for 3 to 4 seconds
         b) Electrocautery: increased risk of perforation and difficult to control in tight space
         c) Complications: septal perforation (avoid bilateral cautery, do not attempt cautery >2 times)
      ii. Hemostatic gel: apply absorbable gelfoam or cellulose
         a) Does not work well with heavy bleeding
      iii. Consider packing if above measures unsuccessful
   b. Anterior packing
      i. Nasal tampon
         a) Lubricated and advanced along the inferior aspect of nasal canal
         b) Tampon will expand when it comes in contact with blood or saline
         c) Results improved if a vasoconstrictor is added to tampon
      ii. Gauze
         a) Ribbon gauze impregnated with petroleum jelly and antibiotic
         b) Gauze is packed posterior to anterior and inferior to superior filling as much of nasal cavity as possible by means of bayonet forceps
      iii. Consider bilateral packing to tamponade septum
      iv. Prescribe antibiotics after packing complete
      v. Complications of anterior packing
         a) Infection
         b) Neurogenic syncope during packing
         c) Septal pressure necrosis
         d) Failed bilateral anterior packing is the definition of posterior epistaxis
4. Management of posterior epistaxis
   a. Inflatable urinary catheter
      i. Foley catheter: 10 to 14 French with 30-cc inflatable balloon
      ii. Insert catheter into bleeding nostril past site of bleed
      iii. Inflate with 5 to 7 cc of air or saline and pull back onto posterior site of bleed
      iv. Inflate catheter additionally until fit is snug
      v. Place anterior nasal packing in both nares to prevent septal deviation
      vi. Secure catheter in place

   b. Posterior nasal gauze pack
      i. Catheter advanced through nostril until visualized in the posterior oropharynx
      ii. Catheter grasped with forceps
      iii. Gauze pack attached to catheter
      iv. Catheter with gauze pack is withdrawn from nostril until gauze pack is firmly against area of bleed
      v. Anterior nose packed with gauze as above
      vi. Catheter secured in place
   c. Dual balloon pack
      i. Anesthetize nostril
      ii. Advance pack past site of bleed
      iii. Inflate posterior balloon with 5 to 7 cc of air or saline and pull back onto the site of bleed
      iv. Inflate catheter an additional 5 to 7 cc or before patient experiences discomfort
      v. Inflate anterior balloon, providing anterior packing
      vi. Pack opposite nare
      vii. Secure in place
   d. Complications
      i. Infection
      ii. Septal deviation, necrosis
      iii. Aspiration
      iv. Neurogenic syncope
      v. Hypoxia and hypercarbia
      vi. Dysphagia
   e. Administer antibiotics after packing
   f. Admit all posterior packed patients to a monitored bed

C. Mandibular dislocation
   1. Condyles lock anterior to eminence
   2. Dislocation may occur unilaterally or bilaterally
   3. Procedure
      a. Benzodiazepines for muscle spasm
      b. Push down and backward with thumbs placed on the lower molar teeth
      c. Take care to prevent injury to heath-care provider's fingers

D. Contact lens removal
   1. Hard contact lens in awake patient
      a. Direct patient to look toward nose and then toward chin
      b. The lower eyelid catches the edge of the contact lens and spontaneously removes it
   2. Hard contact lens removal in unresponsive patient
      a. Use thumbs to retract upper and lower eyelids
      b. Close eyelids with gentle pressure, applying firmer pressure on lower eyelid

E. Lateral canthotomy
  1. General considerations
     a. Used to release pressure and decrease intra-orbital pressure
     b. Returns retinal artery flow
  2. Indications
     a. Orbital compartment syndrome secondary to trauma
        i. Retrobulbar hematoma leading to acute loss of visual acuity, increased intraorbital pressure, and proptosis in the awake patient
        ii. Intraorbital pressure >40 mm Hg in the unconscious patient
  3. Contraindications
     a. Suspected globe rupture
  4. Procedure
     a. Anesthetize lateral canthus with lidocaine with epinephrine
     b. Use small hemostat to crush lateral canthus in order to minimize bleeding
     c. Incise superior and inferior crus of lateral canthal tendon located at edge of outer eye margin
  5. Complications
     a. Inadvertent globe rupture, bleeding, and infection

VI. Procedural Anesthesia

A. Topical
  1. Benzocaine
     a. Mucous membrane anesthesia
     b. Adverse effects: methemoglobinemia
  2. Lidocaine and prilocaine (EMLA cream)
     a. Produce anesthesia over intact skin >60
  3. Ethyl chloride and fluorimethane sprays
     a. Evaporation leads to skin cooling and instant moderate anesthesia for ~1 minute
  4. Tetracaine-adrenaline-cocaine (TAC)
     a. Apply for 10 minutes to wound
     b. Wounds <5 cm in length
     c. Avoid use in end organs (fingers, nose, penis, etc)
     d. Particularly useful for face and scalp
     e. Avoid mucous membranes

B. Local
  1. Decrease pain of infiltration
     a. Use smaller gauge needle
     b. Add sodium bicarbonate (1 in 10 parts)
     c. Room temperature
  2. Plus epinephrine
     a. Prolongs duration of anesthesia
     b. Decreases bleeding

     c. Slows absorption and decreases potential for toxicity
     d. Allows greater volume to be used
     e. Traditionally taught to avoid in areas of end artery supply
        i. "Nose, toes, fingers, and hose (penis)"
  3. Local anesthetics may have antimicrobial properties in vitro
     a. Aspirate culture fluid prior to instilling anesthesia
     b. Bicarbonate addition may increase antimicrobial activity
  4. Complications
     a. Allergic reactions
        i. Analgesics are amides or esters
           a) Amides
              i) Lidocaine
              ii) Bupivacaine
           b) Esters
              i) Procaine
              ii) Tetracaine
        ii. Most allergies result from the metabolite para-aminobenzoic acid (PABA)
           a) PABA is a metabolite of esters
        iii. Pure amides rarely cause allergy
           a) Multidose amide preparations may contain the preservative methylparaben (MPB) which is structurally similar to PABA
        iv. If true or unclear allergy to esters and amides, consider use of antihistamine injection such as diphenhydramine.
     b. Seizures
     c. Respiratory arrest
     d. Maximum dose lidocaine
        i. 5 mg/kg for plain lidocaine
        ii. 7 mg/kg for lidocaine plus epinephrine

C. Regional blocks
  1. General considerations
     a. Alternative to local anesthesia for laceration repairs
     b. Alternative to conscious sedation for reduction of fractures or dislocations
  2. Head and neck
     a. Supraorbital block: forehead (Figure 16–5)
        i. Procedure
           a) 1 to 3 cc of anesthetic placed in the area of the supraorbital notch
           b) If no response, place anesthetic from the lateral to medial aspect of the orbital rim
        ii. Complications
           a) Hematoma and rarely ecchymosis

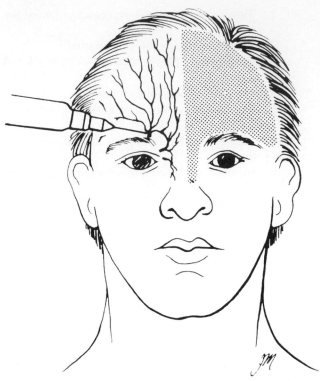

FIGURE 16–5.   Supraorbital regional block. (Reproduced, with permission, from Stone CK, Humphries RI: *Current Diagnosis & Treatment: Emergency Medicine,* 6th ed. Copyright © 2008, New York: McGraw-Hill.)

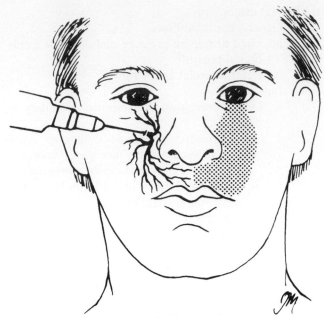

FIGURE 16–6.   Infraorbital regional block. (Reproduced, with permission, from Stone CK, Humphries RI: *Current Diagnosis & Treatment: Emergency Medicine,* 6th ed. Copyright © 2008, New York: McGraw-Hill.)

    b. Infraorbital block: upper lip and midface (Figure 16–6)
        i. Intraoral approach
            a) Needle injected 0.5 cm from the buccal surface along the long axis of the second bicuspid until the needle is palpated along the inferior foramen ~2.5 cm deep
            b) If needle directed too posterior or superior could enter the orbit
            c) Alternative approach is to inject 5 cc of anesthetic in the upper buccal fold and massage the tissue for 10 to 15 seconds
        ii. Extraoral approach
            a) Needle advanced through skin aiming toward infraorbital foramen then massage area for 10 to 15 seconds
            b) Avoid epinephrine because of possibility of infiltrating facial artery
    c. Mental block: lower lip
        i. Intraoral approach
            a) Retract lip with left hand and insert needle at level of canine inferiorly toward the mental foramen
            b) Deposit 3 cc of anesthetic

        ii. Extraoral approach
            a) Inject 2 to 3 cc anesthetic at mental foramen aligned below second premolar
3. Hand and wrist (Figure 16–7)
    a. Digital block
        i. Anesthetic placed on medial, lateral, and dorsal surface of digit as proximal as possible at metacarpophalangeal joint
    b. Median nerve block: lateral two-thirds of the palm, palmar surface of lateral 3.5 digits
        i. Located between palmaris longus and flexor carpi radialis tendons ~1 cm below skin at proximal wrist crease
    c. Ulnar nerve block: medial (ulnar) one-third of the hand
        i. Requires 2 separate injections
            a) Inject 3 to 4 cc of anesthetic underneath flexor carpi ulnaris (FCU) tendon
                i) Nerve runs between FCU and ulnar artery and deep to the ulnar artery
                    (a) Palpate proximal to pisiform bone when patient flexes wrist against resistance
            ii) Lateral needle entry is easier than volar to avoid puncturing ulnar artery
                    (a) Aspirate to avoid arterial injection

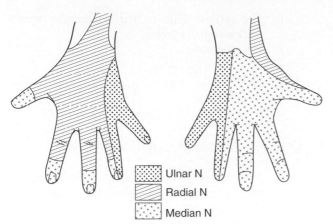

FIGURE 16–7. Sensory innervations of the hand.

(b) Superficial ulnar branches blocked with subcutaneous "wheal" of anesthetic from FCU to mid-dorsum of wrist at proximal crease.

 d. Radial nerve block: lateral two-thirds of the dorsal surface of the hand, dorsal surface of lateral 3.5 digits

  i. Inject wheal of anesthetic subcutaneously just lateral (radial) to pulse around to mid-dorsum of wrist

4. Foot

 a. Sural nerve block: lateral foot

  i. Needle inserted 1 cm above the lateral malleolus injecting anesthetic between the Achilles tendon and lateral malleolus

 b. Posterior tibial block: sole of foot

  i. Needle inserted 1 cm above medial malleolus, posterior-to-posterior tibial artery, injecting anesthetic between Achilles tendon and medial malleolus

 c. Superficial peroneal nerve block: dorsum of foot including the first web space of foot

  i. Anesthetic placed between extensor hallucis longus tendon and lateral malleolus on the anterior surface of the ankle

VII. Urologic Procedures

A. Radiologic imaging

 1. General considerations

  a. Injury to lower urinary tract must be ruled out prior to assessment of injury to upper urinary tract. "down-up evaluation"

  b. This order is necessary to avoid missing injury

2. Retrograde urethrogram

 a. Indications

  i. Performed to assess integrity of urethra

 b. Procedure

  i. Order baseline supine abdominal x-ray

  ii. Advance a Christmas tree adapter attached to 60-cc syringe snugly into distal urethra

   a) May also insert Foley catheter just inside urethra and inflate balloon for snug fit

  iii. Inject 50 to 60 mL of contrast slowly (50 mL diatrizoate sodium-diatrizoate meglumine in 450 mL normal saline)

  iv. Take urethrogram

  v. Flame-like extravasation is a positive test for urethral injury

3. Retrograde cystogram

 a. Obtain baseline supine abdominal radiograph

 b. Fill bladder with contrast material to gravity and then clamp Foley

  i. First check abdominal x-ray after first 100 mL instillation. If extravasation present, study is positive and terminated

  ii. If bladder contraction occurs then stop and slowly administer an additional 50 mL

  iii. Stop if a total of 400 mL is instilled

   a) Volumes <400 mL in adults may have false negatives

   b) Goal is to slightly overextend the bladder

 c. Obtain post-fill abdominal x-ray

 d. Remove clamp and drain by gravity

 e. Obtain post evacuation abdominal x-ray

 f. Interpretation of results

  i. Extravasation of fluid reveals positive bladder injury

  ii. Extravasation may be intra or extraperitoneal

   a) Extraperitoneal

    i) Extravasation flame-like projecting lateral to bladder

    ii) Mostly nonsurgical management unless bladder neck involvement

   b) Intraperitoneal

    i) Extravasation outlines abdominal structures

    ii) Fills paracolic gutters

    iii) Surgical management

4. CT cystogram

 a. Procedure

  i. Place Foley catheter

  ii. Instill 350 mL of diluted contrast material (50 mL diatrizoate sodium-diatrizoate meglumine, 450 mL normal saline)

     iii. Contiguous 10-mm axial images are then obtained from the dome of the diaphragm to the perineum
  b. Interpretation
     i. Interstitial injury: intramural contrast material without extravasation
     ii. Intraperitoneal: same as for retrograde cystogram
     iii. Extraperitoneal
       a) Simple: contrast around the bladder
       b) Complex: contrast dissects beyond the bladder into different pelvic fascial planes

VIII. Vascular Procedures

A. General considerations
  1. Poiseuille law
    a. Flow is related to radius of catheter to the fourth power and inversely related to catheter length
     i. Therefore, if catheter's radius is doubled, flow increases 16-fold
     ii. If length is doubled flow will decrease by half

B. Venous cutdown
  1. Anatomic locations
    a. Saphenous vein at the ankle
     i. Just anterior to medial malleolus
     ii. Elastic and easily dissected out
     iii. Highest rates of infection in comparison with other locations
     iv. May have difficulty infusing fluids quickly secondary to vein valves
    b. Basilic vein
     i. First choice for upper extremity cutdown
     ii. Antecubital fossa 2 cm above and 2 to 3 cm lateral to the medial epicondyle
     iii. Median nerve and brachial artery in close proximity and at risk for injury
    c. External jugular vein
     i. Superficial location along sternocleido-mastoid muscle
  2. Procedure
    a. Sterile preparation and drape
    b. Place tourniquet
    c. Skin incision perpendicular to the course of the vein
    d. Expose vein with blunt dissection
    e. Proximal and distal ties placed around vein to control bleeding
    f. Small incision made in vein with 11 blade
    g. 14- or 16-gauge catheter placed into lumen and attached to IV tubing

    h. The proximal tie is tied around the vessel wall and the catheter
    i. Ligate distal tie
    j. Close skin incision
  3. Complications
    a. Infection
    b. Phlebitis

C. Central venous access (central lines)
  1. Indications
    a. More aggressive volume resuscitation necessary or unable to get peripheral access
    b. Placed if pressors are needed (only dopamine can be used through peripheral line)
    c. Temporary hemodialysis access
    d. Monitoring hemodynamic parameters
    e. Placement of temporary transvenous pacemakers
    f. Peripheral nutrition
  2. General procedure tips
    a. Choose approach and gain access with needle
     i. Patient should be in Trendelenburg position for subclavian and internal jugular access
    b. Hold needle very still while removing the syringes and threading the wire
     i. When access is subclavian or internal jugular vein, the wire should not be threaded more than 10 cm (1 black line on the wire) to avoid contact with myocardium and dysrhythmias
     ii. Never let go of the wire as it may flow into the right heart
    c. Remove needle and dilate
     i. Dilate skin not vessel
     ii. Blunt dilatation: hold skin taught and gently turn dilator while pushing it just beyond the skin
     iii. Scalpel: put dilator against the skin and make a small nick
    d. Remove dilator and push central line until the tip touches the skin, then pull out the wire until it can be grasped form the brown (distal) port
  3. Subclavian central venous access
    a. Approach
     i. Infraclavicular approach: needle is advanced starting at junction of middle and medial thirds of clavicle under clavicle aiming toward suprasternal notch
     ii. Supraclavicular approach: needle is advanced starting 1 cm lateral to clavicular head of sternocleidomastoid muscle and 1 cm posterior to clavicle at 10-degree angle aimed just caudal to the contralateral nipple

b. Right side versus left side
   i. Right side preferred with supraclavicular approach
     a) Avoid injury to thoracic duct
     b) Right subclavian straighter
   ii. Left subclavian is preferred with infra-clavicular approach
     a) Located more medial in comparison with right subclavian
     b) Has a gentle slope into SVC and easier to thread than acute angle of right sub-clavian
c. Advantage: lower infection rate in comparison with other approaches
d. Complications
   i. Pneumothorax
   ii. Hemochylothorax and hydrochylothorax
   iii. Dysrhythmias (usually from wire being threaded too deeply)
   iv. Inadvertent subclavian artery puncture
   v. Venous air embolism
   vi. Subclavian vein thrombosis
   vii. Phrenic nerve injury

4. Internal jugular central venous access
a. Approach
   i. Central approach: needle is advanced starting at apex of triangle formed by clavicle and sternal and clavicular heads of the sternocleidomastoid muscle at a 30- to 40-degree angle to skin lateral to carotid pulsation aiming toward ipsilateral nipple. Depth of vein is usually 1 to 1.5 cm
   ii. Posterior approach: needle is advanced starting at lateral edge of sternocleidomastoid muscle one-third of the way from clavicle to mastoid process aiming toward sternal notch
   iii. Anterior approach: needle is advanced starting at midpoint of medial aspect of sternocleidomastoid lateral to carotid pulsation at angle of 30 to 45 degrees to skin and aimed for the ipsilateral nipple
b. Right internal jugular threads easier than left due to straight course of the vessel
c. Complications
   i. Inadvertent carotid artery puncture (highest incidence with anterior approach)
   ii. Dysrhythmias
   iii. Pneumothorax
   iv. Venous air embolism
   v. Brachial plexus injury
   vi. Jugular vein thrombosis
   vii. Thoracic duct injury
   viii. Tracheal puncture
   ix. Transient Horner syndrome
   x. Inadvertent vertebral artery puncture

5. Femoral central venous access
a. Approach
   i. Locate femoral pulse
   ii. Advance the needle at a 45-degree angle to the skin just medial to the femoral pulsation
b. Complications
   i. Femoral vein thrombosis
   ii. Venous air embolism
   iii. Femoral nerve injury
   iv. Bowel or bladder perforation

D. Pediatric vascular access
1. Central line access
a. Subclavian
   i. The younger the patient, the higher the complication rate
   ii. Smaller, more cephalad location
   iii. Higher rates of pneumothorax
2. Umbilical catherization in the newborn
a. General considerations
   i. Can access either vein or artery for fluid administration
   ii. Cut cord after placing purse string suture
   iii. 1 vein at 12 o'clock and 2 arteries
     a) Vein is larger but thin-walled
     b) Patent urachus may be present and leak urine
   iv. Vein is easier to access and may be more useful in emergency
   v. Difficult to access after 3 days but successful catherization reported in up to 10 days
   vi. Use 3.5 to 5 Foley catheter
   vii. Advance catheter 4 or 5 cm. Deeper insertion may cause liver injury
b. Consider prophylactic antibiotics (controversial)
c. Complications
   i. Arrhythmias
   ii. Air embolism
   iii. Hepatic necrosis
     a) Occurs when sclerosing substances injected into catheter inserted too deeply
   iv. Infection
3. Intraosseous
a. General considerations
   i. Almost every drug and fluid can be administered intraosseously
   ii. Success rate of 85% in children <3 years
   iii. Use specialized intraosseus needles and devices
     a) Standard needles for venous access are **not** adequate

b) 18-gauge spinal needles are too long, bend, and easily occlude

b. Site preparation
   i. Proximal tibia is preferred site
   ii. Avoid sternum as primary site due to risk of osteomyelitis and mediastinitis

c. Proximal tibial administration
   i. Choose flat anteromedial surface 1 to 3 cm below tibial tuberosity
   ii. Direct needle down away from joint
   iii. Advance with twisting or rotary motion
   iv. Typical distance to cortex is only 1 or 2 cm

d. Placement confirmation
   i. Aspirate blood and marrow
   ii. Needle will stand straight unsupported
   iii. Fluids flow easily

e. Complications
   i. Infections in 3%
   ii. Fat embolism rare in children but reported in adults
   iii. Compartment syndrome rarely
   iv. Inadvertent growth plate injury

IX. Wound Care

A. Stages of healing (significant overlap between stages)
   1. Inflammatory stage occurs immediately
      a. Hemostasis
         i. Platelet and coagulation cascade
         ii. Smooth muscle contraction
      b. Neutrophils and macrophages clean up dead tissue, bacteria, and other debris
   2. Proliferation
      a. Epithelialization
         i. Wound is waterproof within 48 hours
         ii. Allow wound to get wet only after this time
      b. Neovascularization
         i. Days 3 to 30
         ii. Reaches peak by days 7 to 10 and erythema can mimic and be mistaken for infection
      c. Fibroplasia and collagen formation
         i. Occurs from day 2 to week 3
         ii. New collagen creation counteracts clearance of damaged collagen
         iii. Above process balanced during days 7 to 10
            a) Wound susceptible to dehiscence
   3. Remodeling
      a. Wound contraction
      b. Collagen remodeled along tension lines
      c. Occurs from 3 weeks to 2 years

B. Wound strength
   1. Scar tissue only 80% as strong as undamaged skin
   2. 50% of ultimate strength by 50 days
   3. 100% of ultimate strength by 150 days
   4. Tenuous during days 7 to 10

C. Wound infection
   1. Epidimiology: 3% to 5% of clean wounds become infected
   2. Risk factors
      a. Crush and puncture wounds
      b. Foreign body retention
      c. Contamination
         i. Saliva
         ii. Soil
         iii. Organic material
      d. Diabetes or steroid usage
      e. Consider prophylactic antibiotics if
         i. Extremity bite wounds
            a) Human and cat bites should receive antibiotics
         ii. Puncture wounds
         iii. Closed intraoral lacerations

D. Delayed primary closure
   1. Because most wounds become infected on days 3 to 5, an uninfected wound can be closed after debridement with good cosmetic results after this time
   2. Keep wound moist until delayed closure

E. Wound healing by secondary intent
   1. Passive healing of wound with minimal intervention
   2. Leaves larger scar compared to primary or delayed primary closure

F. Keys to good healing
   1. Wounds on concave surfaces have better cosmetic results
   2. Good technique
      a. Eversion of would edges
         i. Enter skin with suture needle at or >90 degrees
      b. Avoid tissue strangulation by excessively tight suturing
      c. Avoid tension on wound edges
      d. Use smallest suture material possible
      e. Better to use many small sutures placed closer together than large sutures farther apart
      f. Avoid use of forceps on wound edges

G. Specific suture material
  1. General consideration
    a. Sutures with higher tissue reactivity cause more scarring and infection
      i. Higher for natural products such as silk and gut
    b. Natural materials such as plain gut and silk tend to be more inflammatory and at risk for infection
    c. Polyfilaments have greater infection rates than monofilaments
  2. Classification
    a. Nonabsorbable versus absorbable
      i. Absorbable sutures lose tensile strength <2 months
    b. Monofilament versus polyfilament
      i. Polyfilament (braided suture). handle/tie easily but harbour organisms
      ii. Monofilament: lower infection rate but with lower knot security

H. Suture removal
  1. Suture marks may form if left >7 days
  2. Differential tissue
    a. Face: within 5 days
    b. Extremity: 7 days
    c. Chest, back abdomen: 7 to 10 days
    d. Scalp, hands, feet, joints: 10 to 14 days

BIBLIOGRAPHY

Taryle DA, Chandler JE, Good JT Jr, et al: Emergency room intubations: complications and survival. *Chest.* 1979 May; 75(5):541.

Li J, Murphy-Lavoie H, Bugas C, et al: Complications of emergency intubation with and without paralysis. *Am J Emerg Med.* 1999 Mar;17(2):141.

Gnauck K, Lungo JB, Scalzo A, et al: Emergency intubation of the pediatric medical patient: use of anesthetic agents in the emergency department. *Ann Emerg Med.* 1994 Jun; 23(6):1242.

Roberts J, Hedges J: *Clinical Procedures in Emergency Medicine.* 4th ed. Saunders: Independence Square West Philadelphia, Philadelphia; 2004.

Partin W: *Current Emergency Diagnosis and Treatment.* 6th ed. New York: McGraw-Hill; 2008.

Tintinelli JE, Kelen GD, Stapczynski JS: *Tintinalli's Emergency Medicine: A Comprehensive Study Guide.* 6th ed. New York: McGraw-Hill; 2004.

Brunicardi FC, Andersen DK, Billiar TR, et al: *Schwartz's Principles of Surgery.* 8th ed. New York: McGraw-Hill; 2005.

Hall JB, Schmidt GA, Wood LDH: *Principles of Critical Care.* 3rd ed. New York: McGraw-Hill; 2005.

Simon RR, Brenner BE: *Procedures and Techniques in Emergency Medicine.* Baltimore:Lippincott, Williams and Wilkin;1982.

Vaccaro JP, Brody JM: CT Cystography in the evaluation of major bladder trauma. *Radiographics.* 2000;20:1373.

Chapter 17
DERMATOLOGIC EMERGENCIES

Listy Thomas and Barbara Barnett

I. Rashes

A. Ominous symptoms and signs
   1. Recent travel
   2. History of sexually transmitted disease
   3. Tick bite
   4. Headache
   5. Fever
   6. Non-blanching lesion (diascopy)
   7. Mucosal lesions
   8. Palm and sole involvement
   9. Bullae

B. Definitions (Figure 17–1)
   1. Macule versus patch (macule >1 cm is called a patch)
      a. Flat nonpalpable discoloration
      b. Examples include freckles or flat moles
   2. Papule versus plaque (papule >1 cm is called a plaque)
      a. Solid elevation
      b. Examples include warts and some drug reactions
   3. Nodule versus tumor (nodule >2 cm is called a tumor)
      a. Solid palpable lesion that may or may not be elevated
      b. Examples include erythema nodosum and lipomas
   4. Vesicle versus bulla (vesicle >0.5 cm is called a bulla)
      a. Clear fluid containing raised lesion
      b. Examples include contact dermatitis, blisters from second-degree burns, and pemphigus
   5. Pustule versus abscess (pustule >0.5 cm is called an abscess)
      a. Elevated superficial lesions containing pus
      b. Examples include acne, follicultis, and furuncles

   6. Petechiae versus purpura (petechiae >0.2 cm to 1 cm are called purpura)
      a. Nonblanching lesions of extravasated blood
      b. Examples include meningococcemia and vasculitis related rashes

II. Pediatric Rashes (see Pediatric chapter, Table 1–2)

III. Infectious Dermatology

A. Bacterial
   1. Cutaneous anthrax: *Bacillus anthracis* (see also Infectious Diseases chapter) (Figure 17–2)
      a. Etiology
         i. Animal product laborers
         ii. Terrorist related outbreak: cutaneous lesion should prompt search for inhalation or gastrointestinal anthrax
         iii. Cutaneous anthrax cannot penetrate healthy skin
      b. Symptoms and signs
         i. Initial papule will develop at site of skin break
         ii. Erythematous papule with central vesicle or bulla
         iii. Usually painless but patient may complain of burning
         iv. Transforms into hemorrhagic and necrotic lesion: black eschar
         v. Regional adenitis
      c. Management
         i. Treat with ciprofloxacin or doxycycline
         ii. Good prognosis
   2. Erysipelas
      a. Etiology
         i. Usually group A *Streptococcus* cellulitis
      b. Symptoms and signs
         i. Painful rash preceded by fevers and chills
         ii. Lymphangitis (rapid lymph channel spread)

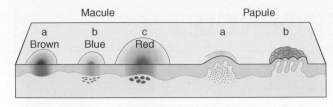

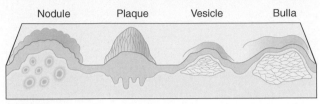

Macule   Papule

a   b   c   a   b
Brown Blue Red

Nodule Plaque Vesicle Bulla

FIGURE 17–1. Skin. (Reproduced, with permission, from Kasper DL et al: *Harrison's Principles of Internal Medicine,* 16th ed. Copyright © 2005, New York: McGraw-Hill.

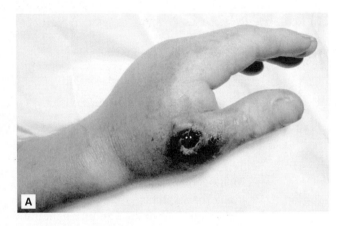

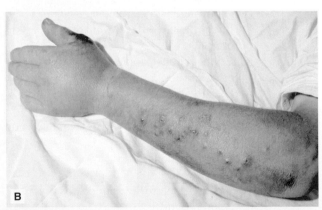

FIGURE 17–2. A, B. Anthrax. (Reproduced, with permission, from Wolff K, Johnson RA, Suurmond D: *Fitzpatrick's Color Atlas and Synopsis of Clinical Dermatology,* 5th ed. Copyright © 2005, New York: McGraw-Hill.)

    iii. Unlike cellulitis, erysipelas has **well-demarcated**, sharp, palpable margins
  c. Management
    i. Gram-positive antibiotic coverage
    ii. Admit if extensive facial involvement or toxic-appearing
3. Staphylococcal scalded skin syndrome (SSSS) (Figure 17–3, see color insert section)
  a. Epidemiology
    i. Children and infants affected, adults rarely
    ii. Mortality in adults (20%) >children (1% to 5%)
  b. Etiology
    i. *Staphylococcal* infection with exotoxin release
  c. Symptoms and signs
    i. Not ill-appearing
    ii. Oral mucosal involvement limited to lip
    iii. Tender warm skin (erythroderma)
    iv. Crusting lesions around mouth and eyes
    v. Bullae with Nikolsky sign
      a) Slight pressure causes superficial layers of epidermis to separate
    vi. Desquamation occurs in 3 to 5 days
  d. Diagnosis
    i. Wound culture
    ii. Toxin detection by PCR
  e. Management
    i. Fluid resuscitation
    ii. Antibiotics for *Staphylococcus aureus*: β-lactamase-resistant penicillin (eg, dicloxacillin)
    iii. Steroids not indicated
    iv. Admit ill-appearing patients, especially infants

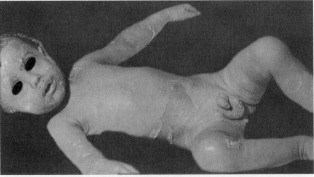

FIGURE 17–3. SSSS. (Reproduced, with permission, from Wolff K, Johnson RA, Suurmond D: *Fitzpatrick's Color Atlas and Synopsis of Clinical Dermatology,* 5th ed. Copyright © 2005, New York: McGraw-Hill.)

4. Toxic shock syndrome (TSS)
   a. Epidemiology
      i. Highest incidence was in 1980, decrease in menstrual form with change in tampon formulation
   b. Etiology
      i. Most commonly *Staphylococcus aureus*
      ii. Similar syndrome with *Streptococcus pyogenes*
      iii. Exotoxin mediated
      iv. Nonmenstrual causes of TSS
         a) Postsurgical
         b) Nasal packing for epistaxis
         c) Nonmenstrual gynecologic procedures (childbirth, abortion, PID, barrier protection, etc.)
         d) Focal infections and skin disruption
   c. Symptoms and signs
      i. Fever >38.9°C (102°F)
      ii. Diffuse macular erythroderma followed by desquamation
      iii. Hypotension
      iv. Multisystem involvement (≥3 of the following)
         a) Gastrointestinal: vomiting or diarrhea
         b) Muscular: myalgias or elevated CPK
         c) Mucous membrane: vaginal, oropharyngeal or conjunctival hyperemia
         d) Renal: pyuria, renal insufficiency
         e) Hepatic: transaminitis twice upper limit normal
         f) Hematologic: thrombocytopenia
         g) CNS: altered mental status, without focal findings
   d. Management
      i. Aggressive supportive care
      ii. Fluid resuscitation, vasopressor support as necessary
      iii. Identification of source, debridement, or removal of foreign body
      iv. Antibiotics
         a) Helpful with bacteremia or occult infection
         b) Clindamycin 600 to 900 mg every 8 hours
         c) Consider IVIG therapy in severe cases
5. Lyme disease: erythema migrans (see also Infectious Diseases chapter) (Figure 17–4, see color insert section)
   a. Etiology
      i. Tick: *Ixodes scapularis*
      ii. Bacterium: *Borrelia burgdorferi*
   b. Symptoms and signs: rash characteristics
      i. Appears 7 to 10 days after infection
      ii. Size increases over days

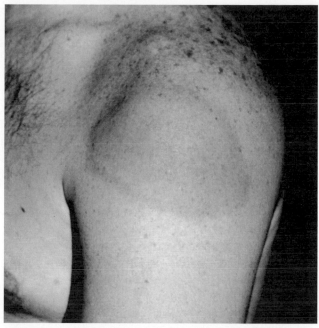

FIGURE 17–4.   Erythema migrans. (Reproduced, with permission, from Wolff K, Johnson RA, Suurmond D: *Fitzpatrick's Color Atlas and Synopsis of Clinical Dermatology,* 5th ed. Copyright © 2005, New York: McGraw-Hill.)

      iii. Often occurs near site of bite
      iv. Multiple lesions occur in up to one-third of patients
      v. Average size is 16 cm in diameter
      vi. May or may not have central clearing ("bull's eye sign")
      vii. Persists 2 to 3 weeks without treatment
6. Rocky Mountain spotted fever (RMSF) (see also Infectious Diseases chapter) (Figure 17–5, see color insert section)
   a. Epidemiology
      i. Most common fatal tick-borne vasculitis caused by *Rickettsia rickettsii*
      ii. Late spring and early summer
      iii. North Carolina, Oklahoma, South Carolina, Tennessee, and Georgia
      iv. Occurs least commonly in Rocky Mountain states (misnomer)
   b. Etiology
      i. *Dermacentor andersoni* (wood tick) or *Dermacentor variabilis* (dog tick)
   c. Symptoms and signs
      i. Fever, rash, myalgias, photophobia, and headache
      ii. Ill-appearing
      iii. Difficult to differentiate from meningitis and meningococcemia

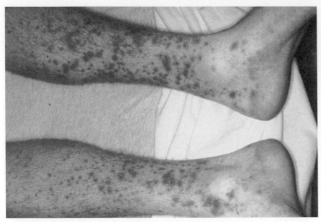

FIGURE 17–5. Rocky Mountain spotted fever. (Reproduced, with permission, from Kasper DL et al: *Harrison's Principles of Internal Medicine,* 16th ed. Copyright © 2005, New York: McGraw-Hill).

    iv. Rash
       a) Peripheral beginning on wrists and ankles then spreads centrally (centripetal distribution)
       b) Initial maculopapular rash that blanch with pressure evolve into nonblanching petechiae and purpura typically over 4 or 5 days
  d. Diagnosis
    i. Clinical diagnosis
       a) Serologic testing not available in clinically timely manner
       b) Treat empirically
       c) Only 50% to 70% report tick bite
  e. Management
    i. Tetracycline
    ii. Chloramphenicol in children
7. Gonococcal (disseminated) infection
  a. Etiology
    i. Sexually transmitted via pharyngeal, rectal, or genital source
  b. Symptoms and signs
    i. Fever, rash, migratory arthritis, and tenosynovitis
    ii. Usually affects women during menstruation or pregnancy
    iii. Initially appears as few red maculopapular lesions with a petechial component that evolve into pustule with necrotic centers
    iv. Hemorrhagic transformation of lesions may occur
  c. Differential
    i. RMSF, meningococcemia, endocarditis, vasculitides, and typhus

    ii. In contrast to RMSF, disseminated GC may present with lesions on wrists and ankles but in a asymmetric distribution
    iii. Patients with disseminated GC are less toxic-appearing in contrast to RMSF and meningococcemia
    iv. Lesions in disseminated gonococcal disease are fewer in number
  d. Diagnosis
    i. Treat empirically if clinically suspected
    ii. Cultures, gram stain of oral, rectal, and genital swabs
  e. Management
    i. Patients with disseminated GC should be admitted for parenteral antibiotics
    ii. Responds well to antibiotics, cephalosporins considered first-line treatment (spectinomycin or erythromycin for pregnant women and children)
    iii. Fluoroquinolones no longer considered first-line therapy as >5% resistance as per 2007 CDC guidelines
8. Endocarditis (see also Infectious Diseases chapter) (Figures 17–6 and 17–7 [see color insert section])
  a. Etiology
    i. Intravenous drug use, immunocompromise, dental work, rheumatic fever, prosthetic valves
    ii. Usually *Staphylococcus aureus* or *Streptococcus viridans*

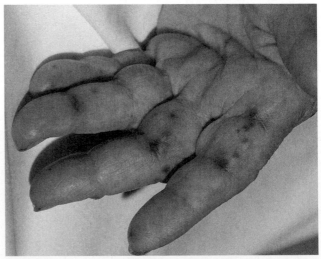

FIGURE 17–6. Janeway lesions. (Reproduced, with permission, from Wolff K, Johnson RA, Suurmond D: *Fitzpatrick's Color Atlas and Synopsis of Clinical Dermatology,* 5th ed. Copyright © 2005, New York: McGraw-Hill.)

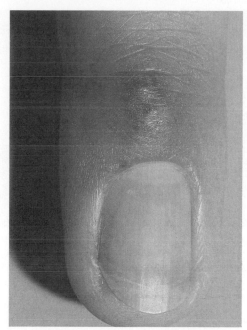

FIGURE 17–7. Septic embolus. (Reproduced, with permission, from Wolff K, Johnson RA, Suurmond D: *Fitzpatrick's Color Atlas and Synopsis of Clinical Dermatology,* 5th ed. Copyright © 2005, New York: McGraw-Hill.)

   b. Symptoms and signs
       i. Roth spots (retinal hemorrhage with central clearing)
       ii. Janeway lesions (painless plaques on palms and soles)
       iii. Osler nodes (painful nodes on tips of fingers and toes)
       iv. Splinter hemorrhages (on fingernails and toenails)
   9. Meningococcemia (see also Infectious Diseases chapter)
       a. Epidemiology
           i. 20% to 40% of young adults are carriers
       b. Etiology
           i. *Neisseria meningitides:* encapsulated Gram-negative diplococcus
           ii. Person to person transmission via respiratory droplets
       c. Symptoms and signs
           i. May be preceded by upper respiratory infection followed by headache, fever, chills, myalgias, and arthralgias.
           ii. Difficult to discriminate from viral syndrome
           iii. Few infections can lead to death so rapidly
           iv. May progress to DIC

           v. Skin lesions
               a) Petechiae or coalescing purpura
               b) May also be macular or maculopapular with necrotic center
               c) Coalescing confluent hemorrhagic lesions
       d. Diagnosis
           i. Positive skin cultures (50%)
           ii. Blood cultures or CSF cultures
           iii. Clinical
               a) Consider in ill patient with fever and rash
               b) Differential includes endocarditis, vasculitis, and RMSF
       e. Management
           i. Antibiotics: ceftriaxone
           ii. Prophylaxis alternatives for close contacts and health-care providers
               a) Cipro single dose
               b) Rifampin 600 mg PO bid × 2 days
               c) Single dose IV/IM ceftriaxone
   10. Necrotizing fasciitis (Figure 17–8)
       a. Definition
           i. Rapidly progressing infection of the deep fascial planes with overlying necrosis of subcutaneous tissues
           ii. Perineal involvement is specifically referred to as Fournier gangrene
       b. Risk factors
           i. Immunocompromise (DM, HIV, and cancer)
           ii. Alcoholism
           iii. Surgical or traumatic wounds

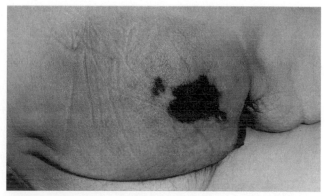

FIGURE 17–8. Necrotizing fasciitis. (Reproduced, with permission, from Wolff K, Johnson RA, Suurmond D: *Fitzpatrick's Color Atlas and Synopsis of Clinical Dermatology,* 5th ed. Copyright © 2005, New York: McGraw-Hill, 2005.)

c. Classification
   i. Type I: polymicrobial infection
   ii. Type II: group A β-hemolytic *Streptococci* ("flesh-eating bacteria")
   iii. Type III: clostridial infection
d. Symptoms and signs
   i. Easily confused for cellulitis
   ii. Pain out of proportion to exam
   iii. May be painless after destruction of cutaneous nerves
   iv. May appear deceptively well early on in disease
   v. External examination may not be as impressive as underlying tissue destruction
   vi. Crepitus from subcutaneous emphysema may be appreciated
e. Diagnosis
   i. Plain film may localize subcutaneous emphysema
   ii. CT scan may help localize area of necrosis
f. Management
   i. Immediate surgical consultation for debridement
      a) Mortality rate decreases from 70% to 12% if surgery within 4 hours
   ii. Fluids
   iii. Broad-spectrum antibiotics
   iv. Hyperbaric O$_2$ therapy controversial

B. Viral
 1. Herpes simplex virus (see also Infectious Diseases chapter)
    a. Crusted erosions in clusters
    b. Evolves into pustules and excoriations over 5 to 7 days
    c. Fever, pain, malaise, and regional lymphadenopathy
    d. Primary lesions typically last 2 to 3 weeks
    e. Lesions typically involve oral, genital, periorbital, and fingers (herpetic whitlow)
    f. Genital lesions may cause urinary retention
    g. Do not drain herpetic whitlow on digits (Figure 17–9)
    h. Precipitating factors
       i. Concurrent infection
       ii. Menstruation
       iii. Stress or local trauma
       iv. Ultraviolet light
 2. Herpes zoster (Figure 17–10)
    a. Etiology
       i. Reactivated dormant virus in dorsal root ganglia
    b. Symptoms and signs
       i. Clustered lesions on erythematous base along dermatome

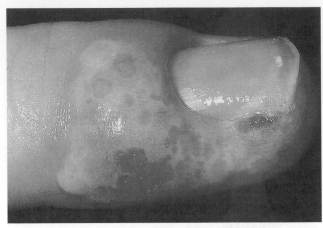

FIGURE 17–9.   Herpetic whitlow. (Reproduced, with permission, from Wolff K, Johnson RA, Suurmond D: *Fitzpatrick's Color Atlas and Synopsis of Clinical Dermatology,* 5th ed. Copyright © 2005, New York: McGraw-Hill.)

       ii. Should not cross far past midline
       iii. Pain 5 to 7 days prior to rash eruption
       iv. Usually lasts 3 weeks
       v. Involvement of multiple dermatomes suggests immunocompromised state and possible need for admission for disseminated disease
       vi. Hutchinson sign
          a) Zoster lesions on the tip of the nose (nasociliary nerve): sign of ocular involvement
          b) Ophthalmic nerve involvement may lead to permanent vision loss (Figure 17–11)

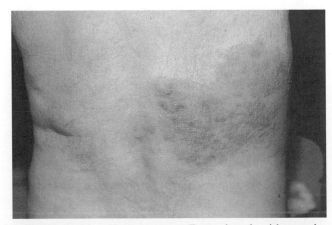

FIGURE 17–10.   Herpes zoster. (Reproduced, with permission, from Wolff K, Johnson RA, Suurmond D: *Fitzpatrick's Color Atlas and Synopsis of Clinical Dermatology,* 5th ed. Copyright © 2005, New York: McGraw-Hill.)

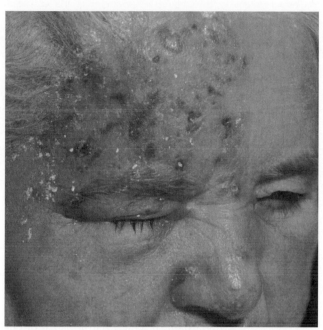

FIGURE 17–11. Zoster on face. (Reproduced, with permission, from Wolff K, Johnson RA, Suurmond D. *Fitzpatrick's Color Atlas and Synopsis of Clinical Dermatology,* 5th ed. Copyright © 2005, New York: McGraw-Hill.)

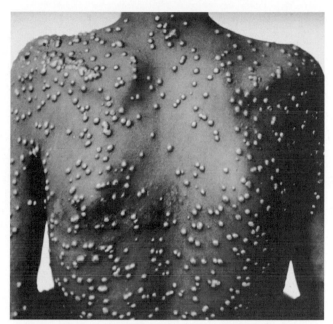

FIGURE 17–12. Smallpox. (Reproduced, with permission, from Wolff K, Johnson RA, Suurmond D: *Fitzpatrick's Color Atlas and Synopsis of Clinical Dermatology,* 5th ed. Copyright © 2005, New York: McGraw-Hill.)

c. Management
    i. Treatment with acyclovir shortens duration of illness
    ii. Give within first 72 hours
    iii. Decreases new lesion formation
    iv. May decrease duration of postherpetic neuralgia (pain >1 month)
3. Variola (smallpox) (see also Infectious Disease chapter) (Figures 17–12 and 17–13 [see color insert section])
    a. Rash
        i. Easily confused with varicella
        ii. Macules >papules >classic pustules
            a) Deep-seated, firm, and well circumscribed
            b) Each stage lasts 1 or 2 days
        iii. Unlike varicella, the rash of variola present uniformly in the same stage
        iv. Centrifugal distribution: face and limbs >trunk
            a) Often forms first on oral mucosa and face
4. Pityriasis rosea (Figures 17–14 and 17–15 [see color insert section])
    a. Etiology
        i. Suspected viral etiology (*Herpesvirus 7*)
    b. Symptoms and signs
        i. Acute self-limiting rash that lasts 4 to 7 weeks

ii. May present with mild malaise, fever, and lymphadenopathy
iii. Oval, salmon-shaped patches
iv. Christmas tree pattern (follows cleavage lines of skin)
v. May be preceded by 2- to 5-cm **herald patch**
    a) Precedes generalized rash by 1 or 2 weeks

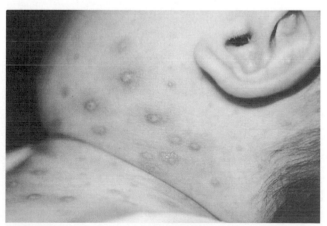

FIGURE 17–13. Chicken pox. (Courtesy of Lawrence B. Stack, MD as reproduced, with permission, from Knoop KJ, Stack LB, Storrow AB. *Atlas of Emergency Medicine,* 2nd ed. New York: McGraw-Hill, 2002.)

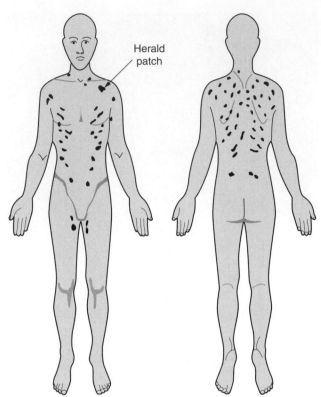

FIGURE 17–14. Pityriasis rosea. (Reproduced, with permission, from Wolff K, Johnson RA, Suurmond D: *Fitzpatrick's Color Atlas and Synopsis of Clinical Dermatology,* 5th ed. Copyright © 2005, New York: McGraw-Hill.)

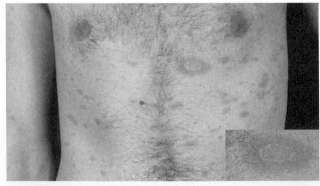

FIGURE 17–15. Pityriasis rosea. (Reproduced, with permission, from Wolff K, Johnson RA, Suurmond D: *Fitzpatrick's Color Atlas and Synopsis of Clinical Dermatology,* 5th ed. Copyright © 2005, New York: McGraw-Hill.)

b) Oval-shaped

c) Salmon-colored with an erythematous periphery

vi. Not contagious

c. Diagnosis

i. Clinical diagnosis of exclusion

ii. An RPR or VDRL should be drawn to rule out the "great masquerader" syphilis

d. Management

i. Self-limiting

ii. Antihistamines

iii. Mild to midpotency topical steroids

C. Fungal

1. Tinea infections

a. Pathophysiology

i. Feed on dead cornified layers of skin, hair, and nails

ii. Does not infect deep but spreads in centrifugal pattern which accounts for circular pattern

iii. Hyperepithelialization in response to infection leads to shedding scales

b. "Id reaction"

i. Sterile reaction at site distant from tinea infection

ii. Vesicles are occasionally painful or pruritic

iii. Can be precipitated by antifungal medication

iv. Occurs typically with tinea pedis but may occur with any dermatophytosis

v. Treatment of underlying infection or dermatitis leads to resolution

vi. Systemic or topical steroids may aid resolution

c. Tinea corporis (body) (Figure 17–16)

i. Etiology

a) Most commonly caused by *Trychophyton rubrum*

b) Transmission from contact with infected soil, animals, and people

ii. Symptoms and signs

a) Scaly plaques

b) Often pruritic

c) Reactive vesicles and papules may form at advancing border

iii. Diagnosis

a) KOH preparation of lesion scrapings

i) Scrapings at lesion border have the highest fungal yield

ii) Sample from unroofed vesicles has the highest yield if present

iii) KOH dissolves the keratin and leaves fungus visible to microscopy

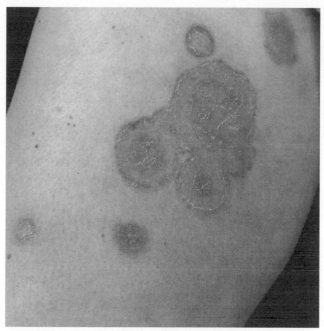

FIGURE 17–16. Tinea corporis. (Reproduced, with permission, from Wolff K, Johnson RA, Surmond D: *Fitzpatrick's Color Atlas and Synopsis of Clinical Dermatology,* 5th ed. Copyright © 2005, New York: McGraw-Hill.)

iv. Management
   a) Topical antifungal medication including area a few centimeters beyond border
   b) Topical steroids for the first few days may decrease inflammation and pruritis
   c) Oral antifungal medication for severe or refractory infections

d. Tinea capitis (scalp) (Figure 17–17)
  i. Epidemiology
   a) Children <10 years
  ii. Etiology
   a) Usually *Trychophyton tonsurans*
    i) Predilection for hair shaft of eyelids, eyelash, and scalp
  iii. Symptoms and signs
   a) May begin as small red papule at base of hair that spreads in typical circular form
   b) Hair becomes brittle and breaks a few millimeters above skin surface leaving classic dotted appearance of fractured hair
   c) Severe deep boggy infection and induration is termed a kerion
  iv. Diagnosis
   a) KOH preparation
   b) Wood light fluoresces select dermatophytes

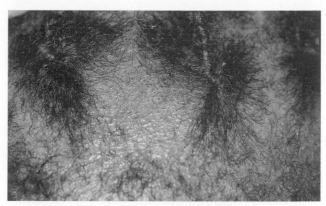

FIGURE 17–17. Tinea capitis. (Reproduced, with permission, from Wolff K, Johnson RA, Suurmond D: *Fitzpatrick's Color Atlas and Synopsis of Clinical Dermatology,* 5th ed. Copyright © 2005, New York: McGraw-Hill.)

  v. Management
   a) Topical therapy rarely successful
   b) Griseofulvin PO bid × 6 weeks
    i) Follow LFTs, CBC, and renal function
   c) Selenium shampoo
   d) Oral steroids used to treat kerion, may decrease risk of permanent hair loss (avoid topical steroids)

D. Parasitic
  1. Scabies (Figure 17–18, see color insert section)
   a. Etiology
    i. Infection by the arthropod *Sarcoptes scabiei* var *hominis*

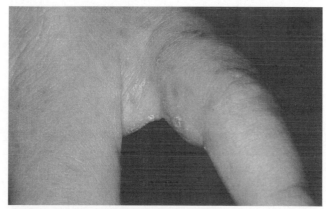

FIGURE 17–18. Scabies. (Reproduced, with permission, from Wolff K, Johnson RA, Surmond D: *Fitzpatrick's Color Atlas and Synopsis of Clinical Dermatology,* 5th ed. Copyright © 2005, New York: McGraw-Hill.)

b. Pathophysiology
  i. Mite transmitted by close person-to-person contact
  ii. Mites/fomites can survive for 3 days away from human skin, so infected sheets and clothing are also infectious
  iii. After mating, females burrow into skin and lay eggs
  iv. Eggs hatch and feeding mites lay trail of feces clinically recognized as linear burrows

a. Symptoms and signs
  i. Intense pruritis worse at night
  ii. Similar symptoms in family members
  iii. Linear burrows
  iv. Distribution differs by age
    a) Adults: wrist flexors, interdigital web space, waist, and buttocks
    b) Children: face, scalp, neck, and palms and soles
  v. Norwegian scabies (crusted scabies)
    a) A severe type of scabies infection
    c) Crusted form of scabies consisting of millions of mites
    d) Associated with immunocompromise, handicapped, and the elderly
    e) Mobidity and mortality associated with bacterial superinfection

b. Diagnosis
  i. Pathognomonic lesion is a linear burrow in web spaces of fingers
  ii. Consider when multiple family members affected
  iii. Scabies preparation by scraping skin lesion with oil immersion and microscopy
  iv. Empiric treatment

c. Management
  i. Permethrin (Elimite) 5% cream
  ii. Lindane (Kwell) lotion
    a) Avoid lindane in children <6 years and pregnant women secondary to neurotoxicity and seizures
  iii. Treat close contacts even if asymptomatic
  iv. Wash clothing and linens with high heat

2. Pediculosis (lice infection) (Figure 17–19)
  a. Etiology: 3 types of louse infections
    i. *Pediculus humanus capitis* (head)
    ii. *Pediculus humanus corporis* (body)
    iii. *Pthirus pubis* (The STD known as "crabs")
    iv. Infest and lay eggs in fabric (corporis), base of hair (capitis), or throughout hair shaft (pubis)
    v. Person-to-person transmission
    vi. Lice may live on clothing and furniture for weeks

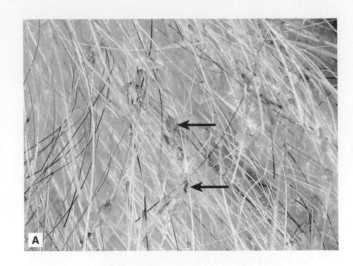

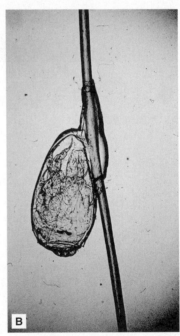

FIGURE 17–19. A, B. Pediculosis. (Reproduced, with permission, from Wolff K, Johnson RA, Surmond D: *Fitzpatrick's Color Atlas and Synopsis of Clinical Dermatology,* 5th ed. Copyright © 2005, New York: McGraw-Hill.)

b. Epidemiology
  i. Capitis infection common in children but uncommon after puberty
  ii. Head louse infection uncommon in African Americans but scalp may be infected with *P. pubis*

c. Symptoms and signs
  i. Intense pruritis during lice feeding
  ii. Lymphadenopathy
  iii. Capitis

a) Inspection may reveal nits firmly attached to base of hair

b) Heaviest infestation typically behind the ears

  iv. Corporis

    a) Louse not attached to hair but to the seams of clothing

    b) Comes out to feed on blood

  v. Pubis

    a) Attached throughout hair and not only on base

    b) Nits attached to eyelashes are evidence of pubic and not head louse infestation

d. Diagnosis

  i. Evidence of nits

    a) ~1 mm in length and flask-like in appearance on microscopy

  ii. Visualization of lice

    a) Use tape to find specimens and view under microscope

    b) Mature lice are the size of sesame seeds

  iii. Nits and lice fluoresce with Wood lamp

e. Management

  i. Capitis and pubis (scalp and pubic)

    a) Permethrin (Elimite) kills the adult louse but not nits

    b) Remove nits with vinegar solution and fine-tooth comb

    c) Wash clothing in hot water and dry with high heat

    d) Carefully sealing clothing for 2 weeks will also starve adult lice and hatched nits, and result in eradication

    e) Reexamine scalp in 1 week

    f) Pubic lice infection in children should raise suspicion of sexual abuse

  ii. Corporis (body)

    a) Discarding infected clothing will result in cure because the body louse does not attach to hair but clothing

    b) Carefully seal clothing for 2 weeks

    c) In case the above is not feasible, hot water laundry and high heat may eradicate infestation

    d) Spraying clothing with permethrin may help although not a labeled use

III. Systemic and Reactive

A. Erythema nodosum

  1. Definition

    a. Hypersensitivity inflammation of deep dermis and subcutaneous fat (panniculitis)

  2. Epidemiology

    a. Women >men (4:1)

  3. Etiology

    a. Systemic disease

      i. Lymphoma, inflammatory bowel disease, sarcoid

    b. Infections

      i. Tuberculosis, group A Streptococcal infections, *Coccidiomyocosis, histoplasmosis, blastomycosis*

    c. Drugs

      i. Sulfonamides, bromides, and oral contraceptives

    d. Idiopathic

  4. Symptoms and signs

    a. Painful red nodules typically found in pretibial region

    b. Fever and arthralgias frequent

    c. Hilar adenopathy less frequent

  5. Diagnosis

    a. Based on clinical presentation

    b. Uncover underlying pathology

      i. CXR for sarcoid and tuberculosis

      ii. Skin testing for tuberculosis

      iii. Throat cultures for streptococcal infections

  6. Management

    a. Identify underlying etiology

      i. Antibiotics if strep infection or tuberculosis

    b. Pain control

    c. Self-limiting

    d. Systemic steroids may mask underlying condition and exacerbate tuberculosis

B. Psoriasis (Figure 17–20)

  1. Definition

    a. Class of chronic and relapsing skin disorder that result in inflammation and thickening caused by epidermal hyperproliferation

  2. Etiology

    a. Strong genetic predisposition

    b. Possibly autoimmune

    c. Triggers

      i. Stress

      ii. Koebner phenomenon: plaque formation on site of prior trauma 1 to 2 weeks after skin injury

      iii. Drugs: steroids, lithium, β-blockers, alcohol

  3. Symptoms and signs

    a. Many clinical variants exist but plaque form most common

    b. Circular or oval erythematous plaques with sharp margins and silvery scales

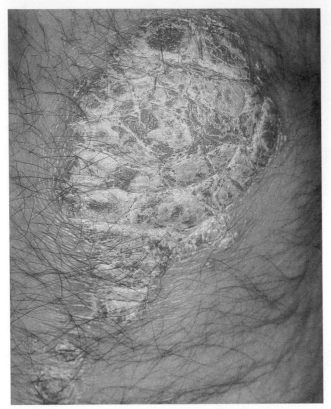

FIGURE 17–20. Psoriasis. (Reproduced, with permission, from Wolff K, Johnson RA, Suurmond D: *Fitzpatrick's Color Atlas and Synopsis of Clinical Dermatology,* 5th ed. Copyright © 2005, New York: McGraw-Hill.)

    c. Most commonly distribute on the scalp and extensor surfaces of elbows and knees
    d. Auspitz sign: removal of silvery scales produces blood droplets
    e. Nail involvement may reveal pitting and hyperkeratosis
    f. Psoriatic arthritis in 10% to 20%
  4. Diagnosis
    a. Clinical diagnosis rarely requiring ancillary testing
    b. Skin biopsy reserved for atypical presentation or concern for superficial basal cell carcinoma
  5. Management
    a. Strategy is to reduce cell turnover
    b. First-line therapy involves topical steroids, coal tar, and keratolytics such as salicylic acid
    c. Phototherapy for widespread disease
    d. Systemic medication for refractory illness
      i. Methotrexate
      ii. Cyclosporine
      iii. Tumor necrosis factor (TNF) inhibitors
    e. Minimize alcohol intake

C. Poison ivy and poison oak
  1. Etiology
    a. Type IV delayed hypersensitivity reaction
  2. Symptoms and signs
    a. Pruritic vesicles
    b. Linear arrangement of vesicles
  3. Diagnosis
    a. Clinical diagnosis
  4. Treatment
    a. Calamine lotion
    b. Mild cases can be treated with antihistamines and topical steroids
    c. Moderate to severe cases treated with long course of tapered steroids to prevent rebound rash

IV. Bullous Lesions

A. Erythema multiforme (EM)
  1. Definition
    a. A self-limiting **hypersensitivity** skin eruption of symmetric, raised macules or papules with concentric color changes
    b. EM major: if mucosal involvement or >10% total body surface involvement (TBSA) (Figures 17–21 and 17–22 [see color insert section])
  2. Epidemiology
    a. Men >women
  3. Etiology
    a. Infection
      i. Herpes simplex (most common overall etiology)

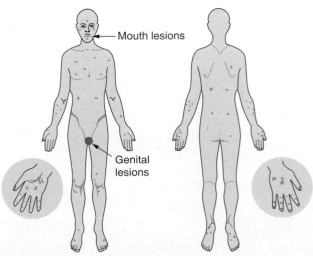

FIGURE 17–21. Erythema multiforme.

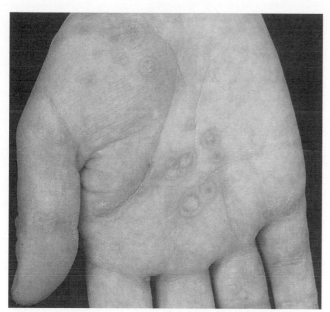

FIGURE 17–22. Erythema multiforme. (Reproduced, with permission, from Wolff K, Johnson RA, Surmond D: *Fitzpatrick's Color Atlas and Synopsis of Clinical Dermatology,* 5th ed. Copyright © 2005, New York: McGraw-Hill)

       ii. Mycoplasma (most common bacterial etiology)

       iii. Tuberculosis

   b. Malignancy (lymphoma)

   c. SOAPS mnemonic (**s**ulfa, **o**ral hypoglycemics, **a**nticonvulsants, **p**enicillin, **N**SAIDs)

   d. Idiopathic 50%

4. Symptoms and signs

   a. Nonspecific prodrome of fever, myalgias, headache, and malaise

   b. Usually nonpruritic

   c. Burning sensation

   d. **Target-shaped** lesions

   e. Papular and vesicobullous lesions (multiple forms)

   f. Lesions may coalesce into generalized erythema

   g. Distribution

       i. Bilateral and usually symmetric on extensor surfaces

       ii. **Palms and soles**

       iii. Centripetal distribution (trunk >extremities)

       iv. Eye involvement in 10%

5. Diagnosis

   a. Clinical diagnosis

   b. Imaging and laboratory panels to uncover suspected underlying etiology

   c. Skin biopsy may aid diagnosis with atypical presentations

6. Management

   a. Treat underlying condition

   b. Remove offending agent or drug

   c. Self-limiting

   d. Steroids not indicated

   e. Acyclovir if herpes simplex infection suspected or not improving

   f. Ophthalmology consult if ocular involvement

   g. Discharge home with follow-up

B. Steven-Johnson syndrome (SJS) and toxic epidermal necrolysis (TEN) (Figures 17–23 and 17–24)

1. Definition

   a. SJS and TEN are variants of a **disease spectrum** with life-threatening mucocutaneous manifestations

       i. SJS <10% to 30% TBSA

       ii. TEN >30% TBSA

2. Epidemiology

   a. Male >female

   b. Affects an older population than EM

3. Etiology

   a. Autoimmune detachment of epidermis and mucous membranes that result in widespread erythema and bullous lesions

   b. Most cases of SJS and TEN are medication related (within the first few months of administration)

   c. Drugs and malignancy more likely in the elderly

   d. Infection more likely in children and younger adults (herpes simplex and mycoplasma)

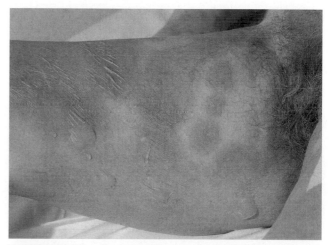

FIGURE 17–23. Stevens-Johnsons syndrome. (Reproduced, with permission, from Wolff K, Johnson RA, Suurmond D: *Fitzpatrick's Color Atlas and Synopsis of Clinical Dermatology,* 5th ed. Copyright © 2005, New York: McGraw-Hill.)

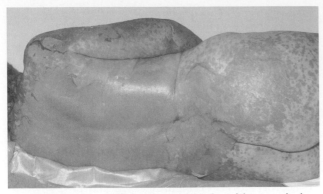

FIGURE 17–24. TEN. (Reproduced, with permission, from Wolff K, Johnson RA, Suurmond D: *Fitzpatrick's Color Atlas and Synopsis of Clinical Dermatology,* 5th ed. Copyright © 2005, New York: McGraw-Hill.)

4. Symptoms and signs
   a. Fever common
   b. Recent upper respiratory infection in ~50%
   c. Purulent sputum common
   d. Rash begins as atypical target-like lesions and progress to **painful** bullae on an erythematous base
   e. Positive **Nikolsky sign**: epidermal separation with slight lateral pressure
   f. Mucous membrane involvement
      i. Dysphagia
      ii. Eye erythema, pain, and discharge
      iii. Dysuria
      iv. Dyspnea secondary to tracheobronchial involvement
      v. Dyspnea from tracheobronchial involvement
   g. Complications
      i. Sepsis is the leading cause of death
      ii. Corneal ulceration, uveitis, and vision loss
      iii. Esophageal strictures
      iv. Penile and vaginal stenosis
      v. Cosmetic deformity
5. Diagnosis
   a. Skin biopsy is definitive and may be required to rule out other deadly bullous diseases such as pemphigus vulgaris (see below)
   b. Imaging and laboratory panel to uncover suspected underlying etiology
6. Management
   a. Supportive management
      i. Hydration
      ii. Treat skin lesions as burns, including possible transfer to burn center
   b. Identify and treat underlying etiology
   c. Steroids **not** indicated

   d. Address tetanus status
   e. Ophthalmology consultation with even minor eye complaints
   f. Mortality depends on degree of TBSA involvement
   g. **Admit** or transfer all patients

C. Pemphigus vulgaris (Figure 17–25, see color insert section)
   1. Definition
      a. Potentially life-threatening autoimmune **mucocutaneous intra**epithelial bullous disease
   2. Epidemiology
      a. Higher prevalence in Jewish and Mediterranean descent
   3. Etiology
      a. IgG against keratinocytes in demosomes causes acantholysis (loss of cell-to-cell adhesion)
      b. A pemphigus-like reaction (subepidermal) can also occur from captopril and D-penicillamine
      c. Associated with myasthenia and thymoma

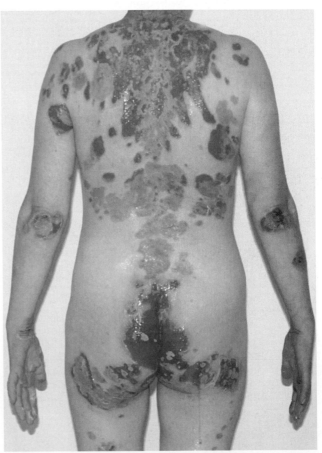

FIGURE 17–25. Pemphigus vulgaris. (Reproduced, with permission, from Wolff K, Johnson RA, Surmond D: *Fitzpatrick's Color Atlas and Synopsis of Clinical Dermatology,* 5th ed. Copyright © 2005, New York: McGraw-Hill.)

4. Symptoms and signs
   a. Mucous membrane lesions **precede** skin lesions
   b. Oral mucous and esophageal membranes most affected
      i. Dysphagia, hoarse voice
      ii. Dehydration
   c. Painful, **flaccid** bullae that easily rupture so that patients may present with only erosions
   d. **Positive Nikolsky sign** (not specific)
   e. Asboe-Hansen sign: gentle lateral pressure on bullae spreads fluid into neighboring unaffected skin
5. Diagnosis
   a. Skin biopsy to discriminate from SJS/TN and bullous pemphigoid (see below)
6. Treatment
   a. Admission for all but the mildest cases
   b. Steroids
   c. Immune modulators (azathioprine, cyclophosphamide, methotrexate)
   d. High mortality rate if untreated (with treatment 5% to 15%)

D. Bullous pemphigoid (Figure 17–26)
   1. Definition
      a. Chronic bullous disease that involves IgG against basement membrane (subepidermal)

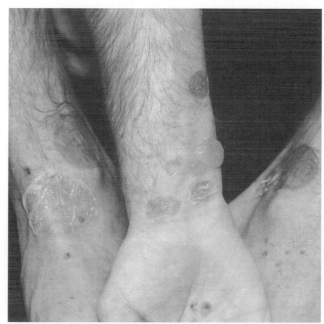

Figure 17–26. Bullous pemhigoid. (Reproduced, with permission, from Wolff K, Johnson RA, Suurmond D: *Fitzpatrick's Color Atlas and Synopsis of Clinical Dermatology,* 5th ed. Copyright © 2005, New York: McGraw-Hill.)

2. Epidemiology
   a. Most common bullous disease
   b. Age of onset: ≥60 years
3. Etiology
   a. Unknown
   b. Repeated skin trauma and presence of other inflammatory skin conditions (eg, psoriasis)
4. Symptoms and signs
   a. **Pruritic** skin rash that evolves into tender **tense** bullae
   b. Mucosal involvement uncommon (10%)
   c. Occurs over legs, forearms, axilla
   d. **Nikolsky negative**
5. Diagnosis
   a. Need biopsy to discriminate from pemphigus vulgaris
   b. Clinically differentiate from pemphigus vulgaris (painful, nonpruritic, flaccid bullae, oral prior to skin lesions)
   c. Cleavage at dermal-epidermal junction on biopsy
6. Management
   a. Consider admission for wound care with severe disease
   b. Often improves and relapses spontaneously
   c. Anti-inflammatory
      i. Steroids, tetracycline, dapsone
   d. Immunomodulators
      i. Azathioprine, methotrexate, cyclosporine
   e. Morbidity related to risks of long-term high-dose steroids
   f. Mortality most commonly caused by sepsis
   g. Relatively good prognosis compared to pemphigus vulgaris

V. Cancers of Skin

A. Basal cell (Figure 17–27)
   1. Definition
      a. Skin tumor arising from basal layer of epidermis or follicular structures (hair, apocrine glands)
   2. Epidemiology
      a. Most common human cancer
      b. Men >women
      c. Less common in dark-skinned individuals
   3. Etiology
      a. Predilection for sun-exposed areas
      b. Associated with remote arsenic ingestion
   4. Symptoms and signs
      a. Raised, smooth, waxy or pearly bump with central umbilication especially in face, head, neck, and upper torso
      b. Nonhealing or bleeding wound

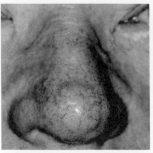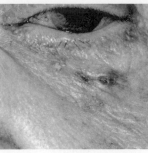

FIGURE 17–27. Basal cell cancer. (Reproduced, with permission, from Wolff K, Johnson RA, Suurmond D: *Fitzpatrick's Color Atlas and Synopsis of Clinical Dermatology,* 5th ed. Copyright © 2005, New York: McGraw-Hill.)

    c. Slow-growing, rarely metastasize
    d. Usually solitary lesions
    e. Ulcerations with raised edges
    f. Mucous membrane sparing
  5. Diagnosis
    a. Clinical
    b. Biopsy
  6. Treatment:
    a. Excision, cryosurgery, topical 5-fluorouracil
    b. Moh surgery (microscopically controlled)
    c. Generally has an excellent prognosis

B. Squamous cell (Figure 17–28)
  1. Definition
    a. Malignancy of epidermal keratinocytes
  2. Etiology
    a. Ultraviolet light exposure or susceptibility (fair skin)
    b. Human papillomavirus (HPV) infection
    c. Arsenic
    d. Immunocompromised individuals have highest risk of metastases
  3. Symptoms and signs
    a. Involves mostly structures in the lip, ear, head, and neck
    b. Well-defined red or brown thickened patch on sun-exposed areas
    c. Actinic keratosis: red or brown patch can develop into squamous cell carcinoma
  4. Diagnosis
    a. Lesions >2 cm diameter and >4 mm deep have high risk of metastases
    b. Biopsy: malignant transformation of keratinocytes
  5. Treatment
    a. 5-fluorouracil ointment
    b. Surgical excision
    c. Cryosurgery

C. Melanoma: metastatic; prognosis depends on depth of lesion (Figure 17–29, see color insert section)
  1. Definition
    a. Highly aggressive malignancy of the pigment-producing cells (melanocytes) of the skin
  2. Epidemiology
    a. Least common skin cancer but highest mortality
    b. White >Hispanic >African American
  3. Etiology
    a. Fair skin
    b. Sun exposure
    c. Family history
    d. Can arise de novo (70%) or from dysplastic nevi (30%)
  4. Symptoms and signs
    a. New or changes to existing mole
    b. ABCDE rule for diagnosing malignant melanoma
      i. **A**symmetry
      ii. **B**order (irregular)
      iii. **C**olor (different shades, not uniform)
      iv. **D**iameter (large, >6 mm)
      v. **E**levation, enlargement
  5. Diagnosis
    a. Skin biopsy

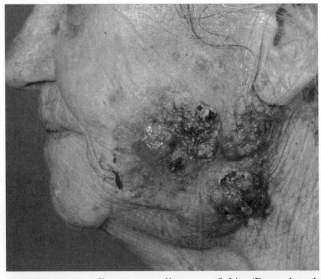

FIGURE 17–28. Squamous cell cancer of skin. (Reproduced, with permission, from Wolff K, Johnson RA, Suurmond D: *Fitzpatrick's Color Atlas and Synopsis of Clinical Dermatology,* 5th ed. Copyright © 2005, New York: McGraw-Hill.)

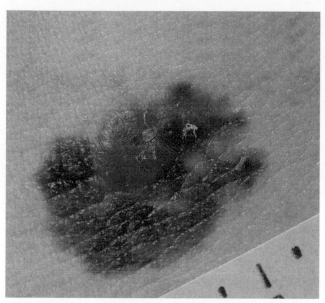

FIGURE 17–29. Melanoma. (Reproduced, with permission, from Wolff K, Johnson RA, Suurmond D: *Fitzpatrick's Color Atlas and Synopsis of Clinical Dermatology,* 5th ed. Copyright © 2005, New York: McGraw-Hill.

6. Management
   a. Early detection and excision is curative
   b. Surgical excision with wide margins
   c. Poor prognosis with lymph node involvement
   d. Chemotherapy for metastatic disease, but no effect on overall survival

BIBLIOGRAPHY

Wolff K, Johnson RA, Suurmond D: *Fitzpatrick's Color Atlas and Synopsis of Clinical Dermatology.* 5th ed. New York: McGraw-Hill; 2005.

Kasper DL, Braunwald E, Fauci AS, et al: *Harrison's Principles of Internal Medicine.* 16th ed. New York: McGraw-Hill; 2005.

Tintinalli JE, et al: *Tintinalli's Emergency Medicine: A Comprehensive Study Guide.* 6th ed. New York: McGraw-Hill; 2004.

Knoop KJ, et al: *Atlas of Emergency Medicine.* 2nd ed. New York: McGraw-Hill; 2002.

Chapter 18
IMMUNOLOGY AND RHEUMATOLOGY

Brad J. Kaufman and Tushar Kapoor

I. Transplant-related Issues

A. Complications of immunosuppressive medications
1. Cyclosporine: nephrotoxicity, neurotoxicity, hyperkalemia, hyperuricemia, hypertension, hyperbilirubinemia, cholestasis, gastric dysmotility, hirsutism
2. Azathioprine: leukopenia, thrombocytopenia, cholestatic jaundice, hepatitis, pancreatitis
3. Prednisone: Cushing syndrome, osteoporosis, adrenal suppression, hypertension, hyperglycemia, peptic ulcer disease, myopathy, cataracts
4. All immunocompromising medications may result in infection
   a. Increase the risk for infection (PCP, CMV, HSV, EBV, VZV, Candida)
      i. Most common infection is CMV
   b. Fever or other signs of infection must be taken seriously
      i. Immunosuppressed patients can rapidly progress to sepsis
      ii. Consider broad-spectrum antibiotics
5. Numerous drug interactions. Check before prescribing new medication

B. Transplant rejection
1. Epidemiology
   a. 30% to 50% of transplant recipients experience an episode of rejection
2. Etiology
   a. Transplanted organ identified as foreign
   b. Injury via cellular (neutrophil, macrophage, T cell, natural killer [NK] cells), humoral (B cell, antibody), and inflammatory (cytokine, prostaglandin) pathways
3. Classification
   a. Hyperacute rejection
      i. Rare event occurring minutes to hours after transplant
      ii. Caused by large amounts of preformed antibodies such as anti-ABO antibodies or human leukocyte antigen (HLA) mismatch
      iii. Also known as "white graft" reaction named for the white color of the graft due to loss of blood supply from arterial spasms
      iv. Most commonly occurs in kidney transplants
   b. Acute rejection
      i. Humoral and T cell-mediated
      ii. Usually occurs 1 to 2 weeks after transplantation
   c. Chronic rejection
      i. Multiple episodes of rejection occurring over months to years
      ii. Exact immunologic mechanism of this rejection is unclear
      iii. Gradual tissue death and transplant ischemia because of vascular injury

C. Transplants types
1. Bone marrow transplant
   a. Indication
      i. Malignant: leukemia, lymphoma, multiple myeloma, and some solid tumors
      ii. Nonmalignant: aplastic anemia and thalassemia
   b. Procedure
      i. Patient's native bone marrow and cancer cells are eliminated with radiation or chemotherapy
      ii. Harvested bone marrow is administered intravenously
      iii. Transplanted cells populate patient's bone marrow and function within 1 to 3 weeks
   c. Types
      i. Allogeneic transplant: bone marrow is from an HLA-matched donor
      ii. Autologous transplant: bone marrow harvested from self

d. Complications
  i. Graft-versus-host disease (GVHD)
     a) Occurs only in allogeneic transplantation
     b) Transplanted marrow cells attack host cells
     c) May present with rash and diarrhea
     d) Fatal without immunosuppressant therapy
  ii. Bone marrow is the only transplant not subject to attack by the host immune system (rejection)

2. Heart transplant
  a. Physiology
     i. The transplanted heart is de-innervated (no vagal tone) and remains slightly tachycardic with patient's heart rate between 90 and 100 beats per minute
        a) Heart rate does not respond to centrally mediated tachycardia but does increase secondary to circulating catecholamines
     ii. Electrical conduction of the transplanted heart
        a) May have 2 functional sinoatrial nodes
           i) One node from donor heart's SA node and one from recipient's SA node if left in place by the atrial suture line
           ii) ECG may have 2 distinct P waves
              (a) Donor heart's P wave correlates 1:1 with QRS complexes
              (b) Recipient's native P wave may march independently
              (c) May be mistaken for atrial fibrillation or atrial flutter
  b. Complications
     i. Rejection
        a) Symptoms and signs
           i) Dysrhythmias, generalized fatigue, or cardiac dysfunction on echocardiogram
           ii) Subtle presentation with nonspecific complaints that require biopsy for diagnosis
        b) Treat with immunosuppressive medications
        c) Rejection rates decrease >1 year but coronary atherosclerosis increases
     ii. Myocardial infarction[1]
        a) Accelerated allograft coronary artery disease post-transplant
        b) Some cardiologists perform yearly "routine" angiography
        c) 50% with coronary artery disease 5 years post-transplant

     d) Presents atypically with nonspecific symptoms
     e) Chest pain is the **exception,** and not the rule[2]
  iii. Sinus rate dysfunction: may require medications or pacemaker placement
     a) Carotid sinus massage and atropine have no effect on heart rate
        i) No vagal innervation
        ii) Isoproterenol, digoxin, calcium channel blockers, lidocaine,

3. Liver transplant
  a. Complications
     i. Biliary tract complications occur frequently (eg, cholangitis, stricture, leakage)
     ii. Acute rejection
        a) Symptoms and signs: fever, right upper quadrant (RUQ) tenderness, lymphocytosis, eosinophilia, and/or elevated liver enzymes
        b) Diagnosis requires biopsy
        c) Treated with high-dose glucocorticoids
        d) Patient should be transferred to transplant center if possible
     iii. Thrombosis of hepatic artery, portal vein, or biliary tract dilation
        a) Diagnose with abdominal ultrasound

4. Lung transplant
  a. Types: single lung, double lung, or heart-lung transplant
  b. Indications: cystic fibrosis, idiopathic pulmonary fibrosis, emphysema, or primary pulmonary hypertension
  c. Complications: infection and rejection
     i. Bronchoscopy may be necessary to discriminate between subclinical rejection and infection
     ii. Acute rejection
        a) Symptoms and signs: cough, chest tightness, fever, hypoxemia, decline in FEV_1, and/or infiltrate on chest x-ray (CXR)
        b) May have multiple episodes in the first year
        c) Treated with high-dose steroids

5. Renal transplant
  a. Complications
     i. Graft failure
        a) Results in acute renal failure defined as 20% rise of creatinine from baseline level
           i) Causes of graft failure
              (a) Nephrotoxicity from immunosuppressive drugs such as cyclosporine and tacrolimus

(b) Urinary tract infection or obstruction

(c) Renal vascular stenosis or thrombosis

(d) Renal disease from hypertension or diabetes

ii. Renal artery stenosis
   a) 10% incidence
   b) Caused by stricture or arteriosclerosis especially in those with hypertension

iii. Renal artery thrombosis

iv. Renal vein thrombosis: occurs within the first post-operative month

v. Hyperacute rejection (most likely with kidney transplant)
   a) Pre-transplant screening has made this a rare complication
   b) Symptoms and signs: range from kidney never functioning, requiring patient to return immediately back to dialysis, to an acute rise in creatinine within hours to days of transplant
      i) Pain and tenderness of graft may or may not exist

vi. Acute rejection
   a) Symptoms and signs: decreased urine output, elevated blood pressure, rising creatinine, and leukocytosis
      i) Severe episodes may present with fever as well as graft swelling, pain, and tenderness

vii. Chronic rejection
   a) Symptoms and signs: gradual rise in creatinine over 4 to 6 months with low-grade proteinuria and progressive hypertension

II. Hypersensitivity Reactions

A. Symptoms and signs
   1. Urticaria, pruritis, angioedema, abdominal pain, vomiting, diarrhea, bronchospasm, and/or conjunctivitis

B. Management
   1. Antihistamines (H_1 and H_2 blockers)
   2. Corticosteroids

C. Types (Table 18–1)
   1. Type 1 hypersensitivity (anaphylactic)
      a. Etiology: IgE-mediated anaphylaxis
         i. Occurs immediately after second exposure
         ii. May result in anaphylaxis
      b. Common triggers
         i. Antibiotics (PCN)
         ii. Peanuts
         iii. *Hymenoptera* stings
   2. Type 2 hypersensitivity (cytotoxic)
      a. Etiology: IgG and IgM reaction to cell-surface antigens that result in complement activation and NK-cell phagocytosis
      b. Examples
         i. Administration of mismatched blood
         ii. Hyperacute transplant rejection
         iii. Acute rheumatic fever (ARF)
   3. Type 3 hypersensitivity (immune complex)
      a. Etiology: soluble antigen-antibody complexes activate the complement system
      b. Symptoms and signs: fever, arthralgias, lymphadenopathy, pain, pruritis, and erythema at injection site
         i. Renal (eg, proteinuria, hematuria), cardiovascular (eg, myocarditis, pericarditis,

TABLE 18–1. Hypersensitivity Reactions

TYPE	MEDIATOR	REACTION
I (immediate, anaphylactic)	IgE	Cross-linking of IgE on mast cell or basophil causes histamine release. Requires two separate exposures to antigen. First exposure causes sensitization. May be triggered by antibiotics, foods, or *Hymenoptera* stings.
II (cytotoxic)	IgG	IgG and IgM react to cell-surface antigens resulting in complement activation and NK-cell phagocytosis. Examples include autoimmune hemolytic anemia, erythroblastalis fetalis, and Goodpasture syndrome.
III (immune complex)	IgG	Soluble antigen-antibody complexes activate the complement system. Example includes "serum sickness."
IV (delayed)	T cell	Activated T lymphocyte mediated. Examples include TB skin test, transplant rejection, contact dermatitis (poison ivy/oak).

vasculitis), neurologic (eg, neuropathy) or pulmonary (eg, dyspnea, cyanosis)

  c. Examples

    i. "Serum sickness" caused by the injection of foreign protein (eg, antitoxin made from horse serum, vaccines, and blood products)

      a) Medications have been implicated in causing serum sickness-like reactions (eg, allopurinol, procainamide, and quinidine)

4. Type 4 hypersensitivity (delayed)

  a. Delayed reaction occurs 24 to 48 hours post-exposure

  b. Mediated by activated T lymphocytes

  c. Examples

    i. TB skin test

    ii. Acute and chronic transplant rejection

    iii. Contact dermatitis (poison ivy/oak)

5. Anaphylaxis (extreme type I hypersensitivity)

  a. Definition: respiratory or cardiovascular compromise (distributory shock) with signs of allergic reaction

  b. Etiology: most common causes include antibiotics (penicillin), radiocontrast agents, and *Hymenoptera* stings

  c. Management

    i. Secure airway if respiratory distress or possibility of worsening angioedema

    ii. Epinephrine

      a) Racemic epinephrine via nebulizer can reduce laryngeal edema but does not replace intramuscular (IM) or intravenous (IV) epinephrine

      b) Epinephrine is indicated for any signs of airway obstruction, respiratory distress or shock. Patients may require continuous epinephrine infusion

        i) Subcutaneous administration discouraged (unpredictable absorption and slower onset)

        ii) IM injection in lateral thigh

          (a) Adults 0.3 to 0.5 mL 1:1000 solution IM q 15 minutes

          (b) Children 0.01 mL/kg (min 0.1 mL) 1:1000 solution IM q 15 minutes

        iii) IV

          a) Adults 1 mL 1:10,000 solution diluted in 10 mL NS

          b) Children 0.01 mL/kg (min 0.1 mL) 1:10,000 solution IV prn

        iv) IV infusion (all ages: 0.1 to 1 mcg/kg/min)

    iii. Consider glucagon for patients on β-blockers

      a) β-blockade may interfere with epinephrine and traditional therapy for allergy and anaphylaxis

    iv. IV fluids

    v. Oxygen

    vi. Antihistamines (H_1 and H_2 blockers)

    vii. Corticosteroids

    viii. Albuterol and epinephrine nebulizer for wheezing or chest tightness

    ix. Aminophylline for refractory severe bronchospasm

  d. Disposition

    i. All patients should be observed for 4 to 6 hours to ensure resolution of symptoms without recurrence

    ii. 6 hours observation for patients treated with epinephrine for rebound anaphylaxis

    iii. Unstable patients should be admitted to the ICU

    iv. If discharged

      a) Corticosteroids and antihistamines should be continued as outpatient

      b) Adult or pediatric epi-pen should be prescribed with clear instructions for use

      c) Follow-up with allergist

6. Angioedema

  a. Definition: edema of cutaneous and subcutaneous tissue secondary to capillary dilation

    i. Can be classified into allergic, idiopathic, and hereditary

  b. Symptoms and signs: painless, nonpruritic, nonpitting edema of skin

    i. May affect abdominal organs and upper airway

    ii. Abdominal involvement may mimic surgical abdomen

  c. Types

    i. Idiopathic

      a) Usually affects tongue, lips, and face

      b) Common triggers

        i) ACE inhibitors

          (a) Inhibits bradykinin degradation

          (b) Occurs in 0.1% to 0.2% of patients taking ACE inhibitors

          (c) Can occur at any time

        ii) Aspirin and NSAIDs

          (a) Any cyclooxygenase inhibitors

        iii) Contrast material

c) Management: supportive, although be prepared for airway management
   i) May be refractory to standard medical therapy with epinephrine, antihistamines, or steroids
  ii. Hereditary angioedema
   a) Epidemiology: 75% have first episode <16 years
   b) Etiology
    i) Autosomal dominant inheritance
    ii) C1 esterase inhibitor deficiency or defect
    iii) Leads to permanently low levels of C4
   c) Management
    i) Consider prophylactic airway management
    ii) Administer standard anaphylaxis therapy, although unlikely to be effective
    iii) Administer fresh frozen plasma (FFP) to replace C1 esterase
    iv) Danazol and stanozolol may be effective prophylaxis for frequent symptoms

III. Arthritis

A. Classification schema: significant overlap among entities
  1. Acute versus chronic
  2. By number of joints involved
   a. Monoarticular
    i. Septic joint (bacterial or gonococcal)
    ii. Crystalline disease (gout or pseudogout)
    iii. Lyme disease
   b. Oligoarticular (1 to 4 joints) and polyarticular (>4 joints)
    i. Seropositive arthropathies (antibody exists)
     a) Rheumatoid arthritis
     b) Juvenile rheumatoid arthritis
     c) Lupus erythematosus
     d) Endocarditis
    ii. Seronegative spondyloarthropathies (HLA-B27)
     a) Reiter syndrome
     b) Psoriatic arthritis
     c) Ankylosing spondylitis
     d) Inflammatory bowel disease (Crohn disease and ulcerative colitis)
  3. Symmetric versus asymmetric
   a. Systemic diseases such as ankylosing spondylitis, lupus, hepatitis, and rheumatoid arthritis tend to cause diffuse symmetric arthritis.

Psoriasis may be an exception to this rule (can present as either)
  4. Migratory versus nonmigratory
   a. Migratory (lasts 2 to 3 days)
    i. Lupus
    ii. Gonococcal
    iii. ARF
    iv. Bacterial endocarditis

B. Putting it all together
  1. Gonococcal arthritis: as a rule, a migratory asymmetric oligoarthritis that becomes monoarticular in 3 to 5 days
  2. Rheumatoid arthritis: a chronic nonmigratory symmetric polyarthritis with testable antibody (rheumatoid factor)
  3. Septic joint: an acute nonmigratory monoarthritis
  4. Lyme disease: multiple presentations in acute and chronic disease (see Infectious Diseases chapter)
  5. Lupus: affects all connective tissue and manifests with chronic symmetric migratory polyarthritis with multiple testable antibodies, most notably antinuclear antibody (ANA), especially anti-DS-DNA and anti-Smith antibodies
  6. Ankylosing spondylitis: chronic symmetric polyarthritis

C. Septic arthritis
  1. Etiology
   a. Joints seeded via hematogenous spread (most common route)
  2. Bacterial pathogens
   a. Described as gonococcal and non-gonococcal
    i. *Neisseria gonorrhea* most common in sexually active young individuals
    ii. *Staphylococcus aureus* most common in other age groups
    iii. Others: *Streptococcus viridans, Streptococcus pneumoniae,* group B streptococci, and aerobic Gram-negative rods
    iv. Nonsuppurative joint infection produced by *Borrelia burgdorferi* (Lyme disease), HIV, *Mycobacteria pneumoniae,* and fungi
   b. Rheumatoid arthritis and systemic lupus erythematosus (SLE) reduce normal defensive mechanism in synovial fluid
    i. More susceptible to infection
  3. Prosthetic joint infections
   a. Early infections (within 3 months of implantation) are caused mostly by *S. aureus*
   b. Delayed infections (within 3 to 24 months of implantation) by coagulase-negative *Staphylococcus* sp. or Gram-negative aerobes

c. Both early and delayed infections are acquired in the operating room. Late infections (>24 months following implantation) are secondary to hematogenous spread from various infectious foci

4. Symptoms and signs
   a. Pain, fever, and decreased range of motion
      i. The knee is the most common infected joint
      ii. Small joints less commonly involved
      iii. Only 41% have fever[4]
      iv. Symptoms may evolve over days to weeks
   b. Atypical presentation in the elderly, immunocompromised or intravenous drug abuse (IVDA)
   c. Gonococcal arthritis may also display skin lesions (dermatitis-arthritis syndrome) that evolve over a few days from papules to vesicles/pustules
   d. Group B streptoccocus most often infects the sacroiliac and sternoclavicular joints
   e. Bursitis causes swelling and pain
      i. Reduced active range of motion
      ii. Full passive range of motion
   f. Prosthetic joint infections may have minimal physical findings
   g. ≥12% mortality if untreated[3]

5. Diagnosis
   a. Arthrocentesis (Table 18–2)
      i. Normal joint fluid
         a) Straw-colored and clear enough to read newsprint through
         b) String sign: drops from a syringe will form a string 5 to 10 cm long between the gloved fingertips
         c) Will form a clot when mixed with 4 parts of acetic acid
         d) Synovial fluid glucose and protein concentrations are nonspecific and do not need to be performed
      ii. Septic joint fluid

         a) Typically white cell count is >50,000 with >75% polymorphonuclear leukocytes
         b) According to one study, 26% of septic arthritis <20,000 WBCs[5]
   b. Blood cultures
   c. If gonococcal infection is considered, obtain cultures from cervix, rectum, urethra, pharynx, and any suggestive skin lesions
   d. Fluid from an infected bursa may resemble that of bacterial joint infection
   e. Elevated C-reactive protein, erythrocyte sedimentation rate (ESR), and WBC unreliable[3]
      i. C-reactive CRP may be normal in up to 12%
      ii. ESR normal in 30%
      iii. Serum WBC normal in 50%
   f. X-rays
      i. May show only periarticular soft tissue swelling

6. Management
   a. Orthopedic consultation
      i. Drainage of infected synovial fluid
      ii. Surgical irrigation and debridement
      iii. Prosthetic joints may require hardware removal
   b. Prolonged course of IV antibiotics
      i. Start antibiotics prior to culture results
      ii. Initial choice of antibiotic is based on suggestive etiology as well as the results of the Gram stain

D. Gout and pseudogout
   1. Epidemiology: most common crystal-induced arthropathies
      a. Increased prevalence in those with a family history
      b. Males >females
   2. Etiology
      a. Gout is caused by monosodium urate monohydrate crystals

TABLE 18–2. Synovial Fluid Analysis

	NORMAL	NONINFLAMMATORY	INFLAMMATORY	SEPTIC
Clarity	Transparent	Transparent	Cloudy	Cloudy
WBC microliter	<200	<200 to 2000	200 to 50,000	>50,000
PMN (%)	<25	<25	>50	>75
Example		Osteoarthritis	Gout	Bacterial
		Trauma	Pseudogout	
		Rheumatic fever	Rheumatoid arthritis	

i. Acute episodes from overproduction or reduced secretion of uric acid

ii. Consumption of foods that contain high levels of purines may increase frequency of attacks (eg, alcohol, fish)

b. Pseudogout is caused by calcium pyrophosphate crystals

   i. Inflammatory response triggered by lysis of polymorphonuclear WBCs that have ingested crystals

3. Symptoms and signs

a. Monoarticular joint red, hot, swollen, and tender

b. Most common site for gout is first MTP joint (podagra)

c. Gout typically occurs more acutely than pseudogout

   i. Gout pain occurs within hours to a day

   ii. Pseudogout has an indolent progression that lasts days

d. May find extraarticular deposit of urate crystals, called tophi with gout

e. May require arthrocentesis to differentiate from septic joint

4. Diagnosis

a. Arthrocentesis

   i. Necessary to rule out septic joint

   ii. Send fluid for cell count, Gram stain, culture, and crystal analysis

   iii. Crystals

     a) Gout: negatively birefringent, needle-shaped monosodium urate crystals

       i) Seen both intracellularly and extracellularly

     b) Pseudogout: positively birefringent, rhomboid-shaped, calcium pyrophosphate crystals

   iv. WBC count in synovial fluid is usually between 50,000 and 100,000 in crystal-induced arthritis

b. X-rays

   i. May show degenerative joint changes with chronic disease

c. Serum uric acid level: cannot establish or negate diagnosis of gout as values range widely during an acute attack

5. Management

a. Acute phase of gout and pseudogout treated identically with ice, NSAIDs, narcotics and

   i. Oral corticosteroids and triamcinolone if patient cannot tolerate NSAIDs

   ii. Removal of crystal-containing fluid may relieve symptoms

b. Gout

   i. Colchicine reduces formation of uric acid crystals in the joint. Narrow therapeutic window. Toxicity causes vomiting and/or diarrhea

   ii. Allopurinol and probenecid used for gout prophylaxis, not for acute episodes

   iii. Avoid high-dose aspirin (increases uric acid levels)

c. Pseudogout

   i. Triamcinolone

   ii. No prophylactic medications for pseudogout

E. SLE

1. Epidemiology

a. Increased association in African Americans and females

b. Significant genetic predisposition

2. Diagnosis (Table 18–3)

3. Differential

a. Lupus-like syndromes

   i. Drug-induced

     a) HIPP (**H**ydralazine, **i**soniazid, **p**rocainamide, and **p**henytoin)

   ii. Lupus-like syndrome is discriminated from lupus by

     a) Lack of renal and central nervous system (CNS) involvement

     b) Resolution of symptoms with drug cessation

     c) Antihistone antibody levels elevated >95% with drug-induced lupus

     d) Normal C3 and C4 complement levels

4. Management

a. Emergency management of complications of SLE (eg, stroke, myocardial infarction [MI], pulmonary embolism [PE], cardiac tamponade, lupus pneumonitis)

b. Arthralgias and myalgias should be treated with NSAIDs

c. Initiation of glucocorticoids or cytotoxic agents with rheumatologic consultation

5. Complications

a. Morbidity and mortality from SLE often caused by infection, nephritis, thrombosis (often secondary to antiphospholipid syndrome), carditis, pneumonitis, pulmonary hypertension, stroke (higher incidence in first 5 years of disease especially if patient has antiphospholipid antibody syndrome), MI or cerebritis

F. Rheumatoid arthritis

1. Epidemiology

a. 1% prevalence in United States

TABLE 18–3.   SLE Diagnosis (American Rheumatism Association Revised Criteria)*

1. Malar rash—butterfly-shaped, fixed erythema over cheeks and bridge of nose
2. Discoid rash—erythematous patches with keratotic scaling over sun-exposed areas
3. Photosensitivity—often to UV light
4. Oral ulcers—painful or painless
5. Arthritis—arthralgias are the initial complaint in many patients
   a. Symmetric polyarthritis, frequently involving proximal interphalangeal (PIP) and metacarpophalangeal (MCP) joints of hands, as well as wrists and knees
   b. Consider septic arthritis if one joint is much more inflamed than others
6. Serositis—pericarditis, myocarditis, pleuritis
7. Renal disorder—may progress to nephrotic syndrome or renal failure
8. Neurologic disorder—most commonly headaches and difficulty with memory and reasoning but seizures or psychosis may also occur
9. Hematologic disorder—may have hemolytic anemia, leucopenia, lymphopenia, thrombocytopenia, or other alterations in blood counts
10. Immunologic disorder—such as vasculitis of intestine, retina, etc
11. Antinuclear antibodies (ANA)—very sensitive but poorly specific
    Anti-Sm—most specific but not sensitive
    Anti-dsDNA—specific but moderately sensitive

* Diagnosis requires at least 4 of 11 conditions at any time during a patient's history

b. Female to male ratio is 3:1
c. Disease leads to joint deformity from destruction of synovial membranes and articular surfaces
d. Prognosis worse with large joint involvement

2. Symptoms and signs
   a. Morning stiffness
   b. Polyarticular and symmetrical joint involvement evidenced by edema, effusion, warmth, tenderness, subcutaneous rheumatoid nodules, swan-neck deformities, ulnar deviation of fingers at metacarpophalangeal (MCP) joints
      i. Distal interphalangeal joints (DIP) usually spared
   c. May involve inflammation of other organ systems (eg, myocarditis, pericarditis, pleuritis, hepatitis, scleritis, and vasculitis)
   d. Arytenoid involvement results in voice change, stridor or respiratory distress
      i. May lead to a challenging intubation
   e. Atlantoaxial subluxation
      i. Cervical spine precautions during endotracheal intubation

3. Diagnosis
   a. Pleural effusions common with uniquely low glucose, low pH, and high LDH
   b. Arthrocentesis usually reveals synovial fluid with WBC count of 2000 to 50,000 per mm^3 and no crystals or bacteria
   c. 4 of the following 7 criteria are required for diagnosis of RA as per the American Rheumatism Association
      i. Morning stiffness that lasts >1 hour before improvement
      ii. Arthritis that involves 3 or more joints
      iii. Arthritis of the hand, particularly involvement of the proximal interphalangeal (PIP) joints, MCP joints, or wrist joints
      iv. Bilateral involvement of joint areas (eg., both wrists, symmetric PIP, and MCP joints)
      v. Positive serum rheumatoid factor (70% of cases)
      vi. Rheumatoid nodules
      vii. Radiographic evidence of RA
   d. Differentiate from osteoarthritis (Table 18–4)

4. Management
   a. NSAIDs and steroids commonly initially prescribed
   b. Patients should be referred to a rheumatologist for management with combination drug therapy, immunosuppressants, or immunomodulating medications

G. Juvenile chronic arthritis (JCA)
   1. Epidemiology: typically diagnosis in early childhood
   2. Etiology: unknown
      a. Not a single disease but a term encompassing a group of diseases manifested by chronic joint inflammation
      b. Disease may progress to other rheumatic diseases such as SLE or scleroderma

TABLE 18–4. Rheumatoid Arthritis versus Osteoarthritis

	RHEUMATOID ARTHRITIS	OSTEOARTHRITIS
Symmetric	Yes	Usually
Polyarticular	Yes	Yes
Involves DIP	No	Yes
Constitutional symptoms	General malaise, weakness, fever of undetermined etiology, weight loss, myalgias, tendonitis, bursitis	None
Multisystem involvement	Myocarditis, pericarditis, pleuritis, hepatitis, scleritis, vasculitis, pleural effusions, pneumonitis	None
Treatment	NSAIDs and/or corticosteroids, narcotics	NSAIDs

3. Symptoms and signs
    a. Morning stiffness and arthralgia
    b. Classified as systemic, pauciarticular, or polyarticular
        i. Systemic
            a) Fever of at least 102.2°F several times a day
            b) Linear evanescent rash on trunk and extremities
            c) Arthralgias
        ii. Pauciarticular (oligoarthritis)
            a) Arthritis affects up to 4 joints
            b) Typically larger joints such as the knees, ankles, or wrists
        iii. Polyarticular
            a) Arthritis affects 5 or more joints and can affect as many as 20 to 40 separate joints
            b) Often affects both large and small joints in a symmetric bilateral distribution
4. Diagnostic criteria
    a. Diagnosis of exclusion
    b. Arthritis (swelling and/or pain) in at least 1 joint >6 weeks
    c. Age <16 years
    d. May have evanescent salmon-pink linear rash on trunk and extremities, hepatosplenomegaly, lymphadenopathy, muscle tenderness, myocarditis
    e. Studies
        i. Elevated ESR and ANA titers
        ii. Radiographic imaging useful to evaluate for other diagnoses in differential
5. Management
    a. NSAIDs, methotrexate, etanercept (TNF inhibitor), corticosteroids
    b. Physical therapy
    c. Treatment requires a team-based approach to consider all aspects of illness (pediatric rheumatologist, physical and occupational therapists, social workers)

H. ARF
    1. Epidemiology
        a. Occurs in 0.5% to 3% of patients infected with group A strepcoccus
            i. Occurs 2 to 6 weeks after group A β-hemolytic streptococcal infection
            ii. Decline in incidence likely because of antibiotic treatment
    2. Etiology: molecular cross-reactivity between streptococcus and host cell proteins resulting in antibody production and a type 2 hypersensitivity inflammatory reaction
    3. Diagnosis (Table 18–5)
    4. Management
        a. Treat for any possible residual group A streptococcus infection
            i. Antibiotics
                a) PCN is the drug of choice
                b) Patients with chorea and preexisting cardiac disease should be on prophylactic antibiotics indefinitely
                c) Antibiotics typically maintained for ~10 years after last episode of rheumatic fever
                d) Antibiotics prevent development of rheumatic fever but do not prevent post-streptococcal glomerulonephritis
        b. NSAIDs, salicylates, or steroids for pain and inflammation
        c. May need to treat heart failure with digoxin
        d. Haldol for control of chorea

I. Ankylosing spondylitis
    1. Definition
        a. Chronic inflammatory disorder of the sacroiliac joints and axial skeleton resulting

TABLE 18–5.   Jones Criteria for Diagnosis of Acute Rheumatic Fever*

MAJOR	MINOR
1. Carditis • May include cardiomegaly, new murmur, CHF, pericarditis, valvular disease • Cause of much of the disability associated with ARF. May lead to mitral stenosis	1. Previous history of ARF
2. Arthritis • Involves large joints • Polyarticular • Migratory (ie, fleeting)	2. Arthralgia
3. Sydenham chorea • Rapid purposeless movements of face and upper extremities	3. Fever
4. Erythema marginatus • Long-lasting serpiginous rash	4. Elevated ESR or CRP
5. Subcutaneous nodules • Firm, painless nodules on extensor surfaces of wrists, elbows, and knees	5. Prolonged PR interval
	6. Rising titer of antistreptococcal antibodies

*Diagnosis requires evidence of previous group A strepcoccal infection as well as 2 major Jones criteria or 1 major and 2 minor criterion

in a tendency to fracture with even minor trauma

2. Epidemiology
   a. Male to female ratio is 3:1
   b. Starts in late teens to early twenties
3. Etiology
   a. Genetic predisposition: seronegative spondyloarthropathy associated with HLA-B27-positive individuals
4. Symptoms and signs
   a. Fever and weight loss may occur during exacerbations
   b. Chronic pain (usually in lower back), stiffness, fatigue
      i. May lead to severe physical disability and problems with mobility
   c. Pain and disability may lead to depression and emotional problems
   d. Associated with C1 on C2 subluxation
   e. Vertebral fractures or spinal stenosis can cause cauda equina syndrome and neurologic deficits
   f. Extra-articular manifestation: iritis, uveitis, aortitis, aortic fibrosis, and pulmonary fibrosis
5. Diagnosis
   a. Spinal x-ray may reveal "bamboo spine"
   b. HLA-B27 antigen positive >90%
   c. ESR, CRP, ANA usually normal
6. Management
   a. NSAIDs for pain control and to decrease inflammation
   b. Physical therapy may reduce symptoms
   c. Refer to rheumatologist

   d. Sometimes surgery can reduce complications (eg, spinal surgery to treat vertebral fusion or for stabilization of vertebral fractures)
J. Reactive arthritis
   1. Definition: sterile reactive inflammatory arthritis, often a consequence of infectious process elsewhere in body. Usually begins several weeks after the underlying infection has resolved
      a. More common in patients with HLA-B27
   2. Etiology: most commonly from gastrointestinal infection (associated with *Salmonella, Yersinia, Campylobacter, Clostridium difficile, Shigella, Entamoeba, Cryptosporidium*)
K. Reiter syndrome
   1. Definition: acute asymmetric oligoarthritis association with *Chlamydia* or infectious diarrhea (*Shigella, Salmonella,* or *Yersinia*)
      a. Association with HLA-B27 and HIV
   2. Symptoms and signs: last 1 to 6 months
      a. Classic triad of conjunctivitis, nongonococcal urethritis, and arthritis (mnemonic: can't see, can't pee, and can't climb a tree)
         i. Joint pains primarily involve knees, ankles, and feet
         ii. Urethritis often presents with frequency, dysuria, urgency, and urethral discharge
         iii. Conjunctivitis presents with discharge, erythema, burning, tearing, photophobia, and pain
   3. May have constitutional symptoms such as fever and malaise

4. Management
    a. Treat joint pain with NSAIDs
    b. Antibiotics for cervicitis and urethritis, but generally not for diarrhea

IV. Vasculitis

A. General
    1. Definition: inflammation of blood vessels
        a. May disrupt blood flow to affected areas (ie, cause ischemia)
    2. Symptoms and signs
        a. Fatigue
        b. Weakness
        c. Fever
        d. Petechiae
        e. Joint pains
        f. Abdominal pain
        g. Renal dysfunction
        h. Nervous system dysfunction
    3. Diagnosis: biopsy of affected tissue often necessary for diagnosis

B. Large vessel vasculitides
    1. Takayasu arteritis
        a. Epidemiology
            i. Peak age is 20 to 30 years
            ii. Male to female ratio is 1:8
        b. Symptoms and signs
            i. Initial systemic illness
                a) Fever, malaise, arthalgias, and fatigue
            ii. Upper extremity claudication
            iii. Jaw claudication
            iv. Bruits over subclavian artery or aorta
            v. Large vessel obliterative changes. stenosis and aneurysms
                a) Left subclavian, superior mesenteric, and abdominal aortic arteries most commonly involved
        c. Management
            i. Steroids
            ii. Angioplasty or surgical revascularization for critical stenosis
    2. Temporal (giant cell) arteritis
        a. Definition: large and medium vessel arteritis that may effect any vessel, but most commonly effects the temporal artery
        b. Epidemiology
            i. Consider in patients >50 years with headache
            ii. Male to female ratio is 1:4
        c. Symptoms and signs
            i. Jaw claudication in 50% (early sign)
            ii. **Visual loss** can occur in 50% of untreated patients

            a) Temporal artery provides blood to the ocular nerve
            b) Many have contralateral eye involvement within 3 weeks
            iii. Associated with polymyalgia rheumatica
                a) Effects up to 50% of patients with temporal arteritis
                b) Definition: inflammatory condition effecting the muscles
                    i) Most commonly neck, shoulders, and hips
                        (a) Results in debilitating pain and weakness
                c) Treatment: NSAIDs and glucocorticoid steroids
        d. Diagnosis
            i. ESR >80 in majority of patients. 10% have normal ESR
            ii. 50% have elevated liver function tests
            iii. Biopsy of effected vessel (most commonly temporal artery) is definitive but not sensitive
        e. Management
            i. Treatment with high dose steroids for 36 to 72 months
                a) Best to attain biopsy within 24 to 48 hours of initiation of steroids since arteritis is rapidly reversed with steroid treatment
            ii. Outpatient workup for most patients

C. Medium-size vessel vasculitides
    1. Polyarteritis nodosa (PAN)
        a. Epidemiology: untreated mortality is 80%
            i. Renal failure is the most common cause of death followed by CNS disease
        b. Symptoms and signs: commonly effects kidneys, nervous system, and heart
            i. Intractable hypertension
            ii. Associated with "locked in syndrome" with brainstem infarction
                a) Quadriplegia with upper facial motor sparing
                b) Preserved vertical eye movement and blinking
        c. Diagnosis
            i. Elevated ESR and C-reactive protein
            ii. May be p-ANCA positive
        d. Management
            i. Corticosteroids plus cyclophosphamide
            ii. Plasmapharesis and antivirals if hepatitis associated
        e. Complications include mesenteric ischemia and perforation

2. Kawasaki disease (see Pediatric chapter)

D. Small vessel vasculitides
1. Churg-Strauss disease
   a. Epidemiology
      i. Peak incidence in fourth decade (younger than most vasculitides)
      ii. Cardiac involvement and CHF is the leading cause of mortality
   b. Symptoms and signs: most commonly effects vessels of the lungs
      i. Adult onset asthma with eosinophilia
      ii. Dyspnea
      iii. Chest pain
   c. Diagnosis
      i. CXR may reveal infiltrates in most patients with advanced disease
      ii. Eosinophilia
      iii. p-ANCA positive
   d. Management: primarily with steroids
2. Wegener granulomatosis
   a. Definition: a vasculitis primarily effecting the upper airway, lungs, and kidneys
   b. Symptoms and signs
      i. Upper and Lungs
         a) Chronic sinusitis
         b) Frequent bronchitis and pneumonias
      ii. Kidneys
         a) Segmental, necrotizing glomerulonephritis
   c. Diagnosis
      i. Biopsy affected organ
      ii. c-ANCA positive
   d. Treatment: initially with steroids and cyclophosphamide
3. Henoch-Schonlein purpura (see Pediatric chapter)

V. Raynaud Disease

A. Definition: vasospasm in small arteries and arterioles
1. Usually in response to a stressor (eg, cold temperature or emotional strain)

B. Symptoms and signs
1. Usually involves hands and fingers
   a. Pain
   b. Pallor
   c. Cyanosis
   d. Numbness
   e. Parasthesias
2. Typically lasts 30 to 60 minutes

C. Management
1. May resolve with rewarming of extremity
2. May improve with calcium channel blockers or α-receptor blockers

VI. Scleroderma (Progressive Systemic Sclerosis)

A. Epidemiology: women to men ratio is 3:1

B. Definition: chronic autoimmune disease of connective tissue thickening and tightening

C. Symptoms and signs
1. May involve fibrosis of multiple organ systems
2. Most patients concurrently afflicted with Raynaud disease
3. May have CREST syndrome: **C**alcinosis, **R**aynaud phenomenon, **E**sophageal dysmotility, **S**clerodactyly, and **T**elangiectasia

D. Management (usually initiated by rheumatologist)
1. Skin lesions treated with phototherapy or minocycline
2. Kidney involvement treated with ACE inhibitors
3. Interstitial lung disease may be treated with cyclophosphamide
4. Pulmonary hypertension may be treated with prostacycline-like drugs
5. Weakness and muscle disease may be treated with glucocorticoids and/or immunosuppressants

REFERENCES

1. Neish AS, Loh E, Schoen FJ: Myocardial changes in cardiac transplant-associated coronary arteriosclerosis: potential for timely diagnosis. *J Am Coll Cardiol.* 1992 Mar 1;19(3):586.
2. Gao SZ, Schroeder JS, Hunt SA, et al: Acute myocardial infarction in cardiac transplant recipients. *Am J Cardiol.* 1989 Nov 15;64(18):1093.
3. Weston VC, Jones AC, Bradbury N, et al: Clinical features and outcome of septic arthritis in a single UK Health District 1982–1991. *Ann Rheum Dis.* 1999;58:214.
4. Schlapbach P, Ambord C, Blochlinger AM, Gerber NJ: Bacterial arthritis: are fever, rigors, leucocytosis and blood cultures of diagnostic value? *J Clin Rheumatol.* 1990;9:69.
5. Coutlakis PJ, Roberts WN, Wise CM: Another look at synovial fluid leukocytosis and infection. *J Clin Rheumatol.* 2002:8:67.

Chapter 19

HEMATOLOGY AND ONCOLOGY

Michael Cassara and Kevin Munjal

I. Introductory Considerations

A. Normal erythropoiesis
1. Differentiation of pluripotential stem cells into reticulocytes influenced by erythropoietin (produced in the kidney)
2. Hemoglobin is incorporated into stem cells
   a. Hemoglobin is a tetramer of four globin chains
      i. Adult hemoglobin consists of two α chains and two β chains
      ii. Each globin chain contains a molecule of heme. Each heme molecule contains ferrous iron (Fe^{2+}) at its center. Heme-containing ferric iron (Fe^{3+}) is known as methemoglobin (hemoglobin M)
      iii. Iron is transported to marrow (for erythropoiesis) and other tissues (for storage) by transferrin
      iv. Iron not incorporated into heme is stored in the liver and other tissues as ferritin
   b. 97% of adult hemoglobin is hemoglobin A ($\alpha_2 \beta_2$)
   c. Hemoglobin A_2 forms the remainder ($\alpha_2 \delta_2$)
   d. Fetal hemoglobin (hemoglobin F) consists of two α and two γ globin chains ($\alpha_2 \gamma_2$)
3. Reticulocytes enter the general circulation for 1 to 2 days before their final maturation
   a. Reticulocytes mature into circulating erythrocytes when they lose their nuclear and ribosomal material
4. Mature erythrocytes circulate for 120 days

B. Review of pathway for heme degradation
1. Macrophages in the spleen remove senescent erythrocytes
2. Porphyrin ring of heme is cleaved into biliverdin
   a. Biliverdin is reduced into unconjugated (indirect) bilirubin
   b. Bilirubin is conjugated in the liver into a water-soluble product (direct bilirubin)
   c. Examples of diseases of bilirubin metabolism
      i. Indirect hyperbilirubinemias
         a) Physiologic jaundice of the newborn
         b) Hemolytic jaundice
         c) Gilbert disease
         d) Crigler-Najjar syndrome
      ii. Direct hyperbilirubinemias (always pathologic)
         a) Dubin-Johnson syndrome
         b) Biliary tract obstruction (eg, cholelithiasis, choledocholithiasis, malignancy)

II. Anemia

A. Physiologic classification of the etiologies of anemia (Figure 19–1)
1. Hypoproliferation of erythrocytes
2. Disorder of erythrocyte maturation
3. Increased erythrocyte loss
   a. Hemorrhage
   b. Hemolysis

B. Analysis of the results of commonly available laboratory tests may assist the emergency physician in determining the etiology of anemia (Table 19–1)

C. Iron deficiency anemia
1. General considerations
   a. Total body iron stores (in descending order): hemoglobin, reticuloendothelial system, myoglobin, bound to transferrin
   b. Women possess less hemoglobin, less myoglobin, and less iron stores within the reticuloendothelial system compared to men
2. Etiology
   a. Iron-store depletion
      i. Growth (infants, adolescents)
      ii. Menstruation
      iii. Inadequate dietary intake

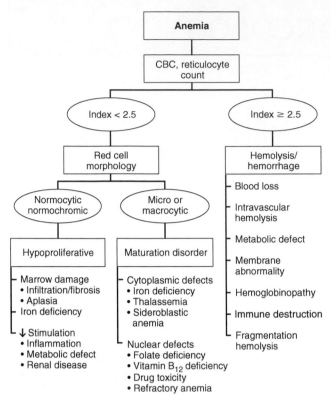

FIGURE 19–1. Etiology of Anemia (Reproduced, with permission, from Fauci AS, Braunwald E, Kasper DL, et al (eds.): *Harrison's Principles of Internal Medicine,* 17th ed. Copyright © 2008, New York: McGraw-Hill.)

TABLE 19–1.   Laboratory Tests in Anemia Diagnosis

I. Complete blood count (CBC)
A. Red blood cell count
1. Hemoglobin
2. Hematocrit
3. Reticulocyte count
B. Red blood cell indices
1. Mean cell volume (MCV)
2. Mean cell hemoglobin (MCH)
3. Mean cell hemoglobin concentration (MCHC)
C. White blood cell count
1. Cell differential
2. Nuclear segmentation of neutrophils
D. Platelet count
E. Cell morphology
1. Cell size
2. Hemoglobin content
3. Anisocytosis
4. Poikilocytosis
5. Polychromasia
II. Iron supply studies
A. Serum iron
B. Total iron binding capacity (TIBC)
C. Serum ferritin
III. Marrow examination
A. Aspirate
1. M/E ratio (ratio of myeloid to erythroid precursors)
2. Cell morphology
3. Iron stain
B. Biopsy
1. Cellularity
2. Morphology

Modified, with permission, from Fauci AS, Braunwald E, Kasper DL, et al (eds.): *Harrison's Principles of Internal Medicine,* 17th ed. Copyright © 2008, New York: McGraw-Hill.

    b. Malabsorption
       i. Sprue
      ii. Gastrectomy
     iii. Inflammatory bowel disease
    c. Hemorrhage
  3. Diagnosis
    a. Fasting serum iron <50 mcg/dL
    b. Percent saturation of transferrin <10%
    c. Serum ferritin <15 mcg/L (correlates with depleted total body iron stores)
    d. Total iron-binding capacity (TIBC) >400 mcg/dL
    e. Decreased mean corpuscular volume (MCV) and mean corpuscular hemoglobin concentration (MCHC)
    f. Microcytic and hypochromic red blood cells (RBCs) on peripheral smear
    g. Decreased reticulocyte count
  4. Management
    a. Search for underlying cause
    b. Emergent blood transfusion (acute, life-threatening, unstable, or symptomatic presentations)
    c. Oral or parenteral iron replacement therapy

D. Sideroblastic Anemia
  1. Pathophysiology
    a. Impaired integration of ferrous iron into the porphyrin ring of heme results in ineffective erythropoiesis and excessive iron accumulation
  2. Etiology
    a. Idiopathic
    b. Hereditary form (rare)
       i. Autosomal
      ii. Sex-linked
    c. Acquired
       i. Lead exposures
      ii. Pyridoxine (vitamin B₆) deficiency (elderly or alcoholics)
     iii. Drug toxicity (chloramphenicol, isoniazid)
     iv. Carcinoma and leukemia
      v. Hemolytic or megaloblastic anemia
     vi. Chronic alcoholism
    vii. Infection

3. Symptoms and signs
   a. Hepatosplenomegaly, pericarditis, lymphadenopathy, and secondary hemochromatosis
   b. Risk for acute myelogenous leukemia
4. Diagnosis
   a. Fasting serum iron is normal or elevated
   b. Percent saturation of transferrin is normal or elevated
   c. Serum ferritin is normal or elevated
   d. Hypochromic, microcytic erythrocytes with inclusion bodies; basophilic stippling may be seen in toxic lead exposures
   e. Lead levels are elevated with toxic exposures
5. Management
   a. Emergent blood transfusion (life-threatening presentations)
   b. Withdrawal of offending agents (drugs, alcohol, lead)
   c. Pyridoxine (vitamin B_6) replacement therapy
   d. Lead chelation therapy (indicated for toxic lead exposures)
   e. Iron chelation to treat secondary hemosiderosis

E. Megaloblastic anemias
   1. Etiology
      a. Vitamin B_{12} deficiency
         i. Inadequate dietary intake (strict vegetarians)
         ii. Malabsorption
            a) Pernicious anemia (intrinsic factor [IF] necessary for B_{12} absorption in ileum)
            b) Gastrectomy (IF produced by gastric mucosa)
            c) Tapeworm infection (*Diphyllobothrium latum*)
            d) Diseases of the ileum (tropical sprue, Crohn disease)
      b. Folate deficiency
         i. Inadequate dietary intake
            a) Alcoholics, drug abusers
            b) Elderly
         ii. Increased metabolic demand
            a) Pregnancy
            b) Chronic hemolytic anemia
            c) Growth spurts in infants and adolescents
         iii. Malabsorption
            a) Tropical sprue, Crohn disease
   2. Diagnosis
      a. Macrocytosis (MCV >100 to 110 fL)
      b. Decreased serum cobalamin levels (vitamin B_{12})
         i. Schilling test for IF deficiency
      c. Decreased serum folate levels
      d. Decreased reticulocyte count
      e. Peripheral smear with characteristic erythrocyte and granulocyte changes
   3. Management
      a. Search for underlying cause
      b. Replacement therapy
         i. Vitamin B_{12} (parenterally if malabsorption-related etiology suspected)
         ii. Folate

F. Inherited hemolytic anemias
   1. Hereditary spherocytosis
      a. Genetic defects of several proteins (eg, spectrin, ankyrin) necessary to maintain normal erythrocyte shape and rigidity
      b. Anemia, splenomegaly, and jaundice develop
   2. Glucose-6-phosphate dehydrogenase (G6PD) deficiency
      a. Etiology
         i. X-linked trait that causes defect in Embden-Meyerhoff pathway
         ii. Patients asymptomatic until exposed to oxidative stress
            a) Viral and bacterial infections
            b) Metabolic acidosis
            c) Drugs and toxins
               i) Antimalarial drugs
               ii) Sulfonamides (sulfamethoxazole, nitrofurantoin)
               iii) Vitamin K
               iv) Methylene blue
               v) Phenazopyridine
               vi) Naphthalene
               vii) Fava beans (*Vicia fava*)
      b. Acute hemolytic crisis develops
         i. Rapidly decreased hematocrit
         ii. Elevated unconjugated bilirubin
         iii. Decreased serum haptoglobin
            a) Serum haptoglobin binds tightly to serum hemoglobin
            b) Saturation and consumption of haptoglobin occurs with acute hemolytic crisis
         iv. Vascular collapse
      c. Management
         i. Withdraw known oxidant stressors
         ii. Treat underlying infection
   3. α-Thalassemias
      a. Etiology
         i. Impaired α-globin chain synthesis
            a) Excess β-globin chains are produced as a result of deletions or mutations in α-globin gene

b) The excess β- or γ-chains form unstable hemoglobin tetramers
  i) Hemoglobin H (β$_4$)
  ii) Hemoglobin Barts (γ$_4$)
c) These hemoglobin tetramers create abnormally shaped erythrocytes unable to transport oxygen

b. Symptoms and signs: depend on severity of α-globin gene defect
  i. Four α-globin loci deletion/mutation
    a) Incompatible with extrauterine life
    b) Few circulating hemoglobin (5% to 10%), most of which are hemoglobin Barts
    c) No circulating hemoglobin A
    d) Hydrops fetalis (Latin meaning "edema of the fetus")
  ii. Three α-globin loci deletion/mutation (hemoglobin H disease)
    a) Presents commonly in childhood
    b) 70% to 95% circulating hemoglobin A
    c) Serum hemoglobin ranges from 6 to 10 g/dL
    d) MCV ranges from 60 to 70 fL (microcytic)
    e) Reticulocytosis, hemolytic anemia, splenomegaly develop
  iii. Defect of two of four α-globin loci (α-thalassemia trait)
    a) Clinical picture similar to that of iron deficiency anemia
    b) Near normal erythropoiesis predominates
    c) 85% to 95% circulating hemoglobin A
    d) Serum hemoglobin ranges from 12 to 13 g/dL
    e) MCV ranges from 70 to 80 fL
  iv. Deletion/mutation of one α-globin loci (silent carrier)
    a) Essentially normal erythropoiesis
    b) Anemia and hypochromia is not present in these patients
    c) Circulating hemoglobin A, MCV, and serum hemoglobin levels are normal

c. Diagnosis based on serologic testing and hemoglobin electrophoresis

d. Management
  i. Four α-globin loci deletion/mutation
    a) Genetic prescreening and counseling of parents
  ii. Three α-globin loci deletion/mutation (hemoglobin H disease)
    a) Symptomatic care
    b) Blood transfusion
    c) Splenectomy

iii. Treatment unnecessary for trait or silent carrier state

4. β-Thalassemias
  a. Etiology
    i. Impaired β-globin chain synthesis (only two β-globin chain genes)
    ii. Excess α-globin chains do not form tetramers, as in α-thalassemia, instead, they attach to and damage erythrocyte cell membranes
  b. Symptoms and signs: depend on the severity of genetic defect
    i. Homozygous β-chain thalassemia (β-thalassemia major; β^0; Cooley anemia)
      a) No β-globin chains formed
      b) Common in Mediterranean populations
      c) Patients exhibit a severe microcytic hypochromic anemia
      d) Bone changes caused by increased marrow expansion retard growth. ("chipmunk" facies)
      e) Hepatosplenomegaly, jaundice, and dark skin (from melanin deposition) may develop as a result of hemolytic anemia due to repeated transfusions
    ii. Heterozygous β-chain thalassemia (β-thalassemia minor or trait; β$^+$)
      a) Some β-globin chains are formed
      b) Mild microcytic, hypochromic anemia, decreased MCV, and normal serum iron
      c) Elevated percentages of hemoglobin A$_2$ (~5%,) and hemoglobin F (1% to 3% to ≥15%)
  c. Diagnosis with serologic testing and Hgb electrophoresis
  d. Management
    i. β-Thalassemia major
      a) Severe untreated β-thalassemia major is fatal
      b) Periodic blood transfusions
      c) Splenectomy (may decrease transfusion requirement)
      d) Iron chelation therapy (with deferoxamine) to prevent secondary hemosiderosis
      e) Bone marrow transplantation
    ii. β-Thalassemia minor
      a) No specific therapy indicated
      b) Genetic prescreening and counseling of parents

5. Sickle cell diseases
  a. Etiology
    i. Valine for glutamate substitution causes distortion of β-globin chain and "sickles" erythrocytes

ii. Variants of sickle cell disease include sickle SC disease in which lysine is substituted for glutamate on the β-globin gene

iii. Patients with sickle SC disease have milder symptoms but may be indistinguishable from sickle SS disease

b. Symptoms and signs

i. Vasoocclusive emergencies

a) Pain crisis

b) Priapism

c) Stroke

d) Acute chest syndrome

i) Fever, chest pain, and pulmonary infiltrates

ii) Etiology unclear (may result from combination of fat emboli, infection, and infarction)

ii. Hematologic emergencies

a) Acute sequestration crisis

i) Typically in children

ii) Sudden massive pooling of blood in spleen

iii) Acute hemoglobin drop

b) Aplastic crisis (also associated with parvovirus B19)

c) Hemolytic crisis

i) Fall in hemoglobin concentration

ii) Jaundice

iii) Gallstones develop from increased bilirubin load associated with chronic hemolysis

iii. Infectious emergency

a) Splenic autoinfarction makes patient susceptible to encapsulated organisms

i) *Streptococcus pneumoniae*

ii) *Haemophilus influenzae*

iii) *Neisseria meningitides*

b) Osteomyelitis

i) *Salmonella* spp. (most common cause in pediatric patients)

ii) *Staphylococcus aureus* (most common cause overall)

iii) *Streptococcus pneumoniae*

c. Diagnosis with serologic testing and Hb electrophoresis

d. Management

i. Supportive and preventative

a) Maintain hydration

b) Avoid low O_2 tension (high altitudes)

ii. Blood transfusions (if severe anemia develops)

iii. Hydroxyurea (increases fetal hemoglobin levels)

iv. Exchange transfusion (with severe symptoms such as refractory priapism, acute chest syndrome, and stroke)

v. Surgical evaluation (for acute splenic sequestration)

vi. Intensive care unit (ICU) admission for severe illness (stroke, acute chest syndrome)

G. Acquired hemolytic anemias

1. Etiology

a. Entrapment (hypersplenism)

i. Normal function of spleen is to remove senescent erythrocytes from circulation

ii. Splenomegaly from infiltrative diseases, splenic congestion, and hypertrophy results in increased erythrocyte sequestration

iii. May cause concurrent granulocytopenia or thrombocytopenia

b. Immune mediated

i. Warm reactive IgG antibody

a) Idiopathic

b) Lymphoma

c) Systemic lupus erythematosis

d) Collagen vascular disease

e) Postviral infections

f) Drugs

ii. Cold-reactive IgM antibody (cold agglutinin disease)

a) Infection with *Mycoplasma pneumoniae*

b) Infectious mononucleosis

c) Lymphoma

d) Idiopathic

iii. Cold-reactive IgG antibody

a) Paroxysmal cold hemoglobinuria

i) Viral infection

ii) Autoimmune

iii) Tertiary syphilis

iv. Drug-dependent antibody

a) Methyldopa

b) Penicillin

c) Quinidine

c. Intravascular trauma

i. Thrombotic thrombocytopenic purpura (TTP) (see Platelet Dysfunction section below)

ii. Hemolytic uremic syndrome (HUS) (see Platelet Dysfunction section below)

iii. Disseminated intravascular coagulation (DIC) (see Disorders of Coagulation section below)

iv. Others: mechanical valves, aortofemoral bypass, structural heart lesion repairs

d. Extravascular trauma
   i. Jogging, marching, karate, playing bongo drums
2. Diagnosis
   a. CBC, reticulocyte count, liver function testing, LDH, haptoglobin
      i. Increased unconjugated bilirubin
      ii. Decreased or absent haptoglobin
      iii. LDH elevation not specific for hemolysis
   b. Peripheral smear
      i. Evaluate for schistocytes and evidence of intravascular hemolysis (eg, TTP and HUS)
      ii. Evaluation of RBC morphology for spherocytosis
   c. Coombs testing
      i. Direct Coombs test
         a) Detects antibodies present on RBCs surface
            i) Washed RBCs are removed from patient's serum and bathed in Coombs reagent
            ii) Clumping indicates a positive test
         b) Positive direct Coombs test seen with active autoimmune hemolytic disease
      ii. Indirect Coombs test
         a) Used for cross-matching blood
         b) Detects presence of antibodies in patient's serum
            i) Patient's blood is separated into plasma and cellular elements
            ii) "Normal" RBCs (not from patient) are added to patient's plasma
            iii) Clumping indicates presence of antibodies
            iv) Clumping indicates that the added RBCs are not compatible for transfusion into the source patient
   d. Urine
      i. Hemoglobinuria
      ii. Urine hemosiderin
         a) Free hemoglobin filtered by the kidney is complexed in the kidney with ferritin or with hemosiderin
3. Management
   a. Treat underlying disease
   b. Avoid transfusion unless absolutely necessary as hemolysis continues
   c. Slow transfusion to prevent complications
   d. Splenectomy indicated in severe cases of sequestration secondary to hypersplenism

III. Selected Disorders of Hemostasis

A. Normal hemostasis
   1. Depends on vasculature, platelets, and coagulation pathway (Figure 19–2)
   2. Intrinsic pathway
      a. Activated when blood comes into contact with injured and exposed subendothelial
         i. Slower than the extrinsic pathway
      b. Defects in the intrinsic coagulation pathway are evident by an abnormally prolonged partial thromboplastin time (aPTT)
         i. Deficiencies of factors VIII, IX, and XI account for 99% of all inherited bleeding disorders
            a) Hemophilia A (factor VIII)
            b) Hemophilia B (factor IX, Christmas disease)
            c) Hemophilia C (factor XI)
         ii. Antithrombin III inhibits factors IIa, IXa, Xa, XIa, and XIIa
            a) Enhanced antithrombin activity (with heparins) inhibits coagulation
   3. Extrinsic pathway
      a. Alternate route for activation of the coagulation cascade
         i. Rapid response following tissue injury (trauma)
         ii. Activates factor X almost immediately
         iii. Augments the intrinsic pathway
      b. Defects in the extrinsic coagulation pathway are evident by an abnormally prolonged prothrombin time (PT)
      c. Chemical reactions to activate factors II, VII, IX, and X require reduced vitamin K as a coenzyme.
         i. Deficiency in vitamin K will lead to impaired coagulation
         ii. Inhibition of vitamin K reduction (with warfarin) inhibits coagulation
   4. Common pathway
      a. Factor Xa converts prothrombin (factor II) to thrombin (factor IIa)
      b. Thrombin converts fibrinogen into fibrin
      c. Abnormal partial thromboplastin and prothrombin times reflect defects in the common pathway
   5. Fibrinolysis
      a. Occurs when plasminogen, tissue plasminogen activator, and fibrin are in close proximity
      b. Cross-linked fibrin is degraded and clot lysis occurs (production of fibrin split products)

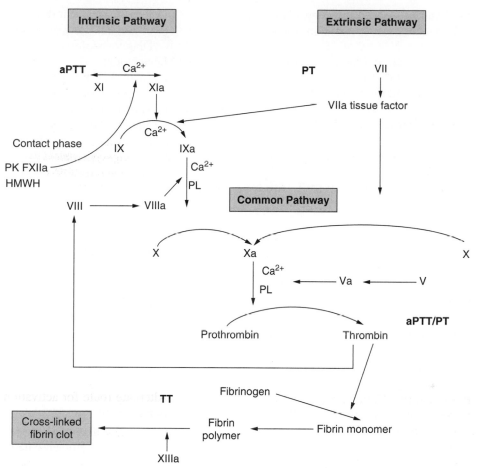

FIGURE 19–2. Coagulation pathway. (Reproduced, with permission, from Fauci AS, Braunwald E, Kasper DL, et al (eds.): *Harrison's Principles of Internal Medicine,* 17th ed. Copyright © 2008, New York: McGraw-Hill.)

B. Platelet dysfunction
   1. Thrombocytopenia
      a. Definition: platelet count <100,000 mm³
      b. Symptoms and signs
         i. Platelet dysfunction presents with mucous membrane bleeding (epistaxis, gingival, and vaginal bleeding), petechiae, and purpura
         ii. Counts <50,000 mm³: variable risk of bleeding
         iii. Counts <10,000 mm³: risk of spontaneous hemorrhage
   2. Heparin-induced thrombocytopenia (HIT)[2]
      a. Type I HIT
         i. Platelet recovery with or without cessation of heparin
         ii. Platelets rarely <100,000
         iii. Benign and not associated with thrombosis
         iv. Occurs within first few days postexposure
         v. 10% incidence

   b. Type II HIT
      i. Autoimmune, consumptive disease
      ii. Women >men
      iii. Occurs in 1% of patients
      iv. Occurs on days 4 to 14 postexposure
      v. Up to 30% incidence of thrombotic events
      vi. Arterial >venous events
      vii. Platelet-rich white clots
   c. Management
      i. Prevention (avoid heparins)
      ii. Use direct thrombin inhibitors (hirudin) when anticoagulation necessary in these patients
      iii. Platelet transfusion contraindicated with type II HIT unless life threatening bleeding present
   3. von Willebrand disease
      a. Epidemiology

i. Most common inherited bleeding disorder (1:1000); autosomal dominant transmission

ii. Role of von Willebrand factor (vWF)

   a) Facilitates platelet adhesion and links platelet membrane receptors to endothelium

   b) Plasma carrier for factor VIII

b. Classification

  i. Type I (most common): mild-to-moderate decrease in vWF

  ii. Type II disease: dysfunctional vWF

  iii. Type III disease: no detectable vWF

c. Symptoms and signs

  i. Mucosal hemorrhage as characteristic of other platelet disorders (epistaxis, gingival, vaginal)

  ii. Gastrointestinal (GI) or genitourinary tract bleeding

d. Diagnosis

  i. Abnormal bleeding time (classically, the best test)

  ii. Normal PT and PTT

  iii. Reduction of vWF activity

e. Management

  i. DDAVP sufficient for most patients

  ii. Factor VIII concentrate (20 to 30 IU/ kg) for rare patient with type II or type III disease

4. Idiopathic thrombocytopenic purpura (ITP)

a. Definition

  i. Acquired autoimmune thrombocytopenia without an identifiable cause

  ii. Autoantibodies attach to circulating platelets signaling for removal by reticuloendothelial system.

b. Symptoms and signs

  i. Thrombocytopenia with normal bone marrow

  ii. Acute form is seen most often in children (2 to 6 years)

    a) Antecedent viral infection (within 3 weeks of onset)

    b) Typically resolves >1 or 2 months

  iii. Chronic form is more common in adults (women >men)

    a) Associated with autoimmune disorder (systemic lupus erythematosus or HIV)

    b) History of epistaxis, gingival bleeding, menorrhagia

c. Diagnosis based on history and clinical presentation

  i. Thrombocytopenia $\leq 20,000$ mm³

  ii. Peripheral smear shows decreased quantity of large, well-granulated platelets

iii. Peripheral smear does not show evidence of mechanical hemolysis or schistocytes

iv. Diagnosis of exclusion

d. Management

  i. Acute ITP has spontaneous remission in >90% although chronic ITP rarely remits

  ii. Transfusion unhelpful as platelets are quickly consumed (not contraindicated however)

  iii. Steroids are mainstay of treatment

  iv. Splenectomy for steroid failure

  v. Immunoglobulin

5. TTP

a. Etiology and associations

  i. Pregnancy, AIDS, lupus, scleroderma, and Sjögren syndrome

  ii. Drugs: cyclosporine, quinidine, and tacrolimus

b. Symptoms and signs

  i. Classic pentad

    a) **F**ever

    b) **A**nemia (microangiopathic, hemolytic)

    c) **T**hrombocytopenia

    d) **R**enal failure

    e) **N**eurologic findings

c. Diagnosis

  i. Difficult diagnosis to make in ED

    a) Microangiopathic hemolysis (meaning schistocytes on smear) necessary for diagnosis

  ii. Laboratory testing

    a) Evidence of intravascular hemolysis

     i) Platelets <20,000

     ii) Decreased haptoglobin

     iii) Increased reticulocyte count

     iv) Increased indirect bilirubin

     v) Schistocytes or helmet cells on peripheral smear

     vi) Increased LDH

    b) **Normal coagulation studies** (helps to differentiate TTP from DIC)

d. Management

  i. Treat prior to definitive diagnosis

  ii. Emergent hematology consultation

  iii. Acquired TTP is treated with plasmapharesis

  iv. Corticosteroids helpful in presence of high autoantibody titers or plasma exchange failure

6. HUS

a. Definition

  i. Triad of microangiopathic hemolytic anemia (MAHA), thrombocytopenia, and progressive renal failure primarily in children aged 6 months to 4 years

    ii. Shares clinical features with TTP

b. Epidemiology

    i. Most common cause of acute renal failure in children

    ii. Primarily in children aged 6 months to 4 years but may occur in adults

c. Etiology

    i. Most cases associated with *E. coli* H7:0157 and production of Shiga-like toxin (verotoxin)

    ii. Less commonly a familial disease (3%)

    iii. Idiopathic

d. Symptoms and signs

    i. Bloody diarrhea in 50% with Shiga-like toxin

    ii. Seizures and lethargy

    iii. Fever

    iv. Hypertension, edema with renal failure

    v. Petechiae

e. Diagnosis

    i. Difficult to differentiate from TTP

      a) Renal dysfunction more pronounced with HUS

      b) Neurologic symptoms more pronounced with TTP

    ii. Urinalysis

      a) RBC casts

      b) Proteinuria

    iii. Laboratory

      a) Thrombocytopenia

      b) Anemia

      c) Evidence of renal dysfunction

    iv. Evidence of MAHA (nonimmune-mediated)

      a) Schistocytes on peripheral smear (RBC fragmentation)

      b) Elevated LDH

      c) Decreased haptoglobin

      d) Negative coombs testing

f. Management

    i. Supportive

    ii. Dialysis

    iii. Antibiotics not indicated

    iv. Consider plasmapharesis if unable to rule out TTP

C. Disorders of coagulation (Table 19–2)

  1. Hemophilia A

    a. Definition

      i. X-linked recessive bleeding disorder secondary to low or absent factor VIII

    b. Classification

      i. Severe (<1% factor activity)

      ii. Moderate (1% to 5% factor activity)

      iii. Mild (>5% factor activity)

    c. Symptoms and signs

      i. Spontaneous bleeding with severe disease

TABLE 19–2. Disorders of Coagulation

DISORDER	GENETICS	LABORATORY FINDINGS	CLINICAL FINDINGS	TREATMENT OF CHOICE
Hemophilia A	X-linked recessive	Normal or ↑ PTT	Hematuria, ecchymosis, hemarthrosis, intracranial hemorrhage	Recombinant factor VIII
Hemophilia B	X-linked recessive	Normal or ↑ PT	Same as hemophilia A	Recombinant factor IX
von Willebrand disease	Autosomal dominant	↑ Bleeding time; ↓ vWF activity; ↓ factor VIII activity	Hemorrhage from multiple sites; spontaneous bleeding in severe cases	DDAVP for responders otherwise factor VIII concentrate
Disseminated intravascular coagulation	N/A	↑ PT; ↑ PTT; ↓ fibrinogen; ↑ fibrin split products	Hemorrhage from multiple sites	FFP, platelets, PRBCs
Polycythemia vera	N/A	HCT >60%; ↓ erythropoietin; ↑ uric acid	Splenomegaly, hypertension, thromboembolism	IVF, phlebotomy
Deficiency of protein C and S	Unknown	↓ protein C; ↓ protein S	Thromboembolism	Anticoagulation, FFP
Factor V Leiden mutation	Autosomal recessive with co-cominance	(+) factor V Leiden DNA test	Thromboembolism	Anticoagulation

ii. Intracranial hemorrhage is a major cause of death

iii. Hemarthrosis

iv. Retroperitoneal hemorrhage

v. Ecchymoses and hematomas of deep muscles

vi. Mucosal bleeding not as common (more common with platelet disorders)

vii. Hematuria

d. Diagnosis

   i. Factor VIII assay

   ii. aPTT

e. Management

   i. Recombinant factor VIII: therapy of choice

      a) Each IU/kg increases factor VIII levels by 2%

      b) Life-threatening bleeding (central nervous system [CNS], GI, trauma) requires replacement to 100% factor activity (dose of factor VIII is 50 IU/kg)

        i) With CNS hemorrhage and head injury, do not delay treatment while awaiting computed tomography (CT) confirmation of hemorrhage

      c) Hemarthrosis and other moderate complexity injuries require replacement using a dose of factor VIII equal to 25 to 50 IU/kg

      d) Minor hemorrhage requires replacement using a dose of factor VIII equal to 12.5 to 25 IU/kg

   ii. Factor VIII concentrates (with risk of disease transmission)

   iii. Cryoprecipitate only if recombinant factor VIII unavailable (better alternatives now available)

   iv. Fresh frozen plasma (FFP) (contains little factor VIII; administration limited by potential for volume overload)

   v. "Bypass products" (eg, recombinant factor VII) may be used if severe allergies or antibodies to factor VIII exist

   vi. Steroids (for hematuria)

   vii. Epsilon aminocaproic acid (helpful for oral mucosal bleeding)

   viii. DDAVP (may benefit mild hemophiliacs by raising factor activity fourfold)

2. Hemophilia B (Christmas disease)

a. Definition

   i. X-linked recessive bleeding disorder secondary to low or absent factor IX

b. Classification and complications similar to hemophilia A

c. Clinically indistinguishable from hemophilia A

d. Management

   i. Recombinant factor IX is therapy of choice

      a) Each IU/kg raises factor IX level by 1%

   ii. Cryoprecipitate **does not** possess factor IX

   iii. DDAVP ineffective with hemophilia B

D. Prothrombotic disorders and hypercoagulable states

1. Deficiencies of protein C and protein S

a. Vitamin K-dependent proteins (made in liver) degrade activated factors V and VIII and terminate fibrin formation

b. Deficiencies are therefore correlated with thromboembolism

   i. Management: warfarin anticoagulation after initial heparin anticoagulation (to prevent theoretical "warfarin necrosis")

      a) Warfarin antagonizes protein C deficiency[3]

2. Factor V Leiden mutation

a. Most common familial thrombophilia in whites

b. May require lifetime anticoagulation

3. Antithrombin III deficiency

a. Mutation of either serine protease or heparin-binding site results in ineffective molecule

b. Treat with oral anticoagulants only after first thrombotic episode

4. Antiphospholipid antibodies (includes lupus anticoagulant)

a. Prothrombotic condition of unclear immune etiology

b. Presence of lupus anticoagulant leads to thrombosis, not bleeding (misnamed)

c. <20% of patients with lupus anticoagulant have systemic lupus erythematosus

d. PTT values may be elevated but hypercoagulable

e. Suspect in women with multiple spontaneous abortions

5. Paroxysmal nocturnal hemoglobinuria

a. Great imitator: thrombosis of large vessels to abdomen, brain, and liver can cause a myriad of symptoms

b. Classic triad

   i. Hemolytic anemia

   ii. Thrombosis

   iii. Pancytopenia

6. HIT

7. Myeloproliferative disorders (including polycythemia vera; see below)

8. Malignancy

E. DIC
1. Etiology
    a. Massive release of tissue factor into the circulation
        i. Obstetrical catastrophes (amniotic fluid embolism, placental abruption)
        ii. Metastatic malignancy
        iii. Massive trauma
        iv. Sepsis
        v. Bacterial endotoxin activation of coagulation cascade
        vi. Snake envenomation
2. Pathophysiology: syndrome of both thrombosis and hemorrhage
    a. Microthrombus formation
        i. Consumption of coagulation factors
        ii. Decreased fibrinogen
        iii. Increased fibrin split products
    b. Systemic hemorrhage (when coagulation factors depleted)
3. Symptoms and signs
    a. Dependent on site and severity of thrombosis and/or hemorrhage
    b. May be difficult to distinguish clinically from TTP and HUS
4. Diagnosis
    a. Abnormal coagulation studies (PT and PTT)
    b. Increased fibrin split products (positive D-dimer)
    c. Decreased fibrinogen
    d. Thrombocytopenia
    e. Schistocytes
5. Management
    a. Supportive care
    b. Bleeding complications
        i. FFP
        ii. Platelet transfusion
        iii. Blood transfusion (if necessary)
    c. Thrombotic complications
        i. Anticoagulation (heparin)

F. Polycythemia vera
1. Definition
    a. Overproduction of normal erythrocytes, granulocytes, and platelets in the absence of appropriate physiologic stimulus (ie, hypoxia)
2. Symptoms and signs
    a. Patients typically asymptomatic; symptoms caused by hyperviscosity and elevated histamine/uric acid levels
    b. Headaches, vertigo, dizziness (hypervolemia)
    c. Splenomegaly
    d. Systolic hypertension

    e. Venous or arterial thrombosis (stroke, myocardial infarction, renal infarction, Budd-Chiari syndrome, pulmonary embolism [PE])
        i. Risk of thrombosis correlates with height of erythrocytosis/hematocrit (not thrombocytosis)
    f. Platelet dysfunction
        i. Epistaxis, bruising, and GI bleeding
3. Diagnosis
    a. Elevated circulating erythrocytes, platelets, and granulocytes
    b. Hematocrit >60%
    c. Negative feedback leads to decrease erythropoietin levels
4. Management
    a. Supportive care
        i. Avoid excessive IV fluids when hypervolemia present (eg, elevated systolic hypertension)
    b. Phlebotomy
        i. Withdrawal of 500 cc of blood; replacement with isotonic saline
        ii. Target hematocrit for 55% to 60%
    c. Hydroxyurea (for elevated uric acid levels)
    d. Prophylactic anticoagulation not indicated
    e. Antiplatelet agents (ie, aspirin) may have a role in preventing thrombotic complications

IV. Selected Blood Component Therapies

A. Whole blood
1. Rarely used today (individual blood components provided separately)
2. Indications
    a. Autologous transfusion
    b. Exchange transfusion (ie, sickle cell anemia)
3. Comments
    a. Risk of transfusion reaction is >2 times than with packed red blood cells (PRBCs)
    b. Risk of allergic reaction is 1%
    c. Requires cross-matching

B. PRBCs
1. Preparation
    a. Plasma removed from whole blood and remaining RBC mass is washed
    b. Washing RBCs removes leukocytes, platelets, proteins, and other antigenic components of whole blood
2. Type and cross-match
    a. ABO blood group antigen system (Table 19–3)
        i. Most important blood classification scheme

TABLE 19–3. ABO Blood Types

	A	B	AB	O
Antigen on cell surface	A	B	AB	None
Antibody in serum	Anti-B	Anti-A	None	Anti-A Anti-B
Comments	—	—	Universal recipient	Universal donor

    ii. Major blood groups are A, B, AB, and O
       a) Erythrocytes possess (or lack) these surface antigens
       b) Individuals possess antibodies to the antigens they lack
    iii. Transfusion of mismatched blood will lead to an acute hemolytic transfusion reaction
  b. Rh system
    i. Second most important classification scheme
       a) Presence of D antigen confers "positivity" (ie, Rh$^+$)
       b) Absence of D antigen confers "negativity" (ie, Rh$^-$)
    ii. Production of anti-D antibody occurs in Rh$^-$ individuals who have exposure to small amounts of D antigen
       a) Maternal-fetal mixing (Rh$^-$ mother and Rh$^+$ fetus)
       b) Anti-D immunoglobulin required in Rh$^-$ mothers with exposure to D antigen within 72 hours of exposure
3. Indications
  a. Severe symptomatic anemia and hemorrhage
  b. NIH does not recommend transfusion for hemoglobin levels >6 g/dL in healthy nonsurgical patients
  c. Transfusion usually recommended prior to major surgery when hemoglobin levels are <10 g/dL
4. Administration
  a. Requires type and cross-match
  b. Unit of PRBCs has approximate volume of 250 mL
  c. In adults, 1 unit of PRBCs increases hemoglobin level by ~1 g/dL and hematocrit by ~2% to 3%
  d. In children, PRBCs increase the hematocrit by 1% for each mL/kg transfused

C. FFP
  1. Preparation
    a. Frozen fluid product of centrifuged and separated whole blood
    b. Contains factors II, V, VII, IX, X, and XI

2. Indications
  a. Clotting factor deficiencies
    i. Hemophilia A
    ii. Hemophilia B
    iii. von Willebrand disease
    iv. Hypofibrinogenemia and other clotting factor deficiencies
    v. Cirrhosis (lack factors II, VII, IX, and X)
  b. Massive blood transfusion (controversial)
    i. Transfuse 1 unit of FFP for every 5 to 6 units of PRBCs
  c. Coagulopathy secondary to super-therapeutic warfarin
    i. Transfusion of 5 to 10 mL/kg of FFP will reverse the effects of supertherapeutic warfarin
3. Administration
  a. Requires ABO-compatibility; not cross-matched
  b. Amount to transfuse: 3 to 10 mL/kg or as needed
  c. Each unit of FFP has a volume of ~200 to 250 mL
  d. Each unit of FFP increases coagulation factor levels by 2% to 3%
  e. 5 to 6 units of platelets contains the equivalent of 1 unit of FFP

D. Cryoprecipitate
  1. Preparation
    a. Cryoprecipitate prepared from precipitants of slowly thawed FFP
    b. Contains factor VIII, factor XIII, vWF, fibrinogen, and fibronectin
  2. Indications
    a. Hypofibrinogenemia (congenital, DIC, cancer, cirrhosis)
    b. Reversal of tissue plasminogen activator
    c. Coagulopathy from massive transfusion
    d. Uremic bleeding
    e. Clotting factor deficiencies (historically)
       i. Hemophilia A (better alternatives exist)
       ii. Factor XIII deficiency
       iii. von Willebrand disease (better alternatives exist)
       iv. **No role** in the treatment of hemophilia B
  3. Administration
    a. Requires ABO-compatibility; not cross-matched
    b. Each bag of cryoprecipitate contains 10 to 25 mL of fluid

E. Platelets
  1. Preparation
    a. Obtained from centrifuged whole blood

2. Indications
   a. Thrombocytopenia <10,000 cells/mm^3 in asymptomatic patients
   b. Thrombocytopenia <20,000 cells/mm^3 with active hemorrhage
   c. Thrombocytopenia <50,000 cells/mm^3 undergoing invasive procedure
   d. Dilutional thrombocytopenia (with massive blood transfusions)
3. Contraindications
   a. Diseases in which ongoing consumption will lead to worsening of thrombosis and ischemia
      i. TTP
      ii. HIT (type II)
      iii. DIC
4. Administration
   a. Amount to transfuse: 1 unit per 10 kg body weight (6 to 10 units of platelets for the average adult)
   b. Cross-matching is unnecessary, but all transfused platelets should be ABO and Rh compatible
   c. 1 unit increases the platelet count by 5000 to 10,000 cells/mm^3
   d. 5 to 6 units of platelets contain the equivalent of 250 to 350 mL of plasma (equivalent to 1 unit of FFP)

F. Transfusion complications
   1. Massive transfusion
      a. Definition
         i. No strict definition but commonly referred as the replacement of entire body blood volume within 24 hours, or >10 units of PRBC transfusions within a few hours
      b. Complications
         i. Metabolic alkalosis and hypocalcemia secondary to citrated blood
         ii. Hyperkalemia or hypokalemia
         iii. Hypothermia
         iv. Dilutional coagulopathy
         v. Thrombocytopenia
         vi. Acute respiratory distress syndrome (ARDS)
      c. Management
         i. Administer via blood warmer (no microwave)
         ii. Factor replacement as necessary based on coagulation studies (no definitive guidelines or formulas)
         iii. Calcium gluconate (if electrocardiographic changes occur)

2. Hemolytic crisis (acute transfusion reaction)
   a. Etiology
      i. Most commonly caused by ABO incompatibility
      ii. May result in activation of coagulation cascade (DIC)
   b. Symptoms and signs
      i. Headache, back pain, joint pain, anxiety, fever, tachycardia, hypotension, wheezing, pulmonary edema, and renal failure
      ii. Delayed reactions occur in extravascular space, most commonly spleen, liver, or bone marrow
      iii. Pink serum or urine
   c. Management
      i. Stop transfusion
      ii. IV fluids
         a) Maintain urine output at 30 to 100 cc/h
      iii. Laboratory analysis
         a) Repeat type and screen and cross-matching, serum haptoglobin, CBC, and chemistry
         b) Direct Coombs testing
3. Febrile transfusion reaction
   a. Etiology: recipient antibody response to donor leukocytes, and release of cytokines that are produced in storage
      i. Difficult to differentiate from hemolytic reaction
   b. Management: stop transfusion until hemolytic reaction excluded
   c. Prevention: use leukocyte poor blood if patient has a history of multiple transfusion or frequent febrile reactions
4. Allergic reaction and anaphylaxis
   a. Etiology: recipient response to donor plasma proteins
      i. Most commonly occur secondary to hereditary IgA deficiency
   b. Symptoms and signs: urticaria, pruritis most common
      i. Bronchospasm, wheezing, and anaphylaxis rare
   c. Management
      i. Severe: stop transfusion, support airway/circulation, administer epinephrine, diphenhydramine, and corticosteroids
      ii. Mild: may not need to stop transfusion
      iii. Suspect IgA deficiency particularly in patients of Arab descent
5. Transfusion-related acute lung injury
   a. Definition: self-limited reaction that resembles ARDS

 i. Noncardiogenic pulmonary edema (bilateral patchy infiltrates) within 4 hours of transfusion
 b. Etiology: thought to be caused by granulocyte and antibody deposition in the lung
 c. Management: stop transfusion immediately, support airway
6. Graft-versus-host reaction
 a. Etiology
  i. Donor blood attacks lymphoid tissue of host
 b. Symptoms and signs
  i. Nonspecific
  ii. Fever
  iii. Abdominal pain
  iv. Vomiting and diarrhea
  v. Rash
  vi. Hepatomegaly and right upper quadrant tenderness
 c. Diagnosis
  i. Clinical suspicion
  ii. Laboratory tests may reveal pancytopenia
  iii. Elevated liver function tests common
 d. Management
  i. Stop transfusion
  ii. Prevention
   a) Use irradiated blood in immunosuppressed patients
7. Infections (United States)
 a. Transmission risk highly variable depending on source[4]
  i. HIV: 1:1,900,000 units
  ii. Hepatitis B: 1:137,000 units
  iii. Hepatitis C: 1:1,000,000 units
  iv. Human-T lymphotrophic virus: 1:500,000
  v. Transmission of bacteria: 1:500,000 (PRBCs), 1:40,000 (platelets)
   a) *Yersinia enterocolitica* (most common; can survive in refrigerated blood products)

V. Selected Drug Therapies

A. Antiplatelet agents
 1. Aspirin
  a. Mechanism
   i. Irreversibly blocks conversion of arachidonic acid into thromboxane A_2 (platelet aggregation agent) by inhibiting cyclooxygenase (COX)
   ii. Effect on platelets irreversible, lasts for entire platelet life span (~7 to 10 days)
  b. Complications
   i. Reye syndrome in children
   ii. Thrombocytopenia

 c. Reversal
  i. Platelets rarely required (for intracranial hemorrhage controversial)
 2. Clopidogrel and ticlopidine
  a. Mechanism
   i. Irreversibly blocks ADP receptor on platelets
   ii. Deforms the fibrinogen receptor on platelet, that renders the platelet unable to aggregate via the GP IIb and GP IIIa pathway
  b. Complications
   i. Dyspepsia, rash, diarrhea
   ii. Ticlopidine is associated with hematologic effects
    a) Neutropenia
    b) ITP
    c) TTP
  c. Reversal
   i. Platelet transfusion

B. Anticoagulants
 1. Heparin
  a. Mechanism
   i. Reduced thrombin and fibrin formation by binding and activating antithrombin III
  b. Preparations
   i. Unfractionated
    a) Derived from bovine lung tissue
    b) Inhibits factors Xa and IIa in roughly equal proportions
    c) Requires frequent monitoring of aPTT (target generally between 1.5 and 2.5 times baseline)
   ii. Low-molecular-weight heparin
    a) Derived from porcine intestinal mucosa
    b) Higher ratio of antifactor Xa to antifactor IIa activity than unfractionated heparin
    c) Activity onset within 3 to 5 hours
  c. Complications
   i. HIT (see above)
  d. Reversal
   i. Reversed with protamine sulfate (derived from fish sperm; beware hypotension and anaphylaxis)
 2. Warfarin
  a. Mechanism
   i. Inhibits synthesis of vitamin K-dependent coagulation factors (factors II, VII, IX, and X)
   ii. Also inhibits the anticoagulants protein C and protein S
   iii. Ingredient in many rodenticides or "superwarfarins"

b. Reversal
   i. Reversed with FFP or prothrombin complex concentrate
   ii. May be reversed with vitamin K
     a) Oral route preferred, unless rapid reversal required (may administer intravenously)
     b) Delay (up to 24 hours) in onset
3. GP IIb and GP IIIa receptor inhibitors (eg, abciximab, eptifibatide, tirofiban)
  a. Mechanism
   i. Inhibit platelet aggregation and activation by preventing activated fibrinogen binding to GP IIb and GP IIIa receptors
   ii. Effects typically last 24 to 48 hours
  b. Complications
   i. Thrombocytopenia
   ii. Hemorrhage
  c. Reversal
   i. Platelet transfusion
   ii. Desmopressin (may be beneficial)

C. Fibrinolytics
1. Mechanism
  a. Convert plasminogen to plasmin
  b. Plasmin dissolves fibrin to fibrin split products
2. Preparations
  a. Streptokinase (SK)
   i. Derived from β-hemolytic streptococci (highly antigenic)
   ii. Do not administer within 6 months of prior usage (common practice was to use only once per patient) or within 12 months of antecedent streptococcal infection
  b. Urokinase
   i. Derived from human neonatal kidney cells
  c. Tissue plasminogen activator (tPA)
  d. Reteplase (recombinant variant of tPA)
  e. Tenecteplase (recombinant variant of tPA)
   i. Higher level of fibrin specificity and increased potency with newer generation preparations
3. Indications
  a. Acute ST-segment elevation myocardial infarction
  b. Acute ischemic stroke (tPA)
  c. Massive PE
  d. Thrombosed arteriovenous shunts
4. Complications
  a. CNS hemorrhage
   i. 0.7% with treatment for myocardial infarction
   ii. In the NINDS trial, rate of intracranial hemorrhage was 6.4% versus 0.6% without tPA
  b. Hemorrhage from other sites

5. Reversal of thrombolytic therapy
  a. Epsilon-aminocaproic acid
   i. Use for life-threatening bleeding only (uncontrolled thrombosis may result)
  b. Cryoprecipitate to replace fibrinogen

VI. Hematologic Neoplasms

A. Leukemias
1. Definition
  a. Proliferation of immature or abnormal cell lines that crowd out bone marrow resulting in neutropenia, anemia, and thrombocytopenia
2. Classification
  a. Acute versus chronic
   i. Acute leukemias
    a) Occur quickly and need rapid treatment
    b) Generally present with more anemia, neutropenia, and thrombocytopenia (cells are arrested in immature stage)
   ii. Chronic leukemias
    a) Can occur over years and be asymptomatic in early disease
  b. Lymphoid versus myeloid
   i. Myeloid cells differentiate into granulocytes that protect against bacterial infections
   ii. Lymphoid cells differentiate into T cells, B cells, and natural killer (NK) cells
    a) T cells are involved in cell-mediated immunity
    b) B cells are involved with humoral immunity and produce antibodies
    c) NK cells protect the host from tumors and viruses
3. Acute myeloid leukemia (AML)
  a. Epidemiology–incidence greater in men and elderly
  b. Risk factors
   i. Down syndrome (trisomy 21), Klinefelter syndrome (XXY), and Patau syndrome (trisomy 13)
   ii. Radiation exposure
   iii. Chemical and toxic exposures
    a) Benzene
    b) Smoking
    c) Herbicides and pesticides
    d) Petroleum products
    e) Antineoplastic drugs (most common)
  c. Symptoms and signs
   i. Constitutional (fatigue, anorexia, weight loss, fever)
   ii. Bone pain
   iii. Lymphadenopathy

d. Diagnosis
  i. Anemia, thrombocytopenia, leukocytosis, or leukopenia
  ii. Bone marrow aspirate/biopsy
e. Management
  i. Supportive care
    a) Transfusion therapy
    b) Infection prophylaxis/treatment
    c) Recombinant hematopoietic growth factors
  ii. Induction chemotherapy
  iii. Bone marrow transplantation
4. Chronic myeloid leukemia (CML; least common of major leukemias)
  a. Epidemiology: incidence increases with age
  b. Risk factors
    i. Translocation of chromosomes 9 and 22 (Philadelphia chromosome)
    ii. Radiation exposure
    iii. Chemical and toxic exposures
    iv. Smoking accelerates the progression to blast crisis
  c. Symptoms and signs
    i. Patients may be asymptomatic
    ii. Constitutional symptoms (as above)
    iii. Splenomegaly
    iv. Bleeding
    v. Thrombosis (with WBC counts >100,000 cells/mm^3)
    vi. Lymphadenopathy
    vii. Inevitably, disease transitions from a chronic phase to an accelerated phase with blast crisis
  d. Diagnosis
    i. Routine laboratory serology
    ii. Bone marrow aspirate or biopsy
    iii. Blast crisis is defined as acute leukemia >30% blasts
  e. Management
    i. Supportive care
      a) Transfusion therapy
      b) Infection prophylaxis/treatment
      c) Leukopheresis
      d) Splenectomy
    ii. Bone marrow transplantation (only potential cure)
    iii. Interferon-α
    iv. Chemotherapy
    v. Median survival of 4 years
5. Acute lymphocytic leukemia (ALL)
  a. Epidemiology: most common leukemia in children and young adults
  b. Symptoms and signs
    i. Of bone marrow failure
    ii. 10% present with DIC

iii. Hepatosplenomegaly
iv. Lymphadenopathy
v. CNS infiltration
vi. Uric acid nephropathy
  a) Rapid turnover of acute leukemic cells
  b) May lead to tumor lysis syndrome (see below)
vii. Infection is leading cause of death
  a) *Staphylococcus* spp., Gram-negative organisms, fungi (*Aspergillus*, *Candida* spp.), opportunistic pathogens (*Pneumocystis juroveci*), viruses (HSV)
c. Diagnosis
  i. Lymph node and tissue biopsy
  ii. Bone marrow aspiration
d. Management
  i. Supportive care
  ii. Chemotherapy
  iii. Bone marrow transplantation
6. Chronic lymphocytic leukemia (CLL)
  a. Epidemiology
    i. Most common adult leukemia in Western countries
    ii. Elder patients
    iii. Males more commonly affected females
  b. Symptoms and signs
    i. Asymptomatic lymphocytosis
    ii. Constitutional symptoms uncommon, unless concurrent infection, extensive bulky disease, or transformation to aggressive lymphoma
  c. Diagnosis often requires ancillary testing, including lymph node or tissue biopsy and/or bone marrow aspiration
  d. Management
    i. Supportive care
    ii. Chemotherapy
    iii. Immunoglobulin therapy
    iv. Splenectomy
    v. Bone marrow transplantation
    vi. Median survival <2 years

B. Lymphoma
  1. Non-Hodgkin lymphoma (NHL)
    a. Leading cause of cancer-related death
    b. Worse prognosis than that for Hodgkin lymphoma (HL)
    c. Symptoms and signs
      i. Persistent, painless, peripheral lymphadenopathy
        a) Epitrochlear nodes, mesenteric nodes, mediastinal nodes, retroperitoneal nodes, pelvic nodes, and enlargement of oral/nasal lymphoid tissue are consistent with NHL

b) Any lymph node >1 cm persistent for >4 weeks and unassociated with a documented infection should be considered for biopsy

c) May mimic infectious mononucleosis

ii. Chest discomfort

a) May present with superior vena cava (SVC) syndrome (see below)

d. Diagnosis often requires specialized ancillary testing, including lymph node biopsy and/or bone marrow aspiration

e. Management

i. Supportive care and observation

ii. Chemotherapy

iii. Radiation therapy

iv. Interferon-α

v. Monoclonal antibodies

vi. Bone marrow transplantation

vii. Surgical resection

2. Hodgkin lymphoma (HL)

a. Epidemiology

i. Bimodal age distribution 15 to 35 and >55 years

b. Symptoms and signs

i. Nontender lymph nodes

a) Cervical or supraclavicular lymphadenopathy

b) Mediastinal adenopathy

c) Nodes may become painful after drinking alcohol

ii. Constitutional symptoms (fever, night sweats, and weight loss)

iii. Persistent cough

iv. Chest discomfort

a) May present as superior vena cava syndrome

v. Bone pain

vi. Sudden spinal cord compression (advanced disease)

c. Diagnosis

i. Lymph node biopsy and/or bone marrow aspiration

ii. Presence of **Reed-Sternberg cells**

iii. Better prognosis than NHL

d. Management

i. Supportive care

ii. Staging laparotomy

iii. Radiation therapy and chemotherapy (mainstay of treatment)

iv. Bone marrow transplantation

C. Multiple myeloma

1. Definition

a. Malignant proliferation of plasma cells derived from a single clone

2. Symptoms and signs

a. Bone pain (most common symptom)

i. Back and ribs

ii. May be associated with pathologic fracture

iii. Spinal cord compression at lytic lesion sites

b. Bacterial infections

i. Hypogammaglobulinemia

a) Decreased production/increased destruction of normal immunoglobulins; poor response in presence of infection

c. Renal failure

i. Hypercalcemia is the most common cause

ii. Tubular damage (excretion of light chains)

d. Anemia

e. Bleeding

f. Hyperviscosity syndrome

g. POEMS syndrome

i. **P**olyneuropathy, **O**rganomegaly, **E**ndocrinopathy, **M**ultiple myeloma, and **S**kin changes

3. Diagnosis

a. Bone marrow aspiration

b. Marrow plasmacytosis >10%

c. Lytic bone lesions

d. Serum immunoglobulin levels

e. Serum protein electrophoresis

f. Bence-Jones (light chain) proteins in urine

G. Incidence increases with age (median age at diagnosis is 68 years)

4. Management

a. Supportive care

i. Glucocorticoid therapy

ii. Calcitonin and bisphosphonates for hypercalcemia

iii. Prophylactic antibiotics and IV γ globulin therapy

b. Allopurinol to prevent hyperuricemia

c. Plasmapheresis to remove serum light chains

d. Chemotherapy/bone marrow transplant

5. Prognosis

a. 15% die within the first 3 months of diagnosis

b. Subsequent death rate is 15% per year

VII. Selected Oncologic Emergencies

A. Neutropenic fever

1. Definition

a. Single oral temperature of ≥38.3°C (101°F) **or** sustained temperature elevation of 38°C (100.4°F) for 1 hour **and**

b. Polymorphonuclear leukocyte count <500 to 1000 cells/mm^3

2. Diagnosis
   a. All neutropenic patients with fever should be managed as if they have a serious bacterial infection
   b. Cultures (blood, urine, and other areas as indicated)
   c. Radiographic imaging as indicated (eg, chest radiographs, CT sinuses, etc.)
3. Management
   a. Admission
   b. Start prophylactic empiric antibiotic therapy
      i. Monotherapy
         a) Imipenem and cilastatin
         b) Ceftazidime
         c) Cefipime
      ii. Combination therapy
         a) Antipseudomonal penicillin + aminoglycoside
         b) Ceftazidime or cefepime or imipenem/cilastatin and vancomycin
            i) This combination is for suspected infection with MRSA (recent hospitalizations) or in patients with indwelling catheters
4. Complications
   a. Untreated neutropenic fever associated with a 20% mortality rate compared to <2% if treated promptly
   b. Infections are the number one cause of cancer death
   c. Although fever may result from the malignancy itself, 55% to 70% of fevers in this patient population will have an infectious etiology

B. Hyperviscosity syndrome (HVS)
1. Definition
   a. Elevated serum viscosity that causes sludging, decreased microvascular perfusion, and vascular stasis
   b. Serum viscosity relative to water 4 to 5 (normal 1.4 to 1.8)
2. Etiologies
   a. Increased serum protein (dysproteinemia) is the most common cause
      i. Waldenström macroglobulinemia
      ii. Multiple myeloma
   b. Marked leukocytosis (>100,000 cells/mm^3) or erythrocytosis
      i. Leukemias, polycythemia vera, other dysproteinemias, and other hemoglobinopathies (eg, sickle cell anemia)
3. Symptoms and signs

   a. End-organ ischemia (myocardial infarction, stroke, or nonspecific neurologic symptoms, renal insufficiency/failure)
   b. Congestive heart failure, respiratory failure
   c. Mucosal hemorrhage
   d. Visual disturbances
      i. Results from retinopathy
      ii. Ophthalmic examination reveals venous engorgement with "sausage-link" or "boxcar" segmentation
      iii. Hemorrhages, exudates, and papilledema
4. Diagnosis
   a. CBC
   b. Serum protein electrophoresis (SPEP) and urine protein electrophoresis (UPEP) abnormalities help to differentiate the various dysproteinemias
   c. Hypercalcemia
   d. Elevated erythrocyte sedimentation rate
   e. Presence of Bence-Jones proteins may indicate multiple myeloma
   f. Pseudohyponatremia (see endocrine and metabolic section) may result from hyperproteinemia
   g. Anemia with rouleaux formation may indicate Waldenström macroglobulinemia
5. Management depends on etiology
   a. Supportive care
      i. Fluid hydration
      ii. Diuresis
   b. Temporizing measure
      i. For patients with known dysproteinemia and coma
      ii. Two-unit phlebotomy, then replacement of the patient's RBCs with physiologic saline
   c. Emergent leukapheresis and plasmapheresis
   d. Phlebotomy for polycythemia vera

C. Tumor lysis syndrome
1. Definition
   a. Electrolyte abnormalities that result from the breakdown products of dying cancer cells
2. Etiology
   a. Typically following chemotherapy of
      i. Leukemias and lymphomas (especially Burkitt lymphoma)
      ii. Small cell lung carcinoma
   b. Following steroid administration
3. Symptoms and signs
   a. Occurs most commonly within 1 to 5 days of initiating chemotherapy or radiation therapy for rapidly growing tumors
   b. Reflect the presenting electrolyte abnormality

4. Diagnosis (constellation of the following metabolic disturbances)
   a. Hyperuricemia (>7 or 8 mg/dL)
      i. Secondary to DNA degradation
      ii. Acute renal failure
   b. Hyperkalemia
      i. Susceptible to arrhythmias
      ii. Exacerbated by renal failure
   c. Hyperphosphatemia
      i. Secondary to protein degradation
      ii. Precipitation with calcium in heart and kidney
   d. Hypocalcemia
      i. Secondary to hyperphosphatemia
      ii. Muscle weakness and cramps
5. Management
   a. Prevention
      i. Delay chemotherapy or radiation therapy if underlying disorders (eg, renal insufficiency) exist
   b. Hyperuricemia
      i. Fluids
      ii. Allopurinol
      iii. Alkalinize urine with acetazolamide
      iv. Monitor electrolytes
   c. Withdraw offending agents
      i. Stop chemotherapy and radiation therapy
   d. Hemodialysis (indications listed below)
      i. Potassium >6 mEq/L
      ii. Uric acid >10 mg/dL
      iii. Creatinine >10 mg/dL
      iv. Phosphorous >10 mg/dL
      v. Volume overload
      vi. Symptomatic hypocalcemia

D. Hypercalcemia
   1. Most common electrolyte disorder associated with cancer
   2. Etiology (in the cancer patient)
      a. Metastatic bone disease
         i. Release of calcium (and phosphate) from osteolysis
      b. Tumor-produced hormone-like substances
         i. Parathyroid hormone
         ii. Prostaglandins and other peptides may increase osteolysis and calcium levels
      c. Commonly associated with breast cancer, lung cancers, head and neck malignancies, multiple myeloma, and leukemia

E. SVC syndrome
   1. Definition
      a. Acute or subacute process caused by obstruction of the SVC caused by compression, infiltration, or thrombosis
   2. Etiology
      a. Malignancy accounts for >90% of all cases of SVC syndrome
         i. Lung cancer (small cell and squamous cell carcinomas) cause 65% of all cases
         ii. Lymphoma
         iii. Breast cancer
         iv. Testicular cancer
      b. Nonmalignant causes
         i. Luetic thoracic aneurysms (tertiary syphilis)
         ii. Tuberculosis
         iii. Indwelling central venous catheters
         iv. Goiter
         v. Mediastinitis
      c. Overall mortality (carcinoma etiology) is 75% at 1 year
   3. Symptoms and signs
      a. Caused by venous hypertension in areas normally drained by the SVC
      b. Dyspnea is the most common symptom
      c. Nonspecific CNS symptoms (confusion, seizures, headache, stroke-like syndrome)
      d. Periorbital edema and facial swelling
      e. Swelling of the upper extremities and trunk
      f. Thoracic and neck vein distension/engorgement ("stokes sign")
      g. Plethora
   4. Diagnosis
      a. Clinical conditions which mimic SVC syndrome are heart failure and pericardial tamponade
      b. Chest radiography may be helpful
         i. Mediastinal mass (75% are right-sided)
         ii. Hilar adenopathy
         iii. Pleural effusions (usually right-sided)
      c. Venography is relatively contraindicated
      d. CT (cervical, thoracic)
      e. Invasive visualization (bronchoscopy, mediastinoscopy, limited thoracotomy, scalene node biopsy)
   5. Management
      a. Supportive care
         i. Obtain intravenous access on the contralateral (unaffected) side
         ii. Head elevation
      b. Diuretic therapy
      c. Corticosteroids
         i. Only if tumor is steroid-sensitive or if compromising the airway
      d. Percutaneous transluminal stent placement

F. Neurologic emergencies
   1. Cerebral herniation (see also Trauma chapter)
      a. Etiology

i. Tumor with mass effect
   a) Primary brain (50%) and metastatic cancers (lung, breast, colon, testicle, kidney)
ii. Intracerebral hemorrhage and edema
iii. Radiation-induced cerebral edema and necrosis

b. Diagnosis
   i. Clinical presentation consistent with herniation
   ii. Head CT or MRI

c. Management
   i. Dexamethasone
      a) Not useful for elevated ICP secondary to trauma
      b) Often given in the context of neoplasm-related edema and elevated ICP
   ii. Modest, short-term hyperventilation (impending herniation)
      a) Avoid prolonged hyperventilation
      b) Avoid reducing $PaCO_2$ <25 mm Hg
   iii. Mannitol (dose is 1g/kg)
   iv. Furosemide
   v. Empiric seizure prophylaxis
   vi. Emergent neurosurgical consultation

2. Spinal cord compression
   a. Etiology
      i. Metastatic cancer (85%)
      ii. Primary spinal tumor in (15%)
         a) Most common—multiple myeloma, lymphoma, carcinoma of the lung, breast, and prostate
   b. Symptoms and signs
      i. Nonspecific back pain (initial presenting symptom in 95% of patients with epidural metastasis)
         a) Thoracic spine >cervical spine >lumbar spine
      ii. Pain precedes motor and sensory deficits
         a) Bowel or bladder dysfunction (acute urinary retention common)
         b) Weakness or paresthesias

      c) Hyporeflexia or hyperreflexia (depending on duration of symptoms)
      iii. Partial spinal cord syndromes (eg, Brown-Sequard syndrome)
   c. Diagnosis
      i. MRI
      ii. Conventional radiographs of the spine show evidence of tumor in the vertebral bodies 50% to 70% of the time
      iii. Assessment for increased postvoid residual volume of bladder (normally <100 cc)
      iv. Maintain high clinical suspicion in any cancer patient with back pain as outcome reflects presenting symptoms
         a) Pain and paresthesias may be the only complaint
         b) Symptoms present for >24 hours rarely resolve
   d. Management
      i. Early aggressive radiation therapy
      ii. Emergent neurosurgical or orthopedic spine consultation
      iii. Dexamethasone (IV)
         a) Initial (loading) dose: 10 to 100 mg
         b) Supplemental doses: 4 to 24 mg

REFERENCES

1. Fauci AS, Braunwald E, Kasper DL, et al (eds): *Harrison's Principles of Internal Medicine,* 17th ed. New York: McGraw-Hill; 2008.
2. Jang I-K, Hursting HJ: When heparins promote thrombosis: review of heparin-induced thrombocytopenia. *Circulation.* 2005,111:2671.
3. Rose VL, Kwaan HC, Williamson K, et al: Protein C antigen deficiency and warfarin necrosis. *Am J Clin Pathol.* 1986, 86:653.
4. Dodd RY, Adverse consequences of blood transfusion: quantitative risk estimates. In: Nance ST, ed: *Blood Supply: Risks, Perceptions and Prospects for the Future.* Bethesda, MD: American Association of Blood Banks, 1994:1-24.

Chapter 20
PSYCHIATRIC EMERGENCIES

Howard A. Greller

I. Suicide

A. Epidemiology
  1. 10 to 40 attempts for every completed act
  2. 1 in 3 individuals consider suicide in their lifetime

B. Risk factors[1]
  1. Determination of risk is imperfect science
     a. Many methods, none 100% reliable
     b. SADPERSONS is a score that can be useful rule of thumb (Table 20–1)
  2. Elderly
  3. White or Native American
  4. Separated or divorced
  5. Psychiatric disorders
     a. Major depression at highest risk
     b. Borderline personality disorder
  6. Alcohol or substance abuse
     a. 25% of all suicides involve alcohol
  7. Chronic illness
  8. Unemployment in 18- to 24-year-old men
  9. Presence of a firearm in household is an independent risk factor
     a. 5 to 10 times more likely for adolescents
  10. Men are more successful (more lethal), women more likely to attempt
     a. 10% to 15% of those that attempt suicide are ultimately successful
     b. 60% to 70% of successful suicide attempts have no prior attempts (first-timers)

C. Decreased risk factors[2]
  1. Pregnancy
  2. Marriage

D. Methods
  1. Most completed suicides involve firearms (70%)
  2. Most attempted suicides involve ingestions (72%)
     a. Antidepressant overdose most common

E. Management[2, 3]
  1. Routine toxicologic screening **not** necessary
     a. Except **acetaminophen**—clinically silent initial presentation
     b. Most present with clinical signs or symptoms
     c. ECG to screen for tricyclic antidepressant overdose
  2. Police have the right to take custody of an individual at risk to self or others
  3. Suicide precautions
     a. Direct observation of patient while in ED
        i. Staff member, not family member
        ii. Patient should be searched by security, disrobed, and placed into a gown
        iii. Room should be free of instruments, equipment, or medications
     b. Physical and chemical restraint as necessary
     c. Err on side of caution, admit when uncertain

II. Schizophrenia[2]

A. Criteria for schizophrenia (*DSM-IV-TR*)
  1. ≥2 symptoms for ≥1 month
     a. Delusions
     b. Hallucinations
     c. Disorganized speech (derailment or incoherence)
     d. Grossly disorganized or catatonic behavior
     e. Negative symptoms
        i. Flat affect, inexpressive facial expressions, monotone speech, etc
     f. Need only 1 symptom if delusions are bizarre or hallucinations are a running commentary
  2. Sharp deterioration from prior level of functioning
  3. Symptoms >6 months
     a. At least 1 month of the above symptoms followed by prodromal or residual symptoms

TABLE 20–1. SADPERSONS Scale[2]

FACTOR	POINTS
Sex (male)	1
Age (<19 or >45 years)	1
Depression or hopelessness	2
Previous attempts or psychiatric care	1
Excessive alcohol or drug use	1
Rational thinking loss	2
Separated, divorced, or widowed	1
Organized or serious attempt	2
No social supports	1
Stated future attempt	2
≤5 points	Questionable outpatient treatment
≥6 points	Emergency psychiatric treatment
≥9 points	Psychiatric hospitalization

4. Schizoaffective disorder and mood disorder ruled out (see schizoaffective disorder and mood disorder section below)
5. Not caused by comorbid medical condition or substance abuse or medication

B. Differential considerations
   1. Exclude organic causes
      a. Organic (medical) versus functional (psychiatric)[2] (Table 20–2)
   2. Schizophreniform disorder
      a. Definition: symptoms of schizophrenia lasting >1 month but <6 months

b. 33% recover
c. 66% go on to be diagnosed with schizophrenia
3. Functional disorders[1]
   a. Definition: physical symptoms with a psychogenic etiology
4. Brief psychotic disorder
   a. Sudden onset of psychotic symptoms (hallucinations, delusions, etc.) lasting several days to 1 month
   b. Postpartum females and major stress predispose
5. Mood disorder with psychotic features
   a. Symptoms of psychosis present only during mood disturbance
6. Schizoaffective disorder
   a. Definition: A condition in which symptoms of a mood disorder and schizophrenia coexist
   b. Mood disorder with the presence of psychotic symptoms for >2 weeks in absence of prominent mood symptoms
7. Delusional disorder
   a. Non-bizarre delusions that dominate lives

III. Mood Disorders[2]

A. Definition(s)
   1. Mood is an "enduring emotional orientation that colors the individual's psychology"
   2. Affect is "the outward and changeable manifestation of an individual's emotional tone"
   3. Dysphoria is depressed mood or feeling

B. Epidemiology
   1. Mood disorders are becoming more common
   2. Lifetime suicide risk for untreated depressive illness is 15%

TABLE 20–2. Organic versus Functional Signs of Schizophrenia

MADFOCS	ORGANIC	FUNCTIONAL
Memory deficits	Recent	Remote
Activity	Psychomotor retardation	Repetitive activity
	Tremor	Posturing
	Ataxia	Rocking
Distortions	Visual hallucinations	Auditory hallucinations
Feelings	Emotional lability	Flat affect
Orientation	Disoriented	Oriented
Cognition	Occasionally lucid, perceptive and attends or focuses periodically	Continuous scattered thoughts, unable to attend
Some other findings	Age >40 years	Age <40 years
	Sudden onset	Gradual onset
	Abnormal physical and vitals	Normal physical and vitals
	Social immodesty	Social modesty
	Aphasia	Intelligible speech
	Impaired consciousness	Awake and alert

C. Major depression
  1. Definition
    a. ≥5 symptoms for at least 2 weeks
    b. Must include either depressed mood or anhedonia (inability to experience pleasure or interest in formerly pleasurable or satisfying activities)
    c. Significant weight loss when not intentional
    d. Insomnia or hypersomnia
    e. Psychomotor agitation or retardation
    f. Fatigue or loss of energy
    g. Feelings of worthlessness or excessive or inappropriate guilt
    h. Diminished ability to think or concentrate, or indecisiveness
    i. Recurrent thoughts of death, recurrent suicidal ideation, or suicide plan or attempt
    j. Do not meet criteria for "mixed episode"
    k. Condition in which criteria are met for both manic episode and major depressive episode (except duration)
    l. Causes clinically significant distress or social impairment
    m. Not caused by substance or medical condition
    n. Not accounted for by bereavement; persist for >2 months and cause marked functional impairment

D. Bipolar disorders
  1. Lifelong, episodic, extreme mood swings
    a. Bipolar I: at least 1 manic and ≥1 major depressive episode
    b. Bipolar II: at least 1 hypomanic, at least 1 major depressive episode
  2. Hypomanic: manic episode without psychosis, marked impairment of function or need for hospitalization
  3. Manic episode (*DSM-IV-TR*)
    a. Abnormally and persistently elevated, expansive or irritable mood for at least 2 weeks (or any duration if requires hospitalization)
    b. ≥3 of the following (4 if mood is only irritable)
      i. Inflated self-esteem or grandiosity
      ii. Decreased need for sleep
      iii. Pressured speech
      iv. Flight of ideas, racing thoughts
      v. Distractibility
      vi. Increased goal-directed activity, psychomotor agitation
      vii. Excessive pleasurable activity (buying sprees, sexual indiscretion, foolish investments, etc.)
    c. Not a "mixed episode"

    d. Marked impairment of function, necessitates hospitalization
    e. Not from substance or other medical condition

E. Seasonal affective disorder (SAD)
  1. Definition: major depression during seasons with less daylight
    a. Resolves or changes to manic episodes with daylight
    b. Present for at least 2 years
  2. Management: phototherapy

F. Postpartum depression
  1. Definition: depression typically affecting women after childbirth.
  2. Risk factors
    a. Underlying mood disorder
    b. Unemployed
    c. No assistance

G. Dysthymic disorder
  1. Long-standing, low-grade depression
    a. Patient gets little pleasure from leisure activities

IV. Complications of Antipsychotic Medications and Dopamine Antagonists

A. Dystonias
  1. Definition: a movement disorder in which muscle contractions cause abnormal repetitive movements and postures
    a. Can occur anytime
    b. Areas effected
      i. Buccolingual (tongue)
      ii. Torticollis (head)
      iii. Oculogyric (eye)
      iv. Opisthotonos (back arching)
      v. Laryngospasm (rare)
  2. Treat with anticholinergic drugs (benztropine or diphenhydramine)
  3. Outpatient oral therapy for 48 to 72 hours

B. Akathesia
  1. Definition: a sensation of inner restlessness manifesting as inability to remain motionless
    a. "Restless legs" syndrome
  2. Management: β-blockers or anticholinergic drugs (diphenhydramine)
    a. Change offending medication or lower dosage

C. Akinesia and drug-induced parkinsonism
  1. Definition: inability to initiate movement
    a. Usually secondary to diminished dopaminergic cell activity
    b. Difficult to differentiate from Parkinson disease

2. Management: anticholinergic agents (eg, benztropine)
   a. Can treat with Parkinson medication
   b. If etiology is antipsychotic therapy, consider switching to atypical antipsychotic agent

D. Tardive dyskinesia
   1. Definition: involuntary movements, especially face and tongue
      a. Usually manifests after several years of treatment with offending agent
      b. Mean prevalence of 24%
         i. Related to duration of treatment, cumulative dose, age
   2. Management: discontinue or lower dose of agent
      a. Switch to new atypical antipsychotic agent
      b. Symptoms may persist for months, years or even remain permanently after discontinuation of offending medication

E. Neuroleptic malignant syndrome (NMS)
   1. Definition: life-threatening neurologic disorder manifesting as muscle rigidity, autonomic dysfunction, and hyperthermia
      a. Etiology: thought to be from depletion of dopamine
   2. Symptoms and signs
      a. High fever, muscular rigidity, altered mental status, autonomic instability
      b. Occurs soon after initiation or recent change in dose of neuroleptic therapy
         i. Subacute onset over days to weeks
   3. Management
      a. Discontinue agent
      b. Aggressive supportive care, active cooling
      c. Sedation with benzodiazepines
      d. Neuromuscular blockade and airway management
      e. Dopamine repletion—slowly acting (eg, bromocriptine)

V. Personality Disorders[1, 3]

A. Paranoid
   1. Distrustful of others
      a. Holds grudges and generally unforgiving
   2. Belief in hidden meanings

B. Schizoid
   1. Limited expression and experience of emotion
      a. Unlike avoidant personality types, does not desire friendship
      b. Indifferent to praise and criticism of others. Cool and aloof
   2. Least likely to be seen in clinical practice

C. Avoidant
   1. Marked social inhibition and sensitivity to criticism
      a. Wants to make friends but afraid of rejection
      b. Feelings of inadequacy

D. Schizotypal
   1. Odd beliefs
   2. Eccentric behavior, dress, style, and thought
   3. "Psychics"

E. Antisocial
   1. No regard for moral or legal ethics of society. Lack of remorse
   2. Unable to get along with others. Physically aggressive
   3. Unable to abide by societal rules
   4. Reckless disregard for the safety of self and others
   5. Sociopaths and criminals

F. Borderline
   1. Pattern of instability of interpersonal relationships, self-image, and affects, as well as marked impulsivity, beginning by early adulthood
      a. Risk for successful suicide, bulimia, posttraumatic stress disorder (PTSD) and substance abuse
      b. Extremely labile mood
      c. Intense and unstable relationships
      d. Splitting
         i. Thinking purely in extremes, eg, good versus bad

G. Histrionic
   1. Pattern of excessive emotionality and attention-seeking, including an excessive need for approval
      a. Marked and inappropriate display of emotion
         i. Often attempts suicide but rarely successful
      b. Risk for somatoform illness (see below)
      c. Seductive and sexually inappropriate

H. Narcissistic
   1. Lack of empathy. Selfish and exploitive
   2. Risk of anorexia nervosa
   3. Grandiosity and need for admiration by others
   4. Unable to see the viewpoints of others
   5. Hypersensitive to criticism

I. Dependent
   1. Extreme need for other people
      a. Unable to make decision on own
      b. Marked submissive behavior and fear of separation

J. Obsessive-compulsive disorder (OCD)
  1. Chronic preoccupation with rules, orderliness, and control
     a. Perfectionist
     b. Inflexible
     c. Uncontrollable pattern of thought or behavior

VI. Eating Disorders[1, 2]

A. Anorexia nervosa
  1. Intense fear of gaining weight and distorted body image
     a. <85% ideal body weight
     b. Amenorrhea for 3 cycles
  2. Perfectionist and narcissistic
  3. Type "A" personality.
     a. "A" student
  4. Symptoms and signs
     a. Cardiac: mitral valve prolapse, brady and tachy arrhythmias, CHF, QT prolongation
     b. Mortality rate 5% to 18%
     c. Constipation, hypothermia, hair loss, dry skin, lanugo
     d. Depression and risk for suicide

B. Bulimia
  1. Recurrent binging and purging eating pattern
     a. "The failed anorexic" (weight is normal or even above normal)
     b. Misuse of laxatives, diuretics, or enemas
     c. Most deaths from cardiac arrhythmia
     d. Associated with borderline personality
     e. Use of diet pills and stimulants
  2. Symptoms and signs
     a. Salivary gland hyperplasia
     b. Tonsilar hyperplasia
     c. Muscle weakness and cramps
     d. Carpopedal spasm
     e. Erosion of tooth enamel without cavities
     f. Russell sign: callus on finger or knuckle
     g. Hypokalemia, hypomagnesemia, and contraction alkalosis

VII. Anxiety Disorders[1, 2]

A. General
  1. Epidemiology
     a. 25% lifetime United States prevalence
     b. Most common psychiatric problem seen by primary care
  2. Definition(s)
     a. Anxiety: unpleasurable state of tension that forewarns the presence of danger
     b. Vigilance: consequence of anxiety that leads to rapid threat recognition
     c. Pathologic anxiety: anxiety that surpasses normal response to "threat" and interferes with normal functioning
     d. Panic attack: sudden onset of intense apprehension, fearfulness, or terror, often with sense of impending doom
     e. Agoraphobia: anxiety about or avoidance of places or situations from which escape might be difficult
     f. OCD: characterized by obsessions that cause marked anxiety or distress and by compulsions that serve to neutralize anxiety
     g. PTSD: (see PTSD below)
     h. Acute stress disorder: characterized by symptoms similar to PTSD that occur immediately in aftermath of traumatic event
  3. Management
     a. Pharmacologic therapy
        i. Benzodiazepines
        ii. Buspirone
           a) Takes weeks for clinical effect
           b) Lower risk for dependence
        iii. β-blockers
           a) Decrease tremor, tachycardia, and stage fright
        iv. Monoamine oxidase inhibitors (MAOIs)
           a) Low therapeutic index, dangerous side effect profile, dietary restrictions
           b) Highly effective for social phobia, panic, OCD, and generalized anxiety
        v. Tricyclic antidepressants (TCAs)
           a) Panic and generalized anxiety, PTSD
           b) Ineffective for OCD, social phobias
           c) Potential for toxicity
        vi. Selective serotonin reuptake inhibitors (SSRIs)
           a) Broad spectrum of efficacy
           b) Safer than other agents

B. PTSD
  1. Epidemiology
     a. United States lifetime prevalence of ~10%
     b. Development is directly related to exposure and re-traumatization
     c. Females at higher risk than males
  2. Diagnosis
     a. *DSM-IVR* criteria for diagnosis
        i. Experiencing, witnessing, or being confronted with an event involving serious injury, death, or a threat to an individual's physical integrity
        ii. A response involving helplessness, intense fear, or horror
        iii. Persistent re-experiencing of the event

  iv. Avoidance of stimuli that are associated with the trauma and numbing of general responsiveness
  v. Symptoms of hyperarousal (ie, difficult sleep, decreased concentration, hypervigilance, etc.)
  vi. Duration of >1 month
  vii. Cause of significant distress or impairment in functioning
3. Complications
  a. Increased risk of impulsive behavior and **suicide**
  b. Increased risk for panic disorder, agoraphobia, OCD, social phobia, specific phobia, major depressive disorder, and somatization disorder
  c. Increased risk for substance abuse and/or dependence

VIII. Somatoform Disorders[1,2]

A. Somatization: to experience physical distress in response to psychosocial stress
  1. Epidemiology
    a. Relatively uncommon (~1%)
    b. Runs in families, rare in men
    c. Associated with anxiety and major depression
    d. Increased suicide risk, often associated with substance abuse
    e. Low socioeconomic groups, alcoholism, poor education
  2. Symptoms and signs
    a. History of unexplained symptoms that start before age 30
      i. Not explained by any medical condition
      ii. Not intentionally produced or feigned
    b. All of the following are required for diagnosis
      i. Pain to at least 4 sites (head, back, joints, etc.) or functions (urination, defecation, menstruation, etc.)
      ii. At least 2 GI symptoms other than pain
      iii. At least 1 sexual or reproductive symptom other than pain
      iv. At least 1 neurologic symptom not limited to pain (paralysis, blindness, etc.)

B. Conversion disorder[1,2]: hysterical neurosis, non-painful neurologic disorders with no physical etiology, but signs of hysteria
  1. Epidemiology
    a. Women > men
    b. Low socioeconomic groups
  2. Symptoms and signs
    a. Sudden onset and dramatic presentation of a single symptom

      i. Motor disturbances
        a) Tremors (worse when attended to)
        b) Pseudoseizures
        c) Paralysis or paresis
        d) Aphonia
        e) Disturbed coordination
      ii. Sensory disturbances
        a) Anesthesia
        b) Blindness
    b. "La belle indifférence"
      i. Lack appropriate concern about profound dysfunction (~50%)
      ii. Not under voluntary control

C. Hypochondriasis[1,2]: excessive preoccupation about having a serious illness
  1. Epidemiology
    a. Common disorder, 4% to 9% of general practice
    b. Men and women in equal proportion
    c. Strong association with major depression
  2. Symptoms and signs
    a. Complains in detail and at length using medical jargon
    b. Physical symptoms disproportionate to demonstrable organic disease
    c. Fear of disease and conviction that one is sick
      i. Leads to "illness-claiming behavior"—compulsive insistence on being considered a physical cripple
    d. Preoccupation with one's body
    e. Persistent and unsatisfying pursuit of medical care (doctor shopping)
      i. History of numerous procedures and surgeries
      ii. Recurrent return of symptoms
    f. Amplification
      i. Heightened awareness of and unrealistic interpretation of normal physical signs or sensations
      ii. Symptoms **do** exist, but are misinterpreted as disease
    g. "Experts at defeating doctors to feel more powerful"
  3. Diagnosis[2]
    a. Diagnosis suggested when physician feels "frustration, helplessness, or anger associated with a wish to be rid of the patient"

D. General management of somatization disorders
  1. Reassurance
    a. Works best with young patients who have no underlying medical or psychiatric illness, presenting in response to clear stressor
  2. Different approach to care
    a. Must appreciate that this disorder is a form of suffering

b. Legitimize symptoms, set limits on behaviors

c. Labels are what somatizers seek—incorporate the relationship of bodily function to psychological stress

3. Medication

a. Avoid medications that lead to dependence or abstinence syndromes

b. Defined, clear intervals and endpoints of medication use

c. Diet, physical therapy and exercise, vitamins

4. Conversion disorder has the best prognosis for resolution

5. Psychiatric consultation

IX. Factitious Disorders and Malingering[1, 2]

A. General considerations

1. Signs that are intentionally produced or feigned without apparent external incentives

a. Patient is unable to refrain from behavior even when risks are known

b. The motivation of securing the sick role is unconscious

c. Patients who readily admit producing their own injuries are not included

2. Patients are willing to undergo procedures to maintain sick role

B. Munchausen syndrome: the affected person exaggerates or feigns illness for personal gain (sympathy, investigation, attention)

1. Epidemiology

a. Onset in the 20's, diagnosed between 30 and 39 years of age

b. Frequently affects those with a history of genuine disease

i. Often exhibit objective physical findings

2. Symptoms and signs

a. Patients see themselves as important people, with exceptional lives

b. Patients may induce dangerous illness to protract lengthy hospitalization

C. Munchausen syndrome by proxy

1. Simulation or production of disease in dependents by parent or caregiver to assume the sick role vicariously

a. Without direct harm in 25%

b. Use of many different methods to produce or simulate disease

i. Administration of drugs or toxins

ii. Asphyxiation

2. Specific criteria

a. Illness or abnormality produced or concocted by caregiver

b. Persistent presentation for medical treatment

c. Cessation of signs and symptoms when child separated from caregiver

d. Excludes straightforward physical abuse or neglect

3. Perpetrator characteristics

a. 98% are biologic mothers from all socioeconomic groups

b. Many have background in health professions or social work

c. Depression, anxiety, and somatization are common

d. Many have had an abusive experience in past

4. Mortality is 9% to 31%

a. Most frequently from suffocation and poisoning

b. Permanent disfigurement or impairment in 8%

D. Malingering: separate from somatization disorders and factitious disorders

1. Simulation of disease for secondary gain

a. Avoiding work, military conscription or duty, evading prosecution

b. Obtaining drugs, room and board, holiday from incarceration

2. Frequently found in association with antisocial personality disorder

E. Differential considerations

1. Factitious disorders unlike malingering have no secondary gain other than masquerading illness

2. Patients with factitious disorders are more convincing and subtle in presentation

3. Malingerers are less likely to participate in painful, expensive or dangerous procedures

X. Delirium versus Dementia[1] (also see Neurology chapter)

A. Delirium

1. Acute mental status change with rapid fluctuation

2. Impaired awareness, perceptual disturbance (illusion, hallucinations, etc.)

3. Orientation is impaired

4. Awareness may fluctuate

5. Speech may impair history taking ability

6. Obtain a current and past history from other source

a. Drug, alcohol, and medication use

b. Endocrine disorders

c. Exposure to toxins or environmental injury

d. Psychiatric illness and similar episodes

B. Dementia

1. Chronic, steady decline in short- and long-term memory

a. Sensorium is clear, unlike delirium

2. Most presentations are exacerbations of previously known condition
   a. Early-stage, new-onset patients may minimize or hide symptoms, manifest as depression
3. Recent onset has a higher likelihood of a potentially reversible etiology
4. History is important
   a. Drug or alcohol abuse, medications
   b. Chronic or acute medical illnesses and psychiatric disorders
5. Depression is an important confounder and co-morbidity

XI. Violence, Abuse and Neglect[2]

A. Epidemiology
   1. Lifetime incidence of ~25% women, 8% men
   2. Rape reported ~8% women, 0.3% men
   3. Physical assault 23% women, 7% men
   4. Women report only 20% of rapes, 25% assaults, 50% stalkings

B. Domestic violence
   1. Definition
      a. Victimization of a person with whom the abuser has or has had an intimate, romantic, or spousal relationship; encompasses violence against both men and women
   2. Specific characteristics
      a. Cycle of violence
         i. Tension building
         ii. Explosion, acute battering
         iii. Absence of tension—"loving respite" or "honeymoon phase"
      b. Learned helplessness
         i. Stress response syndrome
   3. Presentation
      a. Emergency physician is often the first professional from whom a victim seeks help
      b. Presenting complaints often are related to illness or stress rather than injury
         i. Often, the complaint does not correlate with physical examination, or complaints are inconsistent with organic disease
         ii. Be aware of multiple presentations without resolution
      c. Characteristic injuries and patterns of injury
         i. Bilateral injuries, especially the extremities
         ii. Scratches, cigarette burns, rope burns, ligature marks
         iii. Fingernail marks, slap marks, bite marks
         iv. Conjunctival and facial petechiae
         v. Maxillofacial injuries very common
         vi. Defensive injuries (eg, "nightstick" fracture)

d. Sexual assault common
   i. Any evidence of genital injury should prompt screening for domestic violence or sexual assault
   ii. Recurrent STDs should prompt screening as well
4. Screening
   a. Essential to take history in private
      i. Translators must not be family members, relative, or friend
      ii. **Ask direct, simple questions** ("Has your partner ever punched you?")
   b. You must inform the patient of limits of confidentiality imposed by mandatory reporting laws (such as in child abuse situations)
   c. Partner violence screen
      i. Have you ever been hit, kicked, punched, or otherwise hurt by someone within the past year? If so, by whom?
      ii. Do you feel safe in your current relationship?
      iii. Is a partner from a previous relationship making you feel unsafe now?
   d. SAFE questions
      i. **S**tress and **S**afety: What stress do you experience in your relationships? Do you feel safe in your relationships? Should I be concerned for your safety?
      ii. **A**fraid and **A**bused: What happens when you and your partner disagree? Do any situations exist in your relationships in which you have felt afraid? Has your partner ever threatened or abused you or your children? Have you been physically hurt by your partner? Has your partner forced you to have unwanted sexual relations?
      iii. **F**riends and **F**amily (assessing degree of social support): If you have been hurt, are your friends or family aware of it? Do you think you could tell them if it did happen? Would they be able to give you support?
      iv. **E**mergency plan: Do you have a safe place to go and the resources you (and your children) need in an emergency? If you are in danger now, would you like help in locating a shelter? Do you have a plan for escape? Would you like to talk with a social worker, counselor, or physician to develop an emergency plan?
      v. A detailed physical examination is paramount, as patient may attempt to hide abuse
5. Complications
   a. Morbidity and mortality
      i. A home where someone has been hit or hurt in a family incident is 4.4 times

more likely to have a homicide than one without

    ii. Most murders in domestic violence situations are handgun-related

  b. Most dangerous time is during attempts to leave relationship

  c. Higher risk with alcohol and substance abuse

  d. Depression and suicide

6. Management

  a. Know your hospital and regional policies regarding collection and preservation of information and evidence, mandatory reporting, and consent

    i. Nearly all states have mandatory reporting of elder abuse (Adult Protective Services)

    ii. Nearly all states have mandatory reporting of children (Child Protective Services)

    iii. Many have penalties for failure to report

  b. Provide a safe environment

  c. Documentation should be meticulous

  d. Consult liberally and involve appropriate agencies as necessary

  e. Admit, refer, or discharge patient to safe environment

C. Elder abuse[2]

1. Epidemiology

  a. Underreported compared to domestic and child abuse

  b. Occurs among all racial, socioeconomic, and religious backgrounds

    i. Believed to be more common in women

XII. Substance Abuse Screening[1]

A. CAGE screening questions for alcoholism

1. **C** Has anyone ever felt you should **cut down** your drinking?

2. **A** Have people **annoyed** you by criticizing your drinking?

3. **G** Have you ever felt **guilty** about your drinking?

4. **E** Have you ever had an **eye-opener** to steady your nerves or get rid of a hangover?

5. A single response is suggestive of alcohol problem, 2 or more responses is 90% sensitive and specific

B. MAST (Michigan Alcohol Screening Test) (modified)

1. Have you ever had a drinking problem?

2. When was your last drink? (<24 hours is positive)

3. One positive answer is 91% sensitive for a problem with alcohol

REFERENCES

1. Marx JA, Hockberger RS, Walls RM, eds: *Rosen's Emergency Medicine: Concepts and Clinical Practice,* 6th ed. St. Louis, MO: Mosby; 2006.

2. Aghababian RV, Allison EJJ, Boyer EW, et al., eds: *Essentials of Emergency Medicine.* Boston: Jones and Bartlett; 2006.

3. Tintinalli JE, Kelen GD, Stapczynski JS, eds: *Emergency Medicine: A Comprehensive Study Guide,* 6th ed. New York: McGraw-Hill; 2004.

Chapter 21
PREHOSPITAL CARE

Dario Gonzalez and Kinjal Sethuramen

I. Landmark EMS Reports and Legislation

A. 1966 Landmark paper: Accidental Death and Disability: The Neglected Disease of Modern Society[1]
   1. Report presented by the National Academy of Sciences and the National Research Council (NAS-NRC)
   2. Listed 24 proposed recommendations that would serve as a blueprint for EMS development
   3. Called for trained medical personnel, rapid transport, treatment protocols, the creation of statewide trauma registries

B. 1966 Highway Safety Act[2]
   1. Established a cabinet-level Department of Transportation (DOT) post
   2. Gave DOT the financial and legislative authority to develop EMS
   3. Required highway safety programs and EMS system development, providing matching funds

C. 1973 Emergency Medical Services Systems Act[3]
   1. Meant to stimulate the development of regional EMS system
   2. Focused on the project development and project manager
   3. EMS medical direction was not emphasized
   4. Included an intended phase-out of federal funds
   5. Described 15 fundamental components of EMS system development

D. 1981 Omnibus Budget Reconciliation Act[4]
   1. Signed into law by President Reagan
   2. Grouped EMS into Preventative Health Block Grant
   3. Although it provided for some continued funding, that decision was essentially left to the states

II. Components of EMS system: Department of Transportation

A. Training (see EMS Provider Level and Credentialing below)

B. Communication
   1. Emergency medical dispatch (EMD) course trains those answering emergency calls from patients
   2. Priority dispatch—rovides most appropriate EMS response based on information from emergency call-ins
   3. Prearrival instruction—callers are given instruction prior to EMS arrival
   4. Online instruction/aid available to EMS crew when necessary by online physician
   5. EMS radio communication
      a. Very high frequency (VHF) has good transmitting range; ultra high frequency (UHF) has limited range but good penetration
      b. UHF is useful in urban areas

C. Transportation

D. Facilities
   1. Transport usually to the closest hospital or to the hospital with the quickest transport time
   2. Exceptions to above rule occur with hospital with special designations better equipped to care for specific conditions (eg, trauma centers, burn centers, stroke centers)

E. Critical care units
   1. Hospitals with specialized or expertise care should be identified in every EMS system
   2. Specialization includes trauma, burn, high-risk obstetric, snake bite designations.

F. Public safety agencies
   1. Strong ties with fire and police departments should exist

G. Consumer participation
   1. Laypersons should be involved with EMS policies to represent the public interest

H. Access to care for all members of society should be ensured

I. Transfer of care
   1. Transfer agreements and protocols should be established between receiving and sending hospitals

J. Standardization of patients' records

K. Public education
   1. Prepare laypersons to deliver CPR
   2. Understand how to access their local EMS system

L. Independent review
   1. Quality control of all measures of EMS function including but not limited to patient mortality/morbidity, review of response times and patient records

M. Disaster management
   1. Disaster preparedness through mock drills in conjunction with public and private organizations

N. Mutual aid agreements
   1. Cooperation between neighboring EMS systems should be established in case individual systems are overwhelmed

O. Research and development

III. Types of EMS Systems

A. In urban areas, most are private (44.5%), fire department (39%), and third service (12%)
   1. Tiered system: has both EMT-B and EMT-I units and a few paramedic units (see below)
   2. Third service EMS provider: government agencies separate from Fire or Police. They concentrate solely on out-of-hospital patient care
   3. Private contractor EMS provider: no public EMS system in some areas. A private EMS company provides care based on competitive bargaining. First responders provided by fire department in this model
   4. There is no single standard for EMS system design
      a. Private
      b. Hospital-based
      c. Public (municipal)
      d. Volunteer
      e. Hybrid
      f. Fire + Private EMS is a more recent form

B. Characteristics of urban EMS
   1. Short response and transport times
   2. Availability of multiple units (ALS, basic life support [BLS], rescue)
   3. Variety of receiving facilities
      a. Level I: fully equipped and staffed ED with all specialty and surgical services available 24 hours a day
      b. Level II: fully equipped and staffed ED with some specialty and surgical services available 24 hours a day
      c. Level III: fully equipped and staffed ED without specialty and surgical services
      d. Level IV: basic life station
   4. High volume → greater experience base for providers
   5. Paid, professional providers
   6. 911 Access

C. Characteristics of rural EMS
   1. Prolonged response and transport times
   2. Limited units (BLS, ALS)
   3. Limited receiving facilities
   4. Low volume → skill and knowledge deterioration
   5. Paid versus volunteer providers (impact on response times)
   6. 911 and dispatch limitations

IV. EMS Provider Levels and Credentialing

A. 4 Certification levels: hours vary by state and system. DOT sets minimum
   1. First responder: 40 hours
   2. EMT-basic (EMT-B): 100 hours
   3. EMT-intermediate (EMT-I): 160 to 200 hours didactic + 48 hours clinical + internship
   4. EMT-paramedic (EMT-P): 600 hours didactic + 300 hours clinical + 300 hours field internship

B. Certified first responder
   1. Typically trained in first aid, defibrillation, and some aspects of basic life support
   2. Often respond as firefighters, police, corporate employees, or other volunteers
   3. Trained to provide care until the arrival of the first ambulance
   4. Current DOT curriculum (40 hours)

C. Emergency medical technician-basic (EMT-B)
   1. BLS procedures
   2. Limited medication administration, noninvasive airway interventions

3. Trauma care
4. Obstetric care
5. Other nonmedical items (communication, extrication, etc)
6. Current DOT curriculum (100 hours)

D. Emergency medical technician-intermediate (EMT-I)
   1. Most recently revised of all EMS curricula
   2. Contains various modules that may be enacted by individual states (IV, intubation, manual defibrillation, medication administration)
   3. Also referred to as Advanced EMTs, EMT-Cardiac, EMT-IV, etc
   4. Current full DOT curriculum (~325 hours)

E. Emergency medical technician-paramedic (EMT-P)
   1. Trained to perform all skills in the EMT-I curriculum with additional training in:
      a. Advanced medication administration
      b. Surgical airway management
      c. Invasive procedures (needle thoracostomy, central line placement, etc)
   2. Current DOT curriculum (400 to 600 hours)
   3. >2000 hours in many states.

F. EMS dispatch
   1. Call-taking that includes information for call
   2. Typing unit assignment and tracking prearrival instructions
   3. Hospital notifications
   4. Hospital diversion status tracking

V. Medical Oversight

A. EMTs and paramedics are not independent practitioners

B. Role is both clinical and administrative

C. Development of medical standards

D. Provider education and credentialing

E. Quality management

F. Direct patient care

G. On-scene physician
   1. Must provide proof of identity and licensure to EMS staff
   2. Can assist EMS staff with protocol implementation but not direct care beyond the ability or protocol of EMS staff and state regulations
   3. May be given authority and responsibility by online physician

VI. Medical Direction

A. Online
   1. Also known as "direct" medical control
   2. Patient care that is dictated in real time by a medical oversight
   3. ALS orders
   4. Patient care consultations
   5. Narcotics tracking
   6. Transportation decisions
   7. Refusal of prehospital care by conscious, competent adult

B. Offline
   1. Also known as "indirect" medical control
   2. Patient care that is dictated remotely from the actual patient encounter
   3. Protocol development and implementation
   4. Quality assurance and improvement
   5. Individual case reviews
   6. Training and curriculum development
   7. CME activities
   8. Development of dispatch algorithms

VII. Performance Improvement

A. State and local regulatory bodies

B. Quality improvement and offline medical control

C. Compliance

D. Protocol development
   1. Required and variable from system to system
   2. Group effort, requires review, and revisions
   3. Medical director
   4. Clinical coordinator
   5. Education coordinator
   6. Field trainers
   7. Field providers
   8. Members of medical community

VIII. Mass Casualty Incident, Disaster Preparedness, Response

A. Multiple casualty incident
   1. Definition
      a. An incident with 3 or more victims
      b. System is not overwhelmed

B. Disaster
   1. Definition
      a. An incident whose medical demands overwhelm the available resources in an area

2. Classification
   a. Type I: local resources can handle the event
   b. Type II: local response is overwhelmed, regional mutual aid needed
   c. Type III: large event, state and federal aid required

C. Hazard vulnerability analysis: preparedness should focus on local factors—hurricanes, floods, earthquakes, tsunamis, terror, war, irresponsible politicians

IX. Disaster Response Plan

A. Must be simple but flexible, closely aligned with hospital operations and local municipal authorities (police, fire, and public health) and integrated with adjacent municipalities

B. Components
   1. Recognition: usually obvious
   2. Activation: local authorities, EMS system, local hospital
   3. Health-care facility notification
   4. Command organization, chain of command established
   5. Job action sheets: delineate the responsibilities of leaders
   6. Response
   7. Patient care activities: extrication, search and rescue, triage, stabilization, transport
      a. Black: dead or unsalvageable
      b. Red: seriously injured who require immediate treatment (first priority) to critical treatment area
      c. Yellow: seriously injured who require urgent treatment to intermediate treatment area
      d. Green: minor injuries to delayed treatment area
   8. Scene control and containment
   9. Recovery
   10. CISD: critical incident stress recovery
   11. Treatment and support of responder
   12. Assessment of response, lessons learned

REFERENCES

1. National Academy of Sciences, National Research council. *Accidental Death and disability: The Neglected Disease of Modern Society.* Washington, DC: National Academy Press; 1966.
2. The Highway Safety Act of 1966: Public Law 89-564. Washington, DC; 1966.
3. Emergency Medical Services Systems Act of 1973: Public Law 93-154. Washington, DC; 1973.
4. The Omnibus Budget Reconciliation Act of 1981: Public Law 97-35. Washington, DC; 1981.

Chapter 22
EMERGENCY ULTRASOUND

Jacob K. Goertz

I. Scope of Practice

A. Focused emergency ultrasound is a limited examination designed to answer "Yes or No" questions

B. Not a comprehensive study

C. Advantages
1. Rapid
2. Portable
3. Answer time-sensitive questions
4. Repeatable
5. Extension of physical examination
6. Noninvasive

D. Focused emergency ultrasound applications
1. Applications are myriad; new applications continue to be developed, such as the use of ultrasound to evaluate presenting signs or symptoms (eg, shortness of breath)
2. Traditional applications of focused emergency ultrasound
a. Focused assessment with sonography for trauma (FAST)
b. Aorta
c. Cardiac
d. First trimester pregnancy
e. Renal
f. Right upper quadrant/biliary
g. Ultrasound-guided procedures
3. American College of Emergency Physicians (ACEP) has provided guidelines regarding the scope of practice of focused emergency ultrasound
a. ACEP policy statement, Emergency Ultrasound Guidelines
b. ACEP policy statement, Emergency Ultrasound Imaging Criteria Compendium
4. American Board of Emergency Medicine (ABEM), *"The Model of the Clinical Practice of Emergency Medicine"* includes "Bedside emergency ultrasound" in the section, "Procedures and Skills Integral to the Practice of Emergency Medicine"

II. Focused Assessment with Sonography for Trama (FAST)

A. Indication for use of the FAST examination to evaluate blunt thoracoabdominal trauma (Figures 22–1 and 22–2)
1. Penetrating or blunt thoracoabdominal trauma
2. Determine the presence or absence of:
a. Intra-abdominal free fluid
b. Pericardial free fluid
i. Ultrasound evidence of cardiac tamponade
c. Intrathoracic free fluid

B. Principles
1. Significant thoracoabdominal trauma may be associated with intra-abdominal, pericardial, or intrathoracic free fluid or blood
2. Free fluid appears anechoic (black) between echogenic abdominal, pericardial, and intrathoracic structures
3. Defined patterns of movement of free fluid in peritoneal cavity
a. Injury in right supramesocolic space (eg, liver laceration)
i. Fluid into right supramesocolic space flows directly into hepatorenal space (Morrison pouch)
ii. Fluid overflows into right subphrenic space and into right paracolic gutter
iii. Fluid may travel into splenorenal fossa via epiploic foramen
b. Injury in left supramesocolic space (eg, splenic laceration)
i. Fluid into left supramesocolic space flows cephalad into perisplenic and subphrenic space
ii. Fluid overflows caudally into splenorenal fossa and into paracolic gutters
iii. Fluid travels into hepatorenal space via epiploic foramen

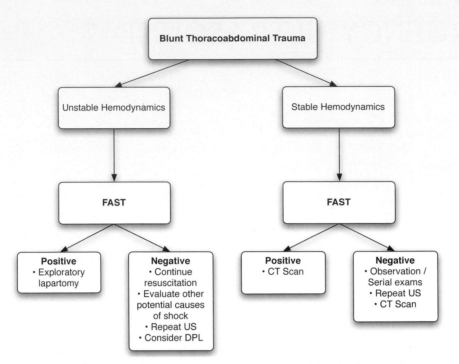

FIGURE 22–1. Algorithm for FAST examination to evaluate blunt thoracoabdominal trauma.

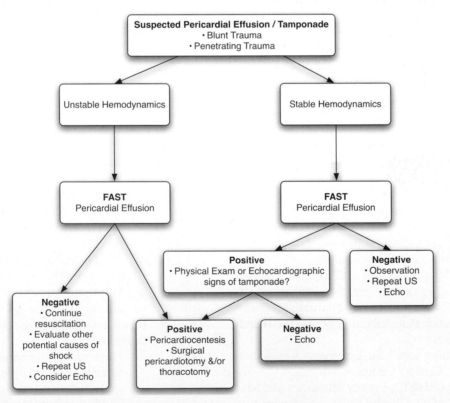

FIGURE 22–2. Algorithm for FAST examination to evaluate suspected pericardial effusion or tamponade in blunt or penetrating thoracoabdominal trauma. (Reprinted, with permission, from Ma OJ, Mateer JR, Blaivas M. *Emergency Ultrasound*, 2nd ed. New York: McGraw-Hill, 2008.)

   c. Injury into inframesocolic space (below transverse colon)
      i. Fluid into inframesocolic space flows directly into pelvis (rectovesicular space in males and rectouterine space in females)
      ii. Fluid extends cephalad into paracolic gutters
         a) Hydrostatic pressure in upper abdomen is less than lower abdomen
         b) Fluid flows preferentially into right paracolic gutter—wider and deeper

C. Views
   1. Right flank (Figure 22–3)
      a. Ultrasound probe in midaxillary line with marker towards patient's head
      b. Visualize hepatorenal interface (Morrison pouch)
      c. Visualize right paracolic gutter inferiorly
      d. Visualize right pleural space superior to the diaphragm
   2. Left flank (Figure 22–4)
      a. Ultrasound probe in midaxillary to posterior axillary line
      b. Visualize splenorenal interface
      c. Visualize perisplenic space
      d. Visualize left paracolic gutter inferiorly
      e. Visualize left pleural space superior to the diaphragm
   3. Pelvis (Figure 22–5)
      a. View suprapubically in transverse and sagittal planes

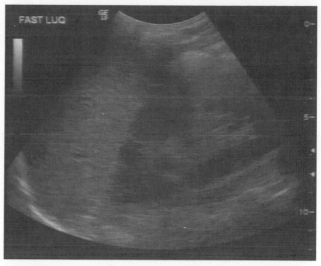

FIGURE 22–4. Normal left flank FAST view demonstrating spleen, kidney, diaphragm, perisplenic space, and splenorenal interface.

      b. Visualize rectovesicular space (in males) or rectouterine space (in females)
         i. Look posterior in transverse view
         ii. Look posterior and superior in sagittal view
   4. Cardiac (Figure 22–6)
      a. Subcostal view
         i. Place probe subcostally
         ii. Flatten probe to look superiorly through heart (parallel to the bed)

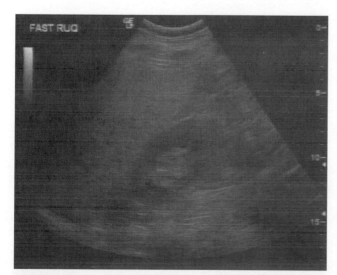

FIGURE 22–3. Normal right flank FAST view demonstrating liver, kidney, diaphragm, hepatorenal space, and paracolic gutter. (Reprinted, with permission, from Ma OJ, Mateer JR, Blaivas M. *Emergency Ultrasound*, 2nd ed. New York: McGraw-Hill, 2008.)

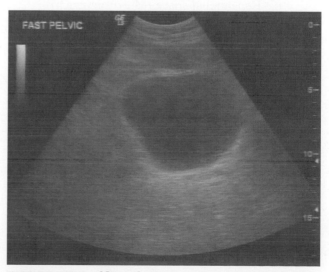

FIGURE 22–5. Normal transverse pelvic FAST view demonstrating bladder.

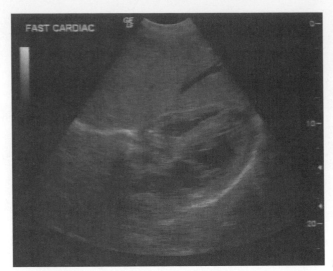

FIGURE 22–6. Normal subcostal cardiac FAST view.

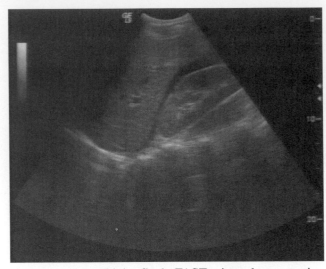

FIGURE 22–7. Right flank FAST view demonstrating free fluid in hepatorenal space.

    b. Heart is imaged anteroinferiorly (near field) to posterosuperiorly (far field)
        i. Right heart (right ventricle) is in near field (closest to the probe)
        ii. Left heart is (left ventricle) in far field (farthest from the probe)
    c. Look for free fluid between the echogenic layers of pericardium
        i. Look for fluid in posterior pericardial space
           a) Effects of gravity with small effusion
           b) Anterior epicardial fat pad may masquerade as pericardial free fluid
    d. Alternative view: parasternal long axis

D. Intraperitoneal free fluid
    1. Free fluid will collect in the following spaces:
        a. Hepatorenal space (Morrison pouch) (Figure 22–7)
        b. Splenorenal space (Figure 22–8)
        c. Perisplenic space (Figure 22–9)
           i. Fluid will collect first in the posterior perisplenic space between the spleen and the diaphragm as this is more posterior than the splenorenal space
        d. Paracolic gutters
        e. Pelvis (Figure 22–10)
           i. Double wall sign: both sides of bladder wall are visualized because of fluid inside bladder (urine) and outside bladder (peritoneal free fluid)
    2. As little as 250 mL of free fluid may be visualized as a thin stripe in Morrison pouch
    3. 500 mL of fluid should be visualized as anechoic stripe in Morrison pouch or perisplenic spaces

    4. Trendelenberg may improve detection
    5. As little as 100 mL of free fluid may be detected in the pelvis

E. Intrathoracic free fluid (Figure 22–11)
    1. As little as 100 mL of free fluid may be visualized in the thoracic cavity

F. Pericardial free fluid (Figure 22–12)
    1. As little as 25 mL of free fluid may be visualized in the pericardial space

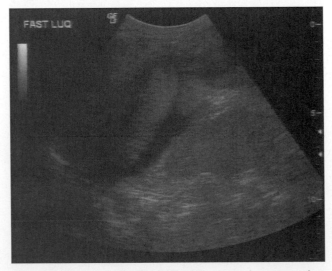

FIGURE 22–8. Left flank FAST view demonstrating free fluid in the splenorenal and perisplenic spaces.

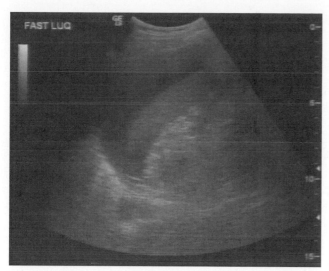

FIGURE 22–9. Left flank FAST view demonstrating the presence of significant free fluid in the perisplenic space without free fluid in the splenorenal space.

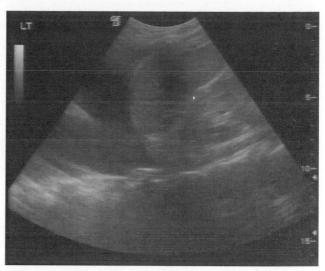

FIGURE 22–11. Left flank FAST view demonstrating free fluid above the diaphragm in the pleural cavity.

2. Tamponade
   a. Dependent upon the rate of fluid collection, not on the fluid volume
   b. Right ventricular diastolic collapse

G. Limitations and pitfalls
   1. FAST does not evaluate solid organ injury (eg, liver lacerations, splenic lacerations)
   2. FAST may miss isolated injuries to solid organs without significant free fluid
   3. FAST may miss injuries to hollow organs without significant free fluid

4. FAST misses diaphragmatic injuries
5. A negative FAST does not exclude intra-abdominal, intrathoracic, or cardiac injuries
6. FAST cannot discriminate blood from other fluid (eg, ascites, pleural effusions)
7. Clotted blood may appear hypoechoic, isoechoic, or hyperechoic
8. Examination may be limited by:
   a. Body habitus and obesity
   b. Bowel gas
   c. Subcutaneous emphysema

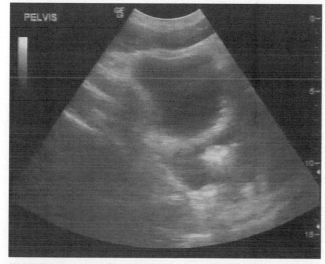

FIGURE 22–10. Transverse pelvic FAST view demonstrating free fluid in pelvis posterior to the bladder.

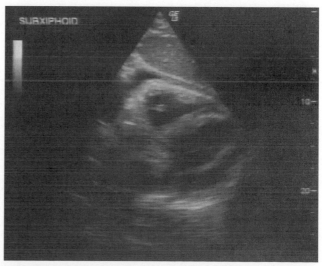

FIGURE 22–12. Subcostal cardiac FAST view demonstrating pericardial free fluid.

III. Aorta

A. Indication
  1. Diagnosis of abdominal aortic aneurysm (AAA)

B. Principles
  1. Types of AAA
    a. Fusiform
      i. Progressive dilation and tapering of aneurysm
      ii. Extend over several centimeters of aorta
      iii. Most common type
    b. Saccular
      i. Outpouching of aorta wall
      ii. Confined to one portion of aorta
  2. Ultrasound is sensitive and specific for detection of the presence or absence of an AAA
    a. Presence of an AAA in a hemodynamically unstable patient warrants emergency vascular surgical consultation

C. Views
  1. Scan the aorta continuously from the diaphragm through the bifurcation in the transverse and sagittal (longitudinal) planes
  2. Landmarks for identification of the aorta
    a. Visualize the spinal shadow in the far field of the picture
    b. The aorta is located anteriorly and to the left of the spinal shadow
    c. The inferior vena cava (IVC) is located anteriorly and to the right of the spinal shadow
  3. Proximal aorta (Figure 22–13)
    a. Place ultrasound probe transversely with the marker to the patient's right immediately subxiphoid in the midline
    b. Landmark: celiac trunk (if visualized)
      i. Common hepatic artery
      ii. Left gastric artery
      iii. Splenic artery
  4. Midaorta (Figure 22–14)
    a. Scan down midline of abdomen with probe positioned transversely
    b. Landmarks (from anterior to posterior)
      i. Splenic vein
      ii. Superior mesenteric artery (SMA)
      iii. Left renal vein
      iv. Aorta
        a) The left and right renal arteries may be visualized branching laterally from the aorta one hand width superior to the umbilicus
  5. Distal aorta
    a. Scan down midline of abdomen to level of bifurcation (usually just above the umbilicus)
    b. Landmark: bifurcation of aorta into right and left iliac arteries
  6. Sagittal aorta
    a. Scan aorta in midline sagittal plane subcostally through bifurcation

D. Measurements
  1. The maximal transverse and anteroposterior diameters of the aorta should be measured at the proximal, mid, and distal portions
  2. Measure from outer wall to outer wall

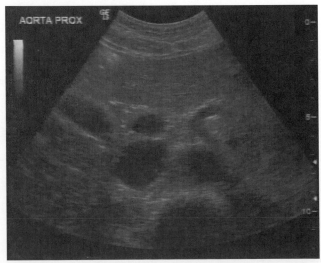

FIGURE 22–13. Proximal aorta view demonstrating *(far-field to near-field)* vertebral shadow, aorta *(patient's left)*, IVC *(patient's right)*, and celiac trunk.

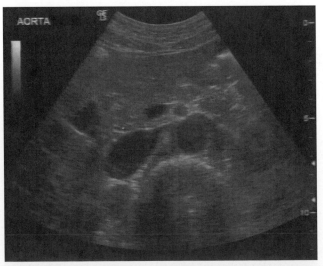

FIGURE 22–14. Midaorta view demonstrating *(far-field to near-field)* vertebral shadow, aorta *(patient's left)*, IVC *(patient's right)*, left renal vein crossing the aorta, SMA, and splenic vien.

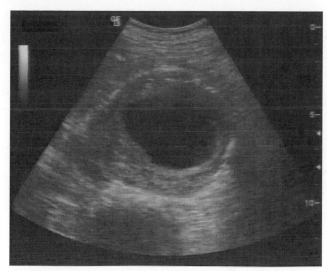

FIGURE 22–15. AAA with diameter >3 cm.

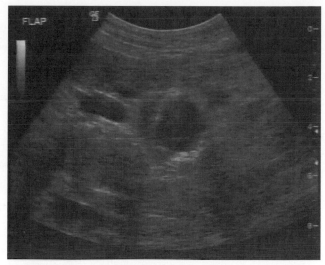

FIGURE 22–17. Aortic dissection demonstrating intimal flap.

E. Abdominal aortic aneurysm (AAA)
　　1. AAA is defined as an aortic diameter ≥3 cm (Figure 22–15)
　　2. Lumenal clot and mural thrombus may be present (Figure 22–16)

F. Limitations and pitfalls
　　1. Leaking and ruptured AAA
　　　　a. Ultrasound is insensitive for detecting ruptured or leaking AAA
　　2. Aortic dissection (Figure 22–17)
　　　　a. Appears as echogenic mobile flap in lumen of aorta
　　　　b. Ultrasound is insensitive for detecting aortic dissection

　　3. Cylinder effect
　　　　a. Measurements made obliquely to the axis of the aorta will result in exaggerated measurements
　　4. Misidentification of aorta
　　　　a. Confusion with IVC
　　5. Examination may be limited by
　　　　a. Obesity
　　　　b. Bowel gas

IV. Cardiac

A. General
　　1. Indications for use of focused cardiac ultrasound in cardiac arrest and during resuscitation (Figure 22–18)
　　　　a. Detection of pericardial free fluid and pericardial effusion
　　　　b. Evaluation for the presence of cardiac tamponade
　　　　c. Evaluation of gross cardiac activity and/or function during resuscitation
　　　　d. Extended indications of focused emergency echocardiography—evaluation of the etiology of cardiac arrest or unexplained hypotension (Figure 22–19)
　　　　　　i. Evaluation of right ventricular dysfunction in the setting of possible pulmonary embolism
　　　　　　ii. Estimation of intravascular volume status and central venous pressure (CVP)
　　2. Anatomy
　　　　a. Heart is located obliquely in the thorax oriented anteriorly, inferiorly, and laterally

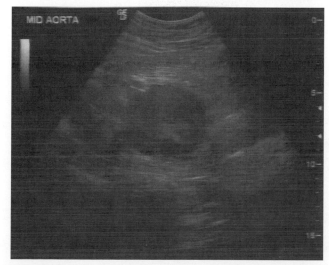

FIGURE 22–16. AAA with mural thrombus in lumen.

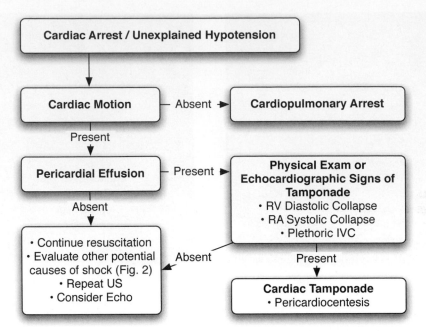

FIGURE 22–18. Algorithm for use of focused cardiac ultrasound in cardiac arrest and during resuscitation.

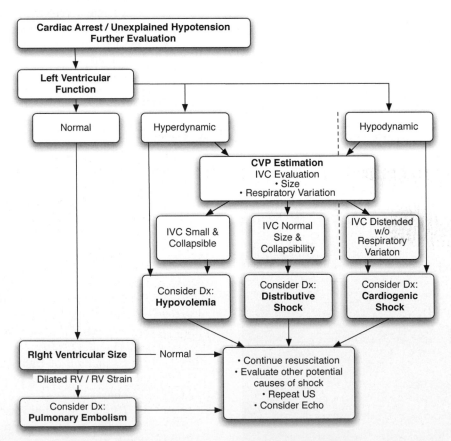

FIGURE 22–19. Algorithm for use of focused emergency cardiac ultrasound for further evaluation of the etiology of cardiac arrest or unexplained hypotension.

b. Right ventricle: located anteriorly
c. Left ventricle: located laterally
d. Apex of heart: located at point of maximal impulse (PMI), fifth intercostal space at mid-clavicular line
e. Base of heart: left atrium

3. Views
a. Orientation
   i. Echocardiography
      a) Scan from left side of patient
      b) Probe indicator to patient's left (except parasternal long axis view)
      c) Marker on right side of screen
   ii. Emergency medicine
      a) Scan from right side of patient
      b) Probe indicator always to patient's right
      c) Marker on left side of screen
      d) Because both indicator and screen marker are reversed, images appear normal ("double negative")
         i) Exception: parasternal long axis is reversed
   iii. Cardiac images on the written board examination will likely have the standard echocardiography orientation—look for the marker on the image
b. Patient positioning
   i. Left lateral decubitus
   ii. Left oblique
   iii. Supine for subcostal
c. Parasternal long axis (Figure 22–20)

i. Probe placed in third or fourth intercostal space with marker directed toward right shoulder
ii. View through heart along long axis
iii. View of the following structures:
   a) Right ventricle
   b) Septum
   c) Aortic valve and aortic outflow tract
   d) Left ventricle
   e) Left atrium and mitral valve
d. Parasternal short axis
   i. Probe placed in third or fourth intercostal space with marker directed towards left shoulder
      a) Probe tilted up to visualize at level of aortic valve
      b) Probe tilted down to visualize at level of ventricle
   ii. View through cross section of heart
   iii. Level of aortic valve (Figure 22–21)
   iv. View of the following structures
      a) Aortic valve
      b) Left atrium
      c) Right atrium
      d) Tricuspid valve
      e) Right ventricular outflow tract
      f) Pulmonic valve
e. Level of ventricle (mitral valve and papillary muscles) (Figure 22–22)
      i) View of the following structures
         a) Left ventricle
         b) Right ventricle

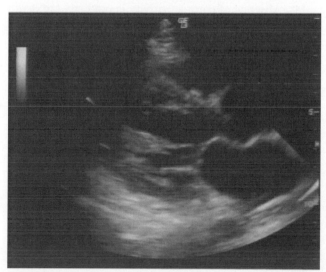

FIGURE 22–20. Parasternal long axis cardiac view demonstrating left atrium, mitral valve, left ventricle, aortic valve, proximal ascending aorta, and right ventricle.

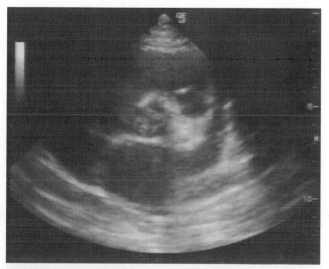

FIGURE 22–21. Parasternal short axis cardiac view at the level of the aortic valve *(center)* demonstrating *(clockwise from bottom)* left atrium, right atrium, tricuspid valve, right ventricular outflow tract, and pulmonic valve.

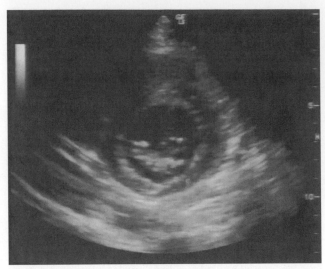

FIGURE 22–22. Parasternal short axis cardiac view at the level of the ventricle demonstrating left and right ventricles.

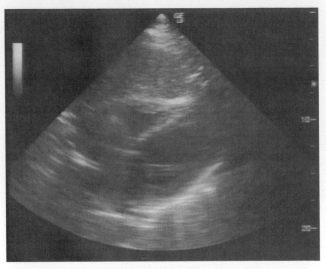

FIGURE 22–24. Subxiphoid cardiac view demonstrating the left ventricle and atrium *(far-field)* and the right ventricle and atrium *(near field)*.

    f. Apical four chamber (Figure 22–23)
        i. View of all four chambers from apex through base of heart
           a) Left ventricle
           b) Right ventricle
           c) Left atrium
           d) Right atrium
           e) Mitral valve
           f) Tricuspid valve
        ii. Probe placed at PMI in fifth intercostal space, marker to left, probe aimed toward right shoulder.

    g. Subcostal (Figure 22–24)
        i. Heart is imaged anteroinferiorly (right-sided structures) to posterosuperiorly (left-sided structures)
           a) Right ventricle
           b) Right atrium
           c) Left ventricle
           d) Left atrium
        ii. Probe placed subcostally, marker towards left hip with probe directed towards left shoulder

B. Resuscitation and cardiac arrest
    1. Absence of cardiac activity is predictive of death
    2. Emergency echocardiography can help elucidate causes of pulseless electrical activity (PEA) and hypotension during resuscitation
        a. Hypovolemia
        b. Cardiac tamponade
        c. Pulmonary embolism

C. Pericardial effusion (Figure 22–25) (see Figure 22–12 for subcostal view of a pericardial effusion)
    1. Visualized as anechoic fluid between two echogenic layers (visceral and parietal) of pericardium
        a. Look for fluid in posterior pericardial space
           i. Effects of gravity with small effusion
          ii. Anterior epicardial fat pad may masquerade as pericardial free fluid
    2. Size of pericardial effusion
        a. Small
           i. Size: <1 cm thick
          ii. Usually localized to posterior pericardial space

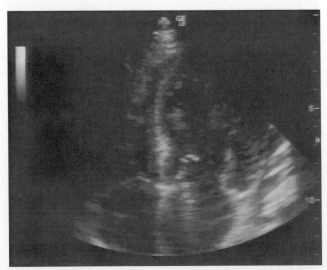

FIGURE 22–23. Apical four chamber cardiac view demonstrating left and right ventricles and left and right atria.

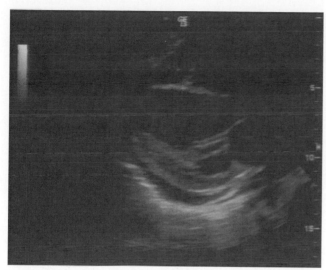

FIGURE 22–25. Parasternal long axis cardiac view demonstrating pericardial effusion located posteriorly between the two echogenic layers of pericardium.

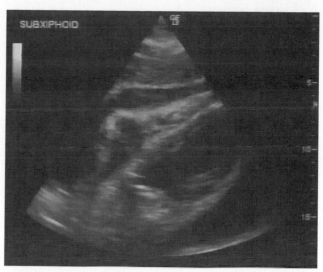

FIGURE 22–26. Subxiphoid view of a pericardial effusion with tamponade demonstrating right ventricular diastolic collapse.

b. Moderate
   i. Size: 1 to 2 cm thick
   ii. Usually wraps around heart in entire pericardial space
c. Large
   i. Size: >2 cm thick
   ii. Heart swings freely in pericardial effusion

D. Cardiac tamponade
1. Physiology
   a. Fluid accumulates in nondistensible fibrous pericardium
   b. Space is limited, therefore pericardial pressures increase
   c. It is the rate of fluid collection not the volume that determines pericardial distensibility
      i. For a given volume, the pericardial pressure will be greater in an acute effusion compared to a chronic effusion
      ii. Chronic effusions allow time for the pericardium to distend
   d. Increased pericardial pressures lead to collapse of right-sided chambers
      i. Right atrial systolic collapse
      ii. Right ventricular diastolic collapse (Figure 22–26)
         a) Look in parasternal long axis, apical four-chamber and/or subcostal views
         b) Tamponade: collapse of right ventricle during diastole
            i) End diastole: immediately prior to mitral valve closure (MV leaflets are still open)
      iii. Distended plethoric IVC

E. Ventricular function
1. Evaluate global function of left ventricle
   a. Evaluate myocardial contractility
   b. Evaluate endocardial thickening
2. Normal
3. Hypodynamic
   a. Poor myocardial contractility and endocardial thickening
   b. Dilated ventricular cavity
4. Hyperdynamic
   a. Increased myocardial contractility

F. Pulmonary embolism
1. Pulmonary embolism leads to increased right-sided pressures causing increased right ventricular pressure and strain
2. Dilated right ventricle (Figure 22–27)
   a. Normal RV-to-LV ratio is ~0.5 to 1
   b. Dilated RV is present when RV-to-LV ratio >1
3. Right ventricular hypokinesis
4. Other causes of right ventricular strain will mimic findings in pulmonary embolism

G. Central venous pressure (CVP)
1. CVP can be estimated from IVC size, distensibility, and respiratory variation
   a. IVC is capacitance vessel and will increase in size with increasing CVPs
      i. Inspiratory force will cause IVC collapse
   b. Normal IVC diameter is ~1.5 to 2 cm and collapses ~50% with inspiration
   c. High CVP will have dilated IVC >1.5 to 2 cm with <50% collapse (Figure 22–28)

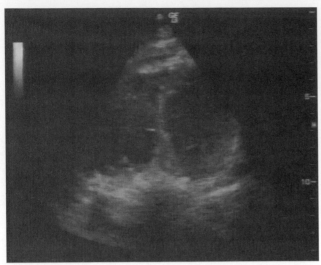

FIGURE 22–27. Apical cardiac view demonstrating dilated right ventricle in a patient with pulmonary embolism.

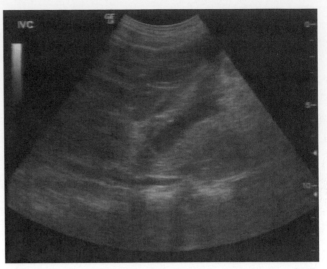

FIGURE 22–29. Collapsed IVC consistent with low CVP.

    d. Low CVP will have collapsed IVC with near or total inspiratory collapse (Figure 22–29)

    e. See Table 22–1 for estimation of CVP based on IVC diameter and respiratory variation

H. Limitations

    1. Focused cardiac ultrasound is a limited examination not intended to evaluate

        a. Segmental wall abnormalities

        b. Valvular disease

        c. Cardiomyopathies

        d. Diastolic dysfunction

        e. Other cardiac manifestations

2. Technical limitations

    a. Bony thorax with small intercostal spaces

    b. Hyperinflated lungs

    c. Abdominal distention

    d. Obesity

I. Pitfalls

    1. Failure to obtain adequate views

    2. Pathologic findings should be visualized in two views

    3. The entire pericardial space should be evaluated for pericardial effusions

        a. Anterior fat pad may masquerade as effusion

        b. Loculated effusions may be present

    4. Pleural effusions may be mistaken for pericardial effusions

        a. Location of effusion in reference to the descending aorta will help differentiate

            i. Pleural effusions will surround descending aorta

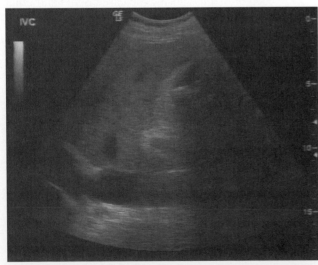

FIGURE 22–28. Plethoric IVC consistent with high CVP.

TABLE 22–1. Estimate CVP from IVC Diameter and Respiratory Variation

IVC SIZE	INSPIRATORY CHANGE	ESTIMATE CVP
<1.5 cm	Total	0 to 5 cm
1.5 to 2.5 cm	>50%	5 to 10 cm
1.5 to 2.5 cm	<50%	10 to 15 cm
>2.5 cm	<50%	15 to 20 cm
>2.5 cm	No change	>20 cm

Adapted with permission, from Ma OJ, Mateer JR: *Emergency Ultrasound.* Copyright © 2003, New York: McGraw-Hill.

5. Pulmonary embolism may be present without evidence of right ventricular strain

6. Right ventricular strain may be present without the presence of pulmonary embolism

V. First Trimester Pregnancy

A. General

1. Indications for use of focused emergency ultrasound in the evaluation of first trimester pregnancy (Figure 22–30)

    a. Evaluation for the presence of intrauterine pregnancy (IUP)

    i. Presence of an IUP minimized likelihood of an ectopic pregnancy in patients without risk factors for heterotopic pregnancies

    b. Other indications for first trimester pelvic ultrasound

    i. Evaluation for ovarian cysts

    ii. Evaluation of the adnexa for identification of suspected ectopic pregnancy

2. Pelvic anatomy

    a. Bladder

    i. Fluid-filled triangular to spherical-shaped structure located anteriorly in the pelvis

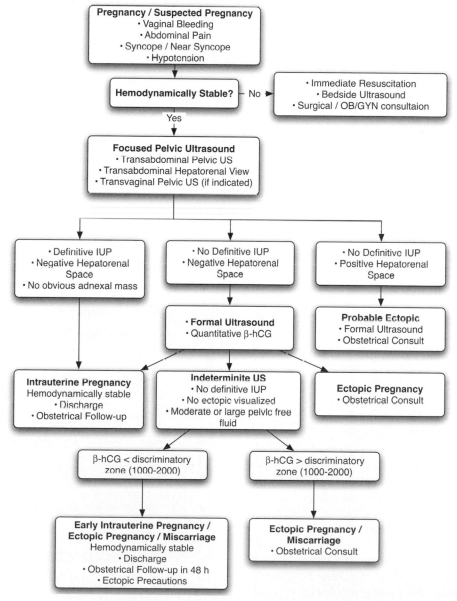

FIGURE 22–30. Algorithm for using focused emergency ultrasound in the evaluation of first trimester pregnancy.

b. Uterus
    i. Located midline in pelvis
    ii. Usually anteverted
c. Rectouterine pouch (pouch of Douglas)
    i. Anatomic space between the uterus and rectum in the female pelvis
    ii. Most dependent portion of the female pelvis
d. Rectum
    i. Located posteriorly in the pelvis
e. Ovaries
    i. Located laterally in the pelvis
    ii. Anterior and medial to external iliac vessels
    iii. Varied ovarian pelvic location in the gravid patient
3. Views
    a. General guidelines on necessary views
        i. Uterus
            a) Long and transverse views
            b) Endometrial stripe (midline)
        ii. IVP
            a) Yolk sac
            b) Fetal pole
            c) Fetal heart motion
            d) Evaluate endometrial mantle surrounding gestation sac
        iii. Adnexa (if they can be visualized)
        iv. Evaluate for free fluid if ectopic suspected
            a) Cul-de-sac (pouch of Douglas)
            b) Hepatorenal space
    b. Transabdominal pelvic ultrasound
        i. Should be performed first before transvaginal ultrasound
            a) Noninvasive
            b) Provides information about orientation of anatomy
            c) Allows visualization of structures outside of field of view of transvaginal ultrasound
            d) May provide necessary answers
        ii. Full bladder technique
            a) Provides sonographic window to evaluate posterior structures
            b) Displaces bowels from field of view
        iii. Sagittal (longitudinal) uterus (Figure 22–31)
            a) Visualize vaginal stripe
            b) Visualize cervix
            c) Visualize endometrial stripe
        iv. Transverse uterus
            a) Visualize endometrial stripe
            b) Scan through entire uterus
        v. Sagittal and transverse adnexa

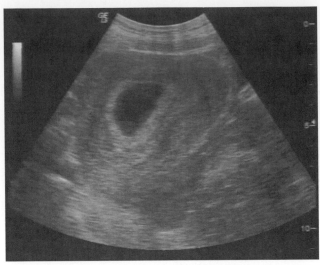

FIGURE 22–31. Transabdominal sagittal view of a gravid uterus demonstrating uterus with gestational sac and endometrial stripe, vaginal stripe, and bladder.

            a) Move transducer laterally and angle through bladder to visualize contralateral ovary
    c. Transvaginal pelvic ultrasound
        i. Improved visualization of pelvic structures
            a) Closer to structures of interest
            b) High-resolution probe provides better resolution
        ii. Empty bladder
        iii. Sagittal (longitudinal) uterus (Figure 22–32)
            a) Visualize vaginal stripe

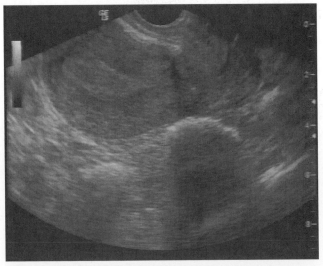

FIGURE 22–32. Transvaginal sagittal view of the uterus demonstrating uterus, cervix, and endometrial stripe.

b) Visualize cervix

c) Visualize endometrial stripe

iv. Transverse uterus (coronal plane)

a) Visualize endometrial stripe

b) Scan through entire uterus

v. Sagittal and transverse (coronal plane) adnexa

a) Ovaries may be easier to locate in transverse plane

B. Ultrasound findings in first trimester pregnancy

1. Intradecidual sign

a. Small endometrial sac imbedded off midline not deforming the midline endometrial stripe

b. Present at 4 to 5 weeks with β-hCG <1000

2. Gestational sac (Figure 22–33)

a. Endometrial sac surrounded by thick chorionic rim

b. Present at 5 weeks with β-hCG 1000 to 2000

c. Seen in most IUPs

d. May see pseudosac in ectopic pregnancy

3. Double decidual sign (Figure 22–34)

a. Two concentric echogenic rings surrounding the gestational sac

i. Inner ring: decidua capsularis = chorionic rim

ii. Hypoechoic endometrial canal

iii. Outer ring: decidua vera = stimulated endometrium

b. Present at 5 weeks with β-hCG 1000 to 2000

c. Considered by some to be the first definitive sign of IUP

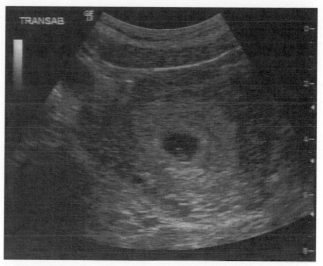

FIGURE 22–34. Transabdominal view of the uterus demonstrating a double decidual sign, yolk sac, and fetal pole.

4. Yolk sac (see Figure 22-34)

a. Symmetric round sac within gestational sac

b. Present at 5 to 6 weeks with β-hCG >2000

c. First definitive sign of IUP

5. Embryo (Figure 22–35)

a. Seen initially as thickening and mass at edge of yolk sac

b. Present at 6 weeks with β-hCG 10,000

c. Grows at rate of 1 mm/day

6. Fetal heart

a. Heart rate should be detectable in embryo that measures >5 mm

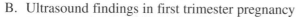

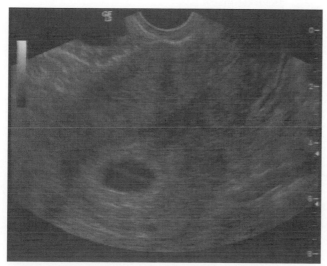

FIGURE 22–33. Transvaginal sagittal view of the gravid uterus demonstrating a gestational sac off-axis of the endometrial stripe.

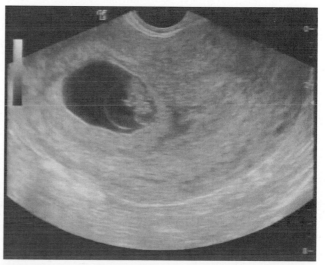

FIGURE 22–35. Transvaginal view of an intrauterine pregnancy with an embryo.

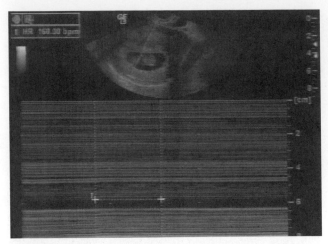

FIGURE 22–36. Fetal heart rate documentation by M-mode ultrasound.

b. Present at 6 to 7 weeks with β-hCG 10,000 to 20,000

c. Normal heart rate 140 to 160

d. Fetal heart rate should be documented using M-mode (Figure 22–36)

7. Correlation of gestational age, β-hCG, and pelvic ultrasound findings (Table 22–2)

   a. In general, findings are visualized with transabdominal ultrasound ~1 week later and with roughly double the β-hCG in comparison with transvaginal ultrasound

C. Ectopic pregnancy

1. Definite ectopic pregnancy

   a. Extrauterine embryo with cardiac activity

   b. Extrauterine gestational sac with embryo or yolk sac

2. Nonspecific signs of ectopic pregnancy

   a. Empty uterus with the following findings (Table 22–3)

      i. Pelvic free fluid

      ii. Pelvic mass/tubal ring (Figure 22–37)

      iii. Hepatorenal free fluid

Table 22–3. Likelihood of Ectopic Pregnancy Based on Empty Uterus and Findings on Ultrasound

ULTRASOUND FINDING	LIKELIHOOD OF ECTOPIC
Any pelvic free fluid	52%
Complex pelvic mass	75%
Moderate or large pelvic free fluid	86%
Tubal ring	>95%
Mass and free fluid	97%
Hepatorenal free fluid	~100%

Adapted, with permission, from Ma OJ, Mateer JR: *Emergency Ultrasound.* Copyright © 2003, New York: McGraw-Hill.

3. Discriminatory zone

   a. Range of β-hCG before which an IUP cannot be definitively confirmed and ectopic pregnancy definitively ruled out

      i. Usually between 1000 and 2000

   b. Dependent upon on criteria used to define IUP

      i. Double decidual sign is present earlier with lower β-hCG than yolk sac but is less definitive than the presence of a yolk sac

   c. Dependent upon method of ultrasound: transvaginal versus transabdominal

   d. Repeat β-hCG in 48 hours and repeat ultrasound

D. Abnormal pregnancies

1. Anembryonic pregnancy (blighted ovum) (Figure 22–38)

   a. Gestational sac diameter >20 mm without evidence of yolk sac or embryo

2. Fetal demise

   a. Deformed gestational sac

   b. Gestational sac low in uterus

   c. Absence of fetal heart motion in embryo >5 mm long

3. Gestational trophoblastic disease (molar pregnancy) (Figure 22–39)

   a. Intrauterine mass with diffuse hypoechoic vesicles ("cluster of grapes" appearance)

TABLE 22–2. Gestational Age, β-hCG, and Pelvic Ultrasound Findings

GESTATIONAL AGE	β-HCG	TRANSVAGINAL ULTRASOUND	TRANSABDOMINAL ULTRASOUND
4 to 5 weeks	<1000	Intradecidual sac	—
5 weeks	1000 to 2000	Gestational sac (± double decidual sign)	—
5 to 6 weeks	>2000	Yolk sac (± embryo)	Gestational sac (± double decidual sign)
6 weeks	10,000 to 20,000	Embryo with cardiac activity	Yolk sac (± embryo)
7 weeks	>20,000	Embryonic torso/head	Embryo with cardiac activity

Adapted, with permission, from Ma OJ, Mateer JR: *Emergency Ultrasound.* Copyright © 2003, New York: McGraw-Hill.

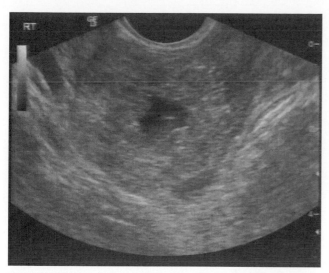

FIGURE 22–37. Ectopic pregnancy demonstrating tubal ring.

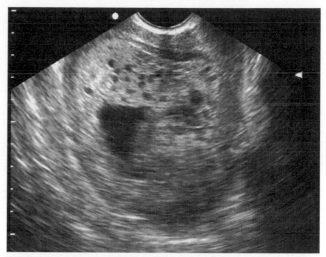

FIGURE 22–39. Molar pregnancy. (Reprinted, with permission, from Ma OJ, Mateer JR, Blaivas M. *Emergency Ultrasound*, 2nd ed. New York: McGraw-Hill, 2008.)

E. Adnexa
   1. Normal ovaries
      a. Ovoid structures measuring 5 cm (L) × 3 cm (W) × 2 cm (D)
      b. Thin-walled
      c. Hypoechoic structure
      d. Ovarian follicles
         i. "Chocolate chip cookie" appearance
   2. Cysts
      a. Simple cyst (Figure 22–40)
         i. Smooth thin-walled
         ii. Anechoic without internal echoes
         iii. Posterior enhancement
      b. Corpus luteum cyst (Figure 22–41)

   i. May have thin or thick walls
   ii. Hemorrhagic corpus luteum cyst will have internal echoes
   iii. "Ring of fire"—increased blood flow to corpus luteum cyst
      a) May also be present with ectopic pregnancy

F. Limitations
   1. Evaluation of patients with risk factors for heterotopic pregnancy (eg, infertility therapy)
   2. Evaluation of fetal anatomy, evidence of fetal well-being, or any maternal-fetal pathology
   3. Evaluation of adnexal pathology

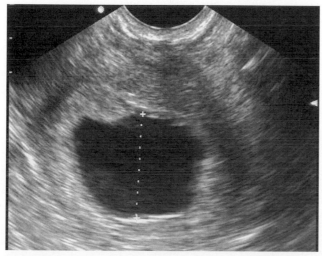

FIGURE 22–38. Anembryonic pregnancy. (Reproduced, with permission, from Ma OJ, Mateer JR: *Emergency Ultrasound*. Copyright © 2003, New York: McGraw-Hill)

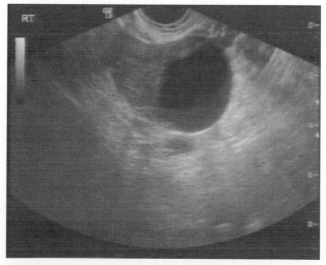

FIGURE 22–40. Simple ovarian cyst.

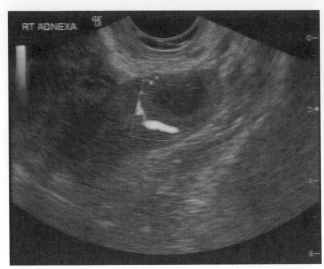

FIGURE 22–41. Corpus luteum cyst demonstrating "ring of fire."

G. Pitfalls
1. Failure to perform ultrasound with β-hCG less than discriminatory zone
   a. Ectopic pregnancies have been reported with β-hCG that ranges from 10 to 1000
2. Interpreting scan as positive for IUP without the presence of a yolk sac
   a. Pseudosac with ectopic pregnancy may be confused with gestational sac of IUP
3. Identification of IUP without ensuring location in uterus
   a. Ectopic pregnancies may be mistaken for intrauterine pregnancy
   b. Scan through entire uterus
   c. Identify endometrial stripe
   d. Ensure that gestational sac is located in midline
   e. Ensure adequate endometrial mantle (>5 mm in all views)
      i. Cornual or interstitial ectopic—rare but high mortality
4. Failure to fully scan through pelvis and attempt to identify ovaries and adnexa
   a. May miss heterotopic pregnancy
   b. May miss other significant pelvic pathology
5. Failure to identify ovaries or misidentifying structures as ovaries
   a. Bowel
   b. Pelvic musculature
6. Bladder
   a. Full bladder in transabdominal ultrasound provides sonographic window and displace bowels

   b. Full bladder in transvaginal ultrasound displaces structures out of field of view

VI. Renal

A. General
1. Indications
   a. Evaluation for the presence of hydronephrosis
   b. Evaluation for bladder distention and urinary retention
2. Principles
   a. Obstructive uropathy will lead to dilation of urinary collecting system (hydronephrosis)
3. Views
   a. Place ultrasound probe in coronal axis at lateral costal margin with marker towards patient's head.
      i. Right kidney—midaxillary line
      ii. Left kidney—posterior axillary line ("knuckles to the bed")
   b. May need to rotate probe to angle between long axis of ribs to visualize kidneys
   c. Both kidneys should be visualized from the upper pole to the lower pole in the long (coronal) and transverse views
      i. Transverse views are obtained by rotating the probe 90 degrees counterclockwise
   d. Ultrasound appearance
      i. Renal cortex appears homogenous and hypoechoic to isoechoic in comparison with liver or spleen
      ii. Renal pyramids are hypoechoic
      iii. Renal sinus is hyperechoic
         a) Dilation of the collecting system (hydronephrosis) will appear as anechoic (black) in the normally hyperechoic renal sinus

B. Hydronephrosis
1. Hydronephrosis is a spectrum from mild to severe
2. Mild hydronephrosis (Figure 22–42)
   a. Distention of collecting system with preservation of calyces and renal papillae
3. Moderate hydronephrosis (Figure 22–43)
   a. Dilation of collecting system with rounding of calyces and obliteration of renal papillae ("bear claw" appearance)
4. Severe hydronephrosis (Figure 22–44)
   a. Calyceal ballooning with cortical thinning

C. Bladder distention (Figure 22–45)
1. Measure bladder size in sagittal and transverse planes

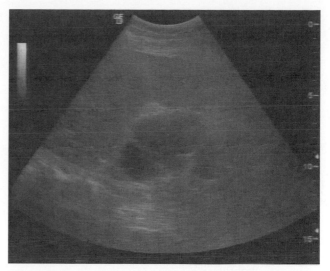

FIGURE 22–42. Mild hydronephrosis.

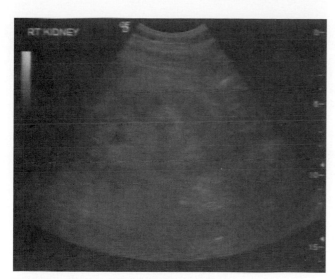

FIGURE 22–44. Severe hydronephrosis.

2. Bladder size (cc) ≈ 0.75 × width (cm) × height (cm) × depth (cm)

D. Limitations and pitfalls
   1. Well-hydrated kidneys may mimic hydronephrosis
      a. Compare nonaffected side to affected side
   2. The full bladder may cause false-positive hydronephrosis
      a. Repeat ultrasound after emptying bladder
   3. Ureteral stones may be present without hydronephrosis
   4. Hypoechoic renal pyramids may be mistaken for hydronephrosis
   5. Renal cysts, especially parapelvic cysts, may be mistaken for hydronephrosis

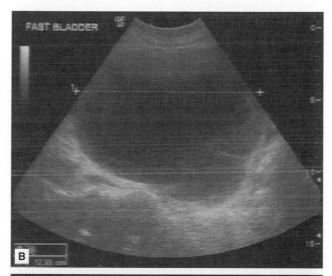

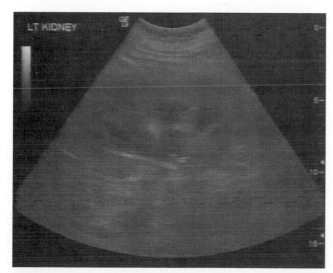

FIGURE 22–43. Moderate hydronephrosis.

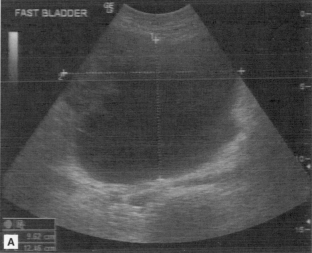

FIGURE 22–45. Distended bladder. (A) Transverse, (B) Sagittal views.

6. Examination may be limited by
   a. Body habitus and obesity
   b. Bowel gas

VII. Right Upper Quadrant (RUQ)

A. General
   1. Indications
      a. Evaluation for cholelithiasis
      b. Evaluation for evidence of acute cholecystitis
         i. Gallbladder wall edema: thickened anterior gallbladder wall
         ii. Pericholecystic fluid
         iii. Sonographic Murphy sign
      c. Evaluation for evidence of choledo-cholithiasis
         i. Dilated common bile duct (CBD)
   2. RUQ anatomy
      a. Gallbladder
         i. Gallbladder is located posteriorly and inferiorly to the liver in gallbladder fossa
            a) Located approximately in right mid-clavicular line
            b) Gallbladder may extend subcostally below the edge of the liver
            c) Most anterior cystic structure in the upper abdomen
         ii. Fundus
            a) Blind terminal pouch extending from the inferior surface of the liver
            b) Phyrigian cap: fold of gallbladder at the fundus
         iii. Body
            a) Contiguous with surface of liver
            b) Inferior surface is contiguous with duodenum
               i) Shadowing from duodenum may interfere and confound imaging of the gallbladder
         iv. Neck
            a) Narrow S-shaped proximal portion of the gallbladder before entering cystic duct
            b) Hartman pouch: fold and sacculation at the neck of the gallbladder
            c) Spiral valves of Heister in neck may cause shadowing
      b. Portal triad
         i. Located at porta hepatis of liver
         ii. Consists of
            a) Biliary system
            b) Portal venous system
            c) Hepatic artery
         iii. Biliary system
            a) Right and left hepatic ducts in the liver form proper hepatic duct proximally
            b) Cystic duct from neck of gallbladder joins proper hepatic duct at the porta hepatis to form the CBD
               i) CBD located anteriorly and laterally in the porta hepatis
            c) CBD courses proximally through the head of the pancreas, is joined by the pancreatic duct (of Wirsung), and empties into the duodenum at the ampulla of Vater
         iv. Portal venous system
            a) Portal vein formed by confluence of splenic vein and superior mesenteric vein
               i) Posterior surface of neck of pancreas
            b) Portal vein courses distally through porta hepatis and divides into right and left portal veins as it enters the liver
               i) Portal vein is located posteriorly in the porta hepatis
         v. Hepatic artery
            a) Common hepatic artery branches off celiac trunk
               i) Common hepatic artery is located anterior and medially in the porta hepatis
            b) Cystic artery branches off common hepatic artery towards the gallbladder
               i) Passes between the CBD anteriorly and portal vein posteriorly
            c) Proper hepatic artery branches into right and left hepatic arteries as it enters the liver
   3. Views
      a. Patient positioning
         i. Supine
         ii. Left lateral decubitus
            a) May provide better imaging
               i) Liver serves as acoustic window
               ii) Bowel gas displaced
         iii. Use patient inspiration and expiration to improve windows
         iv. NPO status may increase gallbladder distention and visualization
      b. Gallbladder
         i. Gallbladder is the most anterior anechoic cystic structure in RUQ
            a) Color Doppler may be utilized to discriminate from anechoic vascular structures
         ii. Gallbladder should be imaged in the long and transverse planes
            a) Place ultrasound probe subcostally in midclavicular line

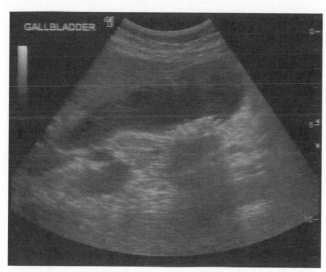

FIGURE 22–46. Long axis view of the gallbladder demonstrating gallbladder neck. Note the presence of small stones with posterior shadowing.

    b) Scan medial to lateral until gallbladder is localized

    c) Rotate probe as necessary to scan through gallbladder in long axis (Figure 22–46)

       i) Visualize gallbladder neck

       ii) Visualize gallbladder fundus

    d) Rotate probe to scan through gallbladder in transverse axis (Figure 22–47)

       i) Scan continuously from fundus through neck

  iii. Neck of the gallbladder should be fully visualized

    a) Evaluate for gallstones impacted in neck of gallbladder (Figure 22–48)

  c. Common bile duct (CBD) (Figure 22–49)

    i. Portal triad most readily identified by following the echogenic linear main lobar fissure from the neck of the gallbladder to the portal triad

    ii. Cross sectional view (Mickey Mouse sign)

      a) Portal vein posterior (head)

      b) Hepatic artery anterior and medially (left ear as Mickey faces you)

      c) CBD anterior and laterally (right ear as Mickey faces you)

    iii. Longitudinal view (parallel channel sign)

      a) Portal vein posterior

      b) CBD anterior

      c) Hepatic artery may be visualized in cross section between portal vein and CBD

    iv. Portal triad may also be located by following the portal system proximally from within liver towards the main portal vein

      a) Portal veins have echogenic walls; hepatic veins do not

    v. Color doppler may be used to discriminate CBD from hepatic artery and portal vein portal vein

      a) Vessels may not demonstrate color flow if angle of incidence is ~ 90 degrees

B. Cholelithiasis

  1. Echogenic gallstone(s) in gallbladder (Figure 22–50)

  2. Posterior shadowing from gallstones

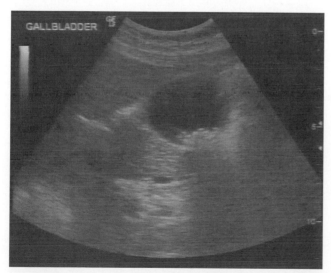

FIGURE 22–47. Transverse view of the gallbladder demonstrating small stones with posterior shadowing.

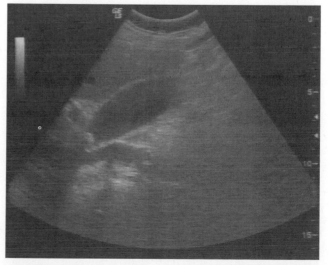

FIGURE 22–48. Long axis view of the gallbladder demonstrating a gallstone impacted in the neck of the gallbladder.

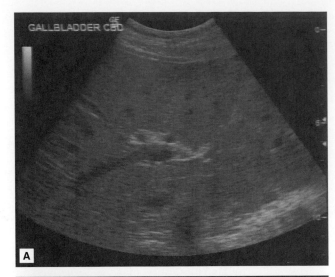

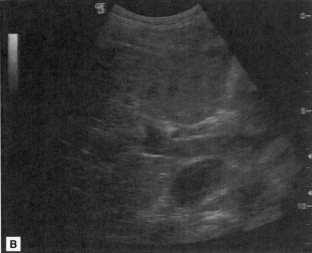

FIGURE 22–49. Portal triad. (**A**) Cross-section (transverse) view. (**B**) Long-axis view.

a. May be only evidence of small stones or gravel

3. Evaluation for stones should be performed in both long and transverse views
   a. Small stones and gravel may be more apparent on transverse view

4. Wall echo sign (WES) (Figure 22–51)
   a. Caused by contracted gallstone-filled gallbladder
      i. Gallbladder **W**all
      ii. **E**choes from gallstones
      iii. **S**hadowing from gallstones

5. Gallbladder polyps
   a. Echogenic mass in gallbladder attached to gallbladder wall
   b. Unlike gallstones
      i. Polyps do not have posterior shadowing
      ii. Polyps are fixed to the wall and do not move with change in patient positioning
   c. The presence of gallbladder polyps with gallstones is suspicious for gallbladder cancer

C. Cholecystis (Figures 22–52 and 22–53)
   1. Evidence of acute cholecystitis
      a. Gallbladder wall edema: thickened anterior gallbladder wall
      b. Pericholecystic fluid
      c. Sonographic Murphy sign
   2. Gallbladder wall thickening and edema
      a. Measure anterior gallbladder wall
         i. Posterior enhancement of posterior wall
         ii. Close apposition of bowel loops

FIGURE 22–50. Gallbladder with echogenic gallstone demonstrating posterior shadowing.

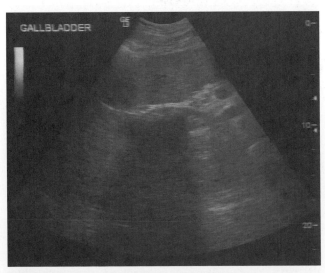

FIGURE 22–51. Cholelithiasis with WES sign

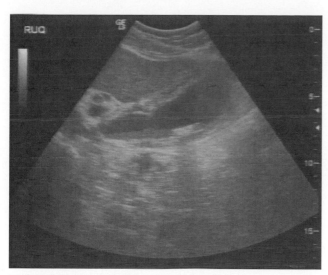

FIGURE 22–52. Cholecystitis with gallbladder wall edema.

b. Normal size ≤4 mm
c. Wall edema may be present
    i. Visualized as hypoechoic stripe between hyperechoic inner and outer gallbladder wall
d. Other causes of gallbladder wall thickening
    i. Contracted gallbladder
        a) Symmetrical thickening of wall with visible muscle layers
    ii. Hepatitis
    iii. Ascites
    iv. CHF
    v. Pancreatitis

3. Pericholecystic fluid
    a. Hypoechoic and anechoic fluid located anterior to the gallbladder surface or within hepatic parenchyma
        i. May be focal or diffuse
4. Sonographic Murphy sign
    a. Tenderness over the gallbladder caused by compression with the ultrasound probe

D. Choledocholithiasis
1. Choledocholithiasis may be evident as a dilated CBD (Figure 22–54)
    a. Rarely, gallstones may be visualized within CBD
2. Measurement of CBD
    a. Measure from inner wall to inner wall
    b. Measurement should be made as close to the edge of the liver as feasible
    c. Normal CBD ≤4 mm
    d. Normal CBD size increases with age
        i. Normal CBD (mm) ≤age/10
    e. Normal CBD after cholecystectomy may be ≥10 mm

E. Gallbladder sludge (Figure 22–55)
1. Non-shadowing echogenic material in gallbladder
    a. Layers with change in patient position
    b. May have small punctate hyperechoic calcifications

F. Limitations
1. Does not evaluate all right upper quadrant pathology including pathology of liver and pancreas
2. Contracted gallbladder may limit visualization
3. Examination may be limited by;

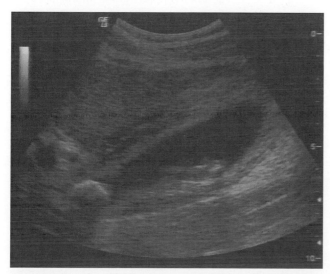

FIGURE 22–53. Cholecystitis with thickened gallbladder wall, pericholecystic fluid, gallstones, and gallstone impacted in the neck of the gallbladder.

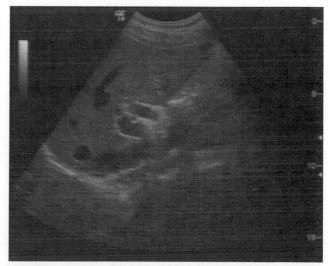

FIGURE 22–54. Dilated CBD demonstrating parallel channel sign.

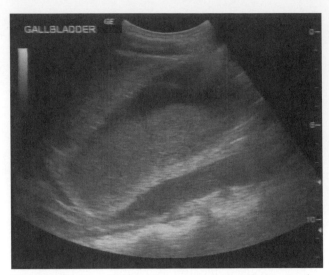

FIGURE 22–55.   Gallbladder demonstrating sludge causing cholecystitis.

    a. Body habitus
    b. Bowel gas

G. Pitfalls
  1. Misidentification of gallbladder with other RUQ structures
    a. Bowel
    b. IVC
  2. Failure to visualize entire gallbladder including the neck and fundus may miss gallstones
  3. Confusion of shadowing from bowel gas with that of gallstones
    a. Duodenum is located adjacent to gallbladder
  4. Misidentification of bile duct with other portal triad structures
  5. Failure to recognized that gallbladder wall thickening may be caused by entities other than cholecystitis

VIII. Ultrasound Guided Procedures

A. Procedural ultrasound utilizes ultrasound to guide procedures that are otherwise performed blindly
  1. Vascular access
    a. U.S. Agency for Healthcare Research and Quality recommends use of ultrasound guidance for placement of central venous catheters
    b. Improves catheter insertion success rates
    c. Reduces the number of venipuncture attempts prior to successful placement
    d. Reduces the number of complications associated with catheter insertion
  2. Localization of fluid and/or anatomic landmarks

    a. Pericardiocentesis
    b. Thoracentesis
    c. Paracentesis
    d. Arthrocentesis
    e. Lumbar puncture
    f. Needle aspirations

B. Methods of performing ultrasound guided procedures
  1. Dynamic guidance
    a. Ultrasound used for direct visualization of needle placement during an invasive procedure
    b. Preferred technique when feasible.
  2. Static guidance
    a. Ultrasound used to determine the proper location for needle insertion during an invasive procedure

C. Performing procedural ultrasound
  1. Scan area of interest and/or appropriate landmarks for the procedure that uses at least two different views
  2. Determine the path of the needle and the location of any significant surrounding structures
  3. Dynamic guidance
    a. The needle should be inserted into the area of interest while continuing to demonstrate both the position of the needle and the area of interest.
      i. Vascular access
        a) Vessel can be localized in either transverse or longitudinal orientation
        b) Confirmation of vessel identity and patency can be performed using B-mode compression ultrasonography and/or Doppler (color and/or spectral Doppler) imaging
    b. Continuous scanning **must** be performed to confirm needle location and prevent complications.
  4. Static guidance:
    a. The location for needle insertion should be marked on the skin and insertion depth ascertained from the ultrasound images.
    b. Scanning should be performed after the procedure for verification and to ascertain the presence of complications.

D. Limitations and pitfalls
  1. Ultrasound guidance is an adjunct only for procedures
  2. Needle artifact must be visualized to determine localization
    a. Short axis imaging (eg, transverse view during vascular access) only visualizes the

cross section of the needle at that point, not the entire path of the needle
  i. Provides information about surrounding structures
 b. Long axis imaging allows visualization of location of needle and area of interest
  i. Does not provide as much information about surrounding structures
3. There is a learning curve in adaptation of blind procedures into ultrasound guided procedures

BIBLIOGRAHY

Abboud PC, Kendal JL: Ultrasound guidance for vascular access. *Emerg Med Clin N Am.* 2004;22:749.

Albayram F, Hamper U: First-trimester obstetric emergencies: spectrum of sonographic findings. *J Clin Ultrasound.* 2002;30:161.

American College of Emergency Physicians: ACEP Emergency Ultrasound Guidelines-2001. *Ann Emerg Med.* 2001;38:470.

Americal College of Emergency Physicians: Emergency Ultrasound Imaging Criteria Compendium. *Ann Emerg Med.* 2006;48:487.

Barkin, AZ, Rosen, CL: Ultrasound detection of abdominal aortic aneurysm. *Emerg Med Clin N Am.* 2004;22:675.

Ciccone TJ, Grossman SA: Cardiac ultrasound. *Emerg Med Clin N Am.* 2004; 22:621.

Cosby KS, Kendall JL: *Practical Guide to Emergency Ultrasound.* New York: Lippincott, Williams & Wilkins, 2006.

Dart RG: Role of pelvic ultrasonography in evaluation of symptomatic first trimester pregnancy. *Ann Emerg Med.* 1999;33:310.

Durham B, Lane B, Burbridge, L, et al: Pelvic ultrasound performed by emergency physicians for the detection of ectopic pregnancy in complicated first-trimester pregnancy. *Ann Emerg Med.* 1997;29:338.

Henderson SV, Hoffner RJ, Aragona JL, et al: Bedside emergency department ultrasonography plus radiography of the kidneys, ureters and bladder vs. intravenous pyelography in the evaluation of suspected ureteral colic. *Acad Emerg Med.* 1998;5:666.

Jehle D, Davis E, Evans T, et al: Emergency department sonography by emergency physicians. *Am J Emerg Med.* 1989; 7:605.

Jehle D, Guarino J, Karamanoukian H: Emergency department ultrasound in the evaluation of blunt abdominal trauma. *Am J Emerg Med.* 1993;11:342.

Jones AE, Tayal VS, Sullivan D, et al: Randomized controlled trial of immediate versus delayed goal-directed ultrasound to identify the cause of non-traumatic hypotension in emergency department patients. *Critical Care Med.* 2004;32:1703.

Kendall JL, Shrimp RJ: Performance and interpretation of focused right upper quadrant ultrasound by emergency physicians. *J Emerg Med.* 2001;21:7.

Kuhn M, Bonnin RL, Dave MJ, et al: Emergency department ultrasound scanning for abdominal aortic aneurysm: accessible, accurate and advantageous. *Ann Emerg Med.* 2000; 36:219.

Lanoix R, Leak LV, Gaeta T, et al: A preliminary evaluation of emergency ultrasound in the setting of an emergency medicine training program. *Am J Emerg Med.* 2000;18:41.

Ma OJ, Mateer JR: *Emergency Ultrasound.* New York: McGraw-Hill, 2003.

Ma OJ, Mateer JR, Keefer MP: Prospective analysis of a rapid trauma ultrasound examination performed by emergency physicians. *J Trauma.* 1995;38:879.

Mandavia D, Hoffner R, Mahaney K, et al: Bedside echocardiography by emergency physicians *Ann Emerg Med.* 2001;38:377.

Mandavia DP, Joseph A: Bedside echocardiography in chest trauma. *Emerg Med Clin N Am.* 2004;22:601.

Mateer J, Plummer D, Heller M, et al: Model curriculum for physicians training in emergency ultrasonography. *Ann Emerg Med.* 1994;23:95.

Mateer JR, Valley VT, Aiman EJ, et al: Outcome analysis of a protocol including bedside endovaginal sonography in patients at risk for ectopic pregnancy. *Ann Emerg Med.* 1996; 27:283.

Miller AH, Roth BA, Mills TJ: Ultrasound guidance versus landmark technique for the placement of central venous catheters in the emergency department. *Acad Emerg Med.* 2002;9:800.

Moore C, Promes SB: Ultrasound in pregnancy. *Emerg Med Clin N Am.* 2004;22:697.

Moore CL, Rose GA, Tayal VS, et al: Determination of left ventricular function by emergency physician echocardiography of hypotensive patients. *Acad Emerg Med.* 2002;9:186.

Noble VE, Brown DFM: Renal ultrasound. *Emerg Med Clin N Am.* 2004;22:641.

Plumer D, Brunelle D, Asinger R, et al: Emergency department echocardiography improves outcome in penetrating cardiac injury. *Ann Emerg Med.* 1992;21:709.

Ralls PW, Colletti PD, Lapin SA, et al: Real time sonography in suspected acute cholecystitis: prospective evaluation of primary and secondary signs. *Radiology.* 1985;155:767.

Rose JS: Ultrasound in abdominal trauma. *Emerg Med Clin N Am.* 2004;22:581.

Rosen CL, Brown DFM, Chang Y, et al: Ultrasonography by emergency physicians in patients with suspected cholecysitis. *Am J Emerg Med.* 2001;19:32.

Rosen CL, Brown DFM, Saganin MJ, et al: Ultrasonagraphy by emergency physicians in patients with suspected ureteral colic. *J Emerg Med,* 1998;16:865.

Rozycki GS, Ochsner MG, Schmidt JA, et al: A prospective study of surgeon-performed ultrasound as the primary adjuvant modality for injured patient assessment. *J Trauma.* 1995; 39:492.

Shah K, Wolfe RE: Hepatobiliary ultrasound. *Emerg Med Clin N Am.* 2004;22:661.

Tayal VS, Graf CD, Gibbs MA: Prospective study of accuracy and outcome of emergency ultrasound for abdominal aortic aneurysm over two years. *Acad Emerg Med.* 2003;10:867.

Thomas HA, Beeson MS, Binder MS: The 2005 model of the clinical practice of emergency medicine: The 2007 update. *Ann Emerg Med.* 2008;52:e1.

Tibbles CD, Porcaro W: Procedural applications of ultrasound. *Emerg Med Clin N Am.* 2004;22:797.

Chapter 23
HIGH YIELD WORD ASSOCIATION

Andrew Webber and Deven Unadkat

Formulas and Doses

Calculation of endotracheal tube (ET) size in children	1 year to 10 years
	$(Age/4) + 4$
ET tube insertion depth in children	$Age(years)/2 + 12$ or
	$3 \times ET$ tube size
Fifth percentile systolic blood pressure in children	$70 + (age$ in years $\times 2)$
Fractional excretion of Na	$(U_{Na} \times P_{Cr}) / (P_{Na} \times U_{Cr})$
	Where U = urine and P = plasma
Osmolar gap	Measured osmolarity – calculated osmolarity
Calculated osmolarity	$2(Na^+) + glucose/18 + BUN/2.8 + EtOH/4$
Winter formula for metabolic acidosis	Predicted $PaCO_2 = 1.5(HCO_3) + 8$
Parkland formula for fluid replacement	(4 mL) (kg) (% BSA of second/third-degree burns)
	Administer 50% over 8 hours and remainder over 16 hours
Alveolo-arterial (A-a) gradient	At sea level: $150 – (1.25 \times PCO_2) – PaO_2$
	Normal range is <10 to 20 mm Hg
Normal age adjusted A-a gradient	$(Age/4) + 4$
	(same as ET pediatric tube size)

Cardiology

Exertional syncope in elderly	Aortic stenosis
Narrow pulse pressure	Aortic stenosis or hypertrophic obstructive cardiomyopathy (HOCM)
Wide pulse pressure	Aortic regurgitation or patent ductus arteriosus
Maneuvers to increase the murmur of HOCM	Valsalva
	Standing after squatting
Maneuvers to decrease the murmur of HOCM	Passive leg raise
	Hand grip
	Squatting
Machine-like murmur	Air embolus or patent ductus arteriosus
Chest pain with neurologic symptoms	Consider aortic dissection
Right ventricular (RV) or right atrial (RA) diastolic collapse on echo	Cardiac tamponade
Endocarditis	Osler nodes: painful nodes on pulp of fingers/toes
	"Sir William Osler could beat you to a pulp"
	Janeway lesions: painless
	"Little Jane couldn't hurt you"
	Roth spots: retinal hemorrhage
	"rOth for central clearing"
Tissue plasminogen activator (t-PA) reversal	Aminocaproic acid and cryoprecipitate
Torsade de pointes treatment	Magnesium, isoproterenol, and overdrive pacing
Rapid wide complex atrial fibrillation	Think Wolf-Parkinson-White syndrome

(Continued)

Cardiology (Cont.)

Regularized atrial fibrillation	Digoxin toxicity
Bidirectional ventricular tachycardia	Digoxin toxicity
Thromboxane A_2 production inhibitor	Aspirin
Irreversible adenosine diphosphate receptor (P2Y12) blockade	Plavix
Treatment of hyperkalemia with digitalis usage	Avoid calcium administration

Dermatology

Herald patch	Pityriasis rosea
Rash and joint pain in young female	Lupus or gonorrhea
Dew drop rash on a rose petal	Varicella
Honey-crusted lesions	Staphylococcus impetigo
Lice found on child's eyelashes	Consider sexual abuse. Louse infection of eyelashes indicates pubic lice, not head lice
Centripetal rash	Rocky Mountain spotted fever, varicella
Centrifugal rash	Smallpox (variola)
Medications that cause erythema multiforme	"Washing skin with SOAPS"
	Sulfa drugs
	Oral hypoglycemics
	Anticonvulsants
	PCN
	NSAIDS
	Mycoplasma and herpes as well
Erythema nodosum	Red, tender anterior tibial nodules (panniculitis)
	Oral contraception
	Sulfonamides
	Ebstein-Barr virus
	Mycoplasma
	Sarcoid, tuberculosis
	Inflammatory bowel disease
	Cancer
Erythema marginatum	Rheumatic fever
Erythema migrans (erythema chronicum migrans)	Lyme disease
Rash in Christmas tree pattern	Pityriasis rosea
Hyperpigmentation and abdominal pain	Adrenal insufficiency
Nikolsky sign	Skin separates with minimal pressure
	Staphylococcal scalded skin syndrome (SSSS) and toxic epidermal necrosis (TEN)
Hypersensitivity reaction types	
Type I	Anaphylaxis
Type II	Transfusion reactions
Type III	Serum sickness and joint pain (Arthus reaction)
Type IV	PPD

Gastrointestinal

Bird beak sign on barium swallow	Achalasia
A-P CXR shows coin in frontal plane	Coin in esophagus
A-P CXR shows coin in sagittal plane	Coin in trachea
Treatment for refractory hiccups	Thorazine (chlorpromazine)
Treatment for food impaction	Glucagon, nifedipine
Most common cause of surgical abdomen in elderly	Biliary colic
Most common cause of small bowel obstruction	Adhesions (followed by incarcerated hernia)
Most common cause of colonic obstruction	Cancer, diverticulitis, and volvulus (in descending order)
Abdominal pain with atrial fibrillation	Mesenteric ischemia

Abdominal distension in marathon runner	Cecal volvulus
Pediatric rectal prolapse	Think cystic fibrosis
Diarrhea and seizures	*Shigella*
Diarrhea and Guillain-Barré syndrome	*Campylobacter*
Diarrhea and shellfish	*Vibrio parahaemolyticus*
Diarrhea and right lower quadrant (RLQ) pain	*Yersinia*
Diarrhea and clindamycin	*C. difficile*
Diarrhea and imported turtles	*Salmonella*
Diarrhea after camping trip	*Giardia*
Diarrhea and fried rice	*Bacillus cereus*
Explosive diarrhea	*Giardia*
Hemolytic uremic syndrome	*E. coli* 0157:H7
Hot-cold sensation reversal and diarrhea	Ciguatera toxin
Peppery-tasting fish	Scombroid toxicity
Pain out of proportion to examination	Mesenteric ischemia
Most common cause of upper gastrointestinal (GI) bleed	Peptic ulcer disease
Rectal bleeding in patient with abdominal aortic aneurysm (AAA) repair	Rule out aortoenteric fistula
Hamman crunch	Pneumomediastinitis

Head, Ears, Eyes, Nose, and Throat (HEENT)

Age at which permanent teeth erupt	Central incisors start to erupt at 6 years
Most common site of sialoadenitis	Submandibular gland (Wharton duct)
Otitis externa in diabetic patient	Rule out malignant otitis externa
Bullous myringitis	Mycoplasma
Anterior nosebleed	Kesselbach plexus or Little area
Posterior nosebleed artery	Sphenopalatine artery
Rheumatoid arthritis and stridor	Stuck arytenoids
Brawny edema	Ludwig angina
Cri de canard (duck cry)	Retropharyngeal abscess
Thumbprint sign	Epiglottitis
Hutchinson sign	Herpes zoster
Cobblestone papillae on upper lid	Allergic conjunctivitis
Conjunctivitis and contact lens	*Pseudomonas*
Dendrites on fluorescein eye exam	Herpes simplex
Teardrop pupil	Globe rupture
Seidel sign	Globe rupture
Hammering metal	Globe rupture
Boxcar vessels	Central retina artery occlusion or temporal arteritis
Cherry red spot	Central retinal artery occlusion
Blood and thunder retina	Central retinal vein occlusion
Floaters, flashing lights, or descending curtains	Retinal detachment
Skier or welder sign with eye pain	Ultraviolet keratitis
Upper lid anesthesia	Supraorbital block
Lower lid anesthesia	Infraorbital block
Lower lip anesthesia	Mental block
Meibomian gland infection	Internal hordeolum
Zoll or Zeis gland infection	External hordeolum
Gingival hyperplasia	Phenytoin, leukemia

Infectious Disease

Home canning	Food botulism
Floppy baby	Infant botulism
Bilateral adrenal hemorrhage	Waterhouse-Friderichsen syndrome and meningoccocemia
Armadillos, cats, and prairie dogs	Bubonic plague

(Continued)

Infectious Disease (Cont.)

Dog bite	Powerful jaws crush—rule out fractures
Cat bite	Pasteurella—puncture wounds
Human bite	*Eikinella corrodens*
Nail puncture through sneakers	*Pseudomonas*
Black water fever	Hemolysis from malaria or babesiosis
Fever and travel	Consider malaria
Multinucleated giant cells	Herpes simplex
Antibiotic that causes orange discoloration of body fluids	Rifampin
Rubella	German measles
	Lymphadenopathy
	Forscheimer spots
Rubeola	Measles
	Koplik spots
Roseola	Rash after defervesence
Painful genital lesion	Herpes simplex
Painless genital lesion	Syphilis, granuloma inguinale
Groove sign	Lymphogranuloma venereum (*Chlamydia trachomatis*)
Antibiotic most associated with oral contraception failure	Rifampin
Rose thorn infection	Sporotrichosis
Transplant patient infection	Cytomegalovirus (CMV)
Marked low glucose levels on cerebrospinal fluid analysis	Tuberculous meningitis

Neurology

Lucid interval after head injury	Epidural hematoma
Sundown eyes—patient unable to look up	Ventricular peritoneal shunt obstruction
Hypotension, hypothermia, bradycardia	Neurogenic shock
Wacky, wobbly, and wet	Normal pressure hydrocephalus
Anterior cord syndrome	Motor weakness, pain/temperature loss below lesion
	Proprioception and vibration intact
Central cord syndrome	Upper >lower extremity weakness
Brown-Sequard syndrome	Ipsilateral weakness and loss of proprioception and vibration. Contralateral pain and temperature loss "If a brown bear bites off half your spine, you can still hop away on contralateral leg because proprioception and strength intact. You can hop away on bare foot since you feel no pain."
Hypertension, bradycardia, and respiratory disturbance	Cushing syndrome and increased intracranial pressure
Urinary retention and back pain	Cauda equina syndrome
Early morning headache	Mass/cancer
Headache in an elderly female	Temporal arteritis
Most common cause of seizure in elderly	Stroke
Most common cause of seizures worldwide	Cysticercosis
Bilateral Bell palsy	Lyme disease, mononucleosis, Guillain-Barré syndrome
Obese female on oral contraception, vitamin A, and minocycline for acne	Pseudotumor cerebri
Diplopia with lateral gaze	Intranuclear ophthalmoplegia associated with multiple sclerosis
Ptosis worse in the evening	Myasthenia gravis
Eaton-Lambert syndrome	Myasthenia-like syndrome associated with lung cancer. Unlike myasthenia, repetitive use increases strength
Ascending weakness	Guillain-Barré syndrome
	Tick paralysis
	Diphtheria
Descending weakness	Botulism
	Myasthenia gravis
	Miller Fisher variant of Guillain-Barré syndrome
	Eaton-Lambert syndrome
Amyotrophic lateral sclerosis	Motor function loss (sensation intact)
Port wine stain and seizures	Sturge-Weber syndrome

Obstetrics and Gynecology

Fetal heartbeat first seen on transvaginal ultrasound	6 weeks' gestation
Fetal heartbeat first seen on transabdominal ultrasound	8 weeks' gestation
Uterus becomes an intraabdominal organ	12 weeks' gestation
Uterine fundus at the umbilicus	20 weeks' gestation
Snowstorm imaged on sonogram and high β-hCG	Molar pregnancy
Persistent hyperemesis gravidarum	Molar pregnancy
Preeclampsia <20 weeks' gestation	Molar pregnancy
Painless third trimester vaginal bleeding	Placenta previa
Painful third trimester vaginal bleeding	Placenta abruptio
Fern, pool, or nitrazine test	(+) presence of amniotic fluid
Most common cause of postpartum bleeding	Uterine atony
Vaginal bleeding in newborn	**Not** child abuse. Due to withdrawal of maternal estrogen in fetal circulation causing endometrial sloughing
Erythromycin estolate in pregnancy	Hepatotoxic to mother
Fetus is most vulnerable to radiation	During 8 to 15 weeks' gestation
Acceptable radiation during pregnancy	5 to 10 rads
Vaginal bleeding in postmenopausal female	Rule out endometrial cancer
Prolapsed cord treatment	Requires emergent cesarean section
	Elevate presenting part
	Knee to chest position
	Arrest delivery
Nuchal cord treatment	Untangle cord around presenting part
	May clamp and sever if nonpulsating
Fitz-Hugh-Curtis syndrome	Perihepatitis in the setting of pelvic inflammatory disease (PID)
Violin string on laparoscopy or ultrasound	PID
Antibiotics and vaginal discharge	Candidiasis
White cottage cheese vaginal discharge	Candidiasis
Thin, green-gray, malodorous, frothy vaginal discharge	Trichomoniasis
Strawberry cervix	Trichomoniasis
Thin gray-white vaginal discharge	Bacterial vaginosis
Positive whiff test	Bacterial vaginosis
Clue cells	Bacterial vaginosis

Orthopedics

Jefferson fracture	C1 fracture (unstable)
Hangman fracture	C2 pedicle fracture (unstable)
Clay-shoveler fracture	Fracture of the C7 spinous process
Teardrop fracture	Fracture of anterior spinal body
Unstable cervical spine fractures	"Jefferson bit off a hangman's thumb
	Jefferson fracture
	Bilateral facet dislocation
	Odontoid type II and type III fractures
	Any fracture dislocation
	Hangman fracture
	Teardrop fracture
C1 on C2 subluxation	Rheumatoid arthritis and ankylosing spondylitis
Priapism after cervical spine injury	C5 fracture
Bennett fracture	Fracture of base of first metacarpal
Boxer fracture	Fracture of neck of fifth metacarpal
Laceration over metacarpophalangeal joint	Rule out "fight bite"
	Consider admission for antibiotics
Swan neck deformity	Flexed distal interphalangeal (DIP) and hyperextended posterior interphalangeal (PIP) joints
Boutonnière deformity	Hyperextended DIP and flexed PIP joints (Opposite of swan neck deformity)
Jammed finger playing basketball	Mallet finger

(Continued)

Orthopedics (Cont.)

Terry Thomas sign	Scapholunate dissociation
Signet ring sign	Scapholunate dissociation
Pizza pie sign	Lunate dislocation
Spilled teacup sign	Lunate dislocation
Smith fracture	Reverse Colles or reverse dinner fork deformity
	Distal radius fracture with volar displacement
Galeazzi fracture	Fracture of distal radius with disruption of radioulnar joint
Monteggia fracture	Fracture of proximal one-third of ulna with dislocation of radial head
Chauffeur or Hutchinson fracture	Radial styloid fracture
Nerve injury from mid/distal humerus fracture	Radial nerve
Nerve injury from proximal humerus fracture	Axillary nerve
Nerve injury and shoulder dislocation	Axillary (deltoid sensation) and musculocutaneous nerve (dorsal forearm sensation)
Vascular injury associated with supracondylar fractures of the elbow	Brachial artery
Chance fracture	Transverse fracture of vertebral body associated with blunt bowel injury
Jones fracture	Fracture of base of fifth metatarsal distal to proximal tuberosity
Pseudo-Jones fracture	Base of fifth metatarsal fractures at proximal tuberosity
Gamekeeper fracture	Ulnar collateral ligament of thumb
Lisfranc fracture	Fracture at base of second metatarsal
Bohler angle	Angle of 28 to 40 degrees normal
	Assess for calcaneal fracture
Nerve and artery injured with knee dislocations	Peroneal nerve and popliteal artery
Unhappy triad in knee	Anterior collateral and medial collateral ligament, and medial meniscus injury
Calcaneal fracture	Rule out lumbar fracture
Back pain in cancer patient	Consider radiation therapy
Needle-shaped negative birefringence	Gout—urate crystals
Rhomboid-shaped positive birefringence	Pseudogout—calcium crystals

Pediatrics

Bleeding baby after home delivery	Consider vitamin K deficiency
Pseudosubluxation of C1 on C2	Spinolaminal line of C2 should be within 1 mm of line drawn between spinolaminal lines of C1 and C3
Bucket handle fracture, posterior rib fractures	Child abuse
Stridor worse with crying	Laryngomalacia
Age cut off for cricothyroidotomy	Contraindicated <8 years
Unilateral purulent nasal discharge	Rule out foreign body
Perioral burn after biting electrical cord	Dealyed labial artery bleeding in 7 to 10 days
Age at which the frontal sinuses develop	Forms at 2 years but not fully developed until 15 years
Neonatal conjunctivitis in the first day of life	Chemical conjunctivitis
Neonatal conjunctivitis in 2 weeks	*Chlamydia*
Hypochloremic metabolic alkalosis	Pyloric stenosis
Bilious vomiting in **first week** of life	Malrotation
NON-bilious vomiting **first month** of life	Pyloric stenosis
Bilious vomiting **first year** of life	Intussusception
Double bubble sign	Consider malrotation/midgut volvulus or duodenal atresia
Currant jelly stools	Intussusception
Corkscrew appearance on abdominal x-ray	Malrotation/midgut volvulus
Cyanosis in week 1 of life	Transposition of the great vessels
Decreased lower extremity pulses	Aortic coarctation
Tetralogy of Fallot	Ventricular septal defect, overriding aorta, pulmonic stenosis (R to L shunt), and right ventricular hypertrophy

Age group to avoid verapamil	<2 years (can cause hypotension and asystole)
Sepsis in the neonate (organisms)	Group B streptococci and *E. coli*
Infectious etiology of croup	Parainfluenza virus
Infectious etiology of bronchiolitis	Respiratory syncytial virus
Shaggy right heart border	Pertussis pneumonia
Lice in children	Do **not** treat with lindane (will cause seizures); use permethrin
Unconscious child morning after New Year's Eve party	Hypoglycemia. Toddler drank left over alcohol from guests

Pulmonary

Kussmaul breathing	Deep respirations secondary to metabolic acidosis classically associated with diabetic ketoacidosis
Pleural-based wedge infarct	Hampton hump (classic for pulmonary embolism [PE] but uncommonly seen)
Vascular cut-off sign	Westermark sign (classic for PE, uncommon)
ECG-finding associated with PE	S1Q3T3 (nonspecific)
Treatment for fat embolus	Steroids (no heparin)
Patient positioning with suspected air embolus	Left lateral decubitus and Trendelenburg (not evidence-based)
Bat wing pattern on CXR	*Pneumocystis* pneumonia (PCP)
When to administer steroids with PCP	$PaO_2 <70$
Safest narcotic for asthmatics	Fentanyl (no histamine release)
Albuterol mechanism	Increases adenylate cyclase to increase cAMP
Currant jelly sputum, alcoholism, bulging fissure	*Klebsiella*
Pneumonia and herpes labialis	*Klebsiella*
Postinfluenza pneumonia	*Staphylococcus*
Staccato cough	*Chlamydia* pneumonia
Pneumonia and cystic fibrosis	*Pseudomonas*
Nursing home resident and cyanosis	*Pseudomonas*
CXR looks worse than patient	*Mycoplasma*
Pneumonia with marked lymphocytosis and shaggy heart border on CXR	*Pertussis*
Cough and widened mediastinum	Pulmonary anthrax
Pneumonia after air travel	*Legionella*
Gram+ paired lancets (diplococci)	*Streptococcus pneumoniae*
Gram+ cocci in clusters	*Staphylococcus aureus*
Small Gram– pleomorphic coccobacilli	*Haemophilus influenza*
Gram– diplococci	*Neisseria meningitides*
Mononuclear cells, no bacteria	*Mycoplasma* (can also see in *Legionella*)
Cavitary lesions on CXR	Tuberculosis or *S. aureus*

Renal/Genitourinary/Electrolytes

Red blood cell (RBC) casts	Glomerulonephritis
Urine+ for blood, but urine– for RBCs	Rhabdomyolysis
Urethritis, iritis, and arthritis	Reiter syndrome
Recurrent balanoposthesis	Rule out diabetes
Renal colic in elderly	Rule out abdominal aortic aneurysm first
Acute renal failure	Rule out bilateral hydronephrosis with ultrasound
Diabetic with perineal rash	Fournier gangrene
Hypermagnesemia	Treat with calcium
Tumor lysis syndrome	Hyperkalemia, hyperuricemia, and hypocalcemia
Nonanion gap acidosis	(**HARDUP**)
	Hyperalimentation/**H**yperventilation
	Acetazolamide
	Renal tubular acidosis
	Diarrhea
	Ureteral diversion
	Pancreatic fistula/**P**arenteral saline

Toxicology and Environmental Emergencies

Smells like ...

Garlic	Organophosphates
Bitter almonds	Cyanide
Pear	Chloral hydrate
Rotten eggs	Hydrogen sulfide
Teen spirit	Nirvana
Moth balls	Naphthalene or Camphor
Wintergreen	Salicylate

Pulse oximetry in ...

Carbon monoxide poisoning	Falsely normal or elevated pulse oximetry
Methemoglobinemia	Pulse oximetry in high 80's
Causes of methemoglobinemia	Dapsone, nitrates, antimalarials, and local anesthetics
G6PD triggers	Bactrim, pyridium, chloroquine, nitrofurantoin, and fava beans
Pinpoint pupils	**POCO**
	Pontine bleed
	Opioids
	Clonidine
	Organophosphates
Maximum dose of lidocaine	5 mg/kg without epinephrine
	7 mg/kg with epinephrine
COPD and intractable seizures	Think theophylline toxicity
Osmolar gap without acidosis	Isopropyl alcohol
Toxins cleared by hemodialysis	**I STUMBLE**
	Isopropyl alcohol
	Salicylate
	Theophylline
	Uremia
	Methanol
	Barbiturates/**B**eta-blockers
	Lithium
	Ethylene glycol
Anesthesiologist altered with negative toxicology screen	Fentanyl
Opioid presenting with dilated pupils	Meperidine (Demerol)
Tinnitus	Salicylates
Found down in industrial fire	Cyanide
Snowstorm vision	Methanol
Tetanus mimicker	Strychnine
Headache in winter	Carbon monoxide
Wrist drop	Lead poisoning
Maltese crosses in urine	Ethylene glycol
Bilateral ischemic basal ganglia strokes	Carbon monoxide poisoning
Bilateral basal ganglia hemorrhage	Methanol intoxication
Vision disturbance—yellow halos	Digoxin toxicity
Wintergreen and Pepto-Bismol	Salicylates
Glass etcher, rust remover, metal cleaner	Hydrofluoric acid
Toxins causing hypoglycemia	EtOH and salicylates
Bullae	Barbiturate overdose
Mixed acid base disturbance	Aspirin toxicity
Bruxism	Ecstasy (MDMA)
Found down in airport	Drug mule/body packer
Rotary nystagmus	PCP
Toxicities treated with serum alkalinization	Salicylate and tricyclic overdoses
Treatment for serotonin syndrome	Benzodiazepines
	Cyproheptadine
Treatment for Lomotil overdose	Naloxone
Antidote for organophosphates	Pralidoxime chloride
Antidote for INH seizures	Pyridoxine
Indications for Digibind	Life-threatening ventricular dysrhythmias
	Bradycardia unresponsive to conventional treatment
	Hyperkalemia >5

Symptoms 6 hours after ingestion of mushroom	Worse prognosis
	Usually amatoxin or *Gyromitra*
Anaphylaxis resistant to epinephrine	Glucagon if patient on β-blockers
Spider bite and abdominal pain	Black widow spider
Wake up to find bat in room	Administer rabies immunization
Bite by spider after lifting a log	Brown recluse spider
Necrotic spider bite	Brown recluse spider
Hourglass shape on spider	Black widow spider
	"It's only a matter of time before she gets you"
Violin shape on spider	Brown recluse spider
	"Lonely spider playing sad violin music"
Coral snake bite victims	Administer antivenin even without symptoms
Coral snakes that are poisonous	When the red and yellow rings touch
	"Red on yellow kill a fellow, red on black venom lack" (applies only to North American coral spiders)
Machine oil urine	Hyperthermia
High-altitude illness and sulfa allergy	**No** acetazolamide
Ferning pattern	Think lightning strike
Unconscious patient pulled from water	Cervical spine precautions

Trauma

Most common intra-abdominal injury in blunt trauma	Spleen
Most common solid organ injury in penetrating trauma	Liver
Most commonly injured cardiac chamber with penetrating trauma	Right ventricle
Covering sucking chest wounds	Tape only 3 sides of the occlusive dressing
Blunt diaphragmatic rupture associated with which other injury	Thoracic aorta rupture
Bicycle handlebar injury	Duodenal hematoma or isolated pancreatic injury
Lap belt sign	Intestinal or mesenteric injury with lumbar spine fracture
Positive diagnostic peritoneal lavage (DPL)	Immediate return of >10 cc blood
	>100,000 RBCs
Saphenous vein cut down location	2 cm anterior and superior to medial malleolus
Battle sign	Ecchymosis behind ear suspicious for basilar skull fracture

Psychiatric and Behavioral

Hypoglycemia with normal or low serum c-peptide	Malingering (self-administration of insulin)
Anorexia and electrolyte disturbance	Hypokalemia
Schizoid versus avoidant personality disorder	Schizoid does not want friends
	Avoidant wants friends but afraid of rejection

Chapter 24
VISUAL SIMULATION

Adam J. Rosh, Corey Long, Michael Cassura, and Aaron Dora-Laskey

Section Editor: David T. Schwartz

QUESTIONS

1. A 54-year-old woman presents to the ED with a complaint of headache after a fall backwards from a bar stool and hitting her head on the ground the previous evening. On examination, you note blood in her right ear canal and an area of ecchymosis as shown (Figure 24–1, see color insert section). Which of the following is the most likely diagnosis?
   A. Le Fort fracture
   B. Basilar skull fracture
   C. Otitis interna
   D. Otitis externa
   E. Tripod fracture

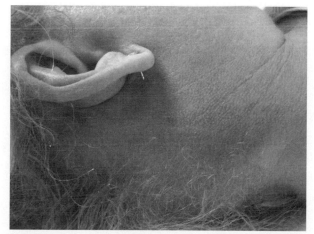

FIGURE 24–1. *(Courtesy of Adam Rosh, MD.)*

2. A 29-year-old woman presents to the ED with a complaint of sudden onset of left facial weakness that was noticed by her coworker. She denies fever, rash, or any other symptoms. On physical examination, she has no other neurologic deficits other than what is shown (Figure 24–2). When asked to shut her left eye, she cannot. Which of the following is the most likely diagnosis?
   A. Bell palsy
   B. Malingering
   C. Ramsay Hunt syndrome
   D. Brain tumor
   E. Cerebrovascular event

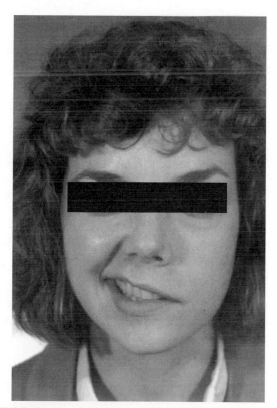

FIGURE 24–2. (Reproduced, with permission, from Lalwani AK: *Current Otolaryngology Head and Neck Surgery,* 2nd ed. Copyright © 2008, New York: McGraw-Hill.)

3. A 33-year-old chef presents to the ED with a complaint of a deformity in his finger. He states that a few weeks ago he sustained a deep laceration over the dorsum of his finger but never sought medical attention for it. On examination, the wound is well-healed, but there is an obvious deformity as shown (Figure 24–3). Which of the following is the most likely diagnosis?
   A. Swan-neck deformity
   B. Boutonniere deformity
   C. Bell-clapper deformity
   D. Mallet finger deformity
   E. Congenital deformity

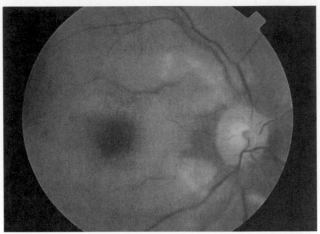

FIGURE 24–4. (Reproduced, with permission, from Tintanalli JE, Kelen GD, Stapczynski JS: *Tintinalli's Emergency Medicine: A Comprehensive Study Guide*, 6th ed. Copyright © 2004, New York: McGraw-Hill.)

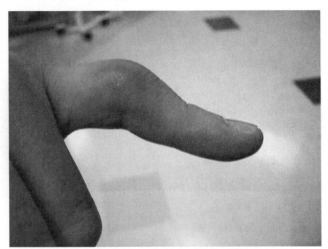

FIGURE 24–3. (*Courtesy of Adam Rosh, MD.*)

5. A 75-year-old man presents to the ED with a complaint of acute-onset vision loss in his right eye. He denies pain. The fundoscopic examination is shown (Figure 24–5, see color insert section). Which of the following is the most appropriate next step in the management of this patient?
   A. Topical β-blocker and acetalzolamide
   B. Ocular massage
   C. Urgent ophthalmic consultation
   D. Steroid injection
   E. Head CT scan and neurology consultation

4. A 71-year-old man presents with a history of diabetes and atrial fibrillation presents with loss of vision in his left eye since he awoke 6 hours ago. On physical examination of the left eye, vision is limited to counting fingers. The fundoscopic examination is shown (Figure 24–4, see color insert section). Which of the following is the most likely diagnosis?
   A. Retinal detachment
   B. Central retinal artery occlusion
   C. Central retinal vein occlusion
   D. Vitreous hemorrhage
   E. Acute angle closure glaucoma

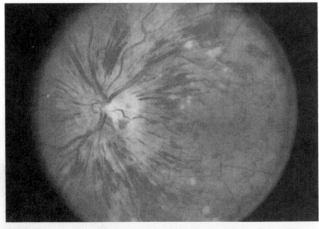

FIGURE 24–5. (Reproduced, with permission, from Knoop KJ, Stack LB, Storrow AB: *An Atlas of Emergency Medicine*, 2nd ed. Copyright © 2002, New York: McGraw-Hill.)

6. A 24-year-old man presents to the ED with a complaint of a rash that developed over the past day. He also complains of pain in his knee, ankle, and wrist. On physical examination his temperature is 100.6°F. You note the rash as shown (Figure 24–6, see color insert section). The lesions are located on his distal extremities. Which of the following organisms is most likely responsible for this patient's presentation?
   A. *Rickettsia rickettsii*
   B. *Treponema pallidum*
   C. *Borrelia burgdorferi*
   D. *Neisseria gonorrhoeae*
   E. *Neisseria meningitidis*

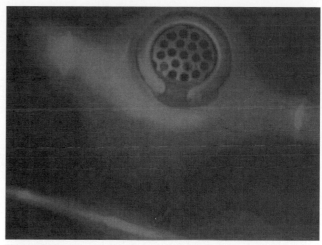

FIGURE 24–7. (*Courtesy of Adam Rosh, MD.*)

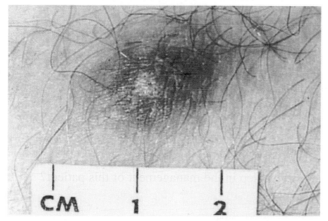

FIGURE 24–6. (Reproduced, with permission, from Kasper DL, Braunwald E, Fauci AS, et al: *Harrison's Principles of Internal Medicine,* 16th ed. Copyright © 2005, New York: McGraw-Hill.)

7. A 31-year-old man is brought to the ED by EMS who states that the man was found lying on the floor of his garage. He is arousable in the ED, speaks with slurred speech, and vomits. Laboratory results reveal serum sodium 139 mEq/L, potassium 3.5 mEq/L, chloride 101 mEq/L, bicarbonate 14 mEq/L, BUN 15 mg/dL, creatinine 1 mg/dL, glucose 105 mg/dL, arterial blood pH 7.27, COHb 4%, and lactate 2.8 mEq/L. Urinalysis shows: 1+ protein, trace ketones, WBC 4/HPF, RBC 2 to 3/HPF, and multiple envelope-shaped and needle-shaped crystals. His urine is placed under a Wood lamp as shown (Figure 24–7, see color insert section). Which of the following conditions would best explain his presentation?
   A. Carbon monoxide poisoning
   B. Ethylene glycol poisoning
   C. Diabetic ketoacidosis
   D. Lactic acidosis
   E. Uremia

8. A 27-year-old man presents to the ED with a rash for 1 week after a trip to Thailand. The rash is shown (Figure 24–8, see color insert section). He denies fever or chills, and states the rash is pruritic. The rash is isolated to his trunk and does not involve the palms, soles, mucous membranes, or genitalia. The most important initial step in management for this patient is
   A. Reassure and discharge home
   B. Send screening serology for syphilis
   C. Steroids
   D. KOH preparation
   E. Antihistamine

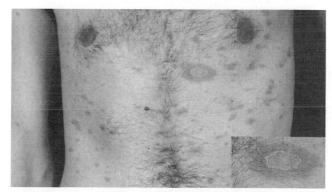

FIGURE 24–8. (Reproduced, with permission, from Wolff K, Johnson RA, Suurmond D: *Fitzpatrick's Color Atlas and Synopsis of Clinical Dermatology,* 5th ed. Copyright © 2005, New York: McGraw-Hill.)

9. A 60-year-old man presents to the ED with a headache and eye pain that is associated with nausea and vomiting. His left eye is shown (Figure 24–9, see color insert section). The pupil is middilated and nonreactive. Which of the following is the most appropriate next step in management?
   A. Administer hydromorphone
   B. Head CT scan
   C. Check intraocular pressure
   D. Check erythrocyte sedimentation rate
   E. Discharge patient

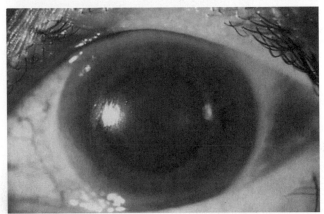

FIGURE 24–9. (Reproduced, with permission, from Knoop KJ, Stack LB, Storrow AB:*An Atlas of Emergency Medicine*, 2nd ed. Copyright © 2002, New York: McGraw-Hill.)

10. A 26-year-old man presents to the ED with a complaint of dysuria for 3 days. He is currently sexually active and uses a condom most of the time. He denies hematuria but notes a yellowish discharge from his urethra as shown (Figure 24–10). You send a clean catch urinalysis to the laboratory that returns positive for leukocyte esterase and 22 WBCs/HPF. Which of the following is the most appropriate next step in management?
   A. Send a urethral swab for culture and administer 125 mg ceftriaxone intramuscularly and 1 g azithromycin orally
   B. Send urine for culture and administer trimethoprim/sulfamethoxazole orally
   C. Discharge the patient with strict instructions to return if his symptoms worsen
   D. Order a CT scan to evaluate for a kidney stone
   E. Have him follow up immediately with a urologist to evaluate for testicular cancer

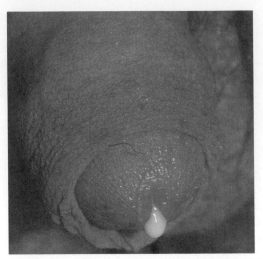

FIGURE 24–10. (Reproduced, with permission, from Wolff K, Johnson RA, Suurmond D: *Fitzpatrick's Color Atlas and Synopsis of Clinical Dermatology,* 5th ed. Copyright © 2005, New York; McGraw-Hill.)

11. A 50-year-old woman presents to the ED with complaints of pain in her right eye and burning sensation over half of her forehead and scalp. On physical examination, you note the rash as shown (Figure 24–11, see color insert section). Which of the following is the most concerning complication of this patient's clinical presentation?
   A. Central nervous system (CNS) involvement leading to meningitis
   B. Ophthalmic involvement leading to anterior uveitis or corneal scarring
   C. Cardiac involvement leading to endocarditis
   D. Permanent scarring of her face
   E. Nasopalantine involvement leading to epistaxis

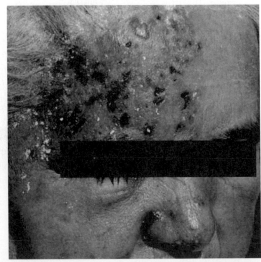

FIGURE 24–11. (Reproduced, with permission, from Wolff K, Johnson RA, Suurmond D: *Fitzpatrick's Color Atlas and Synopsis of Clinical Dermatology,* 5th ed. Copyright © 2005, New York: McGraw-Hill.)

12. A 50-year-old woman presents to the ED with complaints of fever, sore throat, and neck pain for 24 hours. She states that 1 week ago she had 2 molars extracted from her mouth. Her blood pressure is 145/75 mm Hg, heart rate is 102 beats per minute, and temperature is 101.2°F. On examination you notice that the patient is drooling. There is erythema and swelling of her submandibular area as shown (Figure 24–12). Her tongue is swollen and elevated and the floor of her mouth is tender. There is no fluctuant mass in her mouth. Which of the following is the most likely diagnosis?

A. Acute mastoiditis
B. Peritonsillar abscess
C. Ludwig angina
D. Acute necrotizing ulcerative gingivitis (ANUG)
E. *Streptococcus* pharyngitis

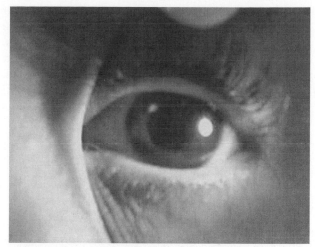

FIGURE 24–13. (*Courtesy of Ami Dave, MD.*)

14. A 32-year-old woman presents to the ED with a complaint of painful lesions as shown (Figure 24–14, see color insert section). Which of the following is the LEAST LIKELY cause of her symptoms?

A. Ulcerative colitis
B. Crohn disease
C. Syphilis
D. Oral contraceptives
E. Pregnancy

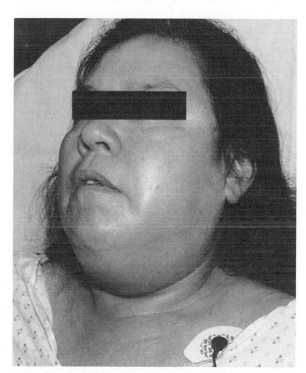

FIGURE 24–12. (Reproduced, with permission, from Knoop KJ, Stack LB, Storrow AB: *An Atlas of Emergency Medicine*, 2nd ed. Copyright © 2002, New York: McGraw-Hill.)

13. A 67-year-old man with a history of atrial fibrillation presents to the ED with a complaint of eye pain after a statue fell off a shelf and hit him in the eye. His eye is shown (Figure 24–13, see color insert section). Which of the following is the most likely diagnosis?

A. Acute glaucoma
B. Globe rupture
C. Hordeolum
D. Hyphema
E. Hypopyon

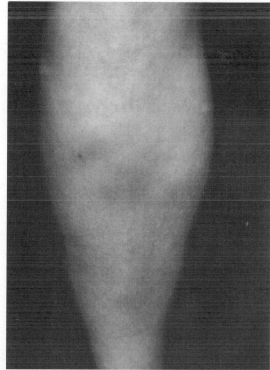

FIGURE 24–14. (Reproduced, with permission, from Wolff K, Johnson RA, Suurmond D: *Fitzpatrick's Color Atlas and Synopsis of Clinical Dermatology*, 5th ed. Copyright © 2005, New York: McGraw-Hill.)

15. A 48-year-old man with a past medical history for hepatitis C and cirrhosis presents to the ED with a complaint of acute onset abdominal pain and chills. You decide to perform a paracentesis as shown (Figure 24–15). You retrieve 1 L of cloudy fluid. Laboratory analysis of the fluid shows a neutrophil count of 550 cells/mm^3. Which of the following is the most appropriate choice of treatment?
    A. Metronidazole
    B. Vancomycin
    C. Discharge home
    D. Neomycin and lactulose
    E. Cefotaxime

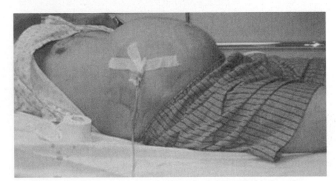

FIGURE 24–15. *(Courtesy of Adam Rosh, MD.)*

16. A 22-year-old college student is brought to the ED by his friends who state they found the patient unresponsive in his bed. Over the past 2 days, the patient complained of high fever, chills, and headache. On physical examination, you note the rash as shown (Figure 24–16, see color insert section). Which of the following is the most likely diagnosis?
    A. Idiopathic thrombocytopenic purpura
    B. Thrombotic thrombocytopenic purpura
    C. Henoch-Schönlein purpura
    D. Meningococcemia
    E. Rocky Mountain spotted fever

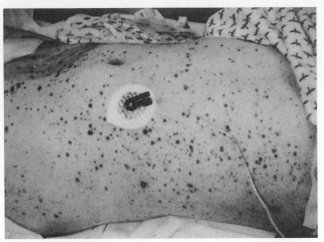

FIGURE 24–16. (Reproduced, with permission, from Knoop KJ, Stack LB, Storrow AB: *An Atlas of Emergency Medicine*, 2nd ed. Copyright © 2002, New York: McGraw-Hill.)

17. A 33-year-old construction worker presents with a complaint of pain over his elbow. The swelling as shown developed over a few days (Figure 24–17). On examination, he is afebrile and has full range of motion without pain. Which of the following is the most likely diagnosis?
    A. Gouty arthritis
    B. Fracture of the olecranon process
    C. Olecranon bursitis
    D. Septic arthritis
    E. Tumor

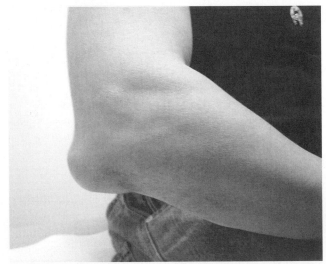

FIGURE 24–17. *(Courtesy of Adam Rosh, MD.)*

18. A 21-year-old man on the college swim team presents with a complaints of right ear pain, pruritis, and discharge. His temperature is 101°F. He withdraws when you retract the pinna of his ear. The external ear is shown (Figure 24–18, see color insert section). Otoscopic examination reveals an edematous, erythematous external auditory canal. Which of the following is the most common organism that causes his diagnosis?

A. *Streptococcus pneumoniae*
B. *Pseudomonas aeruginosa*
C. nontypeable *Haemophilus influenzae*
D. *Moraxella catarrhalis*
E. *Escherichia coli*

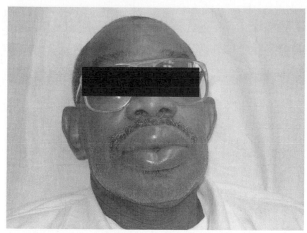

FIGURE 24–19. (*Courtesy of Ami Dave, MD.*)

20. A 33-year-old woman presents to the ED with a complaint of a generalized headache over the last 2 months. She has seen many doctors for it but has yet to get a correct diagnosis. She describes the headache as moderate in intensity and worse with eye movement. She is scared because her vision gets blurry for a few minutes everyday. Her blood pressure, 140/75 mm Hg; heart rate, 75 beats per minute; temperature, 98.9°F; and respiratory rate, 16 breaths per minute. On fundoscopic examination, you see the image as shown (Figure 24–20, see color insert section). Which of the following is the most appropriate next step in management?

A. Call a neurosurgeon for immediate surgery
B. Administer 2 g of ceftriaxone, and place her in isolation
C. Order an MRI to look for a carotid artery dissection
D. Tell her she probably has a migraine and prescribe her a triptan
E. Perform a CT scan and if negative perform a lumbar puncture specifically to measure the opening pressure

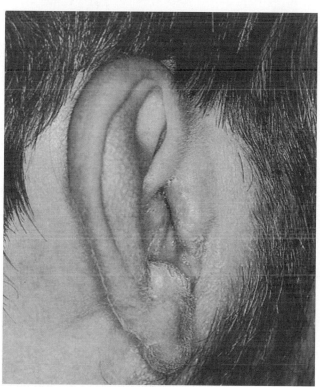

FIGURE 24–18. (*Courtesy of Frank Birinyi, MD.*)

19. Which of the following is most helpful in the treatment of the patient with C1 esterase inhibitor deficiency who presents to the ED with the findings as shown (Figure 24–19)?

A. Acetazolamide
B. Cryoprecipitate
C. Factor VIII
D. Fresh frozen plasma
E. Platelets

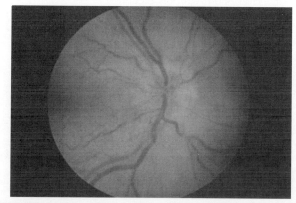

FIGURE 24–20. (Reproduced, with permission, from Knoop KJ, Stack LB, Storrow AB: *An Atlas of Emergency Medicine*, 2nd ed. Copyright © 2002, New York: McGraw-Hill.)

21. A 10 year-old boy presents to the ED with a rash. His parents state that last week the child had a runny nose, headache, and low-grade fever that they treated with acetaminophen. However, the child subsequently developed abdominal pain, blood in his urine, and the rash as shown (Figure 24–21, see color insert section). Which of the following is the most likely diagnosis?
    A. Idiopathic thrombocytopenic purpura
    B. Thrombotic thrombocytopenic purpura
    C. Henoch-Schönlein purpura
    D. Meningococcemia
    E. Rocky Mountain spotted fever

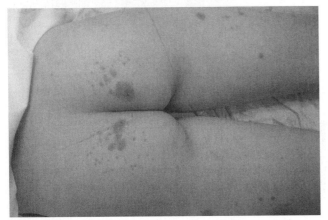

FIGURE 24–21. (*Courtesy of Ami Dave, MD.*)

22. An 18-year-old woman was swimming at a local beach whereupon she felt a sharp sting in her right leg. Subsequently, her leg developed the lesion as shown (Figure 24–22, see color insert section). Which of the following is the most appropriate treatment of choice for this patient?
    A. Fresh water
    B. Vegetable oil
    C. Vinegar
    D. Toothpaste
    E. Household window cleaner

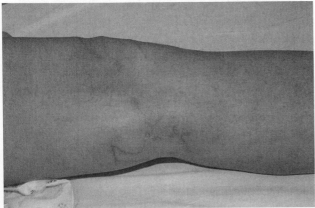

FIGURE 24–22. (*Courtesy of Corey Long, MD.*)

23. A 20-year-old college student presents to the ED with a cutaneous lesion as shown (Figure 24–23). Which aspect of the physical examination of this patient is initially most pertinent to the nature of this type of injury?
    A. Testing of cranial nerves
    B. Otoscopic evaluation of tympanic membranes
    C. Evaluation of gait cadence
    D. Testing of cerebellar deficits
    E. Palpating the cervical spine for tenderness

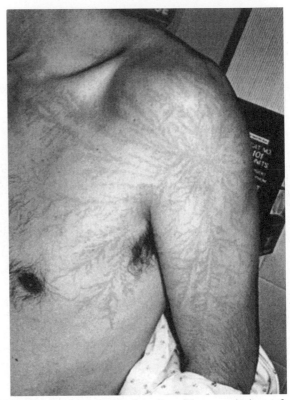

FIGURE 24–23. (Reproduced, with permission, from Tintanalli JE, Kelen GD, Stapczynski JS: *Tintinalli's Emergency Medicine: A Comprehensive Study Guide*, 6th ed. Copyright © 2004, New York: McGraw-Hill.)

24. A 32-year-old woman presents to the ED with a 3-day history of rash, fever, malaise, and mouth sores. She has been unable to eat because of mouth pain. She denies arthralgias, vaginal discharge, new medications, drug allergies, or prior similar episodes. Vital signs are blood pressure, 110/60 mm Hg; heart rate, 107 beats per minute; and temperature, 101.4°F. The patient appears alert but uncomfortable. She has multiple vesiculobullous lesions on her face, conjunctivae, and mouth as shown (Figure 24–24, see color insert section). Visual acuity is 20/20. Target lesions are found on her palms and soles. Which of the following is the most appropriate next step in management?

A. Discharge her with analgesics, antihistamines, and mouth rinses

B. Discharge her with acyclovir, analgesics, antihistamines, and mouth rinses

C. Discharge her after 1 L normal saline IV; prescribe analgesics, antihistamines, oral prednisone, and mouth rinses

D. Admit her and administer 1 to 2 L normal saline IV; analgesics, antihistamines, and transfer to a burn unit

E. Admit her and administer 1 to 2 L normal saline IV; analgesics, antihistamines, and parenteral glucocorticoids

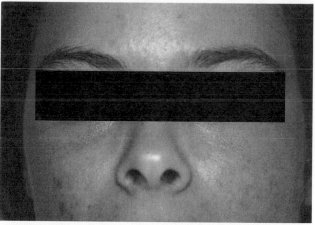

FIGURE 24–25. (Reproduced, with permission, from Wolff K, Johnson RA, Suurmond D: *Fitzpatrick's Color Atlas and Synopsis of Clinical Dermatology*, 5th ed. Copyright © 2005, New York: McGraw-Hill.)

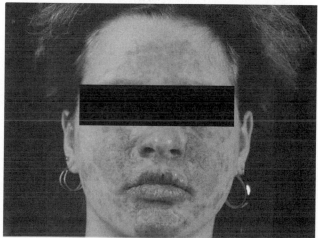

FIGURE 24–24. (Reproduced, with permission, from Wolff K, Johnson RA, Suurmond D: *Fitzpatrick's Color Atlas and Synopsis of Clinical Dermatology*, 5th ed. Copyright © 2005, New York: McGraw-Hill.)

25. A 28-year-old woman presents the ED with complaints of fever, headache, a "sunburn-like" rash, and confusion. A friend states that the patient has complained of nausea, vomiting, diarrhea, and a sore throat over the past few days. Her last menstrual period began 5 days ago. Her heart rate, 110 beats per minute; blood pressure, 95/45 mm Hg; and temperature, 103°F. On physical examination, you note a diffuse blanching erythroderma. Her neck is supple without signs of meningeal irritation. You note a fine desquamation of her skin, especially over the hands and feet, and hyperemia of her bulbar conjunctivae oropharyngeal as shown (Figure 24–25, see color insert section). Laboratory results reveal a CPK of 6000, WBC 14,500 mcg/L, platelets of 90,000/μL, BUN 45 mg/dL, Cr 2.1 mg/dL, and elevated liver enzymes. Which of the following is the most likely causative organism?

A. *Staphylococcus aureus*

B. *Rickettsia rickettsii*

C. *Streptococcus pyogenes*

D. *Neisseria meningitidis*

E. *Neisseria gonorrhoeae*

26. A 55-year-old man presents to the ED with complaints of fever, vomiting, and 2 days of intense epigastric pain that radiates to his back. On physical examination, you note the finding as shown (Figure 24–26, see color insert section). What is the name of this classic sign?

A. Grey-Turner sign

B. Kernig sign

C. McMurray sign

D. Murphy sign

E. McBurney sign

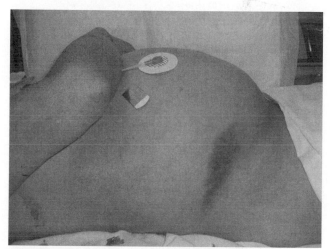

FIGURE 24–26. (*Courtesy of Ami Dave, MD.*)

27. A 31-year-old man presents to the ED with right hand swelling, pain, and erythema as shown (Figure 24–27). The patient's vital signs are significant for an oral temperature of 100.5°F. Upon physical examination, you note an area of erythema and swelling over the right third metacarpalphalangeal joint with localized tenderness. The patient is neurovascularly intact with limited movement due to the pain. Which of the following is the most appropriate disposition for the patient?
    A. Suture and close follow-up with a hand surgeon
    B. Suture and prescription for oral antibiotics
    C. Wound irrigation and prescription for oral antibiotics
    D. Wound irrigation and tetanus prophylaxis
    E. Admission for intravenous antibiotics

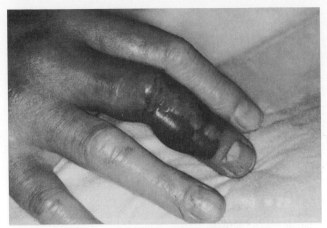

FIGURE 24–28. (Reproduced, with permission, from Knoop KJ, Stack LB, Storrow AB: *An Atlas of Emergency Medicine*, 2nd ed. Copyright © 2002, New York: McGraw-Hill.)

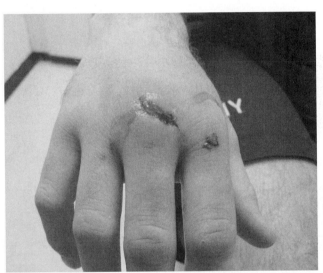

FIGURE 24–27. (*Courtesy of Adam Rosh, MD.*)

28. A farmer in Texas presents to the ED with the condition as shown (Figure 24–28, see color insert section). He describes feeling a sharp pain in his hand that occurred while picking weeds from his farm. Which of the following is the most appropriate initial treatment of choice in this patient?
    A. Antivenin
    B. Tetanus prophylaxis
    C. Antibiotic prophylaxis
    D. Sedation
    E. Atropine

29. A 31-year-old man from Arkansas presents to the ED with a complaint of 8 hours of arm pain. Upon physical examination, there are diffuse petechiae of the mid arm and a small necrotic lesion with surrounding edema as shown (Figure 24–29). Which of the following is the most likely cause of this patient's presentation?
    A. Deep venous thrombosis
    B. Scorpion sting
    C. Brown recluse spider bite
    D. Folliculitis
    E. Thrombocytopenia

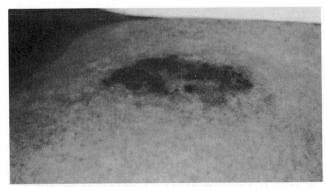

FIGURE 24–29. (Reproduced, with permission, from Knoop KJ, Stack LB, Storrow AB: *An Atlas of Emergency Medicine*, 2nd ed. Copyright © 2002, New York: McGraw-Hill.)

30. A 3-year-old boy is brought to the ED by his mother with complaints of 5 days of rash, fever, and a tender lump on his neck. On examination, you note the findings as shown (Figure 24–30, see color insert section) as well as a 1.5-cm right anterior lymph node. In addition to medical treatment, this boy will require which of the following?

A. Hemodialysis

B. Lumbar puncture

C. Lymph node biopsy

D. Echocardiogram

E. Testing for fluorescent treponemal antibody absorption (FTA-ABS)

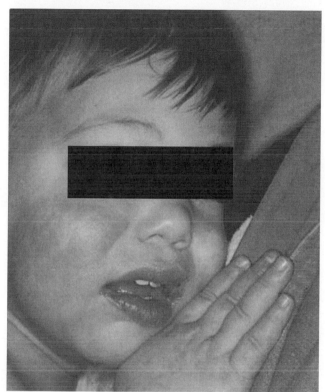

FIGURE 24–30. (Reproduced, with permission, from Wolff K, Johnson RA, Suurmond D: *Fitzpatrick's Color Atlas and Synopsis of Clinical Dermatology,* 5th ed. Copyright © 2005, New York: McGraw-Hill.)

31. A 10-year-old girl is brought into the ED for the rash as shown (Figure 24–31, see color insert section). Over the preceding 3 days, the patient complained of headache, fever, sore throat, and coryza. The patient's mother states that the rash appeared abruptly prior to coming to the ED. On examination, the child is well-appearing and is afebrile. Her neck is supple and oropharynx is normal-appearing. Her lung, cardiac, and abdominal examinations are unremarkable. The facial rash is bright red, raised, with circumoral pallor, and sparing of the nasolabial folds. Which of the following is the most likely diagnosis?

A. Rubeola

B. Rubella

C. Roseola

D. Fifth disease

E. Scarlet fever

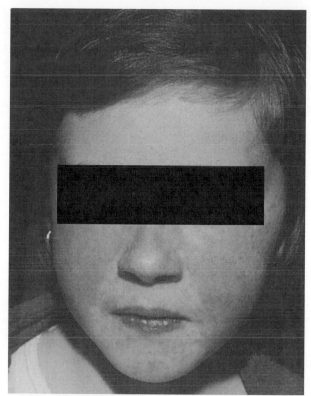

FIGURE 24–31. (Reproduced, with permission, from Wolff K, Johnson RA, Suurmond D: *Fitzpatrick's Color Atlas and Synopsis of Clinical Dermatology,* 5th ed. Copyright © 2005, New Yok: McGraw-Hill.)

32. A 27-year-old man presents to the ED with a complaint of acute-onset penile pain. On examination, you see the condition as shown (Figure 24–32). Which of the following is the most likely diagnosis?

A. Phimosis

B. Paraphimosis

C. Balanitis

D. Priapism

E. Hair tourniquet

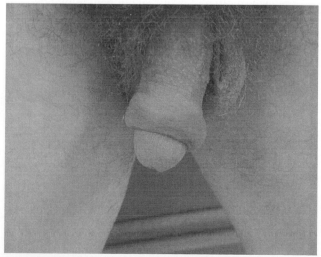

FIGURE 24–32. (*Courtesy of Ami Dave, MD.*)

33. A 20-year-old man was found on the ground beside his car after it hit a tree on the side of the road. Bystanders state that the man got out of his car after the collision but collapsed within a few minutes. A head CT is shown (Figure 24–33). Which of the following is the most likely diagnosis?
   A. Epidural hematoma
   B. Subdural hematoma
   C. Subarachnoid hemorrhage
   D. Intracerebral hematoma
   E. Cerebral contusion

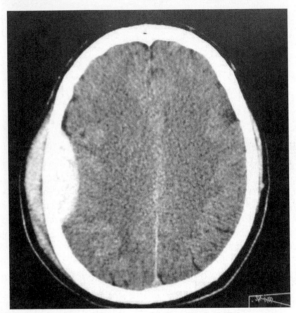

FIGURE 24–33. (*Courtesy of Adam Rosh, MD.*)

34. A 69-year-old man with a history of congestive heart failure and hypertension presents to the ED complaining of dyspnea, cough, and chest tightness for the last 2 days. He takes aspirin and a β-blocker daily and is allergic to penicillin. His vital signs on arrival are blood pressure, 110/75 mm Hg; heart rate 90 beats per minute; respiratory rate, 24 breaths per minute; SaO_2, 92% on room air; and temperature, 37.8°C. He appears well, has bilateral râles, decreased breath sounds on the left, and normal heart sounds on auscultation. The remainder of his physical examination is unremarkable. A complete blood count and serum electrolytes are normal. Figure 24–34 shows his chest radiograph. What is the most appropriate initial treatment?
   A. Albuterol and ipratropium
   B. Ceftriaxone and azithromycin
   C. Furosimide and nitroglycerin
   D. Levofloxacin
   E. Trimethoprim-sulfamethoxazole

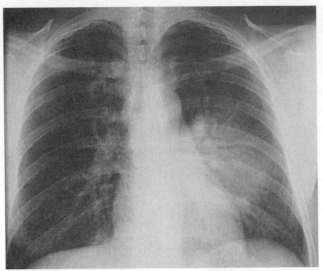

FIGURE 24–34. (Reproduced, with permission, from Schwartz DT: *Emergency Radiology: Case Studies.* Copyright © 2008, New York: McGraw-Hill.)

35. A 40-year-old woman is a restrained driver involved in a moderate-speed motor vehicle collision with airbag deployment. At the scene, she is conscious with complaints of diffuse chest and abdominal pain. At arrival to the ED her vital signs are blood pressure, 140/90 mm Hg; heart rate, 110 beats per minute, respiratory rate, 24 breaths per minute; SaO_2, 100% on 10 L/min supplemental oxygen with a nonrebreather mask. She is speaking in complete sentences, has a midline trachea, no jugular venous distension, nonfocal chest wall tenderness without crepitus or flail segments, decreased bilateral breath sounds, normal heart sounds, a nontender abdomen, and moves all extremities. Based on the chest radiograph (Figure 24–35), what would be the most appropriate intervention?
   A. To the OR for emergent abdominal laparotomy
   B. Needle decompression of the chest in the right second midclavicular intercostal space
   C. Tube thoracostomy of the right chest in the fifth midaxillary intercostal space directed cephalad
   D. Tube thoracostomy of the right chest in the fourth midaxillary intercostal space directed caudad
   E. Rapid sequence intubation with etomidate and succinylcholine

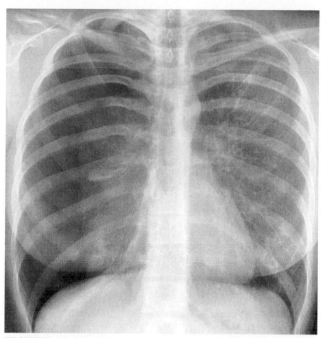

FIGURE 24–35. (Reproduced, with permission, from Schwartz DT: *Emergency Radiology: Case Studies*. Copyright © 2008, New York: McGraw-Hill.)

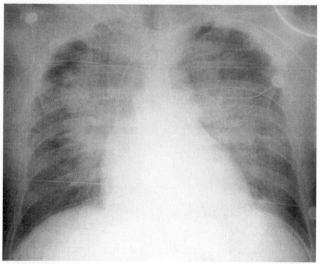

FIGURE 24–36. (Reproduced, with permission, from Schwartz DT: *Emergency Radiology: Case Studies*. Copyright © 2008, New York: McGraw-Hill.)

36. A 75-year-old woman is brought to the ED by ambulance with a complaint of shortness of breath. Her symptoms have been gradually worsening over the past 2 days. She had no fever, cough, or chest pain. She says that she has a "weak heart" and ran out of her medications last week, the names of which she can't remember. Her vital signs are blood pressure, 170/100 mm Hg; heart rate, 110 beats per minute; respiratory rate, 22 breaths per minute; SaO_2, 91% on 4 L nasal cannula; and temperature, 97.7°F (36.5°C). Her examination is remarkable for jugular venous distension, mildly labored breathing with râles half way up both lungs, an audible S_3 heart sound, and 3+ pitting pedal edema bilaterally. Her chest radiograph is shown (Figure 24–36). Which of the following is the first radiographic sign of an acute presentation of this disease process?
A. Alveolar airspace filling
B. Increased interstitial lung markings
C. Kerley B lines
D. Pleural effusion
E. Vasculature cephalization

37. A 56-year-old man with an unknown past medical history presents to the ED with seizures refractory to diazepam and phenytoin. The patient's chest radiograph is shown (Figure 24–37). Which of the following is indicated in the management of this patient?
A. Dantrolene
B. Phenobarbital
C. Physostigmine
D. Pralidoxime
E. Pyridoxine

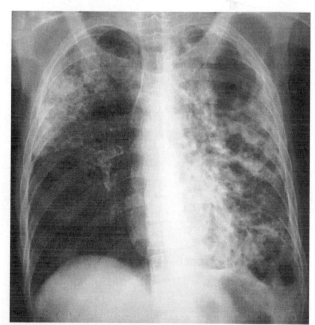

FIGURE 24–37. (Reproduced, with permission, from Schwartz DT: *Emergency Radiology: Case Studies*. Copyright © 2008, New York: McGraw-Hill.)

38. A 29-year-old woman from India, previously healthy, presents to the ED with complaints of dyspnea and a rash. The rash began 5 days ago, is pruritic, and located primarily on the trunk and arms. She has felt increasingly short of breath for the last 2 days and notes a dry cough. She denies fever, chills, hemoptysis, night sweats, and recent travel; she has been in the United States for 5 years. Her temperature is 101.3°F (38.5°C), she has a normal blood pressure and heart rate, but she is mildly tachypneic and has a room air oxygen saturation of 94%. She has numerous subcentimeter erythematous papular and vesicular lesions, some crusted over, which cover her arms, chest, back, and face. Mild bibasilar râles are present at the lung bases. A urine β-hCG test is positive. Based on her clinical and chest radiographic findings (Figure 24–38), what would be the most appropriate initial medical treatment?

    A. Acyclovir
    B. Caspofungin
    C. Ceftriaxone and azithromycin
    D. Isoniazid, rifampin, pyrazinamide, and ethambutol
    E. Prednisone, albuterol, and ipratropium

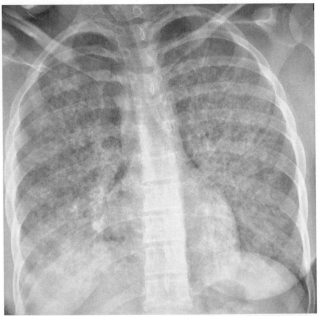

FIGURE 24–38. (Reproduced, with permission, from Schwartz DT: *Emergency Radiology: Case Studies.* Copyright © 2008, New York: McGraw-Hill.)

39. A 64-year-old man is brought into the ED after extrication from a bus that overturned. His vitals on arrival blood pressure, 140/90 mm Hg; heart rate, 110 beats per minute; respiratory rate, 20 breaths per minute; SaO$_2$, 98% on a nonrebreather face mask. He is awake and breathing spontaneously, though will not verbalize any complaints. His portable AP chest radiograph as shown (Figure 24–39). Of the following diagnostic tests or procedures, which would be the most helpful to exclude the injury that should be suspected based on the chest radiographic findings?

    A. Aortography
    B. Diagnostic peritoneal lavage (DPL)
    C. Focused abdominal sonography for trauma (FAST) examination
    D. Pericardiocentesis
    E. Transthoracic echocardiogram

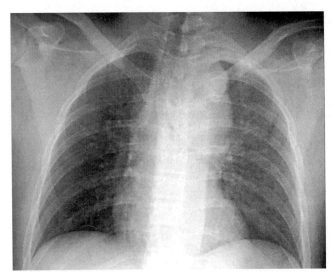

FIGURE 24–39. (Reproduced, with permission, from Schwartz DT, Reisdorff EJ: *Emergency Radiology.* Copyright © 2000, New York: McGraw-Hill.)

40. A 64-year-old man with a history of inguinal hernia repair and colon cancer status-posttumor resection presents to the ED with complaints of nausea, vomiting, and diffuse abdominal pain. Supine and upright abdominal radiographs are shown (Figures 24–40A and 24–40B). Of the following etiologies of this disease process, which is the most likely to result in bowel strangulation?

    A. Adhesion
    B. Gallstones
    C. Hernia
    D. Inflammatory bowel disease
    E. Intussusception

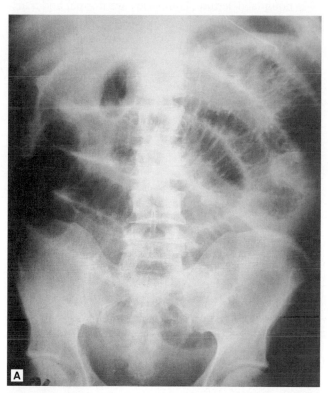

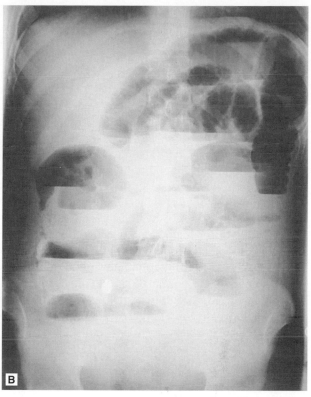

FIGURE 24–40 A, B. (Reproduced, with permission, from Schwartz DT: *Emergency Radiology: Case Studies.* Copyright © 2008, New York: McGraw-Hill.)

41. A 70-year-old man with hypertension presents to the ED with complaints of sudden onset chest and abdominal pain. The pain is constant, diffuse, mainly epigastric, and worse with deep inspiration. He reports no shortness of breath, trauma, or extremity swelling. Based on the history and chest radiograph (Figure 24–41), which of the following represent the most likely diagnosis?
    A. Aortic dissection
    B. Congestive heart failure
    C. Duodenal perforation
    D. Pneumothorax
    E. Pulmonary embolism

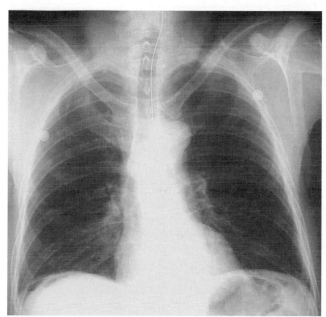

FIGURE 24–41. (Reproduced, with permission, from Schwartz DT: *Emergency Radiology: Case Studies.* Copyright © 2008, New York: McGraw-Hill.)

42. A 33-year-old woman presents to the ED with complaints of nausea, vomiting, and abdominal pain for the past day. She has had a single episode of diarrhea, is unable to tolerate solid food, and denies vaginal bleeding or discharge. Her vital signs are temperature, 100.2°F (37.9°C); blood pressure, 115/85 mm Hg; heart rate, 110 beats per minute; respiratory rate, 16 breaths per minute; SaO_2, 99% on room air. On examination, she is uncomfortable, the lungs are clear, the abdomen tender on the right and around the umbilicus with guarding. There is no costovertebral tenderness, and the remainder of her examination is within normal limits. A β-hCG is negative, urinalysis significant for trace blood and leukocyte esterase, white blood cell count 12,000/μL, and the remainder of the serum complete blood count and chemistries are normal. An abdominal CT scan is obtained. What complication is associated with the pathology as shown (Figure 24–42)?

A. Ectopic pregnancy
B. Hemolytic uremic syndrome
C. Intra-abdominal abscess
D. Pyelonephritis
E. Toxic megacolon

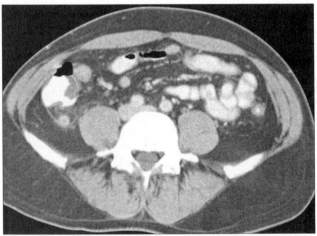

FIGURE 24–42. (Reproduced, with permission, from Schwartz DT Residooff EJ: *Emergency Radiology.* Copyright © 2000, New York: McGraw-Hill.)

43. A 42-year-old otherwise healthy man presents to the ED with a complaint of sudden-onset sharp right lower quadrant pain, nausea, and vomiting for the past 2 hours. He denies fever, dyspnea, and diarrhea, but does note anorexia. On examination he has normal vital signs but appears restless and uncomfortable. His abdominal examination is remarkable for decreased bowel sounds without tenderness, rebound, or guarding. Complete blood count and serum chemistries are normal and a urinalysis reveals trace blood without leukesterase or nitrite. The patient receives pain medication with good effect and undergoes a noncontrast abdominal CT scan. Concerning the disease entity as shown (Figure 24–43), which of the following might be an effective adjunctive treatment?

A. Ampicillin-sulbactam
B. Ciprofloxacin
C. Furosemide
D. Phenazopyridine
E. Tamsulosin

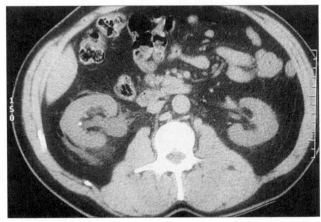

FIGURE 24–43. (Reproduced, with permission, from Schwartz DT, Residooff EJ: *Emergency Radiology.* Copyright © 2000, New York: McGraw-Hill.)

44. A 70-year-old man with a history of hypertension presents to the ED with a complaint of back pain. The pain was relatively abrupt in onset, dull in nature, nonradiating, and not related to any activity. The patient has no paresthesias and no bowel or bladder dysfunction. On examination his vital signs are blood pressure, 105/60 mm Hg; heart rate, 95 beats per minute; respiratory rate, 14 breaths per minute; SaO_2, 99% on room air; temperature, 36.0°C. He is comfortable, his abdomen is nontender, an ill-defined midline abdominal mass is palpable, there is no costovertebral angle tenderness, and he has normal strength, sensation, and reflexes throughout his lower extremities. A section of his abdominal CT is as shown (Figure 24–44). Which of the following is a risk factor for the development of the displayed disease process?

A. Deep vein thrombosis
B. Family history
C. Female sex
D. History of abdominal surgery
E. Obesity

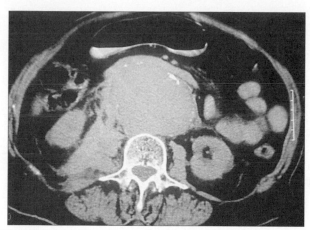

FIGURE 24–44. (Reproduced, with permission, from Schwartz DT Residooff EJ: *Emergency Radiology.* Copyright © 2000, New York: McGraw-Hill.)

45. A 29-year-old man was playing in a pickup football game with friends when he was tackled to the ground. He had immediate pain in his right shoulder and was unable to adduct the shoulder. On examination, there is a visible deformity at the shoulder and the patient holds the arm in external rotation. Radial pulses are equal and ulnar, median, and radial nerve testings are normal at the hand. Figure 24–45 shows the patient's shoulder radiograph. Which of the following would be a common complication of the injury pictured in this patient?
    A. Axillary artery injury
    B. Bankart lesion
    C. Clavicle fracture
    D. Reverse Hill-Sachs deformity
    E. Rotator cuff rupture

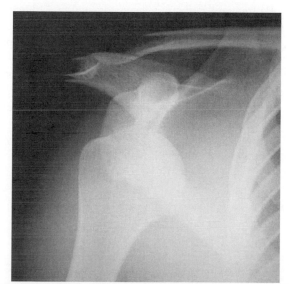

FIGURE 24–45. (Reproduced, with permission, from Schwartz DT: *Emergency Radiology: Case Studies.* Copyright © 2008, New York: McGraw-Hill.)

46. A 25-year-old man presents to the ED with a complaint of right shoulder pain after being shoved laterally into the hard plexiglass boards while playing ice hockey. He has normal pulmonary and neurovascular examinations. The shoulder can be moved through a full range of motion, although with moderate pain throughout, and is held in adduction for comfort. There is tenderness to palpation along the superior aspect of the shoulder. Based on his shoulder radiograph (Figure 24–46), which of the following is the most appropriate disposition for this patient?
    A. Admission overnight for observation
    B. Urgent orthopedic surgery consultation for reduction
    C. Discharge home in sling with expedient orthopedic clinic follow-up
    D. Discharge home in figure-of-eight harness with expedient orthopedic clinic follow-up
    E. Discharge home without immobilization for primary care physician clinic follow-up

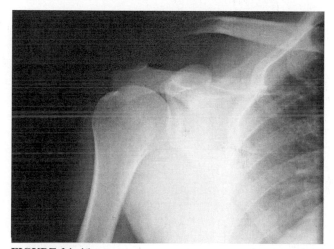

FIGURE 24–46.

47. A 45-year-old woman was rollerblading when she tripped and fell forward onto her outstretched hands. She presents with complaint of mild pain around her left wrist, has no motor or sensory deficits, but winces to axial loading of the thumb. An enlarged version of her wrist radiograph is shown (Figures 24–47A and 24-47B). What is the most common complication of this patient's injury?

A. Avascular necrosis
B. Distal radioulnar joint dislocation
C. Median nerve injury
D. Ulnar collateral ligament injury of the thumb
E. Ulnar nerve injury

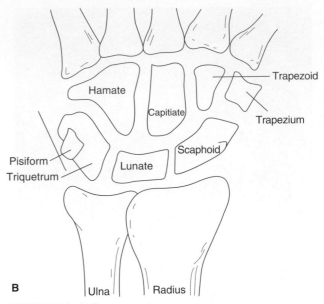

FIGURE 24–47 B.

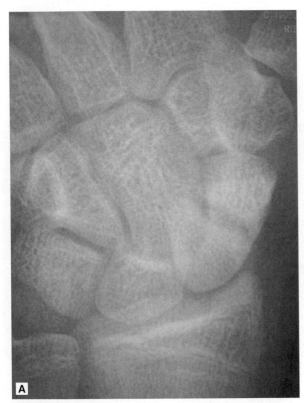

FIGURE 24–47 A.

48. A 54-year-old woman trips and falls while exiting an elevator at work, with immediate complaint of generalized left wrist pain after landing on her outstretched hand. On examination, the wrist is diffusely swollen and tender, and landmarks are difficult to appreciate. There is no evidence of numbness, she has full strength and range of motion of the digits but will not move the wrist secondary to pain. There is good capillary refill in the digits with a strong radial pulse. Figure 24–48 shows the lateral radiograph of the wrist. What is the most appropriate treatment for this patient?

A. Immobilization in a short arm cast, orthopedic follow-up in 1 week
B. Immobilization in a sugar-tong splint, orthopedic follow-up in 1 week
C. Immobilization in a thumb spica splint, orthopedic follow-up in 1 week
D. Immobilization in an ulnar gutter splint, orthopedic follow-up in 1 week
E. Urgent orthopedic consultation for reduction and fixation

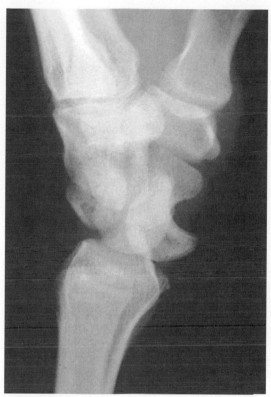

FIGURE 24–48.

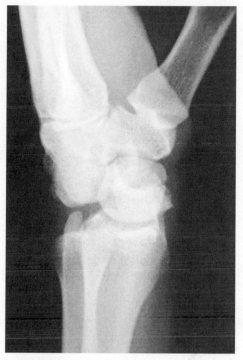

FIGURE 24–49.

49. A 43-year-old man fell onto his right arm while walking down stairs. His only complaint at presentation to the ED is diffuse pain of the right wrist and palm. A radiograph is obtained. Which of the following best characterizes the anatomic disturbance as shown (Figure 24–49)?
    A. Perilunate dislocation
    B. Lunate dislocation
    C. Scaphoid fracture
    D. Scaphoid rotary subluxation
    E. Triquetrum dislocation

50. What is the most common mechanism of injury for the fracture as shown (Figure 24–50)?
    A. Axial load to the thumb
    B. Fall onto pronated hand
    C. Fall onto supinated hand
    D. Forced abduction
    E. Hyperextension

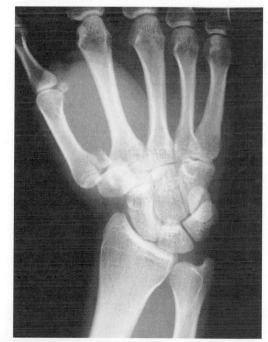

FIGURE 24–50. (Reproduced, with permission, from Schwartz DT Residooff EJ: *Emergency Radiology.* Copyright © 2000, New York: McGraw-Hill.)

51. What is the maximum degree of acceptable angulation for the injury as shown (Figure 24–51)?
    A. 15 degrees
    B. 25 degrees
    C. 35 degrees
    D. 45 degrees
    E. 55 degrees

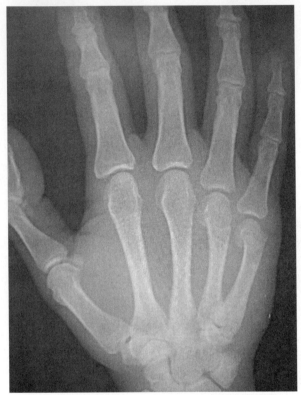

FIGURE 24–51.

52. What is the most common nerve deficit associated with the injury as shown (Figures 24–52A and 24–52B)?
    A. Axillary
    B. Median
    C. Musculocutaneous
    D. Radial
    E. Ulnar

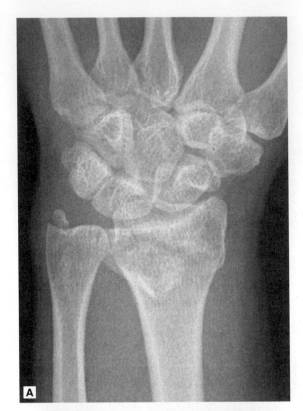

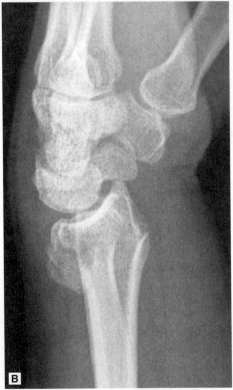

FIGURE 24–52 A, B. (Reproduced, with permission, from Schwartz DT: *Emergency Radiology: Case Studies*. McGraw-Hill, 2008.)

53. A 25-year-old man was skateboarding on a cement half-pipe when he lost control and fell from a 10-foot height, hitting his right arm on the edge of the ramp. Figure 24–53 shows an AP view of his right forearm. Which of the following radiographic signs supports the diagnosis of a Galeazzi fracture?
    A. Distal radioulnar joint dislocation
    B. Intra-articular fracture of the radial styloid
    C. Intra-articular fracture of the distal radial rim
    D. Radial head dislocation
    E. Radial head fracture

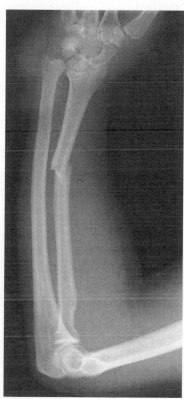

FIGURE 24–53.

54. You are evaluating an 18-year-old woman who was extricated after a high-speed motor vehicle collision. She was restrained with a lap belt. Her vital signs on arrival are remarkable for a heart rate of 124 beats per minute and a blood pressure of 70/40 mm Hg despite 2 L of intravenous saline administered en route. She is pale and diaphoretic, but answers questions appropriately. Examination of the abdomen reveals tenderness and guarding. The pelvis is unstable when gently compressed. A bedside sonogram reveals fluid in Morison pouch. Radiographs are obtained of the chest and pelvis as shown (Figure 24–54). The next step in this patient's management is
    A. Transfusion of platelets
    B. Application of a pneumatic antishock garment (PASG)

C. Transfer to angiography suite for transcatheter embolization
D. Binding of the pelvis by means of a bed sheet
E. Transfer to the operating room for internal reduction and fixation of the fracture

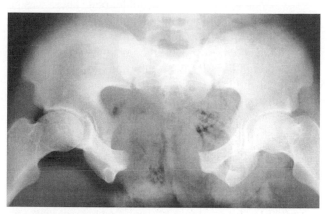

FIGURE 24–54.

55. A 31-year-old dancer twisted her right foot during a recital. She completed the performance, but now complains of worsening pain and ecchymosis along the lateral aspect of her foot, which is exquisitely tender. She is able to bear weight in the ED with moderate difficulty. A radiograph of the affected area is shown (Figure 24–55). Which of the following is true about this injury?
    A. Radionuclide bone scan is indicated for accurate diagnosis if radiographs are negative
    B. Was initially described in marching infantry soldiers, after whom it is named
    C. A soft compression dressing and weight-bearing as tolerated are appropriate pending orthopedic follow-up
    D. Improved outcome is associated with early surgical fixation
    E. Most commonly results from eversion and dorsiflexion

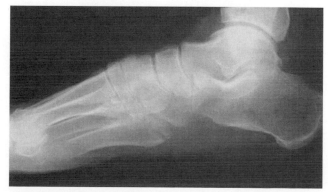

FIGURE 24–55.

56. You are evaluating a 24-year-old police officer with foot pain after the patrol car she was driving at low speed collided with a telephone pole as she swerved to avoid a pedestrian. She has complained only of right foot pain and swelling, and cannot bear weight. She recalls decelerating suddenly, and was restrained with the shoulder belt. There was no airbag deployment, and frontal damage was minimal. Her foot is diffusely swollen, with tenderness and ecchymoses over the metatarsals. Sensation and capillary refill are normal. True statements about the injury as shown (Figure 24–56) include which of the following?

    A. Treatment includes immobilization in a hard-sole shoe and weight-bearing as tolerated
    B. Also known as Chopart injury, after the physician who described amputation at this joint
    C. Frequently associated with injuries to the thoracic spine
    D. May result from rotational forces, axial loads, or crush injuries
    E. Fracture through the base of the first metatarsal is pathognomic for injury to this joint complex

57. A 34-year-old man presents with pain and swelling of the left knee that began after it suddenly "gave way" while playing racquetball. He is unable to walk. He denies any direct trauma, but reports that he had been evaluated by his primary care physician 1 month prior for persistent anterior knee pain that was made worse by physical activity. Radiographs obtained during that earlier visit were interpreted as normal. His examination reveals patellar tenderness and effusion, and he is unable to actively extend at the knee. Radiographs are repeated, and a lateral view of the knee is shown (Figure 24–57). In addition to elevation, ice, and analgesics, appropriate initial management of this injury includes which of the following?

    A. Needle aspiration of joint effusion, compression dressing, and primary care follow-up
    B. Orthopaedic surgical consultation for open reduction and fixation
    C. Consent for general anesthesia and admit for open patellectomy
    D. Closed reduction in the ED and discharge with knee immobilizer and crutches
    E. Emergent MRI to evaluate for quadriceps tendon rupture

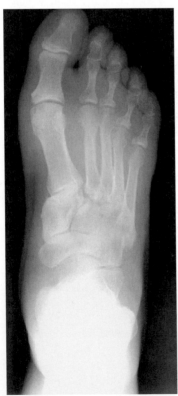

FIGURE 24–56.

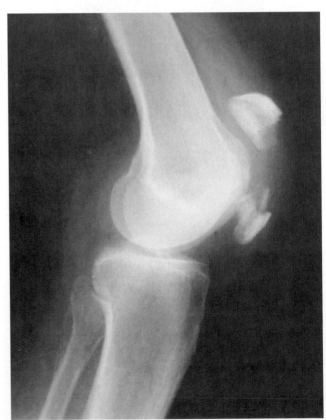

FIGURE 24–57.

58. You are evaluating a 40-year-old martial arts student who sustained a lateral blow to her left knee during practice. She recalls that her leg was extended at the moment she was kicked by her classmate on the lateral side of her knee. She is unable to bear weight. The affected joint is tender and ecchymotic, especially over the proximal tibia, with a small effusion. No instability is appreciated with varus and valgus stress. The Lachman and posterior drawer tests are normal. Distal strength and sensation are normal, and pulses are symmetric. Regarding the injury depicted in the knee radiograph as shown (Figure 24–58), which of the following is true?
    A. Emergent angiography is indicated if the arterial-brachial index is <0.90
    B. Along with medial meniscus injury and damage to the medial collateral ligament, comprises the "unhappy triad"
    C. Associated foot drop may result from stretch on the peroneal nerve
    D. Commonly used grading scales are based on the integrity of the soft tissue envelope and the presence of varus or valgus deformity
    E. All patients should undergo routine CT in the ED

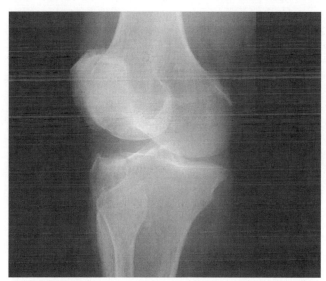

FIGURE 24–58.

59. A 40-year-old man with a history of depression and alcohol dependence is unable to walk after he jumped 10 feet from an elevated train station platform onto the sidewalk below, apparently as a suicidal gesture. He has complaints of pain in his lower back and left foot. Palpation of his lumbar spine and axial loading of the affected heel elicit exquisite tenderness. Radiographs are obtained of his lumbar spine and foot, as well as an axial calcaneus view. Regarding the lateral radiograph of the foot (Figures 24–59A and 24–59B), which of the following is true about this injury?
    A. CT may be useful when planning surgical treatment
    B. Measurement of the talar height on the AP view may be diagnostic when fracture lines are not evident
    C. The most common associated injury is pubic ramus fracture
    D. Treatment is nonoperative
    E. Radiographs of the foot could be omitted in this patient if tenderness over the base of the fifth metatarsal and navicular bone were absent

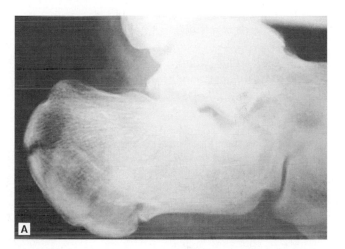

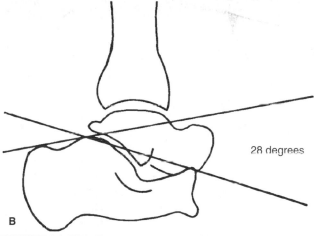

28 degrees

FIGURE 24–59 A, B.

60. A 72-year-old man with a history of diabetes complains of left lower extremity pain that began gradually after awaking. He remembers striking his leg against a coffee table two days earlier, suffering a superficial laceration. He had been evaluated by his primary care physician that afternoon, and sent home with reassurance and analgesics. On examination, a single large bulla suspicious for a fracture blister is noted over the proximal tibial surface, overlying an area of violaceous discoloration. Radiographs are ordered. When the patient returns from the radiology department an hour later, he is noted to be tachycardic and disoriented. Reexamination of the affected leg reveals brawny edema and palpable crepitus below the knee. A likely etiologic agent responsible for the findings as shown (Figure 24–60) is
    A. *Sporothrix schenkii*
    B. *Staphylococcus aureus*
    C. *Clostridium tetani*
    D. *Clostridium perfringens*
    E. *Bacillus anthracis*

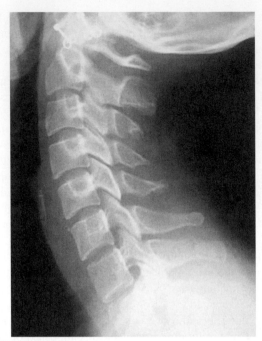

FIGURE 24–61.

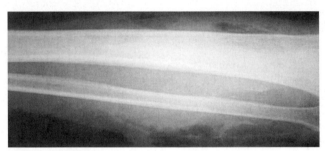

FIGURE 24–60.

61. You are asked to evaluate a 36-year-old man with neck pain who reports that he "pulled a muscle" while weight-lifting. He has tenderness to palpation over the base of his cervical spine. His neurologic examination is normal. A radiograph of his cervical spine is obtained (Figure 24–61). This injury is commonly referred to by the name
    A. Jefferson fracture
    B. Pillar fracture
    C. Hangman fracture
    D. Clay-shoveler fracture
    E. Tillaux fracture

62. A 28-year-old man presents to the ED with severe neck pain after being assaulted with a baseball bat. He had been evaluated in the ED 6 hours earlier, and was treated for a large occipital scalp laceration. He did not complain of neck pain initially, but appeared intoxicated with alcohol. A head CT was read as normal, and he was discharged to home after achieving sobriety. His examination now reveals diffuse marked high cervical tenderness, but no neurologic deficits. Based on the open-mouth and lateral radiographs (Figures 24–62A and 24–62B), what is the most likely diagnosis?
    A. Rotary atlantoaxial dislocation without fracture
    B. Odontoid fracture
    C. Avulsion fracture of the anterior neural arch
    D. Occipitoatlantal dissociation
    E. Occipitoatlantal subluxation

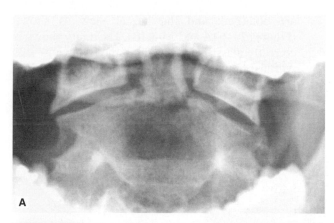

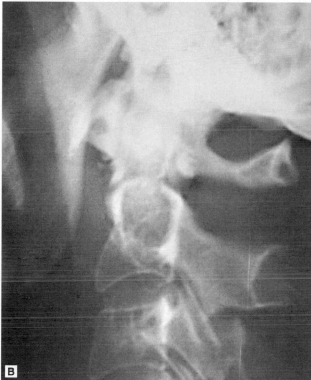

FIGURE 24–62 A, B. (Reproduced, with permission, from Schwartz DT, Reisdorff EJ. *Emergency Radiology*. New York: McGraw-Hill, 2000: 329.)

A. Classified as mechanically stable according to the three-column model
B. Commonly known as an extension-teardrop fracture
C. Routine care includes soft cervical collar for comfort and early mobilization
D. May be associated with acute anterior cord syndrome
E. Typically results from low-speed acceleration-deceleration injuries

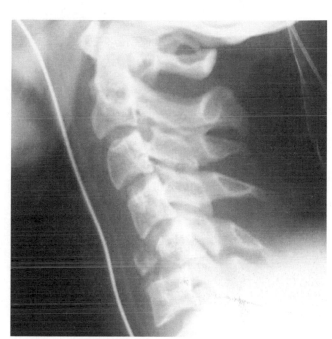

FIGURE 24–63. (Reproduced, with permission, from Schwartz DT, Reisdorff EJ. *Emergency Radiology*. New York: McGraw-Hill, 2000: 329.)

63. A 24-year-old restrained driver arrives to the ED by ambulance after a prolonged extrication following a high-speed motor vehicle collision. She is immobilized on a backboard with a rigid cervical collar. In the ED, she is alert and answers questions appropriately, but tearful. Strength is 0/5 in all four extremities, and there is no sensation to pin-prick below the neck. A lateral radiograph of the cervical spine is obtained (Figure 24–63). Which of the following is true about this injury?

64. A 62-year-old woman is brought to the ED by ambulance after falling backwards from a standing position onto her buttocks. She complains of severe back pain, which limits her ability to raise her legs from the stretcher. Her patellar and Achilles tendon reflexes are diminished but present (1+) in both lower limbs. Perianal and lower extremity sensation to light touch are intact, and rectal tone is normal. There is diffuse tenderness to palpation of the thoracolumbar region. Lumbar spine radiographs are obtained, and the lateral view as shown (Figures 24–64A and 24–64B). The injury shown is correctly classified as which of the following?

A. Burst fracture
B. Wedge compression fracture
C. Chance fracture
D. Spinous process fracture
E. Translational injury

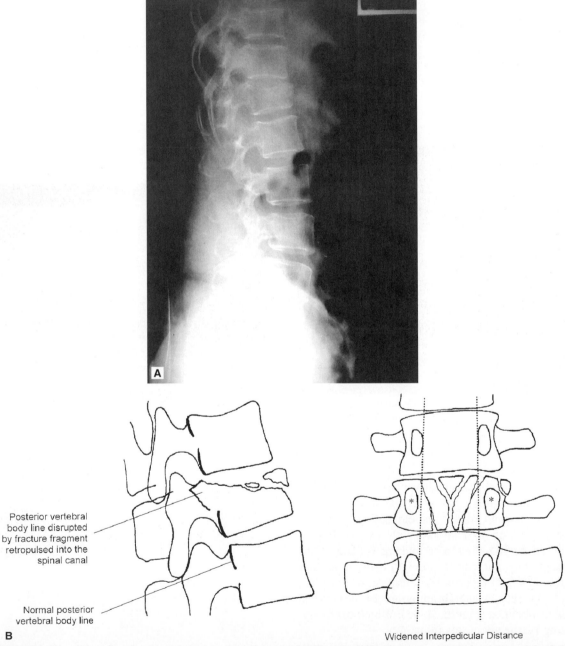

Posterior vertebral body line disrupted by fracture fragment retropulsed into the spinal canal

Normal posterior vertebral body line

Widened Interpedicular Distance

FIGURE 24–64 A, B. (Reproduced, with permission, from Schwartz DT Residooff EJ: *Emergency Radiology*. Copyright © 2000, New York: McGraw-Hill.)

65. A 59-year-old male with a history of alcohol dependence is brought to the ED by ambulance for public intoxication. His vital signs are unremarkable. He is disheveled, malodorous, and responds only to painful stimuli. There is no evidence of head injury. After 4 hours of observation in the hallway, he remains obtunded. Laboratory studies are obtained, and a blood ethanol level is 180 mg/dL. Noncontrast CT of the head is obtained (Figure 24–65). Which of the following statements is true about this diagnosis?

   A. MRI is more sensitive than CT in detecting this lesion acutely
   B. >90% of alcoholic patients who survive this injury will continue to use ethanol regardless of intervention in the ED
   C. Recombinant activated factor VII is indicated for all patients on anticoagulation (eg, warfarin) or antiplatelet agents (eg, aspirin, clopidogrel)
   D. Recognized cause of new-onset seizure within the first 6 months of life
   E. Prognosis correlates most closely with the volume of bleeding

66. A 45-year-old man presents to the ED with complaint of sudden onset headache following sexual intercourse. He has suffered similar episodes in the past, but never of this severity. After an episode of emesis, he is witnessed to have a generalized tonic-clonic seizure lasting 2 minutes that is aborted with intravenous lorazepam. Bedside glucometry is normal. A noncontrast head CT is performed (Figure 24–66). Which of the following is true about this disease?

   A. Lumbar puncture has the greatest sensitivity within 12 hours of symptom onset
   B. The sensitivity of CT is >90% within 24 hours of headache onset
   C. Visual inspection and spectrophotometry are equally sensitive for detection of xanthochromia
   D. Use of clinical grading scale predicts long-term, but not short-term outcome
   E. Coital headache is more common in women

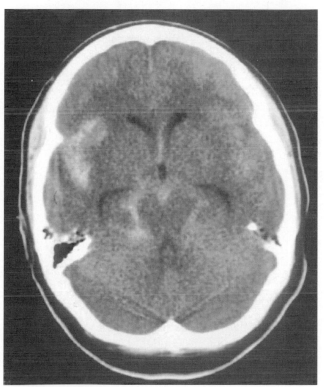

FIGURE 24–66.

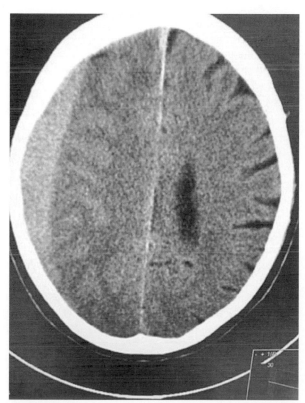

FIGURE 24–65.

67. A 19-year-old man presents with swelling and ecchymoses around his left eye after being punched one time during an altercation. He was briefly dazed but had no loss of consciousness. On examination, he is fully alert and oriented. His neck is nontender and has full range of motion. There is marked left periorbital swelling and ecchymosis without any palpable bony step-off. He refuses to allow you to retract his eyelids, which are swollen closed. A facial CT is obtained. A coronal slice from this scan is shown (Figure 24–67). Which of the following physical examination findings is most likely?
    A. Hypopyon of the injured eye
    B. Contralateral post auricular ecchymosis
    C. Ipsilateral infraorbital anesthesia
    D. Ipsilateral paralysis of downward gaze
    E. Contralateral subcutaneous emphysema

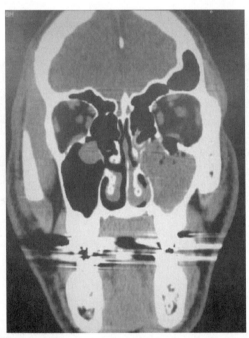

FIGURE 24–67.

68. A 25-year-old woman presents to the ED with a complaint of transient light-headedness after donation of blood at an event sponsored by her local hospital. She denies chest pain, shortness of breath, nausea, vomiting, recent fevers or chills, or any recent travel. She is not taking prescription medications, does not use tobacco or alcohol, and denies illicit substance use. Physical examination is unremarkable; no murmurs, pericardial friction rub, gallop, or adventitious lung sounds are auscultated. Urine HCG levels are negative. Chest radiograph is negative. A rhythm strip is obtained (Figure 24–68). Which of the following represents the best management of this patient's condition?
    A. Administer atropine
    B. Admit for continuous cardiac monitoring
    C. Give intravenous fluid administration, then discharge with instructions to follow up with her primary care provider
    D. Obtain emergent echocardiogram
    E. Perform transcutaneous pacing

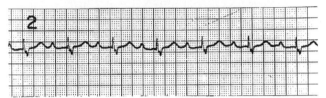

FIGURE 24–68.

69. Which of the following interventions is preferred in the initial management of a 67-year-old woman who presents to the ED with a history of chest pain and lightheadedness of 1-hour duration prior to her arrival and the ECG as shown (Figure 24–69)? She is currently asymptomatic.
    A. Adenosine
    B. Atropine sulfate
    C. Dopamine
    D. Epinephrine
    E. Transcutaneous pacing pad placement

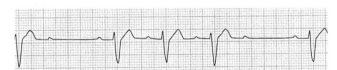

FIGURE 24–69.

70. A 49-year-old man is brought to the ED with altered mental status after being found on the street. You recognize him as one of many "frequent visitors" to your department. He has a history of alcohol dependency, and is often treated for acute intoxication. His ECG as shown (Figure 24–70). Which of the following represents the most likely diagnosis?
    A. Hypocalcemia
    B. Hyperkalemia
    C. Hypokalemia
    D. Hypomagnesemia
    E. Hypothermia

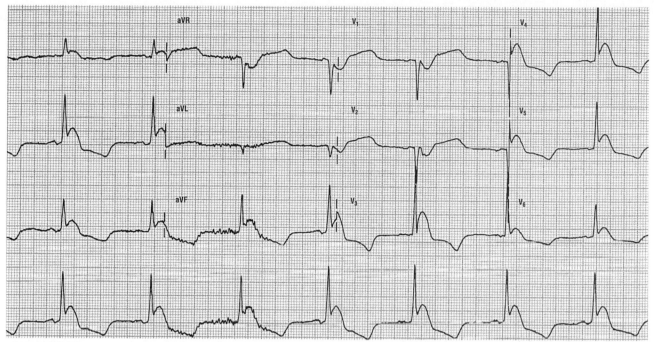

FIGURE 24–70.

71. Which of the following findings increases the likelihood of acute myocardial infarction (MI) in a patient with the ECG as shown (Figure 24–71)?

A. ST segment elevation >1 mm in V5 or V6
B. ST segment elevation >1 mm in V1, V2, or V3
C. ST segment depression >1 mm in V5 or V6
D. Presence of first-degree atrioventricular block
E. Presence of left anterior fascicular block

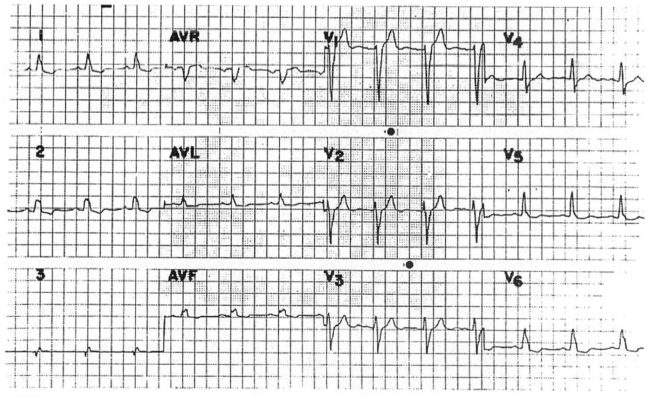

FIGURE 24–71.   (Reproduced, with permission, from Tintanalli JE, Kelen GD, Stapczynski JS: *Tintinalli's Emergency Medicine: A Comprehensive Study Guide*, 6th ed. Copyright © 2004, New York: McGraw-Hill.)

72. A 55-year-old man presents with complaints of acute chest pain and shortness of breath. Physical findings include diaphoresis and a weak distal pulse. Initial vital signs are blood pressure, 80/50 mm Hg; pulse rate, 106 beats per minute; respiratory rate, 22 breaths per minute; and room air pulse oxymetry, 95%. The nurse hands you the ECG (Figure 24–72). Which of the following represents the best therapeutic option for this patient?

A. Administration of a β-adrenergic blocker
B. Administration of dopamine via continuous intravenous infusion
C. Administration of fibrinolytic therapy
D. Immediate percutaneous coronary intervention (PCI)
E. Synchronized cardioversion

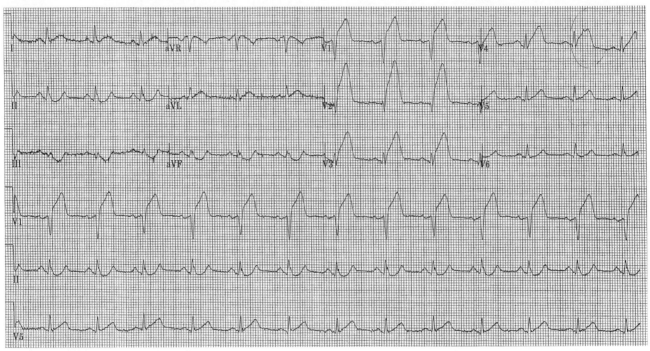

FIGURE 24–72.

73. A 27-year-old man presents to the ED with chest pain. His ECG and chest radiograph are normal at the time of your initial examination. With further questioning, the patient admits to cocaine use 25 minutes prior to presentation. Suddenly, the monitor alarm goes off, and you see the ECG (Figure 24–73). The patient remains awake and alert. Vital signs are blood pressure, 110/70 mm Hg; pulse rate, 170 beats per minute; respirations, 16 breaths per minute; and room air pulse oxymetry, 98%. Which of the following is the best treatment option now?

A. Adenosine
B. Diltiazem
C. Labetalol
D. Procainamide
E. Sodium bicarbonate

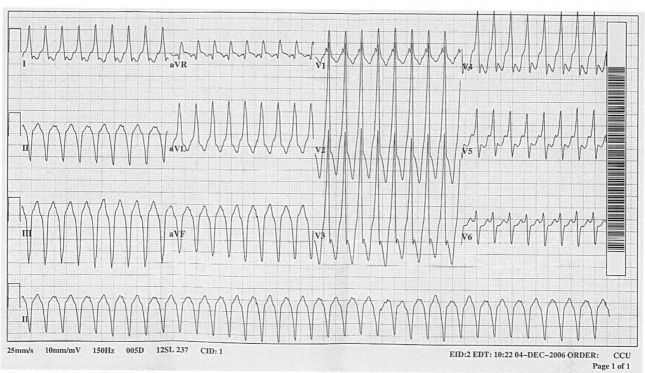

FIGURE 24–73.

74. A 25-year-old man presents 6 hours after smoking crack cocaine. He now has complaint of severe substernal chest pain. Vital signs are blood pressure, 156/86 mm Hg; pulse rate, 120 beats per minute; respiratory rate, 22 breaths per minute; and room air pulse oxymetry, 98%. His ECG as shown (Figure 24–74). Which of the following interventions should be avoided in this patient?

A. Aspirin
B. Diazepam
C. Enoxaparin
D. PCI
E. Propranolol

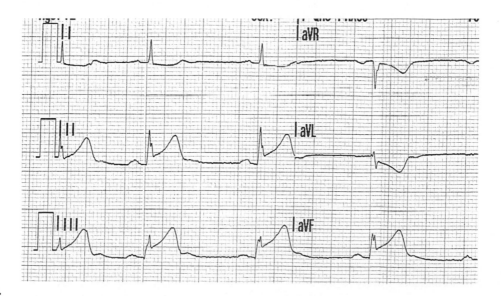

FIGURE 24–74.

75. A 67-year-old man presents to the ED with indigestion, epigastric pain, nausea, and diaphoresis. He states that the discomfort woke him from sleep this morning (~2 hours ago). When compared with prior ECGs from previous ED visits, his ECG reveals new ST segment elevations in leads II, III, and aVF. The patient receives aspirin, clopidogrel, 1 sublingual nitroglycerin tablet, morphine, and low-molecular-weight heparin. After several minutes, you notice that his blood pressure is now 70/30 mm Hg.

A repeat right-sided ECG is obtained (Figure 24–75). Which of the following interventions represents the best therapy for this patient's condition?

A. Administer metoprolol
B. Emergent fibrinolytic therapy with tenecteplase
C. Emergent fibrinolytic therapy with streptokinase
D. Emergent transfer for PCI
E. Fluid bolus of normal saline

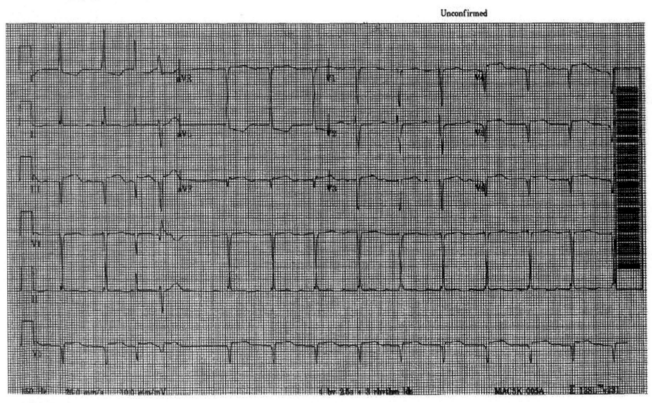

Room: 13

Vent. rate 83 bpm
PR interval 272 ms
QRS duration 96 ms
QT/QTc 412/484 ms
P-R-T axes 66 6 144

Right Sided Leads

Technician: DH
Test ind:

Unconfirmed

FIGURE 24–75.

76. A 42-year-old woman presents to the ED with complaints of palpitations and dyspnea. The nurse hands you her ECG (Figure 24–76). Which of the following most accurately describes the changes shown on her ECG?

A. Acute inferior wall myocardial infarction
B. Nonspecific ST segment depression with idioventricular conduction delay
C. QRS widening with terminal 40 millisecond right axis deviation
D. Shortened PR interval with a delta wave and a widened QRS
E. Sinus rhythm with RBBB and left ventricular hypertrophy

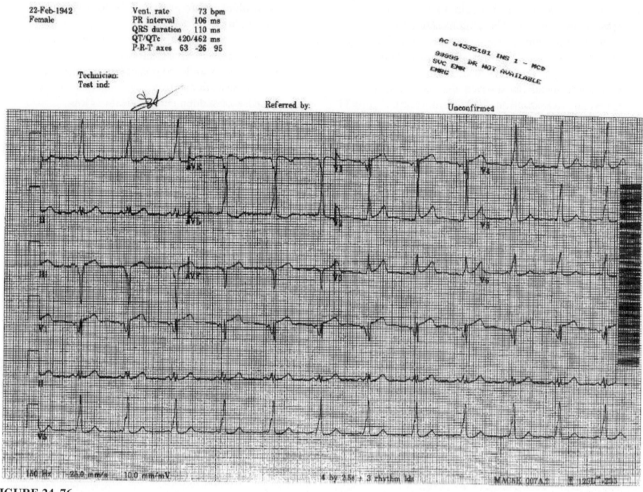

22-Feb-1942
Female

Vent. rate 73 bpm
PR interval 106 ms
QRS duration 110 ms
QT/QTc 420/462 ms
P-R-T axes 63 -26 95

Technician:
Test ind:

Referred by:

Unconfirmed

150 Hz 25.0 mm/s 10.0 mm/mV 4 by 2.5s + 3 rhythm lds MAC5K 007A2

FIGURE 24–76.

77. An 80-year-old man presents to the ED following a syncopal episode. He states that he briefly felt "palpitations," then suddenly "blacked out" without warning. His history is significant for hypertension, for which he takes a diuretic. Vital signs are blood pressure, 108/60 mm Hg; pulse rate, 60 beats per minute; respirations, 12 breaths per minute; and room air pulse oxymetry, 99%. Physical examination is unremarkable. An ECG is obtained (Figure 24–77). Which of the following represents the correct ECG interpretation?

A. First-degree AV block
B. Junctional rhythm
C. Second-degree AV block type I
D. Second-degree AV block type II
E. Third-degree AV block

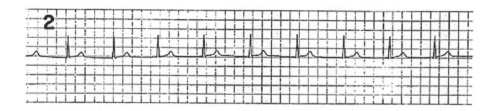

FIGURE 24–77.

78. A 14-year-old girl is brought to the ED after an episode of syncope. The patient states that she had "blacked out" while playing soccer. She also states that she has "fainted" twice previously. The mother adds that her daughter has been complaining of worsening light-headedness over the past few months. Physical examination is unremarkable. β-hCG level is <0.2 mIU/mL. A rhythm strip is obtained (Figure 24–78). Which of the following statements regarding this clinical situation is correct?

A. β-blockers are preferred for this patient's condition
B. Echocardiography confirms the diagnosis in patients with this condition
C. Nitrates should be prescribed to improve cardiac output with exertion
D. Risk of sudden cardiac death is low
E. There is no need to evaluate first-degree relatives

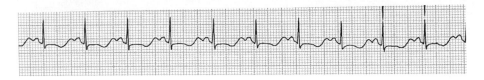

FIGURE 24–78.

79. A 39-year-old man presents with substernal chest pain. The pain had worsened progressively over the past 24 hours. He reports no past medical or surgical history, denies illicit drug or tobacco use, nor recent travel. His ECG (Figure 24–79) is pathognomonic for

I. Acute myocardial infarction
II. Pericardial effusion
III. Pericardial tamponade
IV. Pericarditis
V. Pulmonary embolus

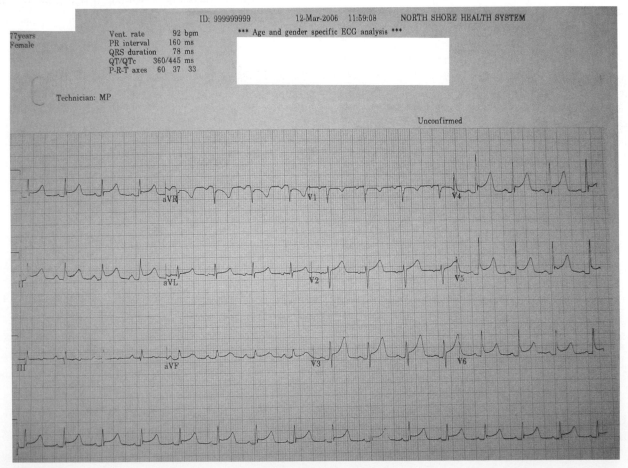

FIGURE 24–79.

The procedure which should next be considered in the evaluation of this patient is
   A. Chest radiograph
   B. CT chest with IV contrast
   C. Echocardiogram
   D. Myocardial biopsy
   E. Pericardiocentesis

80. A 29-year-old woman presents to the ED with complaints of acute dyspnea and chest pain. Vital signs are pulse rate, 120 beats per minute; respiratory rate, 22 breaths per minute; blood pressure, 80/50 mm Hg; and room air pulse oxymetry, 97%. The chest radiograph reveals an enlarged cardiac silhouette but no infiltrate, pulmonary edema, effusion, or pneumothorax. ECG reveals a sinus rhythm with low voltage. An echocardiogram is performed at the bedside (Figure 24–80). Which of the following choices represents the best intervention for this patient's condition?
   A. Afterload reduction with sodium nitroprusside
   B. Emergent thoracostomy
   C. Inotropic support with dobutamine
   D. Ultrasonographically guided pericardiocentesis
   E. Volume expansion with repeated boluses of crystalloid fluid

   Which of the following findings is most consistent with pericardial tamponade?
   A. Decreased left ventricle size
   B. Diastolic collapse of the right ventricle
   C. Presence of pericardial effusion
   D. Rhythmic swinging of the heart
   E. Variation of SVC size with inspiration

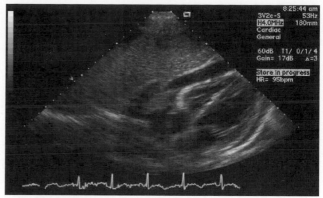

FIGURE 24–80.

81. An 80-year-old woman presents to the ED with acute chest pain. She states that the pain started 1 hour ago, radiates to the left arm and jaw, and is unrelieved with nitroglycerin. As you are evaluating the patient, she suddenly falls unconscious. She has a weak pulse. The monitor shows the rhythm as shown (Figure 24–81). Defibrillation is performed, but the patient rhythm and condition remains unchanged. Which of the following interventions is contraindicated and may worsen this patient's condition?
   A. Amiodarone
   B. Chest thrusts and bag-valve-mask ventilation
   C. Lidocaine
   D. Magnesium sulfate
   E. Procainamide

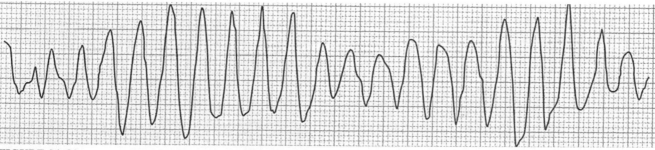

FIGURE 24–81.

82. A 75-year-old man presents to the ED with severe lumbar back pain for 5 hours. Examination of the spine is unremarkable. The abdomen is mildly tender in the epigastrium and periumbilical areas, but is otherwise soft and without rigidity. The patient is without guarding or rebound. Normal bowel sounds are heard. Vital signs are blood pressure, 82/50 mm Hg; pulse rate, 110 beats per minute; respiratory rate, 20 breaths per minute; and temperature, 37°C. Lactate is 2.5 mmol/L. Bedside ultrasound of the abdomen and pelvis is performed (Figure 24–82). Which of the following represents the most likely diagnosis based on the information presented?

    A. Abdominal aortic aneurysm leak
    B. Acute appendicitis
    C. Acute pancreatitis
    D. Mesenteric ischemia
    E. Sigmoid volvulus

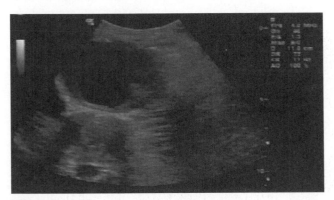

FIGURE 24–82.

83. A 64-year-old man with a past medical history of diabetes presents to the ED with 2 days of increasingly worsening abdominal pain. The pain is associated with nausea, vomiting, and chills. Vital signs are pulse rate, 120 beats per minute; temperature, 103°F (39.4°C); and blood pressure, 110/60 mm Hg. Epigastric and right upper quadrant abdominal tenderness with guarding is noted. Laboratory studies reveal a leukocytosis of 22,500/mm³, an AST 250 units/L, and an ALT 320 units/L. Amylase and lipase are normal. An image from his abdominal ultrasound as shown (Figure 24–83). What is the diagnosis for this patient's condition?

    A. Appendicitis
    B. Cholecystitis
    C. Cholelithiasis
    D. Pancreatitis
    E. Urolithiasis

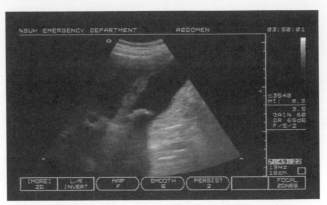

FIGURE 24–83.

84. A 32-year-old woman presents with a complaint of acute right-sided flank pain. The pain is reproducible with percussion over the right costovertebral angle, but is not pleuritic, movement-related, positional, or exertional. She had 2 episodes of vomiting with the onset of pain. She reports no recent fevers, chills, frequency, dysuria, or hematuria. Urine pregnancy test is negative. Hematuria (20 RBCs/HPF) is noted on microscopic analysis of the urine. Abdominal ultrasonography is performed as shown (Figure 24–84). Which of the following represents the correct diagnosis for this patient's condition?

    A. Acute appendicitis
    B. Acute cholecystitis
    C. Acute cholelithiasis
    D. Acute obstructing ureteral calculus
    E. Acute ovarian cyst

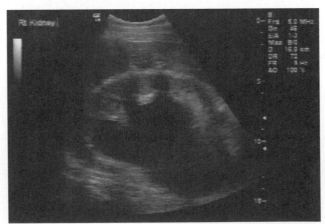

FIGURE 24–84.

85. A 32-year-old woman presents with a history of vague abdominal cramping and vaginal spotting. She reports her last menstrual period as 5 weeks ago. Pelvic examination reveals no cervical motion or adnexal tenderness, no evidence of hemorrhage within the vaginal vault, and a closed cervical os. β-hCG is 1800 mIU/mL. A transvaginal ultrasound is performed as shown (Figure 24–85). Which of the following choices represents the best management of this patient's condition?
   A. Admit for dilatation and curettage
   B. Admit for emergent laparoscopy
   C. Administer methotrexate in ED, then discharge for outpatient follow-up
   D. Administer antibiotics, then discharge with outpatient follow-up
   E. Discharge with instructions to follow-up for a repeat β-hCG in 48 hours

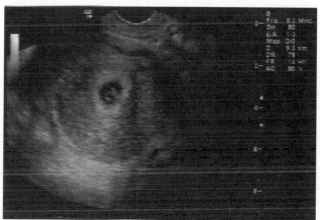

FIGURE 24–85.

86. A 23-year-old man presents to the ED immobilized on a long board and collar. He was a pedestrian struck by a motor vehicle. Vital signs on presentation are pulse rate, 120 beats per minute; respirations, 22 breaths per minute; pulse oximetry, 97%; and blood pressure, 90/60 mm Hg. The patient is awake and alert; Glasgow coma scale score is 15. The patient reports no headache or neck pain, but has chest discomfort and difficulty breathing. He is also experiencing significant bilateral upper quadrant abdominal pain; examination reveals guarding and tenderness in the left upper quadrant with palpation. The pelvis is stable, and palpation does not elicit tenderness. Fluids boluses are administered intravenously. A bedside abdominal ultrasound is performed as shown (Figure 24–86). Which of the following represents the most likely source for this patient's hemorrhage?
   A. Aorta
   B. Diaphragm
   C. Kidney
   D. Spleen
   E. Small intestine

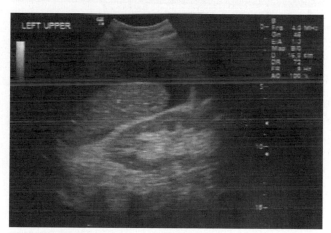

FIGURE 24–86.

87. A 76-year-old woman presents to the ED with a complaint of acute substernal chest pain of 1-hour duration. The patient reports that the pain radiates to her midback (between her scapula), her left arm, and her neck. Her vital signs are pulse rate, 80 beats per minute; respirations, 18 breaths per minute; blood pressure, 110/77 mm Hg; and pulse oximetry, 97%. Her ECG as shown (Figure 24–87). You do not have capability for PCI at your hospital; the closest facility is 2 hours away. Aspirin and a β-adrenergic antagonist are administered. Of the following choices, which is the best intervention to reduce the risk of morbidity and mortality in this patient?
   A. Administration of clopidogrel
   B. Administration of fibrinolytic therapy
   C. Administration of low molecular weight heparin
   D. Administration of unfractionated heparin
   E. Immediate transfer for emergent PCI

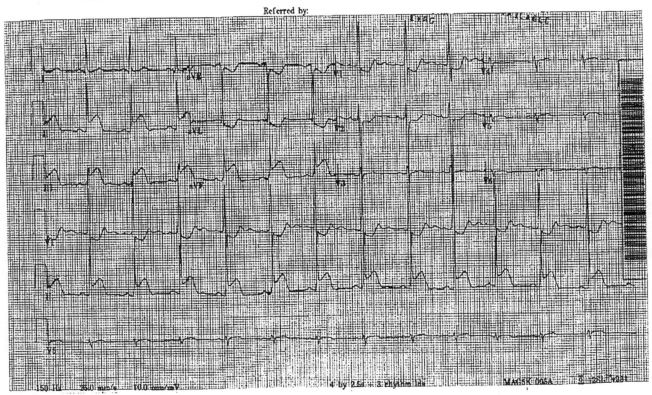

FIGURE 24–87.

88. Which of the following pharmacotherapeutics is associated with the findings in the ECG shown (Figure 24–88)?
   A. Amitriptyline
   B. Digoxin
   C. Enalapril
   D. Phenytoin
   E. Verapamil

Vent	Durations			Axes		
Rate	PR	QRS	QT/QTc	P--QRS--T		
131	0	156	384/461	999	93	43

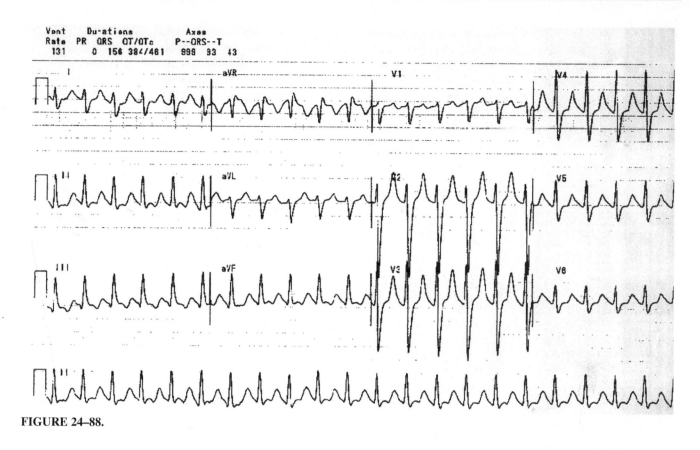

FIGURE 24–88.

89. A 68-year-old man presents to the ED with complaints of acute light-headedness and weakness following a syncopal episode. He reports no history of chest pain, shortness of breath, nausea, vomiting, or diaphoresis. His vital signs are pulse rate, 35 beats per minute; respiratory rate, 16 breaths per minute; blood pressure, 104/76 mm Hg; and room air pulse oximetry, 98%. His rhythm strip as shown (Figure 24–89). Which of the following is the correct interpretation of the findings on this patient's ECG?

A. First-degree AV block
B. Second-degree AV block type 1
C. Second-degree AV block type 2
D. Sinus rhythm with premature atrial contractions
E. Third-degree AV block

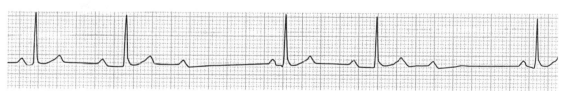

FIGURE 24–89.

90. An 82-year-old woman presents with complaints of profound weakness and fatigue. Her vital signs are pulse rate, 35 beats per minute; respiratory rate, 14 breaths per minute; blood pressure, 80/40 mm Hg; and room air pulse oximetry, 96%. Her rhythm strip as shown (Figure 24–90). Which of the following represents the best initial intervention in the ED?

A. Administration of amiodarone
B. Administration of atropine sulfate
C. Administration of sodium bicarbonate
D. Bolus of 0.9% normal saline
E. Transcutaneous pacing

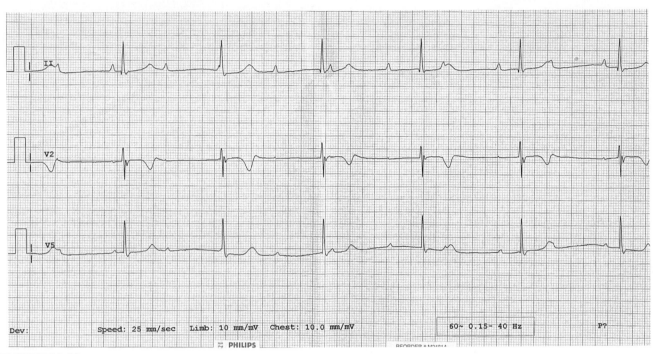

FIGURE 24–90.

91. A 76-year-old man presents with a pulse rate of 48 beats per minute and a blood pressure of 90/60 mm Hg. Serum potassium is 6.7 mEq/L, and a digoxin level is 4.9 mcg/mL. An ECG is obtained as shown (Figure 24–91). Administration of which of the following represents the best treatment for this patient's condition?

A. Calcium chloride
B. Digoxin-specific antibody fragments
C. Magnesium sulfate
D. Procainamide
E. Sodium bicarbonate

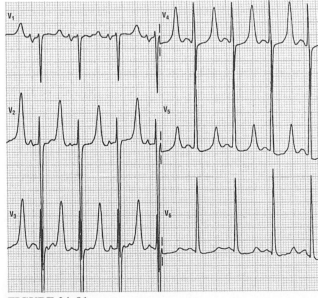

FIGURE 24–91.

92. You are evaluating a 30-year-old woman with acute right-sided abdominal pain. The pain started suddenly, with radiation to the back. Vital signs are pulse rate, 140 beats per minute; respiratory rate, 28 breaths per minute; blood pressure, 80/40 mm Hg; pulse oximetry, 96%; and temperature, 37°C. The patient looks pale. Pelvic and abdominal examinations reveal right lower quadrant tenderness. There is no vaginal bleeding. There is no history of recent trauma, fever, chills, nausea, or vomiting. You perform bedside transvaginal sonography and acquire the image shown (Figure 24–92). After initiating aggressive intravenous fluid resuscitation, you should

A. Request immediate gynecology consultation for presumed ruptured ectopic pregnancy
B. Request immediate gynecology consultation for presumed ruptured hemorrhagic ovarian cyst
C. Request immediate surgical consultation for presumed ruptured abdominal aortic aneurysm
D. Request immediate surgical consultation for presumed ruptured gallbladder
E. Request immediate surgical consultation for presumed ruptured appendix

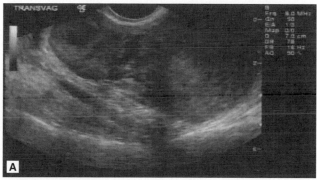
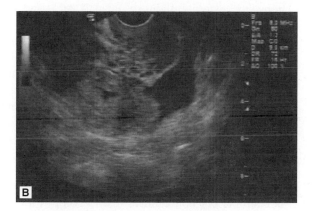

FIGURE 24–92 A, B.

93. A 62-year-old man presents with chest pain. An ECG is obtained (Figure 24–93). The findings on the ECG are consistent with

A. Accelerated idioventricular rhythm
B. Left bundle branch block
C. Right bundle branch block
D. Ventricular tachycardia
E. Wolff-Parkinson-White syndrome

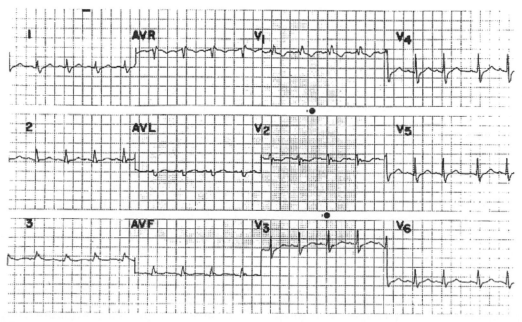

FIGURE 24–93.

1. Answer: B.The skull base comprises the floors of the anterior, middle, and posterior cranial fossae. Fractures in this region typically do not have localized symptoms. However, indirect signs of injury may include visible evidence of bleeding from the fracture into surrounding soft tissue. Ecchymosis around the mastoid bone is often described as Battle sign and periorbital ecchymosis is often described as "raccoon eyes." The most common basilar skull fracture involves the petrous portion of the temporal bone, the external auditory canal (EAC), and the tympanic membrane. It is commonly associated with a torn dura leading to cerebral spinal fluid (CSF) otorrhea or rhinorrhea. Other signs and symptoms of a basilar skull fracture include hemotympanum, vertigo, decreased hearing or deafness, and seventh nerve palsy. Periorbital and mastoid ecchymosis develops gradually over hours after an injury and are often absent in the ED. If clear or pink fluid is seen from the nose or ear and a CSF leak is suspected, the fluid can be placed on filter paper and a "halo" or double ring may appear. This is a simple but nonsensitive test to confirm a CSF leak. Evidence of open communication, such as a CSF leak, mandates neurosurgical consultation and admission (Tintinalli, 1565-1566).

2. Answer: A. The woman in the image demonstrates a Bell smile. Bell palsy is paralysis of the facial nerve and is one of the most common neuropathies of the cranial nerves. It typically occurs with abrupt onset, and is usually unilateral. Cranial nerve VII, the facial nerve, has 2 components, both of which may be affected. One portion comprises efferent fibers that stimulate the muscles of facial expression. The other portion contains taste fibers to the anterior two thirds of the tongue, and secretomotor fibers to the lacrimal and salivary glands. The path of the facial nerve is complex; which makes it vulnerable to injury.

   The definition of Bell palsy is mononeuropathy of the facial nerve, although other cranial nerves are sometimes affected. This paralysis is believed to be a result of inflammation of the nerve, possibly secondary to infection from Lyme or herpes zoster. Weakness and paralysis involves the entire face on the affected side. In supranuclear lesions (upper motor neuron) such as a cortical stroke, the upper third of the face is spared although the lower two thirds are paralyzed. This is because the orbicularis, frontalis, and corrugator muscles are innervated bilaterally. In addition, Bell palsy may cause decreased lacrimation, salivation, and decreased taste (ageusia).

   Treatment includes high-dose steroids in a short burst followed by tapering with lower doses. Treatment is most effective if administered within 48 hours. The addition of acyclovir may decrease resolution time. It is also important to have the patient tape his or her eyelid shut during sleep and to use liquid tears during the day to prevent drying and injury to the cornea.

   (B) Malingering is the intentional production of false or exaggerated symptoms motivated by primary or secondary gain, such as to obtain compensation or drugs, to avoid work or military duty, or to evade criminal prosecution. (C) Acute facial paralysis that occurs in association with herpetic blisters of the skin of the ear canal, auricle, or both is referred to as Ramsay Hunt syndrome, or herpes zoster oticus. (D) Brain tumors typically cause central nervous system (CNS) defects. (E) Because a cerebrovascular event is centrally occurring, sparring of the upper third of the face is seen.

3. Answer: B. Boutonniere deformity may manifest acutely following trauma, but most are found weeks following the injury or as the result of progressive arthritis. The proximal interphalangeal (PIP) joint of the finger is flexed, and the distal interphalangeal (DIP) joint is hyperextended.

   The deformity is due to a disruption of the central slip, which is the main component of the extensor mechanism at the PIP joint. Weakening or disruption of the central slip, with compromise of the triangular ligament results in volar migration of the lateral bands of the PIP joint. As the deformity progresses, the newly dominant flexor superficialis creates constant flexion at the PIP joint. As the intrinsic muscles (lumbrical and interosseous) lose their insertion into the middle phalanx due to the incompetent central slip, their force is diverted entirely through the lateral bands. Over time, these lateral bands migrate palmarly and contract. This is accompanied by secondary shortening of the oblique retinacular ligaments. Subsequently, these changes cause hyperextension at the DIP joint.

   (A) A swan-neck deformity, typically defined as PIP joint hyperextension with concurrent DIP joint flexion that occurs in ~50% of patients with rheumatoid arthritis. (D) A Mallet finger occurs when the extensor tendon of a finger is either forcibly stretched or avulsed from the distal phalanx and the distal portion of the finger hangs in flexion. (C) A bell-clapper deformity occurs when there is failure of normal posterior anchoring of the gubernaculum, epididymis, and testis. The bell-clapper deformity allows the testicle to twist spontaneously on the spermatic cord that causes venous occlusion and engorgement, with subsequent arterial ischemia causing infarction of the testicle. It is not relevant to orthopedic injuries.

4. Answer: B. On fundoscopic examination, the patient has a macular cherry red spot with a pale retina and less pronounced arteries. This is diagnostic of central retinal artery occlusion (CRAO). The cherry red spot represents the fovea that receives its blood supply from the vessels in the choroids. Occlusion of the central retinal blood supply is commonly caused by emboli, thrombi, vasculitis, or trauma. Treatment aims to dislodge the clot from the main artery to one of its branches and includes digital massage, vasodilation, and lowering intraocular pressure (IOP).

   (E) Acute angle-closure glaucoma usually causes painful loss of vision. (C) Central retinal vein occlusion (CRVO) presents similarly to retinal artery occlusion but is caused by thrombosis of the central retinal vein from stasis, edema, and hemorrhage. Fundoscopic examination shows diffuse retinal hemorrhages and optic disc edema, also called the "blood and thunder" fundus. (A) Retinal detachment occurs when vitreous fluid accumulates behind a retinal tear displacing the retina. On fundoscopy, the retina will be hanging in the vitreous. (D) Vitreous hemorrhage is bleeding within the posterior chamber. On fundoscopic examination, these patients have blood obstructing the view of the fundus (Tintinalli, 1460-1462).

5. Answer: C. This patient has CRVO. Additionally, the differential diagnosis for unilateral vision loss includes CRAO, anterior ischemic optic neuropathy, retinal detachment, subretinal neovascularization, and vitreous hemorrhage. The fundoscopic examination can help differentiate between these disorders as it reveals retinal hemorrhages and tortuous retinal veins in CRVO. Hemorrhages involving the whole fundus give a "blood and thunder" appearance and cotton wool spots. There is no known effective medical treatment available for either prevention or treatment of CRVO. Therefore, it is important to identify and treat any systemic medical problems, such as hypertension, diabetes, atherosclerosis, chronic glaucoma, and vasculitis, to reduce further complications. Complications of CRVO develop in a delayed fashion and include neovascularization of the retina and iris and neovascular glaucoma.

   (A and B) are treatments for CRAO. The fundus in CRAO appears pale and sparing of the fovea creates the cherry-red spot, the retinal venules have a boxcar appearance although the arterioles are narrow and irregular. Note that (A) is also part of the treatment for glaucoma. Optic neuritis presents with pain, is retrobulbar and does not change the appearance of the optic disk. Computed tomography (CT) scan of the head and neurology consultation are not indicated.

6. Answer: D. The patient has disseminated gonococcemia, caused by the presence of *Neisseria gonorrhoeae* in the blood stream. The clinical manifestations of this process are biphasic, with an early bacteremic phase consisting of tenosynovitis, arthralgias, and dermatitis, followed by a localized phase consisting of localized septic arthritis. ~75% of patients experience a dermatitis that varies from macular or papular to vesicular or pustular to necrotic or hemorrhagic erythema. The skin lesions are commonly in multiple stages of development. They are generally located on the distal extremities with sparing of the face, scalp, palms, soles, and trunk. Lesions can be painful but are usually asymptomatic, and they resolve in 4 to 7 days even without treatment.

   (A) *Rickettsia rickettsii* is the causative organism of Rocky Mountain spotted fever (RMSF). Most often the rash begins as small, flat, pink, nonitchy macules on the wrists, forearms, and ankles. The rash involves the palms or soles in as high as 50% to 80% of patients; however, this distribution may not occur until later in the course of the disease. As high as 10% to 15% of patients may never develop a rash. (B) *Treponema pallidum* is the causative agent of syphilis. Typically, early lesions are round, discrete, nonpruritic, and symmetric macules distributed on the trunk and proximal extremities. Red papular lesions also may appear on the palms, soles, face, and scalp and may become necrotic. (C) *Borrelia burgdorferi* is the causative agent of Lyme disease. Classic erythema migrans rash is an erythematous papule or macule that occurs at the site of the tick bite and often involves a central punctum. The rash is described as a "bulls-eye" rash. (E) *Neisseria meningitidis* is the causative agent in meningococcemia. Lesions commonly begin on the trunk and legs. The confluence of lesions results in hemorrhagic patches, often with central necrosis.

7. Answer: B. Ethylene glycol is a colorless, odorless, slightly sweet-tasting liquid that is found in antifreeze. Ingestions of antifreeze are either accidental, suicidal, or in substitute of ethanol. Ethylene glycol is metabolized to glycolic acid, which results in a profound anion gap metabolic acidosis. Glycolic acid is subsequently metabolized to oxalic acid, that combines with calcium to form calcium oxalate crystals, which then precipitate in renal tubules, brain, and other tissues. The finding of crystalluria is considered the hallmark of ethylene glycol ingestion, however, its absence does not rule out the diagnosis. Another useful test in the ED involves examining freshly voided urine for fluorescence with a Wood lamp. Sodium fluorescein is added to antifreeze to aid in the detection of radiator leaks (Marx, 2129-2133).

(A) Carbon monoxide poisoning can cause a metabolic acidosis. However, this patient's CO level is within normal limits. (C) Diabetic ketoacidosis can cause a metabolic acidosis. Patients usually have a history of diabetes, elevated blood glucose (>200 mg/dL), and ketones in their urine. (D) Lactic acidosis can cause a metabolic acidosis. In normal aerobic metabolism, glucose is generated into 2 molecules of pyruvate, which are transferred into the mitochondria and metabolized into CO_2 and H_2O. Lactic acid is generated when pyruvate is produced in an anaerobic environment. Lactic acidosis results when lactate production exceeds the bodies buffer systems. This occurs when tissue oxygenation does not adequately meet metabolic requirements. Classically, very high lactic acid levels represent ischemic gut or sepsis, but clinical impression is important because the causes are variable. This patient's lactate is within normal limits. (E) The patient has a normal creatinine level.

8. Answer: B. The picture suggests pityriasis rosea. A herald patch can be identified in this image on the patient's left sternal boarder inferior and medial to the left areola. The differential for pityriasis includes secondary syphilis, tinea versicolor, and drug eruptions. The most important disease to rule out in this case is secondary syphilis. Pityriasis rosea may have prodromal symptoms (eg, malaise, nausea, anorexia, fever, joint pain, lymph node swelling, and headache) that may precede the appearance of the herald patch. No bacteria, virus, or fungus has been isolated as a definite causative agent, although human herpes virus (HHV)-6 and HHV-7 may play a role. Although antihistamines will relieve the patient's symptoms, the question asks for the most important management step. Steroids are the treatment of choice for drug eruption, and KOH will help diagnose tinea versicolor.

9. Answer: C. This patient has acute angle-closure glaucoma, when the aqueous humor production in the posterior chamber of the eye is unable to drain through the anterior chamber and the resultant obstruction causes acutely increased IOP. This condition is precipitated by abrupt pupillary dilation either secondary to use of sympathomimetics and anticholinergics, or, more commonly, going from daylight into a darkened room. On examination, patients with increased IOP have a middilated, nonreactive pupil with corneal clouding and decreased vision. The diagnosis is confirmed by checking the IOP with a tono-pen or tono-meter. Checking IOP is a simple, rapid test that should be performed on all patients with headache and orbital pain. Normal IOP is 10 to 21 mm Hg. If this test is negative, other causes of headache and eye pain should be investigated. Patients with increased IOP should be treated with medications to decrease production of aqueous humor. Treatment includes placing the patient supine, which may cause the lens to pull away from the iris. Pharmacologic intervention aims to decrease IOP by decreasing aqueous humor production and increasing out-flow. Decrease in production is achieved using topical β-blockers, α-agonists, and carbonic anhydrase inhibitors. A miotic like pilocarpine may be used to contract the iris sphincter opening the trabecular meshwork and facilitating the exit of the aqueous humor. Topical steroids may reduce inflammation (Tintinalli, 1459, 1461-1462).

10. Answer: A. Dysuria in young males is often due to urethritis, which is commonly caused by a sexually transmitted disease. Urethritis is classically divided into gonococcal (GU) and nongonococcal (NGU) types. GU is caused by *Neisseria gonorrhoeae*, although the major pathogen in NGU is *Chlamydia trachomatis*. Nearly all males with GU have purulent urethral discharge. NGU may be asymptomatic or with a yellow, mucopurulent discharge. Multiple studies have demonstrated that the two pathogens coexist in males with urethritis up to 50% of the time. Therefore, antibiotics should be directed at eliminating both organisms. A third-generation cephalosporin or azithromycin (2 g) as a single dose is used to treat GU. The use of fluoroquinolones is no longer recommended as first-line agents because of increasing resistance. Common antibiotics used

to treat NGU include azithromycin (1 g) as a single dose **or** doxycycline or erythromycin for 7 days (Marx, 1413-1414).

(B) This choice might be correct if you suspect a patient has a urinary tract infection. However, a young male with dysuria and urethral discharge needs to be treated for a sexually transmitted disease. (C) The patient should not be discharged prior to treatment and culture. In addition, the patient should refer all of their sexually partners for evaluation and treatment. (D and E) There is no clinical suspicion for a kidney stone or testicular cancer.

11. Answer: B. The patient has herpes zoster, or shingles, an infection caused by the varicella-zoster virus. The patient's rash most likely involves the ophthalmic division of the trigeminal nerve. In addition, the vesicles found on the tip of the patient's nose correlate strongly with viral involvement of the eye (Hutchinson sign). Ocular complications that involve the ophthalmic division of the trigeminal nerve occur in 20% to 70% of patients. Severity varies from mild conjunctivitis to panophthalmitis, retinitis, and blindness. In addition, the patient is at risk for anterior uveitis, secondary glaucoma, and corneal scarring. ED care includes local wound care, adequate analgesia, starting antiviral agents, and antibiotics for secondary bacterial infection. When the blinking reflex and eyelid function are compromised, an eye lubricant is needed to prevent corneal desiccation injury. Treatment with antivirals is optimal if started within 72 hours of rash onset. Antivirals are also required if there is any suspicion for eye involvement. If a patient complains of severe pain at or beyond the appearance of crusted vesicles, the clinician should strongly suspect that postherpetic neuralgia has developed. Treatment of postherpetic neuralgia is complex. A multifaceted, patient-specific approach is important. Clinical trials have demonstrated that opioids, tricyclic antidepressants, and anticonvulsants (ie, carbamazepine, gabapentin) may reduce the severity or duration of postherpetic neuralgia, either as single agents or in combination (Marx, 1656-1657).

12. Answer: C. Ludwig angina is a potentially fatal disease that can progress to death within hours. It is a progressive cellulitis of the floor of the mouth and neck that begins in the submandibular space. A dental cause, such as an extraction or dental abscess, is present in ~90% of patients. The most common symptoms include dysphagia, neck pain, and swelling. Physical findings include bilateral submandibular swelling, tongue swelling, and protrusion. A tense edema and induration of the neck may occur that is described as a "bull neck." Management involves securing an airway in either the ED or operating room depending on the progression of symptoms and starting intravenous antibiotic therapy immediately. There is debate on whether these patients should be managed surgically with incision and drainage or medically with antibiotics.

(A) Acute mastoiditis usually presents with swelling of the mastoid, fever, and earache. (B) Peritonsillar abscess typically presents with a fluctuant soft palate mass. (D) ANUG (acute necrotizing ulcerative gingivitis) is an infection of the gingival, typical caused by the anaerobic *Fusobacterium* and spirochetes. Poor oral hygiene, stress, smoking, and immunocompromised states contribute to the predisposition to ANUG. Treatment is typically supportive with the addition of antibiotics that cover oropharyngeal bacteria. (E) Pharyngitis is limited to the oropharynx and should not involve the tissues of the neck (Marx, 977-978).

13. Answer: D. A hyphema is a collection of blood in the anterior chamber of the eye. Blunt or penetrating trauma to the globe is the most common cause. Hyphemas are graded according to the amount of blood that is visible in the anterior chamber. Minimal blood (<30%) is grade 1 and may be managed as an outpatient. Grade 4 is referred to as an eight-ball hyphema and represents hemorrhage that completely fills the anterior chamber.

Symptoms of hyphema include pain, blurry vision, and photophobia. Predispositions for hyphemas include sickle-cell disease, glaucoma, and anticoagulation with warfarin or aspirin. Thorough examination of the eye and appropriate consultation with an ophthalmologist should be obtained to exclude a penetrating globe injury, retained ocular foreign body, and acute glaucoma. Rebleeding is one of the most common complications. Therefore, patients should receive close follow-up by an ophthalmologist if they are discharged from the ED.

Treatment traditionally involves bed rest, head elevation, and application shield to the injured eye. Additionally, patients may be treated with corticosteroids, cycloplegics, miotics, and aminocaproic acid; aimed at decreasing inflammation, increasing absorption of pooled blood and prevention of rebleeding. Sedation is recommended only in the extremely apprehensive individual. Surgical intervention is necessary only if the IOP is >50 mm Hg or (35 mm Hg with sickle-cell disease) or if there is inadequate resolution >4 days.

(A) Acute angle-closure glaucoma occurs when the aqueous humor production in the posterior chamber of the eye is unable to drain through the anterior chamber and the resultant obstruction causes increased IOP. On examination, patients with increased IOP have a middilated, nonreactive pupil with corneal clouding and decreased vision. (B) Globe rupture occurs when the integrity of the outer membranes of the eye is disrupted by blunt or penetrating trauma. This may be detected by a Seidel test, which is positive if streaming of aqueous fluid is noted after placing fluorescein in the eye. (C) A hordeolum is a localized infection or inflammation of the eyelid margin that involves hair follicles of the eyelashes or meibomian glands. A hordeolum is typically painful, erythematous, and localized. (E) A hypopyon is accumulation of pus in the anterior chamber of the eye. This condition is most often seen following a penetrating trauma to the eye.

14. Answer: C. The picture is consistent with erythema nodosum. These are smooth, shiny, red, tender inflammatory nodules that usually appear on the anterior tibia. They result from a hypersensitivity reaction to the subcutaneous fat causing panniculitis. Erythema nodosum may be precipitated by drugs, systemic illness, or infection. Drugs that lead to erythema nodosum include oral contraceptive pills and sulfa-containing medications. Common infectious etiologies include *Streptococcus*, *Mycoplasma*, Epstein-Barr virus, tuberculosis, and fungal infections; although autoimmune etiologies include inflammatory bowel disease (IBD) and Behcets. Most patients are idiopathic or secondary to a recent streptococcal infection. Treatment is supportive and includes NSAIDs, compressive leg dressings, and elevation of the effected extremity. Corticosteroids are not recommended as they may exacerbate underlying TB, lymphoma, or mycoses. Syphilitic gummas should be considered in patients with painful nodular lesions; however, it does not lead to erythema nodosum.

15. Answer: E. Analysis of abdominal fluid and clinical presentation are consistent with spontaneous bacterial peritonitis (SBP). This entity occurs in up to 33% of patients with liver disease and ascites. You should suspect this diagnosis in patients with liver disease who present with fever, abdominal tenderness, progressive ascites, and declining hepatic function. The condition is diagnosed by paracentesis and evaluation of the ascetic fluid. It is recommended to start antibiotic treatment for SBP if the neutrophil count is >250 cells/mm^3. An ascites lactate level of >25 mg/dL was found to be 100% sensitive and specific in predicting SBP in a recent retrospective analysis. Moreover, the combination of an ascites fluid pH of <7.35 and polymorphonuclear count of >500 cells/mL was 100% sensitive and 96% specific. A positive culture is diagnostic. Causative organisms include Gram-negative enterics such as *E. coli, Streptococcus sp., Klebsiella,* and *S. pneumoniae.* Therefore, the most appropriate antibiotic for treatment is a third-generation cephalosporin such as cefotaxime or ceftriaxone (Marx, 1261).

16. Answer: D. The rash shown in this patient is a petechial rash. In some areas, the petechiae coalesced to form small purpura. With progression of meningococcemia, pustules, bullae, and hemorrhagic lesions with central necrosis can develop. Stellate purpura with a central gunmetal-gray hue is characteristic and should be considered highly suggestive of meningococcemia. This rash is the sine qua non of meningococcemia. Meningococcemia is caused by the bacteria, *Neisseria meningitidis.* The early clinical presentation is vague with flu-like symptoms. However, symptoms progress rapidly over hours. If the rash is overlooked and the diagnosis missed, patients with meningococcemia progressively worsen to shock, disseminated intravascular coagulopathy, and multiorgan failure, culminating in seizures, coma, and death. Therefore, management requires prompt diagnosis, isolation, early antibiotic coverage with a third-generation cephalosporin such as ceftriaxone, which penetrates sufficiently into the CSF from blood and has a potent action against meningococci. The patient should be placed in intensive care with supportive management and anticipation of complications such as hypotension and coagulapathy. Prophylaxis of contacts should be provided with rifampin or ciprofloxacin.

(A) Idiopathic thrombocytopenic purpura (ITP) is defined as isolated thrombocytopenia with normal bone marrow and the absence of other causes of thrombocytopenia. Patients with ITP may present with petechiae, bruising, nosebleeds, and bleeding gums. However, bleeding normally does not occur unless the platelet count is below 10,000/mm^3. Treatment for ITP is generally supportive. A red blood cell transfusion is indicated for anemia or hypotension. Steroids can be administered with recent studies demonstrating better efficacy of high-dose dexamethasone for initial treatment. Intravenous immunoglobulin G (IVIG) is recommended for platelet counts <5000 in patients who have received steroids. For life-threatening bleeding, a platelet transfusion may be indicated. In patients with chronic refractory ITP, splenectomy can be performed. (B) Thrombotic thrombocytopenic purpura (TTP) is a syndrome characterized by microangiopathic hemolytic anemia, thrombocytopenia, neurologic abnormalities, fever, and renal dysfunction. The recommended first-line treatment is plasmaphoresis and infusion of fresh frozen plasma. In addition, the patient can receive corticosteroids. Antiplatelet agents such as aspirin or dipyridamole are controversial, but have been used with variable outcomes. Platelet transfusion should be avoided except for life-threatening hemorrhage as platelets may increase thrombus formation in the microcirculation. (C) Henoch-Schonlein purpura (HSP) is a vasculitis that results with a classic clinical triad that includes a characteristic palpable purpuric rash, typically on the buttock and lower extremity, migratory arthritis, and colicky abdominal pain. This condition occurs most commonly in school-aged children and young adults. (E) RMSF is caused by *Rickettsia rickettsii*, which is transmitted by ticks. The organism multiplies in endothelial cells lining small vessels that cause generalized vasculitis as well as headache, fever, confusion, rash, myalgias, and shock. The rash usually appears on day 2 to 3, initially on the wrists, ankles, palms, and soles, and spreads rapidly to the extremities and trunk. Treatment with doxycycline results in resolution of this infection.

17. Answer: C. Bursitis is inflammation of a bursa caused by repetitive use, trauma, infection, or systemic inflammatory disease. Bursae are flattened sacs that serve as a protective buffer between bones and overlapping muscles tendons and skin. These synovial-lined sacs are filled with minimal amounts of fluid to facilitate movement during muscle contraction. Symptoms of bursitis may include localized tenderness, edema, erythema, and/or reduced movement. This patient has **olecranon** bursitis. This condition is relatively common, particularly in those who spend significant amounts of time with flexed elbows. This is commonly referred to "student's elbow." Treatment includes NSAIDs and compressive dressings. Aspiration is rarely recommended as fluid often reaccumulates and there is an increased risk of infection associated with the procedure.

Another form of bursitis is septic bursitis, which occurs from introduction of microorganisms through traumatic injury or through contiguous spread from cellulitis. Trauma of the skin and surrounding tissues makes the olecranon a frequent location for infectious bursitis. Patients with fever, bursa tenderness, erythema, warmth, and peribursal cellulitis should be suspected to have septic bursitis. These patients should undergo aspiration of their bursal fluid for cell count and culture to distinguish septic bursitis from aseptic bursitis. In addition, they should be treated with antibiotics while awaiting culture results. The most common causative organism is *Staphylococcus aureus* followed by *Streptococci*. Superficial septic bursitis can be treated with oral outpatient therapy. Those with systemic symptoms or who are immunocompromised may require admission for intravenous antibiotics.

(A) Gout is inflammation caused by monosodium urate monohydrate (MSU) crystals. The classic picture is of excruciating and sudden pain, swelling, redness, warmness, and stiffness in the joint. Low-grade fever may also be present. Evaluation of synovial fluid reveals needle-shaped crystals that exhibit negative birefringence under polarized light. (B) Typically, a fracture presents with pain. (D) Septic arthritis is an infection of a joint space, most commonly the knee, followed by the hip, shoulder, and wrist. Patients present with a warm, tender, erythematous, swollen joint, and pain with passive range of motion. Fever and chills are common. Arthrocentesis is diagnostic with joint fluid demonstrating a WBC count >50,000/μL with >75% granulocytes. *S. aureus* remains the predominant pathogen for all age groups. In young adults gonococcal septic arthritis is common. If there is any concern for a septic joint, arthrocentesis must be performed. Albeit, if a coincident cellulitis is present over the involved joint, arthrocentesis may need to be delayed since aspiration through cellulitis will seed the joint with the infectious microorganism. (E) Tumors generally do not grow this rapidly.

18. Answer: B. This patient suffers from otitis externa (OE), or "swimmer ear." This is an infection of the EAC, characterized by pain, pruritis, and tenderness of the external ear. Signs and symptoms include erythema and edema of the EAC, which may spread to the tragus and auricle. Likewise, patients may complain of fever, pruritis, clear or purulent otorrhea, and crusting of the EAC. The most common organisms responsible for OE are *Pseudomonas aeruginosa* and *Staphylococcus aureus,* although these organisms are often not isolated from suspect water samples. Treatment

includes cleansing the ear canal of debris by means of suction, irrigation, or gentle curettage. Mild nonpurulent infections can be treated with acetic solution with hydrocortisone. More progressed infections can be treated with a combination of polymyxin B and neomycin sulfate with hydrocortisone. It is important to use a suspension of these antibiotics if there is suspicion or confirmation of a ruptured tympanic membrane as it is less toxic to structures of the middle ear. If significant edema is present, a wick should be inserted to facilitate even distribution of local medications into the external ear canal. The patient should avoid getting fluid into his ear for up to 3 weeks. If cellulitis is present, a systemic antibiotic should be prescribed.

(A), (C), and (D) *S. pneumoniae,* nontypeable *H. influenzae,* and *Moraxella catarrhalis* are the three most common bacterial causes of otitis media. In children aged 6 months to 3 years an infection of the middle ear is usually secondary to a viral upper respiratory infection (URI). (E) Newborns can get supporative otitis media with *E. coli*, but it is not a common pathogen for otitis externa (Tintinalli, 1466-1469).

19. Answer: D. Angioedema is swelling that occurs in response to allergic or inflammatory triggers. Edema typically develops in the periorbital and perioral regions, but may involve other areas. It differs from urticaria because it involves deeper layers of skin. Clinically, this results in less pruritis than is seen with urticarial eruptions. Regardless of the etiology, the common final pathway to angioedema is increased levels of bradykinin, a potent vasodilator.

You recall that C1 activates the classic pathway of the compliment system, ultimately leading to activation of C3 that activates formation of the membrane-attacking complex (MAC), as well as increasing levels of bradykinin. C1 levels and activity are controlled by C1 inhibitor protein. Individuals who suffer from hereditary angioedema (HAE) lack C1 inhibitor and thus have a predisposition to angioedema. In individuals with HAE triggers include trauma, heat and cold exposure, and exercise.

Angioedema may result from allergic triggers such as foods (particularly shrimp), drugs, and insect stings. ACE inhibitors uniquely result in angioedema by inhibiting enzymatic activity of ACE which functions in part to inactivate bradykinin. As such, this medication directly causes increased levels in bradykinin.

Empiric therapy may include antihistamines, corticosteroids, epinephrine, and glucagon. Although, the response is variable if HAE is the underlying condition. In this situation, C1 esterase concentrate should be provided. If not available, fresh frozen plaza, which contains C1 esterase inhibitor, should be given.

20. Answer: E. The image illustrates papilledema. The patient most likely has idiopathic intracranial hypertension (pseudotumor cerebri), a neurologic disease seen primarily in young obese women of childbearing age. Clinically, patients complain of a generalized headache of gradual onset and moderate severity. It may worsen with eye movements or with the valsalva maneuver. Visual complaints are common and may occur several times a day and can become permanent in 10% of patients. Patients typically have papilledema and may develop visual field defects on physical examination. Diagnosis is made by a normal neuroimaging scan and an elevated intracerebral pressure (>200 mm H_2O) measured by the opening pressure from a lumbar puncture. Management involves lowering intracerebral pressure and treating the headache with analgesics. Acetazolamide, a carbonic anhydrase inhibitor, in combination with a loop diuretic or alone can be used to decrease CSF production. Repeat lumbar punctures is another option but many patients find this undesirable. Visual field testing is an important part of the management of these patients. Those with impending visual loss or incapacitation symptoms should have a ventricular shunt or optic nerve sheath fenestration performed (Marx, 1463-1464).

21. Answer: C. HSP is a vasculitis that results in a characteristic palpable purpuric rash, typically on the buttock and lower extremity, in school-aged children and young adults. Often, there is an antecedent URI. In addition to the rash, other symptoms include arthralgias, hematuria, abdominal pain, headaches, malaise, and fever. The emergent concerns in patients with HSP include recognition of significant gastrointestinal bleeding, evaluation for intussusception, and determination if there is significant renal involvement. Most cases are self-limited; however, severe cases with systemic manifestations require admission for supportive care including corticosteroids and cytoxic immunosuppressive therapy. If the vasculitis follows an infection, antibiotics should be administered.

(A) The sudden appearance of petechiae and ecchymosis in no particular distribution over the body may signal a decrease in platelets. ITP is a common cause of an acute low platelet count in children. ITP is thought to be caused by IgG antiplatelet antibodies that develop in response to a viral infection. The antibodies fix to normal platelets that are subsequently destroyed. Many children have mild, self-limited illnesses. Ecchymosis appears spontaneously on areas of the body that are not prone to trauma such as the abdomen and chest. In severe cases, internal bleeding can occur with intracerebral hemorrhage being the most serious complication. Most cases are self-limited and require only supportive care. With more severe cases, steroids have been used to decrease abnormal antibodies. Intravenous γ globulin is also given to interrupt the platelet destruction. Splenectomy is a management strategy for patients who have recurrent or episodes or whose illness does not remit spontaneously. (B) TTP is caused by increased platelet destruction. In TTP, platelet-fibrin thrombi deposit in vessels and cause injury to RBCs and platelets, resulting in microangiopathy hemolytic anemia (resulting in schistocytes on peripheral blood smear) and thrombocytopenia. Patients tend to be females aged 10 to 45 years. Risk factors include pregnancy, autoimmune disorders (eg, SLE), infection, allogenic bone marrow transplantation, malignancy, and medications. The pentad can be recalled with the mnemonic FAT RN: **F**ever, hemolytic **A**nemia, **T**hrombocytopenia, **R**enal failure, and **N**eurologic change (waxing and waning mental status). Treatment includes daily plasmaphoresis until platelet count normalizes. RBCs may be transfused in patients symptomatic from anemia. All patients with TTP should be admitted to an ICU for close monitoring of acute bleeds. (D and E) Meningococcemia and RMSF are both life-threatening illnesses that if not diagnosed early, have a high mortality. The rash of meningococcemia is petechial in nature with areas that coalesce to form small purpura. The rash of RMSF typically begins around the wrists and ankles, but it may start on the trunk or be diffuse at the onset. Classic distribution of the rash on the palms and soles occurs relatively late in the course. Up to 80% of patients may not exhibit this classic distribution.

22. Answer: C. The image demonstrates the pathology associated with envenomations caused by coelenterates, which are responsible for many marine envenomations. Some familiar coelenterates include the Portuguese man-of-war, fire coral, true jellyfish, box jellyfish, and sea anemones. This patient was stung by a true jellyfish. Each of these organisms has toxins present in nematocysts located in tentacles or near the mouth opening. Upon mechanical trauma or chemical stimulation, the jellyfish release its toxin into the skin of its victims. Most toxins contain histamine, catecholamines, hyaluronidases, kinins, and various other hemolytic, cardiotoxic, and dermatonecrotic toxins. The most common clinical manifestation of marine envenomations is the development of a painful, pruritic, papular-urticarial rash. Rarely, these stings lead to anaphylaxis, cardiovascular collapse, and even death. Management of these conditions in the ED includes inactivation of nematocysts with the use of dilute acetic acid or salt-water, removal of nematocysts with forceps or a razor, and administration of antihistamines and corticosteroids. Tetanus prophylaxis should also be administered. Antibiotics are not typically recommended.

23. Answer: B. The ferning, dendritic, feathering rash shown in the image is a characteristic burn associated with a lightning strike. Lightning injuries are brief, high-intensity bursts of direct current (DC). Lightning causes injuries through several mechanisms: a direct strike (high mortality), flash discharge (splash of lightning from a nearby object struck by lightning, such as a tree), direct contact (direct transmission of lightning from touching an object directly struck, such as a light post), flashover (lightning conducted over the surface of the body), ground contact, and secondary blunt trauma. These injuries may inflict fractures, cardiovascular collapse, burns, blunt abdominal injuries, and neurological damage. Rupture of the tympanic membranes is a common associated injury due to the outflow tract of the lightning strike and it is important to check for blood in the ear canals of these patients. It is important to quickly assess the ABCs of these patients and establish an airway. Immobilization of the cervical spine is often indicated as well as close ECG monitoring for ventricular arrhythmias. The most common cause of death is asystole. Patients should be admitted for observation after obtaining baseline laboratories. A noncontrast head CT scan should be ordered for patients with altered mental status. Although 50 to 300 people die each year in the United States caused by lightning strikes, most injuries sustained are not lethal.

24. Answer: D. The patient has signs suggestive of erythema multiforme (EM), an acute inflammatory skin disease that ranges from a localized

eruption (EM minor) to a severe multisystem illness (EM major) with extensive vesiculobullous lesions and erosion of the mucous membranes known as Stevens-Johnson syndrome (SJS). It affects all age groups with the highest incidence in males aged 20 to 40 years. Death is usually a result of infection and dehydration. As in this case, patients with severe disease should be admitted. Therapy consists of intravenous fluids, cessation of suspected inciting agent, analgesics, antihistamines, mouth rinses, and skin care. Although no causative factor can be found in 50% of cases, known triggers include infection, especially *Mycoplasma* and herpes simplex virus, drugs (especially, sulphas and sulphonylureas), anticonvulsants, and antibiotics (especially penicillin), and malignancies. It is important to get an ophthalmology consult if there is ocular involvement to evaluate for corneal adhesions and ulcerations. Because of the significant fluid loss and susceptibility to infections, these patients are treated analogously to burn patients and should be transferred to a burn center. Death is most often due to fulminant sepsis.

(A), (B), and (C) Because of the high morbidity and mortality, patients with EM, especially the more severe form, SJS, should be admitted to the hospital. Outpatient therapy of EM minor with topical steroids is possible. Patients with extensive disease, systemic toxicity, or mucous membrane involvement require hospitalization, optimally in an intensive care unit or a burn unit. (E) Systemic steroids provide symptomatic relief but this benefit must be weighed against the increased risk of infection. There is no proven benefit of systemic steroids in altering the duration and outcome of SJS, as such, this should not be included in the ED management, but may be added to the patients treatment regimen once stabilized (Tintinalli, 1513).

25. Answer: A. This patient suffers from toxic shock syndrome (TSS), a severe, life-threatening syndrome characterized by high fever, diffuse macular erythroderma, hypotension, and desquamation. TSS can rapidly progress to multisystem dysfunction and shock. TSS was initially recognized as a disease of young, healthy, menstruating women, in which tampon use increased the risk 33 times. With increased awareness and changes in tampon composition, cases of TSS declined over the past 20 years. *Staphylococcus aureus* is the causative organism. An exotoxin produced by *S. aureus* is the presumed cause in menstrual-related TSS (MRTSS) and two endotoxins have been implicated in nonmenstrual-related TSS (NMRTSS). TSS should be considered in any unexplained febrile illness associated with erythroderma, hypotension, and diffuse organ pathology. Patients with MRTSS usually present between the third and fifth day of menses. In severe cases, headache is the most common complaint. The rash is a diffuse, blanching erythroderma, often described as a painless "sunburn" that fades within 3 days and is followed by desquamation, especially of the palms and soles. For severe cases, treatment includes aggressive IV fluid resuscitation, IV oxacillin or cefazolin, and hospital admission in a monitored setting. For all patients, the tampon needs to be removed. For patients with epistaxis who receive a nasal tampon, antibiotics are administered to prevent a similar syndrome (Tintinalli, 870-871, 913-918, 1517-1519).

(B) RMSF is caused by *Rickettsia rickettsii*, which is transmitted by ticks. The organism multiplies in endothelial cells lining small vessels, causing generalized vasculitis as well as headache, fever, confusion, rash, myalgias, and shock. The rash usually appears on day 2 to 3, initially on the wrists, ankles, palms, and soles, spreading rapidly to the extremities and trunk. Lesions begin as small, erythematous blanching macules that become maculopapular and petechial. The location and type of rash, in addition to the history distinguish RMSF from TSS. Serologic tests are confirmatory, but treatment with doxycycline or chloramphenicol should be started prior to confirmation. (C) Streptococcal scarlet fever is an acute febrile illness primarily affecting young children, caused by *Streptococcus pyogenes* (group A streptococci [GAS]). The "sandpaper" rash of scarlet fever differs from the macular "sunburn" rash of TSS. Rheumatic fever is a rare complication of Group A streptococcus infections and can be prevented by treatment of the infection within 1 to 2 weeks of the infection. Glomerulonephritis, another complication, is not prevented by treatment of the infection. The treatment is penicillin or a macrolide in penicillin-allergic patients. Although *S. aureus* is the causative organism of TSS, a less common, but more aggressive, TSS-like syndrome, streptococcal TSS (STSS), has emerged recently. The treatment is similar to TSS, with aggressive fluid management along with IV penicillin and clindamycin. These patients may progress to a necrotizing fasciitis or myositis, requiring surgical intervention. (D) Meningococcemia is an infectious vasculitis caused by disseminated *Neisseria meningitides,* a Gram-negative diplococcus. Fever, headache, arthralgias, altered mental status, and abnormal vitals may also be found, in addition to neck stiffness. There is no indication of meningeal irritation in this patient. Furthermore, the rash of meningococcemia is distinctly different from that of TSS, as it presents as petechial, hemorrhagic vesicles, macules, and papules with surrounding erythema, especially on the trunk and extremities. The treatment is IV ceftriaxone. (E) Disseminated gonococcemia, usually seen in young, sexually active females, is caused by *Neisseria gonorrhoeae*. The rash of gonococcemia is pustular with an erythematous base, rather than petechial and hemorrhagic, as are the lesions of RSMF and meningococcemia. It can also be associated with fever and arthralgias. The treatment is with a cephalosporin.

26. Answer: A. The image shows a classic physical examination finding known as Grey Turner sign. The sign most often refers to the presence of ecchymosis in the patient's flank region, which is traditionally seen 2 to 3 days after acute hemorrhagic pancreatitis. It is also associated with significant retroperitoneal bleeding. Cullen sign refers to ecchymosis and induration in the periumbilical area.

    (D) Murphy sign occurs when the patient takes a deep inspiratory breath during palpation of the right upper quadrant (RUQ). If the gallbladder is inflamed, the descending diaphragm forces it against the examiner's fingertips, causing pain and often a sudden pause to inspiration. (B) Kernig sign may be seen in patients with meningitis; patients cannot extend the leg at the knee when the thigh is flexed because of stiffness in the hamstrings. (C) McMurray sign is present when manipulation of the tibia with the leg flexed produces pain and a pronounced click when the meniscus has been injured. If the click occurs when the foot is rotated inward, the tear is in the lateral meniscus. (E) McBurney sign represents maximum tenderness and rigidity over McBurney point, which may be indicative of appendicitis.

27. Answer: E. This patient sustained a clenched-fist injury. These injuries are associated with high infection rates. Wounds sustained by punches to the jaw and human bites, also known as "fight bites," classically occur over the metacarpal joints. Penetration deep into the joint space and infection is common given the positioning of the hand during the injury, exposure to human oral flora, and delay in seeking treatment. Infected wounds are polymicrobial and include *Eikenella corrodens*, a facultative anaerobic

Gram-negative rod harbored in human dental plaque. It acts synergistically with aerobic organisms to increase the morbidity of these injuries. The joint spaces must be examined during full range of motion to detect any tendon lacerations or presence of foreign bodies. Hand radiographs should also be obtained to examine for any bony involvement. Intravenous antibiotics and admission is the appropriate disposition. The antibiotics of choice are penicillin and second-generation cephalosporins with broader coverage in the immunocompromised patient. The wounds should be left open with a sterile dressing, splinted in the position of function (hand-holding-glass position) and elevated. Human bites have resulted in the transmission of hepatitis B, hepatitis C, syphilis, and herpes. Although HIV is present in human saliva, it is in relatively small amounts and considered a low risk of transmission. Appropriate antivirals and testing should be considered in these patients.

(A and B) You should never suture these lacerations. (C and D) Wound irrigation and tetanus prophylaxis is warranted in conjunction with intravenous antibiotics (Marx, 780-783).

28. Answer: A. This patient suffered a venomous snakebite. Pit vipers, such as rattlesnakes, copperheads, and water moccasins, are the most prevalent and are present in all states except Alaska, Maine, and Hawaii. Coral snakes are the second most prevalent and are present mainly in the southern states. *Red on yellow, kill a fellow; red on black, venom lack* is a mnemonic to recall which of these snakes are dangerous. Venomous snakes can also be recognized by their triangular-shaped heads, elliptical pupils, fangs, and the presence of a pit between the eye and nostril—characteristics that the victim may not notice initially. For pit vipers, there is a snakebite grading system, which requires antivenin with progressive symptoms of edema, coagulopathy, and neurologic manifestations. The amount of antivenin is dependent on the severity of these symptoms. For the coral snake bite, local signs may be misleading, because the venom is neurotoxic. The patient may have impending neuromuscular respiratory failure with minimal local signs from the bite. As such, anitvenom is recommended for all signs of a bite from a coral snake.

Venom has a number of substances including proteolytic enzymes and polypeptides, which promote coagulation, neuromuscular blockage, cell lysis, and death. Anaphylaxis may also occur. Airway, breathing, and circulation (ABCs) must always be assessed initially. Tetanus prophylaxis should be given at some point in treatment, but it is not the initial treatment of choice. Antibiotic prophylaxis is not clinically indicated in these patients. Antivenins derived from horse serum are associated with allergic reactions and serum sickness. The newer antivenins are derived from sheep serum and have a lower incidence of allergic reactions (Marx, 786-792).

29. Answer: C. This patient's necrotic lesion and residence in a south-central state is classic for a brown recluse spider bite. This envenomation from this bite may present with systemic symptoms such as fever, chills, myalgias, hemolysis, petechiae, and eventually seizure, renal failure, and death. The brown recluse spider can be distinguished by the violin-shaped marking on its cephalothorax. Its venom contains hemolytic enzymes and substances that cause local vasoconstriction. Initial lesions may appear targetoid, as blood supply to the central area is diminished and becomes necrotic. Lesions have been shown to cause significant scarring and infection. Initial treatment should include the ABCs, wound care, analgesia, and tetanus prophylaxis. Patients may be observed in the ED for a period of 6 hours for signs of envenomation. Antibiotics may become warranted if infection ensues. Loxosceles reclusa antivenin is manufactured in Brazil, but is not currently available in the United States (Marx, 795-796).

30. Answer: D. This patient presents with the classic symptoms of Kawasaki disease, an acute febrile childhood disease and one of the leading causes of acquired heart disease worldwide. The diagnostic criteria include fever for ≥5 days, **and** at least 4 of the following 5 clinical signs: bilateral conjunctival injection, oral mucous membrane changes (injected pharynx, injected or fissured lips, or strawberry tongue), peripheral erythema or edema or periungal desquamation, polymorphous rash, and cervical lymphadenopathy ≥1.5 cm. The cardiac sequelae, which may occur during the acute or latent stage of Kawasaki disease, represent its most serious complications. An echocardiogram should be performed as part of the diagnostic workup and as part of the 2-month follow-up plan once the clinical diagnosis has been established (Paller, 566-571).

31. Answer: D. Fifth disease (erythema infectiosum) is a mild illness caused by Parvovirus B19. It typically occurs in school-aged children in the spring and

winter. Viremia occurs about 1 week after exposure to the virus and lasts 3 to 5 days. Symptoms include headache, fever, sore throat, coryza, pruritis, abdominal pain, and arthralgias. The characteristic rash develops abruptly with bright red cheeks giving the "slapped cheek" appearance. Subsequently, a maculopapular faintly pink rash develops in the trunk and the extremities, then clears in a lacy pattern. The rash fades over several days but can reappear intermittently for several weeks, particularly when the skin is exposed to sun or a warm bath. Fifth disease is self-limited in children and requires only supportive care. In children with sickle cell anemia, Parvovirus is associated with bone marrow suppression and aplastic crisis. Additionally, infection during pregnancy can result in fetal death or red blood cell aplasia with fetal hydrops.

(A) Rubeola (measles) is caused by the measles virus, a single-stranded RNA paramyxovirus. The virus is highly contagious. Typically measles begins with prodromal upper respiratory symptoms including cough, conjunctivitis, and coryza. Koplick spots are tiny red spots with a white/bluish hue center that appear on the buccal mucosa opposite the lower molars. These appear during the prodrome and last for ~1 day. The exanthem appears ~2 weeks after exposure. It begins at the hairline behind the ears and then spreads from the head to the feet over ~3 days. It is erythematous and maculopapular. (B) Rubella (German measles), a mild viral illness is significant for its teratogenic effects. Clinically, patients experience slight fever and marked lymphadenopathy with prominent postauricular and suboccipital lymph nodes. A nonspecific rash develops that is diffusely erythematous and maculopapular. The most significant complication is fetal malformation following a maternal rubella infection during the first or second trimester of pregnancy. (C) Roseola (exanthema subitum) is thought to be caused by human herpes virus C. It is a common illness that rarely occurs <6 months of age or >2 years. The most characteristic feature of roseola is a well-looking child despite high fever. The fever comes on suddenly and persists for 3 to 4 days. The rash appears as the fever vanishes and resolves within 48 hours. Management is supportive. (E) Scarlet fever is caused by a reaction to an erythrogenic toxin produced by group A β-hemolytic *Streptococcus*. It can develop in association with *Streptococcus* pharyngitis and also can be seen in impetigo or cellulitis. The characteristic sandpaper rash begins in the skin folds such as the groin, axillae, and antecubital areas. The rash generally develops within 12 to 48 hours after the onset of fever and chills with subsequent desquamation. It is treated with penicillin.

32. Answer: B. This patient's condition is known as paraphimosis. It is often confused with phimosis, a distinct condition. Both conditions involve the foreskin (prepuce) and the glans of the penis. With paraphimosis, the retracted prepuce is not able to be reduced over the glans of the penis. The most common cause is iatrogenic retraction of the prepuce during penile examination, Foley catherization, or cystoscopy. The retracted prepuce forms a band that compresses blood and lymphatic flow to the distal portions of the prepuce and the glans, which results in swelling and engorgement of these structures. Urinary retention, penile gangrene, and autoamputation may occur if this condition remains untreated. ED management involves reducing the penile edema and performing emergency manual reduction of the prepuce over the glans. Patients often require parenteral analgesics in addition to local, topical, or regional anesthesia. Use of granulated sugar over swollen muscosal areas (causes osmotic gradient) is also described as a noninvasive adjunct. To retract the foreskin back over the glans the physician should apply continuous, firm pressure to the glans penis for 5 minutes to reduce the edema and then pull the foreskin over the glans. If manual reduction is unsuccessful, you can anesthetize the constricting ring with local anesthetic and make a superficial vertical incision dorsally in the midline. This should be done in consultation with an urologist.

(A) With phimosis, the patient is unable to retract the prepuce proximally over the glans penis. The glans is difficult to visualize directly as the prepuce covers it completely ("buried meatus"). A common cause of phimosis is poor hygiene of an uncircumcised penis. This condition is less worrisome than paraphimosis and only occasionally requires dorsal slit of the foreskin. (C) Balantitis is an infection of the glans penis that is more common in uncircumcised males. Patients complain of swelling, erythema, penile discharge, dysuria, bleeding, and sometimes ulceration of the penis. Phimosis can occur, but is uncommon. It is treated with warm soaks and topical antibiotics. The addition of oral antibiotics is reserved for more severe cases. (D) Priapism is a prolonged painful erection unaccompanied by continual sexual stimulation. It is important to exclude penile foreign bodies that mimicks priapism. There are two forms of priapism, a low-flow or

ischemic priapism that is painful, and a high-flow or nonischemic priapism that is rare and typically painless. Ischemic priapism is a surgical emergency as irreversible damage occurs between 24 and 48 hours. Some management options include dry aspiration, aspiration with irrigation, and intracavernous injections of phenylephrine. (E) Hair-tourniquet syndrome occurs when a strand of hair, thread, or fiber wraps around any appendage of a young child. This can result in local ischemia, necrosis, and autoamputation. In any infant with inconsolable crying, this syndrome must be excluded.

33. Answer: A. Epidural hematoma is the result of blood collecting in the potential space between the skull and the dura mater. Most epidural hematomas result from blunt trauma to the temporal or temporoparietal area with an associated skull fracture and middle meningeal artery disruption. The classic history of an epidural hematoma is a lucent period following immediate loss of consciousness after significant blunt head trauma. However, this clinical pattern occurs in a minority of patients. Most patients either never lose consciousness or never regain consciousness after the injury. On CT scan, epidural hematomas appear lenticular or biconvex (football-shaped), typically in the temporal region. The high-pressure arterial bleeding of an epidural hematoma can lead to herniation within hours after injury. Therefore, early recognition and evacuation is important to increase survival. ED trephination (burr holes) is rarely, if ever, performed and should be considered only if definitive neurosurgical care is not available, or if there is no CT scanner available and there is a high clinical suspicion for increasing intracerebral pressure.

(B) Subdural hematoma (SDH) appears as a hyperdense, crescent-shaped lesion that crosses suture lines. It results from a collection of blood below the dura and over the brain. To differentiate the CT finding from an epidural hematoma, think about the high pressure created by the arterial tear of an epidural that causes the hematoma to expand inward. Whereas, the low pressure venous bleed of a SDH layers along the calvarium. (C) Traumatic subarachnoid hemorrhage (SAH) is possibly the most common CT abnormality in patients with moderate to severe traumatic brain injury. (D and E) Intracerebral hematomas and contusions occur secondary to traumatic tearing of intracerebral blood vessels. Contusions most commonly occur in the frontal, temporal, and occipital lobes; and may occur at the site of the blunt trauma or the opposite site of the brain, known as a contrecoup injury (Tintinalli, 1566-1567).

34. Answer: D[1-6]. This patient has pneumonia that involves the superior segment of the left lower lobe, and has an allergy to pencillin; therefore a respiratory fluoroquinolone is a good initial therapeutic choice. Symptomatically, pneumonia can present in a variety of ways, most classically with a productive cough, dyspnea, and fever. Additional symptoms may include chills, chest pain which can be pleuritic, abdominal pain (in lower lobe pneumonia), and dyspnea with exertion. Examination may be notable for rales, rhonchi, decreased breath sounds, egophany, and fremitus.

Chest radiography is the mainstay of diagnosis. Bacterial and viral pneumonias may demonstrate air bronchograms, segmental or lobar consolidation, interstitial infiltrates, or pleural effusions. Fungal pneumonias can cause hilar adenopathy, diffuse nodules, and cavitation. Aspiration often leads to consolidation of the upper segments of the lower lobes, most notably the right lower lobe. Tuberculosis produces a range of abnormalities, from apical consolidations to a heterogeneous miliary pattern.

Sputum examination is of limited value, especially in the ED, because of the low yield, false positives, and difficulty in procuring a suitable specimen. Blood cultures obtained before antibiotic administration can be helpful to identify a specific organism, mainly in more critically ill patients, but rarely affect treatment decisions.

The pneumonia severity index (PSI or PORT score) predicts mortality in patients based on a number of historical, physical, and laboratory variables that assist in determination of which patients may be treated as outpatients. This is a scoring system whereby the patient's age (age -10 in females) is added to a number assigned to coexisting characteristics found to be significant in predicting 30-day mortality. Point assignment ranges from 10 to 30. The greater the correlation with poor outcome the higher the value assigned. Important characteristics include; age >50 years; history of malignancy, congestive heart failure (CHF), cerebrovascular disease, renal disease, liver disease, or compromised immune status; vitals, change in mental status; and acidosis, BUN >30, or hyponatremia. This score is placed into a risk class I to V, with higher score translating to a higher class and higher mortality. Patients with a PORT score of ≥ 90 (class IV), absolutely require hospitalization as mortality ranges from 8% to 9%. The patient in this question would have a score of 79 (age + CHF =

69 + 10), that puts him in class III for a 30-day mortality of <3%. The index is summarized in Tables 24-1, 24–2, and 24–3. As with all clinical decision rules, exceptions exist and physician judgment of patient safety is fundamental.

TABLE 24–1. Pneumonia Severity Index Assignment to Risk Class I

Age ≤50 years
No comorbid conditions including:
Neoplastic disease
Congestive heart failure
Renal disease
Liver disease
No physical examination abnormalities including:
Altered mental status
Pulse <125
Systolic blood pressure >90 mm HG
Temperature >35°C (95°F) or <40°C (104°F)

TABLE 24–2. Pneumonia Severity Index Assignment to Risk Classes II to IV

CRITERIA	POINTS
Demographics	
Female gender	−10
Nursing home resident	10
Coexisting illness	
Neoplastic disease	30
Congestive heart failure	20
Cerebrovascular accident	**10**
Renal disease	10
Liver disease	10
Physical examination	
Abnormal mental status	20
Pulse ≥125	20
Respiratory rate ≥30	20
Blood pressure ≤90 mm Hg	15
Temperature <35° (95°F) or >40°C (104°F)	10
Ancillary studies	
pH <7.35	30
Blood urea nitrogen ≥30 mg dL	20
Na ≤130 mEq L	20
Glucose ≥250 mg dL	10
Hematocrit <30%	10
PaO_2 <60 mm Hg	10
Pleural effusion	10

TABLE 24–3.   Pneumonia Severity Index Prediction of Mortality from Pneumonia

CLASS	POINTS	MORTALITY (%)	TREATMENT RECOMMENDATION
I	No predictors	0.1	Outpatient
II	<70	0.6	Outpatient
III	71 to 90	2.8	Inpatient (briefly)
IV	91 to 130	8.2	Inpatient
V	>130	29.2	Inpatient

Antibiotic therapy should be started promptly and be tailored to suspected pathogens. Organisms covered should include Gram-positives (especially *Streptococcus pneumoniae*) and atypicals (classically, *Mycoplasma, Legionella,* and *Chlamydia* species). Current guidelines encourage administration within four hours of patient arrival to the ED. Outpatient therapy for healthy patients <60 years can include a macrolide or doxycycline. Respiratory fluoroquinolones (levofloxacin, moxifloxacin, gatifloxacin) are reserved for patients with recent antibiotic therapy or more serious disease. Outpatients with significant medical comorbidities or >60 years should be treated with either a respiratory fluoroquinolone or a second- or third-generation cephalosporin **and** a macrolide. Hospitalized patients should be treated with intravenous antibiotics: a β-lactam **and** macrolide **or** a respiratory fluoroquinolone. Immunocompromised patients and those destined for the ICU should receive broader coverage, such as an antipseudomonal extended spectrum β lactam; double coverage for Gram-negative organisms (adding an aminoglycoside) should be considered if sepsis is suspected, and vancomycin should be administered if the patient is from a nursing home or other residence where MRSA may be prevalent. Aspiration pneumonia treatment should include agents active against Gram-negative and anaerobic organisms (clindamycin), and immunocompromised and AIDS patients at risk for *Pneumocystis* pneumonia should receive trimethoprim-sulfamethoxazole.

(A) Nebulized bronchodilator therapy with a β$_2$ agonist and an anticholinergic agent would be the appropriate initial treatment for an asthma or COPD exacerbation. However, this patient has no history of pulmonary disease, good air exchange, and no wheezing on examination. (B) Ceftriaxone and azithromycin is a typical pneumonia regimen for hospitalized patients, which would be appropriate for this patient, but an allergy to penicillin precludes the use of ceftriaxone in this patient because there is considerable cross-reactivity. (C) Althoughe this patient has a history of CHF and a history which might be compatible with an exacerbation, his chest radiograph clearly demonstrates a lobar consolidation rather than pulmonary edema. Acute CHF with pulmonary edema would best be medically managed by sitting the patient upright, providing oxygen, and administering diuretics and nitrates to reduce the cardiac afterload. Additional treatment adjuncts include morphine to reduce the catecholamine surge, ACE inhibitors, and noninvasive positive pressure ventilation. (E) Trimethoprim- sulfamethoxazole is the treatment of choice for pneumonia caused by *Pneumocystis jiroveci* (previously *carinii*). Patients with such infections may present in a similar fashion (fatigue, dry cough, dyspnea), but they are uniformly immunocompromised. An LDH may be elevated and patients can become hypoxic with exertion. Radiographs in such patients can be normal or demonstrate a diffuse or patchy interstitial or airspace-filling infiltrate. Steroids are indicated for patients with room air PaO$_2$ <50 mm Hg.

35.   Answer: C[7]. This patient sustained blunt trauma to the chest, is hemodynamically stable, and has a >50% right-sided pneumothorax. Pneumothorax is a common disease entity in moderate to severe chest trauma. A simple pneumothorax, often caused by a broken rib piercing the pleura or rupture of a subpleural bleb or bulla allows air to escape into the pleural space. A communicating pneumothorax results from a penetrating injury to the chest wall with contiguous communication to the pleural space. A "sucking" chest wound results in which air enters the pleural space during inspiration, and escapes on expiration. Functional impairment of the "good" lung often results secondary to compression by the mediastinum during inspiration secondary to increased contralateral pressure.

A tension pneumothorax occurs when an injury to the chest wall and/or lung causes a functional one-way valve, allowing air to enter the pleural space with inspiration but trapping it during expiration. This leads to increasing pressure in the pleural space, which can eventually cause tracheal deviation to the contralateral side, decreased venous return, and a precipitous drop in cardiac output. Spontaneous pneumothoraces, those without an antecedent history of trauma, are usually caused by rupture of a subpleural bleb or bulla, but may also occur secondary to a variety of respiratory conditions, such as emphysema, asthma, bronchitis, tuberculosis, and pneumonia. Patients often present with abrupt-onset pleuritic chest pain and shortness of breath. Treatment varies based on the size of the pneumothorax, as well as the presence of underlying disease.

Diagnosis of a medium or large pneumothorax (>20%) is often clinical, with decreased breath sounds and increased tympany on the affected side. Chest radiography is necessary to confirm the diagnosis in any stable patient. An upright, inspiratory chest radiograph is standard. An expiratory view may be helpful since intrapleural air may be easier to see with reduced lung volumes. A thin, white line without pulmonary markings peripherally demarcates the visceral pleura in a partial pneumothorax. Other findings include hyperlucency, subcutaneous air, altered diaphragm heights, a deep sulcus, and an accentuated cardiac border. However, small pneumothoraces are easily missed, particularly on supine chest radiographs. Ultrasound is developing an increased role in diagnosis of pneumothoraces in the ED, as demonstrated by the absence of sliding lung against the pleura. CT is very sensitive but not the initial test of choice. In unstable patients, diagnosis and treatment cannot wait for radiologic confirmation, so when there is a reasonable suspicion of pneumothorax in a patient with unstable vitals signs, tube thoracostomy should be performed. This is especially a concern in the setting of endotracheal intubation because of the increased risk of development of a tension pneumothorax. Immediate needle decompression in the second midclavicular intercostal space should precede tube thoracostomy if the patient exhibits signs of tension pneumothorax.

Tube thoracostomy should be performed at the fourth or fifth midaxillary space. After proper anesthesia, a 3 to 4 cm transverse incision is made one rib level inferior to the desired interspace. Blunt dissection with a Kelly clamp should lead superiorly, over the lower rib to avoid the neurovascular bundle, until a "pop" signifies penetration of the parietal pleura; a rush of air or fluid is common. As a gloved finger holds the place and checks for adhesions, the tube is introduced and directed posterior and superior so that no holes are visible on the tube. The tube may be directed inferiorly if primarily for fluid drainage, though this is not usually necessary. The tube is then secured with sutures, an occlusive dressing, tape, and connected to a water seal or suction circuit.

In addition to tube thoracostomy, a hemodynamically stable major blunt trauma victim such as this patient will generally need a CT scan of the chest, as well as of the abdomen and pelvis, to rule out other traumatic injuries.

(A) Emergent abdominal surgery is indicated in a trauma patient with severe intraperitoneal hemorrhage or hollow viscus perforation. Hollow viscus perforation can cause free intraperitoneal air visible on CT or occasionally on chest radiography as free air under the diaphragm. (B) Tension pneumothorax is a critical condition as demonstrated clinically by hypotension, jugular venous distension, absent breath sounds and hyperresonance on the affected side, tracheal deviation away from the affected side, and radiographically by mediastinal shift away from the affected side. (D) Hemothorax is common in thoracic trauma and indicated by decreased breath sounds, dullness to percussion. Chest radiography shows a hazy, ill-defined opacity in the dependent portions of the affected lung, often with costophrenic angle blunting on upright radiographs. A chest tube directed inferiorly most efficiently drains a simple hemothorax, but a chest tube directed in the traditional superior direction is usually sufficient and entails less risk of hepatic or diaphragmatic injury. (E) Intubation is indicated in chest trauma for a number of reasons, including airway protection, hypoxemia, and inadequate ventilation. Chest tube thoracostomy must accompany intubation in cases of even small pneumothoraces because of the potential of positive pressure ventilation to force air into the pleural space, resulting in a tension pneumothorax.

36. Answer: E[8-11]. This patient has alveolar pulmonary edema caused by CHF. Heart failure may be due to a broad range of pathologic processes such as coronary artery disease, hypertension, cardiomyopathy, valvular disease, and pulmonary disease. The renin-angiotensin-aldosterone system initially helps the heart to maintain perfusion before the adaptive response is harmful, perpetuating the disease. Additionally, CHF may be categorized by high-output versus low-output, systolic versus diastolic, and right versus left. Chronic heart failure can be graded by the New York Heart Association (NYHA)

classification as follows: asymptomatic with ordinary activity (I), symptomatic with ordinary activity (II), symptomatic with limited activity (III), and symptomatic at rest (IV). CHF exacerbations are commonly secondary to uncontrolled hypertension, cardiac ischemia, acute valve dysfunction, arrhythmia, noncompliance with medications, diet, infection, anemia, pregnancy, thyroid disease, and pulmonary embolus. Exacerbations of CHF may present with dyspnea (at rest or with exertion), orthopnea, jugular venous distention, dependent edema, râles, or wheezing, in addition to symptoms of the precipitant.

Chest radiography remains the main diagnostic tool. Pulmonary venous pressures progressively rise due to left ventricular failure. Initially, the lungs are able to divert the blood to vessels in the superior portions of the lung (cephalization). When this mechanism is overwhelmed, the increasing pressure causes fluid to enter the pulmonary interstitium, often first in the right lung. This causes an increase in (B) interstitial lung markings and (C) Kerley B lines may be present. Finally, the fluid may enter (D) the pleural space and (A) alveoli that cause diffuse or patchy airspace filling with a central distribution and classic "bat wing" appearance. Chest radiography may be normal in some patients and often lags hours behind the clinical status of the patient.

Brain natriuretic peptide (BNP) is a protein released into the blood in response to cardiomyocyte stretch. Studies have demonstrated that levels >500 pg/mL correlate with active heart failure and levels <100 pg/mL make heart failure an unlikely source of dyspnea. However, it is important to note that any condition that leads to increased myocyte stretch, such as a large pulmonary embolism or decompensated cardiac valvular disease, can cause BNP levels to rise. Most other serum laboratory tests are not diagnostically useful but may elucidate the underlying precipitant of the episode. Echocardiography can be used to evaluate cardiac wall motion and valves but is normally not necessary in the acute setting.

Treatment of an acute CHF exacerbation starts with the patient seated upright and administration of supplemental oxygen. Medical treatments are aimed at reducing preload and afterload, decreasing the excess fluid load, and increasing cardiac contractility. Both intravenous and sublingual formulations of nitrates (nitroglycerin) quickly and effectively reduce preload and afterload. Nitroglycerin given intravenously can be easily titrated to effect; large doses may be necessary. Loop diuretics (furosemide) reduce preload and

plasma volume initially by means of direct vasodilation and ultimately by increasing excretion of sodium and water. β-blockers and ACE inhibitors, mainstays of chronic treatment, have unclear roles in the acute setting, but evidence suggests parenteral ACE-inhibitor treatment may be beneficial. Nesiritide, recombinant human BNP, is a recent agent that reduces preload through natriuresis and inhibition of aldosterone. Though indicated to work as well as nitroglycerin, its use may lead to increased mortality and risk of renal failure, and so its clinical value is uncertain. Morphine reduces afterload, heart rate, and the anxiety associated with hypoxia and circulating catecholamines.

Hypotensive patients (cardiogenic shock) present a particular problem, as they leave no reserve for preload or volume reduction. If there is no response to a fluid bolus, vasopressors (norepinepherine) should be started to maintain the systolic blood pressure >90 mm Hg. Inotropic agents such as dobutamine may then be started to maintain adequate cardiac output. Invasive therapies (intubation, intra-aortic balloon pump) may be necessary and mortality is high. Noninvasive respiratory support (CPAP, BIPAP, NIPPV) decreases preload, afterload, and work of breathing in addition to improving oxygenation. These techniques should be started early for signs of respiratory compromise, as they not only give the pharmacologic therapies time to work, but have been shown to significantly decrease intubation rates.

37. Answer: F.[12] Tuberculosis is caused by infection with *Mycobacterium tuberculosis*, an acid-fast bacillus. Primary infection usually occurs via droplet inhalation of bacteria, which results in infection within the respiratory tract. Chest radiography remains the most valuable tool for diagnosing primary pulmonary tuberculosis, but a positive sputum Gram stain or culture remain the gold standard of definitive diagnosis. Classically, primary tuberculosis appears as an infiltrate of any lobe on chest radiography; hilar or mediastinal lymphadenopathy, and pleural effusions may be seen. This patient demonstrates reactivation tuberculosis as predominantly upper lobe infiltrates, greatest on the right, with cavitation best seen on the left. Other necrotizing pneumonias such as *S. aureus* may look similar, but would likely not affect the upper lobe. Chest radiography in immunocompromised patients with pulmonary tuberculosis can often be atypical or normal.

A positive purified protein derivative (PPD) skin test, signified by 5 to 15 mm of induration (based on the patient's immune status, risk factors, and country of origin), indicates exposure to the disease and not necessarily active infection. The PPD skin test is an example of a type IV hypersensitivity reaction, and so requires an adequate host immune response to generate a positive result. This reaction can, however, dissipate with time. A "booster effect" may occur because the PPD enhances the hypersensitivity reaction; a second skin test 1 to 2 weeks after the first may indicate previous infection.

Active tuberculosis is normally treated initially with isoniazid, rifampin, ethambutol, and pyrazinamide for 2 to 3 months, followed by at least an additional 4 months of isoniazid and rifampin, based on the antibiotic susceptibility of the organism. *M. tuberculosis* has developed resistance to fluoroquinolones, and so patients with tuberculosis risk factors who are undergoing treatment for community-acquired pneumonia should not be treated with fluoroquinolone monotherapy to avoid inducing further resistance. Direct-observed therapy (DOT) improves compliance and is an important option for treatment given the treatment complexity, duration, and public health impact. Latent tuberculosis, a positive PPD without signs or symptoms of active infection, is treated with isoniazid for 6 to 12 months to decrease the incidence of reactivation. Isoniazid interferes with the metabolism of pyridoxine (vitamin B_6) and GABA which can lead to peripheral neuropathy and, in the case of overdose, seizures refractory to standard anticonvulsants. In such patients, pyridoxine should be administered in large doses; if the amount of isoniazid is known, a milligram-for-milligram dose is appropriate. Otherwise 70 mg kg to a total dose of 5 g should be given and repeated until the seizure breaks.

(A) Fever, muscle rigidity, and autonomic instability characterize both malignant hyperthermia and neuroleptic malignant syndrome (NMS). Malignant hyperthermia is induced by volatile halogenated anesthetics and depolarizing paralytics, although NMS is secondary to any agent (often typical or atypical antipsychotic medications) which blocks central dopamine pathways. NMS normally occurs 1 to 2 weeks after initiation of a neuroleptic medication, but has occurred even years later. Dantrolene is used to treat both conditions. (B) Phenobarbital is a barbiturate which can be used in status epilepticus should benzodiazepines and phenytoin fail. (C) Physostigmine is a cholinesterase inhibitor that is used to treat anticholinergic toxicity which can be caused by a diverse number of medications, most often antihistamines, antipsychotic medications, anticholinergics, and tricyclic antidepressants. Symptoms are easily remembered by *red as a beet, dry as a bone, blind as a bat, mad as a hatter, and hot as a hare*, which correspond to flushing, dry skin and mucous membranes, mydriasis, altered mental status, and fever. (D) Pralidoxime is an organophosphate antidote which is useful in cases of nerve gas poisoning (such as Sarin) and cholinesterase inhibitor overdose.

38. Answer: A[13-15]. This patient's chest radiograph and papulovesicular rash with lesions in different stages of evolution are classic for varicella pneumonia. Varicella (chickenpox) is a largely benign illness of childhood caused by the varicella-zoster virus, but its occurrence in adults is increasing. Pneumonia is a rare but dangerous complication of the disease, occurring most often in patients with a history of smoking, immunocompromise, or pregnancy. Cough, shortness of breath, and pleuritic chest pain are usually seen within 1 week of the onset of the rash. Chest radiographs demonstrate bilateral reticular or nodular interstitial patterns. Intravenous acyclovir is the mainstay of treatment and is relatively safe in pregnancy. Adjunctive steroids have been used with unclear efficacy, ventilatory support may be necessary in severe disease, and varicella-zoster immunoglobulin (VZIG) is useful if given very early in the disease course. Mortality is low (~6%) with proper treatment, but long-term morbidity may include restrictive lung disease and impaired diffusion capacity. Although varicella pneumonia can occur in immunocompetent adults, testing for underlying immunocompromise, particularly HIV infection, should be undertaken.

(B) Pneumonia may be caused by a number of fungi, most often *Histoplasma* (Ohio and Mississippi river valleys), *Coccidioides* (southwest desert), and *Blastomyces;* clinical presentations vary from indolent to acute. Other organisms, such as *Aspergillus, Cryptococcus,* and *Mucorales*, may cause disease in immunocompromised patients. Radiographic findings include a focal or diffuse infiltrate (as in this patient), often associated with hilar lymphadenopathy. Antifungal medications include itraconazole, fluconazole, and amphotericin B. (C) Empiric inpatient treatment of uncomplicated community-acquired pneumonia should consist of either a β-lactam and macrolide or a respiratory fluoroquinolone. Radiographically, bacterial pneumonia usually produces focal airspace-filling. (D) Tuberculosis should be initially treated with the four-drug RIPE regimen (rifampin, isoniazid, pyrazinamide, ethambutol) for 2 months until mycobacterial antibiotic sensitivity can be determined, and is most often followed by isoniazid and rifampin for at least an additional 4 months. Disseminated pulmonary tuberculosis, especially in an immunocompromised host, may produce a diffuse reticulonodular infiltrate as in this patient, but typically causes a micronodular or miliary pattern. (E) An asthma exacerbation should be initially treated with both an inhaled β agonist and anticholinergic agent; subsequent treatments can utilize a β agonist alone and should continue until symptomatic relief and improvement of peak-flow measurements are achieved. Treatment with a short steroid pulse (3 to 6 days) has been demonstrated to reduce treatment failure and relapse.

39. Answer: A[16-19]. This chest radiograph shows a widened mediastinum, defined by a mediastinum >8 cm or >25% of the chest width above the level of the carina. In a patient with blunt thoracic trauma, an aortic injury must be excluded. Blunt aortic injuries are associated with a number of findings on chest radiographs: widened mediastinum, rightward deviation of the trachea or nasogastric tube, inferior displacement of the left mainstem bronchus, left pleural effusion, obscuration of the aortic knob, widened right paratracheal stripe, displaced left or right paraspinal lines, a left apical pleural cap, and opacification of the aortopulmonary window. These findings are result of hemorrhage into the mediastinum. The chest radiograph serves as an initial screening tool for aortic injury. If findings on the chest radiograph suggest an aortic injury, or the mechanism of injury is sufficiently severe despite a normal or suboptimal chest radiograph, a CT of the chest, aortography, or transesophageal echocardiography should be performed. The most common mechanism of injury associated with blunt aortic injury is a motor vehicle collision. Most victims of trauma with blunt aortic injury die at the scene or during transport to the ED caused by aortic rupture and exsanguination. Patients who initially survive have incomplete aortic wall injuries. Prompt diagnosis and surgical repair is necessary for patient survival.

Aortography has been the gold standard in the diagnosis of blunt aortic injury. However, improvement in CT scanner technology has lessened the need for aortography. CT of the chest, particularly multirow detector scanners with multiplanar reformatted images, is now used to diagnose definitively or exclude aortic injury. The intravenous contrast is timed for maximal aortic opacification. CT is often undertaken in trauma patients to evaluate for other injuries, making this the most commonly used imaging modality today for hemodynamically stable patients. Transesophageal echocardiography can also detect aortic injury and is most useful in patients too unstable to undergo CT.

(B) Diagnostic peritoneal lavage (DPL) is a sensitive test to detect intraperitoneal blood after trauma. The DPL is considered positive if >10 mL of gross blood is immediately aspirated from a catheter inserted into the peritoneal cavity or the cell count of fluid withdrawn from the cavity after infusion of 1,000 mL normal saline or lactated Ringer is >100,000 RB/ mm^3 with blunt trauma or >50,000 RBC/mm^3 with penetrating trauma. Although largely replaced by the focused abdominal sonography in trauma (FAST) examination, a DPL can help to determine which patients are in need of emergent laparotomy, taken in conjunction with patient stability and CT scan results. DPL does not evaluate for traumatic aortic injury. (C) The FAST examination, which has largely replaced the DPL and takes place in the secondary survey of trauma patients, consists of 4 sonographic windows that look for free intraperitoneal and pericardial fluid. A positive examination is the presence of a dark anechoic stripe representing fluid (likely blood) in Morison pouch, the splenorenal space, the pericardial space, or the retrovesicular space. The RUQ is the most common place to detect fluid, though 250 to 500 mL of peritoneal fluid is often necessary to be visualized and results are dependent on examiner skill. Although the FAST examination can readily detect a pericardial effusion, it has no role in evaluation for traumatic thoracic aortic injury. (D) Pericardiocentesis is a diagnostic and therapeutic maneuver to remove fluid from the pericardial space. In the setting of blunt chest trauma, the fluid would likely be blood and this procedure, which may be ineffective if the blood has clotted, should be considered only as an emergency temporizing measure until the patient can receive definitive care. An ECG lead can be attached to a long, large-bore needle, which is inserted under the xiphoid at a shallow angle until fluid is aspirated or the ECG lead indicates that the needle is touching the myocardium. Pericardiocentesis has no role in evaluating for damage to the aorta. (E) Transthoracic echocardiography cannot be used to evaluate the aorta for traumatic injury, although it is useful in trauma patients to detect blood in the pericardium and cardiac tamponade.

40. Answer: C[20,21]. This patient has the classic presentation of a small bowel obstruction, with multiple air-fluid levels in a step-like pattern and small bowel dilatation. Primary lesions leading to a small bowel obstruction include postoperative adhesions (most common), tumors, hernias, Crohn disease, intussusception, gallstones, foreign bodies, and congenital malformations. Symptoms typically include intermittent crampy abdominal pain, obstipation, and vomiting. Abdominal distension may be prominent. Mild diarrhea is occasionally present and does not alone exclude obstruction.

    Abdominal radiography may demonstrate distended loops of bowel proximal to the obstruction. Multiple air-fluid levels may be seen on an upright view. The string of pearls sign involves a small amount of air trapped in intestine when it is filled with fluid, which looks like pearls in cross-section. Abdominal CT is more sensitive than abdominal radiography. In addition, CT can often show the cause and location of the obstruction.

    Treatment depends on the severity and cause of obstruction but always includes bowel rest, intravenous fluids and electrolytes, and nasogastric tube decompression. Early surgical consultation is necessary because operative intervention is needed if there is suspicion of bowel ischemia.

    (A) Adhesions are the most frequent (50% to 70%) cause of small bowel obstruction, although increasing use of minimally invasive surgery is decreasing this number. (B) Rarely, a large gallstone causing chronic gallbladder inflammation may pass through a fistula into the duodenum and then lodge at, most often, the ileocecal valve causing bowel obstruction. This is known as gallstone ileus. It does not often result in bowel ischemia but does usually need surgical treatment both to extract the obstructing gallstone and to close the cholecystoenteric fistula. (D) IBD, specifically Crohn disease, is a risk factor for the development of small bowel obstruction. This form of obstruction rarely leads to strangulation. (E) Intussusception is primarily a disease of childhood, although it may present in adults who have a bowel wall lesion (eg, polyp). Intussusception occurs when a segment of bowel "telescopes" into the adjacent bowel. This disease process may rarely result in bowel ischemia.

41. Answer: C[22-26]. The posteroanterior chest radiograph demonstrates free air under the right hemidiaphragm consistent with a perforated hollow viscous. Peptic ulcers, gastric or duodenal, usually occur in the setting of *Helicobacter pylori* infection or nonsteroidal anti-inflammatory drug use, but may also be due to Zollinger-Ellison syndrome, oncologic radiation, or certain chemotherapeutic agents. Peptic ulcer disease may be complicated by UGI hemorrhage or perforation. Peptic ulcer perforation releases enteric gas into the peritoneum, where it may be visible by radiography. Patients too ill to sit upright should have a left lateral decubitus view of the abdomen performed, which would then show a dark stripe adjacent to the liver representing free intraperitoneal air. Perforations may also be caused by a gastric ulcer or carcinoma, bowel obstruction, IBD, diverticulitis, colonic malignancy, appendicitis, trauma, ischemia, foreign body ingestion, infection, or be iatrogenic (ERCP, endoscopy, laparoscopy). Treatment is aimed at the underlying problem and almost always requires surgery. Peritonitis is a common and serious complication of any perforation. Patients should be kept NPO and receive intravenous fluids and antibiotics that cover Gram-negative organisms and anaerobes.

    (A) Aortic dissection is a difficult diagnosis to make on a chest radiograph, but the entity is suggested when the mediastinum appears widened. Patients usually have a history of hypertension and imaging of the aorta is necessary to make the diagnosis. (B) CHF is suggested in chest radiography by the presence of cephalization of the pulmonary vasculature, interstitial pulmonary edema (peribronchial cuffing, septal thickening), alveolar edema, cardiomegaly, and pleural effusions. (D) Upright chest radiography is an excellent test for determination of the presence of a pneumothorax. A thin pleural line should be observed, peripheral to which no pulmonary markings are visible. Supine radiographs may show a deep sulcus depressing the diaphragm on the affected side. Lateral decubitus views may be useful if the patient is unable to sit upright. A tension pneumothorax should be suspected if there is tracheal deviation away from the affected side or ipsilateral diaphragmatic flattening. (E) Although many chest radiographs in the presence pulmonary embolism are abnormal, the findings are nonspecific, subtle, and usually not diagnostically helpful. Classical signs include a wedge-shaped infarct at the periphery of the lung (Hampton hump) and focal decreased pulmonary vascularity distal to a prominent pulmonary artery (Westermark sign). Additional nonspecific abnormalities include plate-like atelectasis, pleural effusion, and hemidiaphragm elevation.

42. Answer: C[27,28]. The CT shows acute appendicitis demonstrated by an enlarged tubular appendix unfilled by contrast with a thickened enhancing wall and periappendiceal fat stranding. Appendicitis may lead to an intra-abdominal abscess, especially if perforated. The appendix is a small tubular structure arising from the cecum just inferior to the ileocecal valve. About 7% of individuals will develop appendicitis, usually initiated by obstruction of the lumen by a fecolith or undigested foreign body. Inflammation and necrosis follow increasing lumen pressures. Patients typically present with nausea, vomiting, anorexia, and abdominal pain. The pain typically starts periumbilically then migrates to the right lower quadrant as the peritoneal inflammation becomes more localized. Fever and localized tenderness at McBurney point (2 cm from the anterior superior iliac spine toward the umbilicus) are classic. Localized rebound tenderness can often be elicited. Rovsing sign refers to rebound tenderness referred to the right lower quadrant when the left lower quadrant is palpated and released. The psoas sign refers to abdominal pain with hip extension and the obturator sign to pain with hip flexion and external rotation. Sterile pyuria may be seen when the inflamed appendix abuts the bladder or ureter. An elevated leukocyte count is often but not always seen.

  A classic history and examination should bring a prompt surgical consultation, and patients should be provided pain medications, intravenous fluids, and kept NPO. Though not always necessary, many patients undergo radiologic evaluation. Ultrasound has a sensitivity of 75% to 90% and is a good imaging option in children and pregnant women. Abdominal CT is superior to ultrasound, but entails a greater exposure to radiation. Findings of appendicitis include an appendiceal diameter >6 mm, appendiceal wall thickening, an appendicolith, periappendiceal fat stranding, and periappendiceal abscess or phlegmon formation. Acute appendicitis mandates surgical intervention, and intravenous antibiotics should be initiated to cover anaerobes and Gram-negative organisms.

  (A) A predisposition toward ectopic pregnancy is a complication of pelvic inflammatory disease (PID). PID is most commonly caused by *Neisseria gonorrhea* and *Chlamydia trachomatis*, which should be treated with intramuscular ceftriaxone and azithromycin or doxycycline, respectively. Other risk factors for ectopic pregnancy include any tubal surgery, smoking, advanced age, prior abortion, history of infertility, the use of an intrauterine device, in vitro fertilization, or a prior ectopic pregnancy. (B) Gastroenteritis caused by *E. coli* serotype 0157:H7 is transmitted by inadequately cooked meat and causes bloody diarrhea without mucosal invasion. Treatment is supportive. Hemolytic uremic syndrome (microangiopathic hemolytic anemia, thrombocytopenia, and acute renal failure) is a complication of such infections, more common among children, the elderly, and infections treated with antibiotics. (D) Pyelonephritis is a potential complication of a urinary tract infection or an obstructing ureterocalculus. Symptoms are often those of a urinary tract infection with flank/back pain, fever, chills, or white cells on urine microscopy. (E) Toxic megacolon may occur as a consequence of inflammatory bowel disease or infectious colitis. The condition is defined by nonobstructive colonic dilation confirmed by radiography with evidence of systemic toxicity. Treatment consists of hydration, antibiotics, steroids, and treatment of the underlying condition.

43. Answer: E[29-38]. A midrenal slice of the noncontrast-enhanced abdominal CT scan demonstrates right-sided hydroureter and perinephric stranding consistent with urolithiasis, although the causative stone is not visualized. Renal colic typically presents with sudden-onset flank pain radiating to the groin, a constant dull pain between episodes of severe pain; nausea and vomiting are common. Patients appear restless, writhing, and unable to find a comfortable position. Urinalysis often reveals hematuria. Calculi are often composed of calcium, although a far smaller amount are made of uric acid or struvite, which occur in the setting of a urinary tract infection caused by urea splitting bacteria such as *Proteus* or *Klebsiella*.

  Noncontrast abdominal CT is the test of choice for diagnosis of urolithiasis, with both a sensitivity and specificity >95%. Identification of a calculus within the ureter is the primary diagnostic finding; stones as small as 1 mm can be detected. Calculi are commonly impacted into the ureteropelvic junction, pelvic brim, or ureterovesicular junction. Associated findings are seen in >90% of patients, such as perinephric stranding, ureter wall thickening, hydronephrosis, and hydroureter. Ultrasound is effective in visualizing hydronephrosis but lacks the ability to directly detect ureteral stones. Intravenous pyelography is outmoded but a viable imaging option when CT is unavailable. Because ≥ 80% of stones are radiopaque, abdominal radiography is not generally helpful except for following the transit of a stone identified by other imaging. 90% of stones <5 mm pass spontaneously.

Treatment of renal colic initially consists of analgesic medications. NSAIDs are effective pain relievers, in part by relief of ureterospasm and decrease of glomerular filtration rate. In particular, parenteral ketorolac is valuable in patients who are vomiting. Opitate analgesics are used if NSAIDS alone are insufficient.

Recently, several randomized comparative studies have supported the use of nifedipine and tamsulosin as agents which speed the expulsion of ureteral stones and relieve the pain associated with ureteral spasm. Tamsulosin, an α-blocker used to relieve the urinary symptoms associated with an enlarged prostate, is used "off-label" in cases of renal colic; the FDA has not evaluated this indication.

All patients discharged should be instructed to strain their urine for stones (for later analysis) and follow-up with a urologist. Larger stones (>5mm) often require urologic intervention, such as lithotripsy or ureteroscopy, usually as outpatients. Patients with renal colic should be admitted for intractable pain, inability to tolerate oral fluids, increasing creatinine, or infection.

(A) Broad-spectrum penicillin treatment, often ampicillin-sulbactam, is indicated in cases of suspected intra-abdominal infection, such as appendicitis or cholecystitis. The CT of this patient does not contain any evidence of infection. (B) Ciprofloxacin is a reasonable first-line treatment for urinary tract infections, bacterial gastroenteritis, or mild diverticulitis, none of which is present in this patient. (C) Furosimide is not indicated in the treatment or prevention of urolithiasis. On the contrary, since loop diuretics increase calcium excretion in the kidneys, they may increase stone formation in individuals susceptible to calcium stones. Thiazide diuretics and citrate therapy have been mainstays in the prevention of stones caused by calcium. Allopurinol may be effective in preventing uric acid stones. (D) Phenazopyridine is effective in some patients at decreasing the pain and bladder spasm which accompanies urinary tract infections.

44. Answer: B[39-41]. This patient has a ruptured abdominal aortic aneurysm (AAA). An enlarged aorta is visible in the midfield of the scan (demarcated by mural calcification) with extravascular hemorrhage seen on the right. In addition to family history, other risk factors for AAA include age, hypertension, male sex, hypercholesterolemia, iliac or popliteal aneurysm, stroke, tobacco use, and occlusive peripheral vascular disease. Unruptured aneurysms are usually asymptomatic, occasionally identified as a nontender, supraumbilical mass. Rupture of the aneurysm leads to the classic triad of pain, hypotension, and tender pulsatile mass. The pain may be in the abdomen, back, or flank, and radiate to the legs or groin; ruptured aneurysms are commonly first misdiagnosed as renal colic. Rupture is often into the retroperitoneum, so bleeding may initially be contained. Aortoenteric and aortocaval fistulae are uncommon but dangerous complications of an AAA.

The diagnosis of an AAA depends on the patient's clinical stability. Ultrasound is an excellent test to confirm the presence or absence of an AAA, although is does not directly visualize leakage. Bedside ultrasonography is the test of choice in an unstable or potentially unstable patient with a suspected leaking AAA. However, a convincing clinical scenario in an unstable patient with or without bedside ultrasonography mandates emergent surgical consultation.

CT of the abdomen is an accurate way to identify a leaking AAA, and intravenous and enteric contrast are not needed to make the diagnosis. Intravenous contrast can help to define the aneurysm lumen and mural thrombus. CT is commonly used because it is readily available, fast, and can detect other abdominal disorders. Signs of rupture on CT include retroperitoneal hematoma, contrast extravasation, discontinuous aortic wall, and a high-attenuation crescent within the aneurysm (best seen on noncontrast CT). Nonetheless, no unstable patient should leave the ED for a lengthy diagnostic test when a leaking AAA is a diagnostic consideration. Conventional radiography can detect aortic aneurysm wall calcification in ≥80% of patients although has a very limited role and should only be obtained if ultrasound and CT are unavailable.

The abdominal aorta is normally <2 cm in diameter; an increased risk of rupture occurs at diameters >4 to 6 cm, and surgeons often use a diameter of >5.5 cm or yearly increase of >0.6 to 0.8 cm as a cutoff for elective repair. Because of aortic wall strength and turbulent blood flow, aneurysms are most often infrarenal in location. No patient with a ruptured AAA should ever be considered stable, and surgical repair (open or endovascular) is necessary. Prompt surgery has been shown to increase survival, but mortality remains high.

(A) Deep vein thrombosis is not a risk factor for the development of an AAA, but remains a significant risk factor for conditions such as pulmonary embolism. (C) Females have a lower incidence of AAA than males, thus making this trait relatively protective. (D) History of prior abdominal surgery is an important risk factor for small bowel obstructions secondary to adhesions but has no effect on the incidence of AAA in any population. (E) Obesity is a risk factor for many disease processes, from diabetes, heart disease, and hypertension to sleep apnea and osteoarthritis. There is, however, no direct association between obesity and AAA.

45. Answer: B[42-44]. This radiograph displays an anterior glenohumeral dislocation. The humeral head appears inferior and medial compared to its usual articulation with the glenoid. As a consequence of its great mobility, the shoulder is the most frequently dislocated joint in the body. The vast majority of dislocations are anterior, often from either a fall onto an outstretched arm or forced abduction/extension and external rotation. Such dislocations are usually subcoracoid (80%), subglenoid, or subclavicular. Posterior dislocations account for <5% of all dislocations, classically occurring after either a seizure or lightning strike.

Diagnosis is made by conventional radiography and should include either a "scapular Y" or axillary view in order to confirm and characterize the dislocation. Radiography may also reveal associated injuries. A Hill-Sachs fracture is seen as a depression of the posterolateral aspect of the humeral head, caused by impact with the anterior glenoid, and may be best visualized with an internal rotation AP view. A Bankart deformity is a corresponding disruption of the anteroinferior glenoid labrum or fracture of the bony rim. Avulsion fractures of the greater tuberosity of the humerus are also common. Axillary nerve injury is present in up to 50% of anterior shoulder dislocations. Nerve function may be tested by assessing sensation over the lateral deltoid or testing abduction against resistance. Injuries to other branches of brachial plexus occur less commonly. Injuries are often self-limited neurapraxia, but any deficit should prompt specialist referral.

Reduction of the dislocation should be carried out quickly, as the probability of neurovascular injury and difficulty with the reduction increase with time. Overcoming the forces of muscle spasm is the principal problem in reduction. Conscious sedation is often necessary to successfully reduce a shoulder, and intra-articular anesthesia can aid as well. A number of reduction maneuvers are available. Traction-countertraction involves laying the patient supine and applying traction to the arm in abduction, as countertraction is applied through a sheet around the patient's chest. External rotation involves slowly adducting the arm with the elbow flexed and then externally rotating the shoulder. Another method involves laying the patient prone and hanging a weight from the affected arm; the gentle constant traction often relocates the shoulder within 20 minutes. Finally, scapular manipulation reduces the joint by repositioning the glenoid. The patient lies prone with the affected arm hanging off the side as gentle traction is applied. The inferior aspect of the scapula is then rotated medially while stabilizing the scapular spine with the other hand. Once reduced, patients should be discharged in a sling and swath. Younger patients require a longer term of immobilization (3 to 6 weeks) than older patients (1 to 2 weeks). Early range of motion exercises are necessary in both groups to prevent adhesive capsulitis. Surgery should be considered in young patients with recurrent dislocations.

(A) Axillary artery injury is a rare complication of anterior or inferior shoulder dislocation, normally in older patients with underlying atherosclerotic vascular disease. (D) A reverse Hill-Sachs fracture is a deformity of the anterior portion of the humeral head from impaction on the posterior portion of the glenoid as a result of a posterior shoulder dislocation. (E) Tears of the rotator cuff are relatively common with shoulder dislocations in patients >40 to 50 years. Such injuries are often difficult to diagnose and are a cause of long-term morbidity.

46. Answer: C[42,45,46]. The patient demonstrates a classic presentation of acromioclavicular (AC) joint separation (grade III) as demonstrated by the superior displacement of the distal clavicle and lack of articulation at the AC joint. AC separations occur most commonly after direct blows to the point of the shoulder or falls onto outstretched hands. Several classification systems for this injury exist. The most practical is that of Tossy and Allman: grade I (sprain) involves only stretching or a partial tear of the AC ligament; grade II (subluxation) involves a complete disruption of the AC ligament; grade III (dislocation) involves compete disruption of the AC and coracoclavicular ligaments. Physical examination is significant for tenderness and swelling over the AC joint; the distal clavicle may be palpable and tenting of the skin can be present in grade III injuries. Radiographs of the shoulder are usually normal in grade I injuries,

exhibit AC joint space widening and mild superior clavicle displacement in grade II injuries, and AC disruption with superior clavicle displacement and increased coracoclavicular distance (normally 11 to 13 mm) in grade III injuries. Concurrent fractures of the clavicle or coracoid process are occasionally seen. Stress views of the AC joint are not necessary for management.

Management of most injuries is conservative. Patients with grade I and grade II injuries are discharged home with slings for comfort and may follow up with their primary care provider (PCP). Range of motion exercises should be undertaken as early possible to prevent adhesive capsulitis. Grade III injuries are largely treated in a similar fashion, but operative management is considered in athletes, young patients, and those with particularly severe injuries, so timely referral to an orthopedist is necessary. Adequate analgesia is a component of the treatment of all grades of AC separations.

(A) Admission is not indicated unless severe concurrent pathology (skin puncture, multiple fractures, neurovascular deficit, pneumothorax) is present. (B) Immediate orthopedic consultation is unnecessary when the diagnosis is certain and the injury is isolated. (D) Figure-of-eight harnesses are not normally prescribed currently, as they cause more pain than slings with no therapeutic benefit. (E) Immobilization with a sling is largely for comfort, especially in grade I and grade II AC separations, but is highly recommended in grade III injuries. Specialist referral is indicated for severe injuries.

47. Answer: A[47,48]. The radiograph (Figure 24–47A) shows a fracture through the midportion (waist) of the scaphoid, which classically occurs secondary to a fall on an outstretched hand. The scaphoid is the most commonly fractured carpal. Patients typically present with tenderness between the extensors pollicis brevis and longus (the anatomic "snuff box") and pain with axial loading of the thumb. Radiographic diagnosis can be difficult because the findings can be subtle, and in ≥20% of patients, the radiographs are normal—an occult fracture. To improve visualization, a dedicated scaphoid view with the wrist in ulnar deviation can be obtained. All patients with suspected fractures, whether or not confirmed by radiography, should be immobilized in a thumb spica splint and reevaluated with repeat radiographs in 7 to 10 days. At that time, fractures are more apparent on the radiographs because of bone resorption at the fracture site. It is important to correctly diagnose and treat scaphoid fractures because they are prone to be complicated by avascular necrosis and nonunion, which can lead to chronic wrist pain and disability. The blood supply of the scaphoid enters distally, such that the proximal portion of the scaphoid is vulnerable to avascular necrosis. See Figure 24–47B for a diagram of the carpal bones.

(B) Distal radioulnar joint dislocation may occur in distal radial fractures and Galeazzi fractures, or as an isolated injury following a fall on an outstretched hand. The ulna may dislocate in the volar or dorsal direction, depending on the mechanism, leading to an absence or prominence of the ulnar styloid, respectively, in addition to swelling and pain with pronation/supination. Specialist referral is necessary because treatment usually requires surgical fixation or long-term immobilization. (C) The median nerve is vulnerable to injury as a complication of distal radius fractures as well as lunate and perilunate dislocations. Carpal dislocations include a variety of ligamentous injuries centered on the lunate. Median nerve function is assessed by testing thenar muscle strength—palmar abduction of the thumb against resistance—and sensation of the radial aspect of the index finger. (D) Gamekeeper or skier thumb results from forced abduction of the thumb and tearing of the ulnar collateral ligament. Partial tears are treated with a thumb spica splint, but complete tears require surgical fixation. (E) The ulnar nerve is susceptible to injury as a complication of pisiform, hamate, and severe ulnar fractures. Ulnar nerve function is tested by abducting the fingers against resistance, radial deviation of the index finger, or crossing the fingers. Sensation is tested along the ulnar aspect of the fifth digit. An established distal ulnar nerve palsy may evolve into a "claw hand" caused by the unopposed action of the extensor digitorum communis on the fourth and fifth MCPs and flexor digitorum profundus on the PIPs. Elbow dislocation and medial epicondyle fractures can cause ulnar nerve injury at the elbow.

48. Answer: E[47,48]. This patient has suffered a lunate dislocation, the final stage in the continuum of carpal instability injuries. These injuries most commonly occur following a fall onto an outstretched hand or any other forced wrist extension, ulnar deviation, and carpal supination. A progression of ligamentous injury centered on the lunate ensues that proceeds in stages from scapholunate dissociation (stage I) to perilunate dislocation (stage II) and triquetral fracture or triquetolunate ligament tear (stage III), until finally the lunate itself becomes dislocated (stage IV). Concurrent fractures of the scaphoid, triquetrum, ulnar styloid,

and radial styloid are common. The median nerve is vulnerable to injury, particularly with lunate dislocations.

Radiographically, a lunate dislocation can be seen on the posteroanterior radiograph. Volar rotation of the lunate causes it to appear triangular, known as the "piece of pie sign." On lateral radiographs, the same volar rotation accounts for the "spilled teacup sign" as the lunate appears to be spilling into the palmar side of the wrist, disrupting its articulation with the radius. Carpal dislocations require urgent reduction, warranting orthopedic consultation in the ED or by the next morning because of the potential complexity of injury and high number of injuries that require operative intervention.

(A) Short arm casts are often appropriate for immobilization of nondisplaced carpal fractures. Second in frequency to those of the scaphoid, triquetral fractures may occur by direct trauma or fall onto the hand. Lunate fractures are rare but occur by the same mechanism and may be complicated by Kienbock disease, or posttraumatic avascular necrosis. Fractures of the pisiform, hamate, trapezium, capitate, and trapezoid are all very rare and amendable to treatment by short arm cast immobilization. (B) A sugar-tong splint would be useful to immobilize a distal radius fracture, but only after adequate reduction. A hematoma block helps with anesthesia and fracture reduction, the goals of which are the restoration of radial height and preservation of volar tilt. Finger traps may aid the reduction by decreasing distracting muscle spasm. (C) Thumb spica splinting is the treatment of choice for confirmed or suspected fractures of the scaphoid, the most frequently fractured carpal bone. Scaphoid fractures are associated with posttraumatic avascular necrosis due to compromise of the blood supply. (D) Fractures of the fourth and fifth metacarpals and digits may be treated with an ulnar gutter splint. The splint should run from distal to the midforearm to just beyond the DIP of the fourth to fifth digits. The wrist should be placed in slight extension, the MCPs in moderate (30 to 60 degrees) flexion, and the interphalangeal joints in mild flexion. Fractures of the metacarpal neck (boxer fractures) should be splinted with the MCPs in 90 degrees of flexion.

49. Answer: A[47,48]. The radiograph shows a perilunate dislocation, part of a pattern of carpal instability centered on the lunate. These most commonly occur after a fall on an outstretched hand, often with hyperextension and ulnar deviation. Mayfield et al. organized these injuries into four stages, the first of which is scapholunate dissociation, resulting in scaphoid rotation in a volar direction, which is also known as rotary subluxation of the scaphoid. Stage II injuries, as shown in Figure 24–49, involve further ligamentous damage such that the capitate is dislocated dorsally to the lunate—a "perilunate dislocation." Triquetral dislocation or ligamentous injury is seen in stage III injuries and stage IV injuries are complete lunate dislocations in a volar direction.

(B) A lunate dislocation is the final stage of the above classification, and is classically illustrated by the "spilled teacup" sign on the lateral radiograph of the wrist. There is volar dislocation and rotation of the lunate, which seems to spill forward. The lunate may appear to have a triangular shape on the AP wrist radiograph. This represents a significant ligamentous injury, and may be associated with carpal fractures and median nerve injury. Lunate dislocations must be quickly reduced and often require operative fixation. (C) Scaphoid fractures are often associated with stages II, III, and IV carpal instability injuries, but one is not present in this case. (D) Scaphoid rotation and subluxation represent stage I carpal instability. Such injuries are caused by scapholunate dissociation, which appears on the AP radiographs as scapholunate joint widening (the gap between the front incisor teeth, commonly known as the Terry-Thomas or David Letterman sign). The distal pole of the scaphoid is seen end-on overlying the scaphoid, and appears as a circle known as the signet ring sign. (E) Triquetrum dislocation represents a stage III carpal instability injury, following the perilunate dislocation. This injury may be appreciated on lateral radiographs. The triquetrum may be fractured in injuries of this stage.

50. Answer: A[47,48]. The radiograph displays an intra-articular fracture of the base of the thumb with carpal-metacarpal (CMC) dislocation (Bennett fracture). The mechanism of injury is most commonly an axial load to the thumb, often while the thumb is slightly flexed, such as striking a rigid object with a closed fist. Rupture of the CMC ligaments leads to joint instability and subluxation/dislocation in a dorsal direction. Treatment consists of a thumb spica cast, but even slight displacement of the fracture after closed reduction requires operative intervention.

A Rolando fracture occurs by a similar mechanism but is far less common and results in a comminuted intra-articular fracture at the base of the thumb, often in a "Y" or "T" pattern. These fractures frequently require surgery and lead to arthritis more often than Bennett fractures.

(B) Falls onto an outstretched, pronated hand occur frequently and are associated with fractures of the distal radius (Colles) and carpal bones, as well as lunate and perilunate dislocations. The scaphoid is the most commonly injured carpal bone, followed by the triquetrum. (C) Falls onto an outstretched, supinated hand may result in distal radius fractures with volar angulation (Smith fracture). (D) Forced abduction of the thumb can result in a tear of the ulnar collateral ligament, also known at gamekeeper or skier thumb. A complete tear is likely if >35 degrees laxity in MCP valgus stress (done in extension and 30 degrees flexion), or >15 degrees difference in comparison with the other hand. Partial tears are sufficiently treated with a thumb spica splint, but complete tears usually require operative intervention. (E) Hyperextension of the thumb may lead to a tear of the volar plate and subluxation or dislocation of the first MCP. Such dislocations are reduced by flexing and adducting the metacarpal and applying pressure onto the base of the phalanx.

51. Answer: D[47,48]. The radiograph displays a fifth metacarpal neck fracture, commonly known as a boxer fracture. Such injuries usually result from striking a hard object with a closed fist. These fractures often display volar displacement, but the great mobility of the fourth and fifth digits allows for a large degree of acceptable angulation. Care must be taken to evaluate for rotational deformity, by seeing that all fingers point toward the scaphoid when closing the fist. Reduction of a boxer fracture is accomplished by means of the "90-90" method: after axial countertraction to disimpact the fracture, the DIP, PIP, and MCP are flexed to 90 degrees,, followed by simultaneous dorsal pressure to the PIP and volar pressure to the metacarpal shaft. An ulnar gutter splint is then applied and prompt orthopedic follow-up arranged, as such fractures can lose their reduction.

From the index finger to the fifth digit, the degree of acceptable metacarpal fracture angulation is 15-25-35-45 degrees, owing to differences in digit mobility. (A) 15 degrees corresponds to the index finger. (B) 25 degrees corresponds to the middle finger. (C) 35 degrees corresponds to the ring finger. (E) 55 degrees is excessive displacement for any metacarpal fractures.

52. Answer: B[47,48]. The radiograph shows a Colles fracture, or a distal radius fracture with dorsal displacement. This is the most common fracture about the wrist, usually occuring after a fall onto

an outstretched hand. Smith fractures may result by a similar mechanism but are defined by a distal radial fracture with volar displacement. Injuries associated with distal radius fractures include ulnar styloid fractures and carpal fractures. Median nerve injury may ocucur secondary to impingement by fracture fragments or the reduction of the fracture. ED treatment consists of prompt reduction after a hematoma block; finger traps may aid reduction efforts, which should focus on normalization of radial length and volar tilt. The tip of the radial styloid should extend 9 to 12 mm beyond the articular surface of the ulna and form an angle of 15 to 25 degrees with the ulna, both of which help to assess radial length. The typical amount of volar tilt is 10 to 25 degrees.

A neurologic examination of the hand should be documented before and after the reduction. Median nerve testing is performed by having the patient move the thumb in a palmar direction while the examiner palpates the thenar muscles. Sensation is assessed along the radial edge of the index finger. The radial nerve is examined by thumb or wrist extension and assessing sensation of the dorsal web space between the thumb and index finger. Ulnar nerve function is examined by spreading or crossing the fingers and checking sensation over the ulnar aspect of the fifth digit.

(A) The axillary nerve innervates the deltoid muscle and may be injured by shoulder dislocations. (C) The musculocutaneous nerve is part of the brachial plexus and innervates the biceps muscles. (D) The radial nerve spirals around the humerus and is vulnerable to injury by fracture or compression resulting in a wrist drop. (E) The ulnar nerve may be injured by fractures to the medial epicondyle or elbow dislocations.

53. Answer: A[47,48]. A Galeazzi fracture is characterized by a fracture of the distal third of the radial shaft and disruption of the distal radioulnar joint. The mechanism of injury is normally a fall onto an outstretched hand with forced pronation or, less commonly, a direct blow to the forearm. Although the radial fracture is usually obvious both clinically and radiographically, the distal radioulnar joint can appear normal on radiographs despite subluxation or dislocation. A concurrent ulnar styloid fracture is common. Because of instability of the fracture, operative fixation is almost always required.

(B) A Hutchinson fracture (chauffeur fracture) is an isolated fracture of the radial styloid which extends to the radiocarpal joint. It is usually caused by a fall or direct blow to the wrist. Nondisplaced injuries may be treated with immobilization alone, but displaced fractures need reduction and expedient orthopedic follow-up because many require operative fixation. (C) A Barton fracture involves an intra-articular fracture of the dorsal rim of the distal radius with dorsal displacement. This fracture type is relatively rare and almost uniformly requires prompt operative reduction. (D) A Monteggia fracture is a fracture of the proximal to midulnar shaft with concurrent dislocation of the radial head. Similar to a Galeazzi fracture, the mechanism of injury is often a fall onto the outstretched hand or direct trauma. The radial head may be palpated in the antecubital fossa and the entire forearm shortened. Treatment requires operative fixation, except in some pediatric patients in whom closed reduction may be sufficient. (E) A radial head fracture is also associated with a fall on an outstretched hand, although nondisplaced fractures are often not seen directly on the radiographs. Tenderness over the radial head coupled with a visible posterior fat pad or an enlarged anterior fat pad ("sail sign") on the lateral elbow radiograph are indicative of a fracture and necessitate treatment. Nondisplaced fractures can be immobilized with a sling, whereas displaced and comminuted fractures may be treated with a hematoma block, closed reduction, splint immobilization, and consideration for surgical fragment excision.

54. Answer: D. "Open-book" fractures of the pelvis, as shown in Figure 24–54, result from high-energy anteroposterior compressive forces. This causes separation of the pubic symphysis and rotational instability resulting from disruption of sacroiliac and sacrospinous ligaments. They are associated with a mortality rate of up to 25% because of concomitant visceral injuries. Mortality is even higher when an open injury or shock is present. Bleeding may result from disruption of the venous plexus, hemorrhage from fracture surfaces or injured branches of the iliac arteries. Patients with open-book fractures may have tenderness or deformity over the pubic symphysis, and instability of the pelvis when manually compressed. Examination may reveal blood at the meatus from urethral injury, vaginal bleeding from open pelvic fracture, or decreased rectal tone resulting from injury to the sacral nervous plexus. Frank hypovolemic shock may occur. Injuries to the diaphragm and thoracic aorta occur frequently in high-energy pelvic fractures.

Diagnosis is made by standard anteroposterior (AP) radiography. Stable patients should undergo CT of the abdomen and pelvis to detect associated visceral injuries and visualize the major elements of the pelvic fracture. In hemodynamically unstable patients, the site of bleeding must be identified as either pelvic or abdominal.

When there is disruption of the pelvic ring, ED care should prioritize aggressive resuscitation (including early transfusion of blood), identification of intra-abdominal bleeding (using FAST or DPL), and fracture stabilization. Candidates for angiographic embolization should be identified early (discussed below). Mechanical stabilization is a critical first step when treating high-energy pelvic fractures in the ED. A simple and readily accessible method for fracture reduction—circumferential pelvic antishock sheeting (CPAS)—is achieved by wrapping a longitudinally folded bed sheet around the pelvis and securing it with clamps. The sheet should be positioned between the iliac crests and greater trochanters, leaving free access points for angiography and laparotomy. Another technique is to internally rotate both legs and bind them together. Some authorities recommend application of an external fixator in the ED, but this is time-consuming, requires an orthopedic surgeon, and has not been shown to reduce mortality.

(A) Early blood transfusion is recommended in high-energy (especially open-book) pelvic fractures. These patients may require an average of up to 15 units of packed red blood cells. There is no role for early transfusion of platelets in the nonthrombocytopenic patient. (B) Use of the pneumatic antishock garment (PASG) is controversial. Although historically external compression by the PASG was thought to reduce diastasis in open-book fractures, no proven outcome benefit in blunt abdominal trauma exists. There is evidence to the contrary that it may worsen morbidity by increasing the risk of compartment syndrome, and restricting access to the abdomen and groin. (C) Pelvic angiography and embolization of bleeding vessels may be life-saving when arterial hemorrhage is suspected. In a patient with a major pelvic fracture who has hypotension without evident hemoperitoneum (eg, negative FAST or DPL) emergency angiography is indicated. Other indications for pelvic angiography include blood transfusion requirements >4 units, or contrast blush on CT. The management approach is based on the presence of intra-abdominal bleeding. Hemodynamically unstable patients with negative ultrasound or DPL should undergo angiography and embolization if hemodynamic instability is present, although those with positive findings for intra-abdominal hemorrhage should undergo laparotomy with follow-up angiography if brisk bleeding or hypotension persists. External fixation may also be applied in the operating room in a attempt to reduce pelvic bleeding. (E) Operative reduction of an open-book pelvic fracture is indicated when pubic diastasis >2.5 cm. This may be accomplished by external fixation or open reduction and internal fixation. Stabilization by anterior external fixation may provide definitive treatment of open-book fractures if the posterior arch is intact. However, the first step in this case is to resuscitate and stabilize the critically injured patient before definitive orthopedic treatment is undertaken.

55. Answer: C. Figure 55 demonstrates a fracture of the tuberosity of the fifth metatarsal base. This injury is often referred to as a pseudo-Jones fracture, to distinguish it from the more serious Jones fracture, defined as a transverse fracture of the fifth metatarsal occurring at least 15 mm from its proximal end and involving the articular surface between the bases of the fourth and fifth metatarsals. (The fracture named for Sir Robert Jones was the one he sustained himself, and reported in 1902, as well as 3 similar injuries and 2 avulsion fractures of the tuberosity.) The pseudo-Jones fracture is an avulsion of the fifth metatarsal tuberosity and may involve the articulation with the adjacent cuboid, but does not extend into the articulation between the fourth and fifth metatarsals.

Patients present with swelling and tenderness over the base of the fifth metatarsal, and difficulty bearing weight. Pain may be elicited by inversion of the foot. Management of the pseudo-Jones fracture is primarily symptomatic, with immobilization for 2 to 3 weeks in a compression dressing, hard-sole shoe or walking cast, and weight-bearing as tolerated. Prognosis is excellent. In contrast, true Jones fractures may be complicated by malunion or nonunion, and therefore may merit greater immobilization in a splint or cast and non-weight-bearing for at least 6 weeks.

(A) Diagnosis is made by standard views of the foot: AP, lateral, and oblique. The fracture is sometimes seen on ankle radiographs when only an "ankle sprain" is suspected. The base of the fifth metatarsal should therefore always be palpated in all patients with apparent ankle sprains. If there is tenderness in that region, foot radiographs should be

obtained. (B) The "march" fracture is a stress fracture of the metatarsal shaft, usually the third metatarsal, initially described by the Prussian military physician Breithaupt in 1855. Nondisplaced metatarsal shaft fractures may be treated with a walking cast or hard sole shoe. Displaced midshaft metatarsal fractures require reduction (especially in patients where >3 mm of displacement or 10 degrees of angulation occur), casting, and non-weight-bearing for 6 weeks. The first metatarsal, which has greater load-bearing function, requires more aggressive surgical management. Fractures of the metacarpal neck are treated similarly to shaft fractures, although open fixation may be required in the case of post-reduction instability. (D) Most pseudo-Jones fractures can be successfully treated without surgery. Fixation may be required for intra-articular tuberosity fractures displaced >2 mm or involving >30% of the articular surface. (E) The pseudo-Jones fracture results typically from inversion of the plantar flexed foot, and is believed to involve the lateral band of the plantar aponeurosis (not the insertion of the peroneus brevis tendon, as previously believed).

56. Answer: D. Tarso-metatarsal fracture-dislocation, commonly referred to as a Lisfranc injury, is uncommon because of the substantial force typically required to disrupt this joint complex. Common mechanisms include motor vehicle collisions and sporting injuries. Patients typically present with severe midfoot pain, inability to bear weight, and paresthesias of the toes. Physical examination findings may range from ecchymosis and soft tissue swelling to gross deformity. Plantar ecchymosis is highly suggestive. Vascular compromise may result from injury to the dorsalis pedis artery or its branch between the first and second metatarsals.

(A) Treatment typically includes closed reduction and internal fixation, followed by cast immobilization, and non-weight-bearing for the first 12 weeks. Open injuries or evidence of vascular compromise or compartment syndrome require emergent surgical evaluation. Inadequately or untreated injuries may result in degenerative arthritis, loss of the metatarsal arch, and reflex sympathetic dystrophy (RSD). (B) Francis Chopart described disarticulation at the midtarsal joint, which includes the talonavicular and calcaneocuboid joints. Although rare, injury to this complex may occur from forced dorsiflexion and should be suspected in the presence of isolated midfoot fractures, especially injury to the navicular tuberosity. Nondisplaced Chopart fracture may heal with cast immobilization, but operative treatment is usually required. (C) Associated fractures of the foot are common. These include fractures of the base of the second metatarsal (the **fleck sign**), navicular, cuboid, and cuneiforms. Thoracolumbar injuries are associated with calcaneus fractures that are due to an axial loading mechanism of injury. (E) A fracture through the base of the second metatarsal is pathognomonic of injury to the tarsometatarsal joint complex. Radiographic evaluation should include three standard views, looking for alignment of the medial margins of the second metatarsal base and the second cuneiform on the AP view, and the medial margin of the cuboid and fourth metatarsal base on the internal oblique view. The radiographic findings may be subtle. Displacement of the first or second metatarsals relative to each other on the lateral view may also indicate injury to the Lisfranc joint complex. The Lisfranc joint takes its name from Jacques Lisfranc, a field surgeon in Napoleon's army who initially described a technique of amputation at this joint.When suspicion persists despite initial negative radiographs, consider stress (eg, weight-bearing) views or CT.

57. Answer: B. Patellar fractures occur as the result of direct trauma (eg, falls, dashboard injuries) or forces transmitted indirectly through muscular or tendonous attachments. They are classified by location (upper or lower pole), orientation (transverse or vertical), and degree of displacement and comminution. Transverse and vertical fractures are most common, accounting for 50% to 80% of patellar fractures, with comminuted or stellate fractures representing most of the remainder. Avulsion fractures and isolated osteochondral injuries are less common. Displaced transverse fractures, as shown in Figure 24–57, result from forceful contraction of the quadriceps muscle, and are seen more frequently in young adults. Rarely (as in this case of this patient) they result from the propagation of nondisplaced stress fractures from overuse or athletic injury.

Patients with patellar fractures typically present with pain, swelling, and hemarthrosis, and may be unable to extend at the knee. Although most patellar fractures can be diagnosed by standard AP and lateral radiographs, an axial view (aka, merchant or sunrise view) may be necessary to detect vertical patellar fractures.

Management of patellar injuries depends on the type of fracture and the degree of displacement. Widely displaced transverse fractures (>2 to 3 mm) require open reduction and internal fixation, typically by tension wire banding. Earlier surgical correction is associated with better outcome. Surgical repair is indicated for any injury associated with disruption of the extensor mechanism. If definitive surgical treatment will be delayed, immobilization with a posterior splint or knee immobilizer is acceptable until orthopedic follow-up can be arranged.

(A) Joint aspiration is not routinely indicated, but may be considered along with injection of lidocaine or bupivicaine if knee extension is limited by pain. (C) Partial or complete patellectomy may be required for treatment of displaced comminuted fractures. Surgical correction involves repair of the retinaculum and suturing of the patellar ligament to the quadriceps femoris tendon. (D) Closed reduction in the ED is appropriate for isolated, closed patellar dislocations, and involves gently extending the affected leg while applying anterior and medial force on the lateral aspect of the patella. (E) The extensor mechanism of the knee may be disrupted by displaced transverse patellar fractures and is diagnosed on physical examination. Magnetic resonance imaging (MRI) is not routinely indicated for this purpose. MRI is useful, however, in diagnosing nondisplaced patellar fractures that might not be visible radiographically, as well as associated meniscal or ligamentous injuries.

58. Answer: C. Figure 24–58 shows a fracture of the lateral tibial plateau. The lateral plateau is most commonly fractured (75%), and may cause injury to the peroneal nerve when displaced. Tibial plateau fractures are the second most common fracture about the knee after patellar fractures. They usually result from axial loading with a valgus (medially directed) component. In young individuals, they usually result from high-energy forces (eg, falls, motor vehicle collisions), although elderly patients with osteoporosis may suffer fractures following minor trauma. Patients typically present with knee pain, inability to bear weight, swelling, ecchymosis, and effusion. Varus (laterally directed) or valgus deformity suggests depression of the affected condyle.

Management of plateau fractures varies based upon severity, but always entails precise reduction and non-weight-bearing for 6 to 8 weeks, in addition to early range of motion to prevent joint stiffness. Conservative treatment may include the use of a knee immobilizer and compression dressing, immobilization in a hinged knee fracture brace, or skeletal traction without tibial pinning. Prognosis is dependent upon the degree of depression, displacement, and comminution, and whether the injury is open or closed. Orthopedic consultation is required to determine the need for and timing of open reduction of internal fixation. Complications include compartment syndrome, popliteal artery injury, deep venous thrombosis, and osteoarthritis. (A) There is no defined role for measuring ankle-brachial index (ABI) in patients with fracture of the tibial plateau if the knee is not dislocated. However, accurate determination of neurovascular status must be made promptly, as the popliteal artery may be injured by bone fragments from either condyle. Displaced fractures of the lateral condyle may impinge on the anterior tibial artery. In the setting of knee dislocation, the presence of an ABI <0.9 has been shown to be up to 100% sensitive and 100% specific for vascular injury. (B) Ligamentous injury, especially of the anterior collateral ligament (ACL) and medial collateral ligament (MCL), may occur in up to 25% of tibial plateau fractures. The "unhappy triad" refers specifically to the combination of injuries to the ACL, MCL, and medial meniscus that result from a medially directed force. (D) Several systems have been proposed for classifying tibial plateau fractures (eg, Schatzker classification). These systems describe fractures by their anatomic location and magnitude of displacement, and may be useful in the ED to estimate clinical outcome. (E) Diagnosis can usually be made on routine AP and lateral knee radiographs, although oblique views may be necessary to show subtle fractures. A lipohemarthrosis (fat-fluid level in the suprapatellar bursa) seen on a cross-table lateral view can serve as a clue to the presence of a subtle or occult tibial plateau fracture. CT is used to determine the degree of displacement or in detecting a tibial plateau fracture when the radiographs are equivocal.

59. Answer: A. Fracture of the calcaneus is the most common tarsal fracture, and is typically associated with direct axial compression. Falls or jumps landing on the feet are the most common mechanism. Patients present with heel pain and an inability to bear weight. They may have deformation of the heel or ecchymoses over the sole (which is not seen in isolated malleolar fractures). Diagnosis can usually be made by standard radiographs. Standard foot and ankle radiographs are required; an axial (Harris) view to image the calcaneal tuberosity and subtalar joint is recommended. CT is used to define the extent of calcaneal injury, and is frequently used for surgical planning. Calcaneal fractures are commonly classified as extraarticular or intra-articular, based on whether they involve the subtalar joint. The latter are frequently associated with poor functional outcome (≥75%). (B) When the diagnosis is suspected but distinct fracture is not evident, determination of Boehler angle may be helpful in detecting a calcaneal fracture. As shown in Figure 24–59B, Boehler angle is determined by measuring the angle between 2 intersecting lines: the first crossing the posterior tuberosity and apex of the posterior facet, and the second connecting the apex of the posterior facet and the apex of the anterior process. Boehler angle is classically defined as 28 degrees, though any measurement between 20 degrees and 40 degrees within the range of normal. An angle <20 degrees strongly suggests the presence of a compression fracture. However, a normal Boehler angle does not exclude a fracture. (C) The presence of a calcaneal fracture should prompt the search for associated injuries, such as other lower extremity injuries (25% of patients) and spinal injuries (10% of patients). These commonly include fractures of the tibial plateau and compression fractures of the vertebrae, most commonly at the thoracolumbar junction. ≥7% of calcaneal fractures occur bilaterally. Compartment syndrome of the foot may also complicate a calcaneal fracture. Accurate diagnosis may require measurement of compartment pressures, because tissue ischemia can occur before definitive physical findings appear. (D) Management of calcaneal fractures remains controversial. Generally, conservative therapy is appropriate for most extraarticular fractures of the body, anterior process, or tuberosity. Closed reduction may be preferred for elderly or neuropathic patients. Most intra-articular or displaced calcaneal fractures require open reduction and fixation. Early orthopedic consultation is therefore advised. (E) The Ottawa ankle rules are used to select patients for radiographic imaging who present to the ED with ankle or midfoot pain following trauma. Radiographs of the ankle are required if the patient has bony tenderness over the distal 6 cm of the tibia or fibula (including the malleoli). Radiographs of the foot are required if there is bony tenderness over the navicular or the base of the fifth metatarsal. Ankle and foot radiographs are also indicated if the patient is unable to bear weight for four steps immediately after the injury and in the ED. These rules, however, are not applicable to calcaneal injuries.

60. Answer: D. Clostridial myonecrosis, or gas gangrene, results from inoculation with the ubiquitous

spore-forming bacillus of the genus *Clostridium*. Although historically associated with trauma or surgery, the number of spontaneous cases is increasing. *Clostridium perfringens* is the most frequently implicated species (80% to 95%), followed by *C. septicum*. Mixed aerobic and anaerobic infections may also occur.

The incubation period of *Clostridium* may be <3 days, and the disease progresses rapidly to involve deep tissue layers. Patients may present with altered sensorium and signs of systemic toxicity. Tachycardia may be marked despite minimal elevations in body temperature. The most ominous and important symptom is pain, which is classically out of proportion to examination findings. Because early skin changes may be minimal, a high level of suspicion must be maintained to make an accurate and timely diagnosis. Cutaneous manifestations vary from normal to tense to dusky bronze. As the infection progresses, vesicles with foul-smelling brown exudate may occur. Muscle necrosis, mediated by the elaboration of multiple exotoxins, results in the "cooked flesh" appearance when surgically explored.

Management of clostridial myonecrosis includes fluid resuscitation and broad-spectrum antibiotics (penicillin G plus clindamycin). The mainstay of therapy is aggressive surgical debridement. Although the benefits of hyperbaric oxygen (HBO) therapy have not been shown in controlled trials, many authors recommend early HBO to reduce clostridial growth, inhibit toxin production, and enhance both immune response and wound healing. (A) Lymphocutaneous sporotrichosis results from inoculation of the dimorphic fungus *Sporothrix schenkii* into injured skin. High-risk groups include rose gardeners, horticulturalists, and armadillo hunters. (Armadillos have frequent contact with the *S. schenkii* from digging soil in which the fungus grows.) Cutaneous manifestations are typically painless smooth or verrucous papulonodular lesions up to 4 cm in diameter. They may be erythematous, and frequently ulcerate. Diagnosis is made by culture, preferably of biopsied tissue. Treatment is with itraconazole. (B) Skin manifestations associated with the Gram-positive coccus *Staphylococcus aureus* may result from direct infection (eg, folliculitis) or indirectly from exfoliative toxins, as in the staphylococcal scalded skin syndrome (SSSS). SSSS (aka Ritter disease) is seen most commonly in infants as the result of skin or mucosal colonization. This infection occurs rarely among adults, though when it does, it is associated with a much higher mortality

rate (>50%, versus <5% in children). Patients present with localized disease (bullous impetigo) or generalized skin scalding, often accompanied by fever and malaise. Subcutaneous air is absent. Treatment includes general supportive care, antibiotics, and decontamination of close contacts. (C) The spore-forming anaerobic bacillus *Clostridium tetani* is not associated with a gas-forming soft tissue infection. *C. tetani* is noninvasive, and typically requires a deeply penetrating wound for inoculation (although in some patients the injury may be either innocuous or unapparent). Although *C. tetani* is ubiquitous in soil and feces, successful vaccination has made tetanus rare. When it does occur, it is most often generalized, marked by debilitating trismus, opisthotonus, laryngeal spasm, and autonomic dysregulation. Localized, cephalic, and neonatal forms occur less frequently. Supportive treatment consists of airway management, sedation with benzodiazepines (and in some patients paralysis), and sympathetic blockade. Tetanus immunoglobulin (TIG) binds circulating toxin, and should be administered promptly in addition to tetanus toxoid. Antibiotics (preferably metronidazole) and wound debridement prevent further toxin production by bacteria, but because they may be associated with transient toxin release, they should be preceded by TIG administration when feasible. (E) Cutaneous anthrax results from inoculation with spores of *Bacillus anthracis*, usually as a result of direct or indirect contact with infected animals or their hides. Person-to-person spread is extremely rare. The characteristic lesion begins as a pruritic papule that gradually enlarges and is surrounded by a ring of vesicles, which may contain hemorrhagic exudate. Eventually these vesicles rupture, and a central eschar of necrotic tissue develops. Fever, toxemia, extensive tissue edema, and painful adenopathy may occur. ~10% to 20% of untreated cases result in death. Diagnosis should be suspected clinically, and confirmed by polychrome methylene blue staining (McFadyean reaction). *B. anthracis* is sensitive to penicillin G. Tetracycline and ciprofloxacin are acceptable alternatives.

61. Answer: D. The clay-shoveler fracture is an avulsion fracture of the spinous process of one of the lower cervical vertebrae (classically the seventh) resulting from sudden head flexion against the supraspinous ligament. It was reported as an occupational injury among both Australian drain diggers and German autobahn laborers in the 1930s. Today it is more commonly caused by a direct blow

to the C7 spinous process. When isolated, this injury is mechanically stable and not associated with neurologic injury. Diagnosis is usually evident on the standard lateral view, although it can be missed when C7 is not adequately visualized. Outpatient management may be appropriate if no neurologic deficits or ligamentous laxity is present and pain can be controlled with oral analgesics.

(A) Geoffery Jefferson described burst fracture of the atlas (C1) resulting from compressive axial forces. It may be associated with disruption of the transverse ligament. On the lateral radiograph, this fracture typically causes widening of the predental space (>3 mm in adults or 5 mm in children). On the open-mouth view, the lateral masses appear laterally displaced. If the sum of this displacement is >7 mm, rupture of the transverse ligament is likely. CT may be required for confirmation, especially when displacement is minimal. (B) A pillar fracture results from extension and rotation forces that cause impaction of a vertebra on the articular mass one level below it. The adjacent pedicle and lamina remain intact. This injury is considered to be mechanically stable. (C) The hangman fracture, or traumatic spondylolisthesis of C2, results from combined axial loading and hyperextension. Originally described in judicial hangings—in which a knot was placed under the angle of the mandible and the individual dropped from a height of 5 to 8 feet—the fracture is now commonly seen in motor vehicle collisions. It is characterized by bilateral neural arch fractures of the axis, usually through the pars interarticularis, and may be associated with atlantoaxial dislocation. The relatively large diameter of the spinal cord at this level makes spinal cord injury uncommon. (E) The Tillaux fracture is not an injury of the cervical spine, but an avulsion fracture of the distal tibial epiphysis seen in adolescents resulting from forces on the anterior talofibular ligament.

62. Answer: B. The open-mouth cervical radiograph as shown in Figure 24–62A is a fracture through the base of the odontoid. The lateral view reveals anterior displacement of C1 on C2. Fractures of the first and second cervical vertebrae are frequently unstable, because of their relative lack of mechanical (ie, ligamentous and muscular) support. Type I odontoid fractures occur above the transverse ligaments, and are stable. Type II fractures (see Figures 24–62A and 24–62B) are common, and involve disruption through the base of the odontoid process. They are unstable, and may be complicated by nonunion. Extension of the

fracture into the body of the axis defines type III odontoid fractures. Patients with injury to the axis may have pain referable to the occiput.

The diagnosis is usually evident on standard lateral and open-mouth view radiographs. Axial CT can occasionally miss this fracture because it lies in the plane of the CT slice; coronal and sagittal reformatted CT images may be needed. A common pitfall in the management of patients with head or neck trauma is failure to image the cervical spine based on mechanism alone when intoxication or associated injury masks pain or tenderness.

(A) Rotary atlantoaxial (C1 to C2) dislocation is an unstable flexion-rotation injury. It is diagnosed on the open mouth view which reveals asymmetry of the lateral masses. However, a rotated or obliquely oriented view may result in a false-positive diagnosis. (C) Avulsion fracture of the inferior pole of the anterior tubercle of the atlas (C1) may occur from hyperextension, and is best seen on the lateral view. It is unstable when the entire C1 arch is involved. (D) Occipitoatlantal dissociation may result in anterior or posterior displacement of the skull, and is usually obvious on lateral radiographs. It is frequently fatal. (E) Unlike occipitoatlantal dissociation, occipitoatlantal subluxation may not be radiographically apparent. One method for detecting this injury involves measuring the distances between the basion (the tip of the clivus) and a line extending from the posterior cortex of C2 of the lateral radiograph, and the distance between the basion and the superior cortex of the dens. Both the basion-axial and basion-dental intervals should be <12 mm. This injury is extremely unstable.

63. Answer: D. The flexion-teardrop fracture, as its name implies, results from flexion forces causing anterior displacement of a triangular-shaped fragment from the affected vertebral body. Neurologic injury frequently results from retropulsion of the vertebral body fragment into the spinal canal. The classic manifestation of neurologic injury from the flexion-teardrop fracture is anterior cord syndrome, characterized by paralysis and loss of pain and temperature sensation below the level of the lesion with conservation of posterior column functions (position, touch, and vibratory sense).

In addition to demonstration of the triangular vertebral fragment, radiographs may show abrupt kyphosis, posterior displacement of the vertebral body, widening of the facet joint, and widening of the interspinous and interlaminar processes.

(A) The flexion-teardrop fracture is mechanically unstable. Both two- and three-column models of cervical stability have been developed experimentally. The three-column model divides the spine into anterior, middle, and posterior columns. If two of the three columns are fractured, the injury is considered mechanically unstable. Although clinical scoring systems have been developed to predict instability of the lower cervical spine based on such models, there is no defined role for these tools in the ED. All patients with suspected cervical spinal trauma should be treated as having unstable injuries until proven otherwise, with appropriate immobilization, imaging, and consultation by a spinal surgeon. (B) In contrast to the flexion-teardrop fracture, the extension-teardrop fracture is usually stable in flexion, though it may be unstable in extension. It is associated with motor vehicle accidents and results when sudden neck extension causes the anterior longitudinal ligament to avulse the corner of the vertebral body. Extension-teardrop fractures most commonly affect C5 through C7. They may result in a central cord syndrome as a result of buckling of the ligamentum flavum into the spinal cord. This manifests as weakness which is greater in the upper extremities than in the lower extremities, with some loss of pain and temperature sensation. Bowel and bladder dysfunction are uncommon. (C) Treatment of potentially unstable cervical spinal fractures includes immobilization in a rigid collar, attention to the ABCs (which may be compromised by associated neck injury, disruption of diaphragmatic innervation, or neurogenic shock), and prompt neurosurgical consultation. There is no evidence-based role for soft cervical collars in the ED treatment of neck injury. (E) Flexion-teardrop fracture typically results from high-energy forces that cause severe flexion (eg, head-on motor vehicle collisions). Common mechanisms include motor vehicle collisions, diving into shallow water, and falls.

64. Answer: A. Figure 24–64A shows a burst fracture of the thoracolumbar spine at L1. The thoracic spine is stabilized by its articulation with the rib cage. This stabilizing mechanism is absent at the thoracolumbar junction, resulting in the frequency of this entity being surpassed only by cervical spine injuries. Injuries of the thoracolumbar spine are classified as major (implying mechanical instability and the potential to cause neurologic injury) and minor. Major injuries include wedge compression fractures with >50% loss of vertebral body height, Chance fractures, flexion distraction injuries, translational injuries, and burst fractures. Thoracolumbar burst fractures result from axial loading, and are most commonly associated with motor vehicle collisions. The degree and pattern of neurologic injury depends on the extent of impingement on the spinal cord by fracture fragments. Injury at the level of L1 to L2 may result in a **conus medullaris syndrome** characterized by bowel and bladder incontinence, saddle anesthesia, and upper motor neuron signs. Nerve root compression caudal to L1 manifests classically with distal lower extremity weakness and decreased deep tendon reflexes, in addition to bladder and bowel dysfunction (known as the **cauda equina syndrome**). Conus medullaris and cauda equina lesions may present in combination that make clinical differentiation difficult. Diagnosis of thoracolumbar burst fracture by plain radiography is characterized by disruption of the posterior vertebral body cortical line on the lateral view, and an increased distance between pedicles on the AP view (see Figure 24–64B). Patients with thoracolumbar burst fractures should undergo CT scanning to better characterize vertebral injury and spinal cord involvement. Burst fractures with or without signs of neurologic damage (eg, from nerve root compression) require emergent surgical evaluation.

(B) Thoracolumbar wedge compression fractures result when flexion forces compress the anterior vertebral body. Loss of anterior height is demonstrated by plain radiographs, though—unlike burst fractures—the posterior vertebral body height and posterior cortex remain intact. However, CT is recommended to evaluate the posterior elements and to rule out involvement of the neural canal when >33% of the anterior vertebral body height is lost. Like all major thoracolumbar injuries, wedge compression fractures that involve >50% should be treated with spinal immobilization until imaging with CT and evaluation by a spinal surgeon occur. (C) The Chance fracture is a fracture that extends anteriorly though the spinous process, pedicles, and vertebral body, that results from flexion-distraction forces around an axis anterior to the vertebral bodies. It is most commonly associated with lap-type seat belt restraint, particularly those without a shoulder strap. The incidence of associated intra-abdominal injuries ~50% (especially in children), often involving the pancreas. The lateral radiograph reveals horizontal fractures through the posterior elements and vertebral body. The diagnosis may be missed on axial CT if the fracture lies in the same plane as the scan. Neurologic injury is uncommon. Treatment is generally by closed reduction and immobilization. (D) Fractures of the thoracolumbar transverse and spinous processes are classified as minor fractures, as are wedge fractures that involve <50% loss of vertebral body height. In the absence of neurologic damage, they are considered stable, although CT may be required to exclude the presence of other spinal or visceral injuries. (E) A translational injury refers to the translation of one or more vertebral segments on lower segments that result in complete spinal disruption. It results from shearing forces, and is almost always associated with neurologic injury.

65. Answer: D. Figure 24–65 shows an acute SDH. There are clotted collections of blood between the dura and arachnoid membrane that result from sudden acceleration-deceleration injuries. They may complicate as ≥30% of severe head trauma cases. SDHs are more common in alcoholic and elderly patients whose brains are atrophic and the superficial bridging veins are more susceptible to injury. SDH are classified based on the timing of symptom onset as acute (within the initial 24 hours), subacute (within 1 to 2 weeks), or chronic (>2 weeks). Patients may present with altered level of consciousness, pupillary asymmetry, or motor weakness. The patient may manifest a lucid interval before decompensating, similar to epidural hematoma (EDH). Immediate loss of consciousness with a SDH is a poor prognostic sign, as these patients often have diffuse axonal injury (DAI). SDH diagnosed after infantile seizure may be attributable to birth trauma, but the possibility of child abuse must be considered. The management of SDH requires supportive care and prompt neurosurgical evaluation. The treatment for most SDHs is evacuation, although observation may be appropriate for small bleeds in stable patients.

(A) Noncontrast head CT, rather than MRI, is the imaging modality of choice to detect an acute SDH. CT may also reveal associated injuries and evidence of herniation. SDH appears as a crescent-shaped hyperattenuating lesion interposed between the skull and cerebral cortex. By contrast, an epidural hematoma has a lentiform morphology. Unlike epidural hematomas, SDH may cross suture lines. Subacute SDHs appear isoattenuating, and may only be visible on a contrast-enhanced study. Chronic SDHs are hypoattenuating as a result of iron phagocytosis. (B) The use of drugs or alcohol has been implicated in ≥50% of all patients treated for trauma. For injured patients with histories of

substance use, standardized short bedside interventions have been shown to decrease injury recurrence by 47% over a 3-year period. (C) Although several studies showed a benefit to the off-label use of recombinant-activated factor VII in reducing traumatic intracerebral hemorrhage, a phase III trial by its manufacturer failed to show improvements in mortality and severe disability. (E) Prognosis of SDH is dependent on associated intracranial injuries and the pressure exerted on brain tissue by the expanding hematoma, rather than the absolute size of the hematoma itself. Overall survival ranges from 35% to 50%, with worse outcome associated with greater age, decreased level of consciousness, evidence of herniation on initial presentation, and posterior fossa SDH.

66. Answer: B. Spontaneous SAH has an overall morbidity and mortality rate of 50%. Up to 12% of all patients presenting to the ED with sudden onset, severe headache will be diagnosed with SAH. The majority (80%) occur from rupture of saccular aneurysms of the circle of Willis. Risk factors include age, hypertension, and the use of tobacco, alcohol, and cocaine, as well as heritable connective tissue disorders, and autosomal dominant polycystic kidney disease.

Patients classically present with a "thunderclap headache," often described as the worst headache of their life. Nausea and vomiting are common (≥75%). Examination may reveal meningismus in 50% of patients, and 20% demonstrate focal neurologic findings (eg, ocular palsies). Patients may occasionally present with isolated neck pain without headache. ~50% of patients suffering SAH will demonstrate an altered level of consciousness, and 17% are complicated by seizure.

Noncontrast CT of the brain is the initial test of choice for acute SAH, with >90% sensitivity when performed within initial 24 hours. Its sensitivity wanes with time, however, with ~80% of bleeds detected at 48 hours, and only 50% detected 1 week postevent. Treatment of SAH includes attention to airway, breathing, and circulation, prompt neurosurgical consultation, and the use of the calcium channel blocker, nimodipine, to prevent ischemic stroke due to post-hemorrhage vasospasm. Patients should receive analgesics and antiemetics as needed. The use of prophylactic anticonvulsants is controversial. Angiography is indicated to locate the anatomic source of bleeding. Treatment of an aneurysm consists of surgical clipping or endovascular coils depending on the location of the aneurysm and surgical expertise.

(A) Lumbar puncture (LP) is indicated when SAH is suspected and the CT scan is normal. Diagnosis is made by detection of red blood cells and xanthochromia (presence of yellow pigmentation from metabolized hemoglobin) in CSF supernatant. Xanthochromia may not be detectable within the first 12 hours posthemorrhage, and controversy exists regarding the practice of delaying LP to improve the sensitivity of this test. The practice of comparing RBC counts in the first and last tubes collected is not a reliable means to distinguish a traumatic tap from SAH. (C) Despite its proven superiority in comparison with visual inspection in detecting CSF xanthochromia, only 1% of U.S. laboratories use this technique according to a 2001 survey. Regardless of the assay used, however, the absence of xanthochromia cannot be used to rule out SAH. (D) The Hunt and Hess scale grades patients with SAH based upon initial clinical status, principally the level of consciousness, and ranges from asymptomatic (grade 0) to mild or severe headache (grades 1 and 2) to comatose (grade 5), with higher grades portending worse outcomes. Patients with lower grades are more appropriate candidates for angiography and surgery. (E) Coital cephalgia is a benign headache syndrome associated with sexual intercourse, and is more common among men. In patients who experience sudden, severe headaches during orgasm, the possibility of SAH must be investigated.

67. Answer: C. Blow-out fracture of the orbital floor is one of the most common facial fractures, resulting from increased intraorbital pressure transmitted by a blow to the orbit by a projectile (eg, softball) or closed fist. It may occur alone or in concert with other facial fractures (eg, Le Fort fractures or fractures of the zygomatic arch or orbital rim). Patients may complain of decreased visual acuity, pain, diplopia, or epistaxis. There is a high incidence of ocular injury (25%). The infraorbital nerve passes through the orbital floor, which, when injured, may result in infraorbital anesthesia. Concurrent retroorbital hematoma may manifest as exophthalmos. Swelling and ecchymosis around the orbit are typical, and palpation may reveal tenderness or crepitus due to subcutaneous air.

The role of radiographs in diagnosis of facial fractures has been supplanted by CT when readily available. CT is more able to detect fractures, and may reveal entrapment of extraocular muscles, retrobulbar hematomas, and ocular injuries. MRI may be useful in some instances to evaluate the soft tissues and optic nerve.

Medical therapy includes prophylaxis with oral antibiotics, decongestants, and recommendations against nose-blowing (which might create or aggravate orbital emphysema). Some authors recommend a brief course of oral prednisone to reduce orbital edema. Surgical treatment of an orbital blow-out fracture is typically delayed 1 to 2 weeks postinjury, and is usually limited to patients with persistent diplopia or enophthalmos. Operative fixation with plating is the preferred approach.

(A) The presence of orbital fractures should increase suspicion for ocular injury. Evaluation may be limited by soft tissue swelling, and ophthalmologic consultation should be considered. Associated injuries may include corneal abrasion, traumatic iritis, hyphema, optic neuropathy, or globe rupture. Hypopyon, which represents purulent exudate layering in the anterior chamber, is more commonly associated with infectious or inflammatory conditions, although it may result from penetrating trauma. (B) Ecchymoses around the eyes (raccoon eyes) or the mastoid process (Battle sign) are suggested of basilar skull fracture. Other signs of basilar skull fracture include hemotympanum, CSF rhinorrhea, and CSF otorrhea. (D) Entrapment of the inferior rectus muscle in the fractured orbital floor may result in paralysis of upward (not downward) gaze. Diplopia is typically binocular vertical or oblique in orientation. (E) Subcutaneous emphysema indicates sinus fracture or violation of the nasal antrum. Rarely, emergent cantholysis may be indicated to relieve increased IOP on the optic nerve or retina caused by tension orbital emphysema.

68. Answer: C[49]. First-degree atrioventricular (AV) block is defined as the prolonged transmission of an electrical impulse originating from the sinus node without losing ("dropping") the impulse. The ECG manifestations of first-degree AV block include prolongation of the PR interval >200 milliseconds (0.2 seconds; 1 "big" box on ECG paper), and the presence of a P wave that precedes each QRS waveform. Etiologies for first-degree AV block include idiopathic, intrinsic conduction pathway disease, increased vagal tone, myocardial ischemia/infarction, infection (eg, myocarditis), electrolyte disturbance, and therapeutic/toxic drug effect. The most common site of electrical transmission delay is the AV node, although signal delay may also occur within the atria or, less commonly, in the His-Purkinje system. The management of first-degree AV block is usually supportive; no specific therapy is indicated. Serious sequelae resulting

solely from this dysrhythmia are uncommon. Patients with first-degree AV block but without syncope, murmurs, or unstable signs or symptoms do not require emergent echocardiography, pharmacotherapy, pacing, or continuous cardiac monitoring.

The transient light-headedness in this patient was likely due to the phlebotomy and blood donation, and the first degree AV block was an incidental finding. The patient should be reassured and referred for follow-up to her PCP.

69. Answer: E[50]. The rhythm pictured is second-degree AV block type II (eg, Mobitz II AV block). ECG manifestations of type II second-degree AV block include an absent ("dropped") QRS complex following a P wave. Preservation of the PR interval in all beats preceding and following the non-conducted impulse is noted. QRS complexes are often of normal duration (<120 milliseconds), but may be prolonged if infranodal conduction disorders coexist. Type II second-degree AV block is an example of a "high-grade" AV block, and its presence is always considered pathologic.

The significance of type II second-degree AV block, especially when it occurs in the context of myocardial ischemia and myocardial infarction (MI), is that it represents derangement of the infranodal conduction system. Type II second-degree AV block is most commonly associated with anterior wall MI, in contrast to type I second-degree AV block, which is associated with inferior wall infarctions. Type II second-degree AV block is associated with an increased incidence of deterioration into complete AV block (third-degree AV block).

Stable patients who present with type II second-degree AV block should be monitored continuously. In stable, asymptomatic patients in whom acute coronary syndrome is suspected or confirmed, transcutaneous pacing electrodes should be applied; both temporary transcutaneous and transvenous pacing modalities should be available at the bedside should the patient's condition deteriorate. In unstable or symptomatic patients, transcutaneous or transvenous pacing is the most appropriate initial intervention. Intravenous infusions of dopamine or epinephrine are pharmacologic adjuncts for hemodynamically unstable patients when pacing is not immediately available.

There is no role for atropine in the management of patients with high-grade (infranodal) AV blocks; it is most effective for supranodal AV blocks or blocks that occur at the level of the AV node. In patients with supranodal or nodal AV blocks in the context of acute coronary syndromes, atropine may cause harm by increasing heart rate, myocardial workload, and myocardial oxygen consumption. These effects will worsen ischemia and increase the zone of MI. Adenosine, an AV nodal blocker, is indicated in the management of supraventricular tachycardias (except those in association with Wolff-Parkinson-White syndrome).

70. Answer: E[51]. When encountering an R-S-R' type QRS waveform on an ECG, one reflexively thinks of a right bundle branch block (RBBB). The abnormal ST segments throughout the precordial leads may also suggest to some that this patient is having an acute MI. A closer look at this figure, however, reveals that a bundle branch block is not the condition pictured here. The portion of the QRS which appears to be an R' wave is actually a "J wave," also known as an Osborn wave. The bradycardia and the presence of the Osborn wave indicate that this patient has significant hypothermia. Hypothermia is classified as mild, moderate, or severe. Mild hypothermia is defined as core body temperatures >34°C (93.2°F). Moderate hypothermia is defined as core body temperatures between 30°C (86°F) and 34°C (93.2°F). Severe hypothermia is defined as core body temperatures <30°C (86°F).

Patients with moderate or severe hypothermia should be handled carefully (hypothermic hearts have a low threshold for sudden deterioration to ventricular tachycardia or ventricular fibrillation). Therapy for hypothermic patients depends on the severity of the presentation and on the presence (or absence) of a perfusing rhythm. Techniques for passive rewarming (eg, warm blankets, warm environment), active external rewarming (eg, heating blankets, forced warmed air, warmed IV infusions), and active internal rewarming (eg, cardiopulmonary bypass, peritoneal lavage, endotracheal intubation with humidified warmed air, pleural lavage with warmed fluids, bladder irrigation with warmed fluids) should be initiated in the ED. "Afterdrop," the drop in core temperature seen when extremities are rewarmed faster than the body core, and cold blood redistributes from the periphery to the core, should be avoided. Conventional ACLS-related therapies may also be required, but have limited efficacy in terminating dysrhythmias and restoring perfusion in the hypothermic heart. Other underlying co-morbid conditions and injuries should also be considered when treating patients with hypothermia.

(A, B, C, D) The other choices presented in this question are associated with different ECG findings that are classic and which should be remembered. Hypokalemia, hypocalcemia, and hypomagnesemia produce QT interval prolongation; with severely low electrolyte levels, deterioration into ventricular fibrillation, ventricular tachycardia, or torsade de pointes is likely. Hyperkalemia is associated with hyperacute T waves, progressive distortion of the QRS and QT intervals, and (with extremely elevated potassium levels) a sinusoidal waveform at high risk for deterioration into ventricular fibrillation or asystole.

71. Answer: A[52,53]. Left bundle branch blocks (LBBBs) are commonly found in patients with new or pre-existent coronary artery disease. The mere presence of a new LBBB in a patient with symptoms consistent with acute MI is sufficient criteria for emergent percutaneous coronary intervention (PCI) or fibrinolytic therapy. When LBBB is pre-existent in a patient with symptoms suggestive of an acute MI, the ECG can be difficult to interpret.

Sgarbossa, et al, reported several findings that can be used to predict the presence of MI in patients with preexistent LBBB. These include the following: concordant (lateral lead) ST segment elevation of at least 1 mm; ST segment depression of at least 1 mm in leads V1, V2, or V3; or discordant ST segment elevation of at least 5 mm. Concordance refers to elevation or depression of the ST segment in the same direction as the major QRS vector. Discordance refers to elevation or depression of the ST segment in the direction opposite the major QRS vector.

For example, LBBB in the lateral leads usually manifests with a prominent R wave (QRS complex appears upright and is above the isoelectric line); the ST segment and T waves are usually below the isoelectric line. When ST segment elevations above the isoelectric line and upright T waves occur in the lateral leads (as in a patient with an acute MI), this finding is known as concordance, and is one indicator of myocardial injury. The specificity for MI is >90% when 1 or more of these waveform characteristics are present in a patient with symptoms of acute MI.

72. Answer: D[53]. The findings shown represent an acute anterior wall myocardial infarct (AWMI). MIs classically manifest with ST segment elevations in 2 or more contiguous leads; ST segment elevations occur in the leads corresponding with the location of the occluded coronary artery. ST segment elevation AWMIs produce elevations in the precordial leads (V1 through V4), and most commonly result from thrombosis of the left anterior descending coronary artery or one of its major branches. ST segment elevation inferior wall MIs (IWMIs) produce elevations in leads II, III, and aVF; these infarctions most commonly result from thrombosis of the right coronary artery (RCA) or one of its major branches. ST segment elevation lateral wall MIs produce elevations in leads I, aVL, V5, and V6; these infarctions result most commonly from thrombosis of the left circumflex artery. The only MI which is not associated with ST segment elevations with conventional ECG lead placement is the posterior wall MI (PWMI) (horizontal ST segment depressions in V1 and V2 in association with prominent R waves and an R/S wave ratio of >1 in V2 are the most common findings; ST segment elevations may be seen with additional precordial leads, [V7 through V9]). Posterior wall MIs usually result from thrombosis of the right circumflex branch of the RCA.

The focus of treatment strategies for an acute ST segment elevation MI (STEMI) is to rapidly identify patients with acute events upon presentation to the ED, stratify them according to their risk factors and presenting signs and symptoms (eg, hypotension), and quickly provide them with the best definitive reperfusion therapies. Aspirin is considered standard-of-care intervention when there is no history on allergy. Likewise, β-adrenergic antagonist should be given immediately upon arrival to stable patients provided no contraindications exist (eg, cocaine toxicity, CHF, cardiogenic shock, relative/absolute hypotension). The scientific literature supports administration of unfractionated or low-molecular weight heparins, clopidogrel (most studies support a 300-mg loading dose), and an ACE inhibitor (usually within 24 hours of infarct). Other commonly used therapies include administration of supplemental oxygen, morphine, nitroglycerin, HMG coenzyme A reductase inhibitors (eg, statins; within 24 to 48 hours) and diuretics (if pulmonary edema without cardiogenic shock is evident). Glycoprotein IIb and IIIa inhibitors are commonly used in patients who receive PCI for acute STEMI. In addition, the literature supports the use of these agents in the ED in "high-risk" patients with unstable angina or NSTEMI, in conjunction with aspirin, heparin, and clopidogrel, who are scheduled to receive PCI (high-risk patients are defined as those patients with persistent chest pain, hemodynamic/rhythm instability, diabetes, acute/dynamic ECG changes, elevated cardiac marker serology). There is no evidence supporting the routine use of glucose-insulin-potassium (GIK) infusions or calcium channel blockers in patients with STEMI.

The definitive therapies for acute STEMI are either PCI—preferably with stent placement—or fibrinolytic therapy. Fibrinolytic therapy is universally available in most EDs, but has decreased efficacy in patients with delayed presentations (>12 hours) or with signs and symptoms of cardiogenic shock. Extensive evidence supports PCI with stent as superior to fibrinolysis with regard to the combined end-points of death, stroke, and reinfarction. However, PCI is limited to specialty centers; the best patient outcomes are seen in centers with high case volumes, with skilled personnel, and with cardiac surgery capabilities.

73. Answer: E[54]. Toxin-induced tachyarrhythmias are common complications following the use of cocaine and other sympathomimetic substances (eg, amphetamines). These tachyarrhythmias may deteriorate into ventricular tachycardia (VT) and ventricular fibrillation (VF), or may cause myocardial ischemia/infarction. The management for drug-induced VT and VF is not the same as for ischemia-induced VT and VF; some "standard" approaches to rhythm termination may cause harm. For toxin-induced monomorphic VT, lidocaine (a Vaughn-Williams type I_B antiarrhythmic) is probably the safest antiarrhythmic agent. Type I_A (eg, procainamide), type I_C, and type III antiarrhythmics (eg, sotalol, amiodarone) are fast sodium channel blockers, and may potentiate the effects of cocaine toxicity and worsen the dysrhythmia.

An acceptable alternative for the management of toxin-induced VT or VF is sodium bicarbonate. Sodium bicarbonate, as a hypertonic fluid with a high sodium load, counteracts the poisoning of fast sodium channels caused by cocaine. In addition, sodium bicarbonate administration alkalinizes the serum, and assists with the elimination of some toxins (eg, tricyclic antidepressants) which may have cardiotoxic effects similar to those described for cocaine. Patients with toxin-induced ventricular tachyarrhythmias may also require treatment with benzodiazepines as part of their overall management. Agents that should be avoided in patients with cocaine toxicity, in addition to those previously mentioned, include β-adrenergic antagonists.

74. Answer: E[55]. The findings pictured represent an acute IWMI. These are evident in leads II, III, and aVF, and most commonly result from thrombosis

of the right coronary artery (RCA) or one of its major branches (eg, posterior descending artery [PDA]). The RCA and PDA are responsible for supplying blood to the inferior portion of the intraventricular septum/wall in 85% of the population (this is known as right-sided "dominance"). In 15% of the population, blood supply to this area of the myocardium is derived either from a PDA which arises from a "dominant" left coronary artery or from a codominant pattern of coronary circulation (PDA from the RCA and branches from the left circumflex artery contribute equally to the inferior wall).

Management principles for uncomplicated IWMIs are the same as for other MIs.

Complications associated specifically with IWMIs are concomitant right ventricular infarction and dysrhythmia secondary to sinus and AV node dysfunction. A significant number of IWMIs ($\geq$50%) are associated with right ventricular extension. Patients with IWMI with right ventricular extension and hypotension have worse outcomes. Care should be taken to exclude the presence of right ventricular extension (by performing a right-sided ECG) in patients with IWMIs before use of pharmacotherapeutics that decrease preload (eg, nitroglycerin, morphine).

In the patient described in the question, vasospasm of the coronary artery caused by cocaine toxicity is the likely etiology for MI. However, patients with a history of chronic cocaine use are also known to be at risk of development of early atherosclerotic changes within the coronary circulation; a thromboembolic etiology for MI, therefore, is possible.

The use of β-adrenergic antagonists (even labetalol) is contraindicated in the patient with MI secondary to cocaine toxicity as it may worsen hypertension and decrease coronary perfusion (the mechanism is unopposed peripheral α stimulation that results from β-receptor blockade and leads to vasoconstriction.

Assuming no contraindications are present (eg, right ventricular infarction), nitroglycerin, benzodiazepines, and phentolamine (second-line agent) have been shown to decrease tachycardia, improve hypertension, and reverse cocaine-induced coronary vasoconstriction. PCA is "strongly" preferred over fibrinolysis therapy because of the increased risk of intracranial bleeding in cocaine abusers.

75. Answer: E[56]. Right ventricular (RV) infarction is a common complication (up to 50%) of IWMI, and, like IWMI, occurs most often in the context of

thrombosis to the RCA. RV infarction should be suspected in the patient with an IWMI who presents with hypotension without pulmonary edema or who develops findings consistent with right ventricular failure (eg, hypotension) after administration of pharmacotherapeutics which decrease preload. RV infarction is best diagnosed in the ED by performing a right-sided ECG. Any ST segment elevation in the fourth right-sided precordial lead (V4R) is sensitive for RV infarction. Management of patients with RV infarction should include standard therapies used in patients with MIs in other locations, with the caveat that agents which decrease preload (eg, nitroglycerin, morphine, ACE inhibitors) can make the patient hypotensive, and, therefore, should be avoided. The first-line intervention to correct hypotension seen with RV infarctions is to increase preload by administering boluses of isotonic fluids. Patients with IWMIs with RV extension and hypotension have considerably increased morbidity and mortality when compared with patients with isolated IWMIs. These patients should be considered for reperfusion therapies. Fibrinolytic therapies and PCI are both effective; PCI is preferred for patients in shock.

76. Answer: D[57,58]. The findings pictured in the ECG are consistent with Wolff-Parkinson-White syndrome (WPW). WPW syndrome occurs when impulses travel through an accessory pathway and bypass the normal AV conducting fibers. The most common accessory pathway seen in patients with WPW syndrome is the bundle of Kent. Under normal circumstances, impulses travel from the atria (usually originating in the sinus node) to the AV node, down the bundle of His, through the bundle branches, and finally to the Purkinje fibers imbedded in the ventricular myocardium. In WPW syndrome, the presence of the accessory pathway allows impulses that originate in the atria to be conducted through an alternate pathway. WPW classically produces a shortened PR interval and a "delta wave." The delta wave is a slurring upstroke from the PR segment to the beginning of the QRS complex. These findings result from conduction through the accessory pathway.

An impulse may initially bypass the AV node and travel in an antegrade manner down the accessory pathway. After an impulse depolarizes the ventricles, it then may travel in a retrograde manner up the bundle branches, the bundle of His, and the AV node, returning to the atria. When the impulse reaches the atria, they depolarize again, and a tachydysrhythmia is created. Continuous

antegrade movement of impulses down the accessory pathway and then up the intrinsic conduction pathways (in a retrograde fashion) sustains the tachydysrhythmia. This method of conduction is known as antidromic conduction (reversed conduction up the AV node).

Alternatively, an impulse may travel from the atria down the intrinsic conduction pathways (in an antegrade fashion through the AV node) to the ventricles. Once the ventricles are depolarized, the impulse may travel up the accessory pathway in a retrograde manner, returning to the atria. When the impulse reaches the atria, they depolarize again, and a tachydysrhythmia is created. Continuous antegrade movement of impulses down the intrinsic conduction pathways and then up the accessory pathway (in a retrograde manner) sustains the tachydysrhythmia. This method of conduction is known as orthodromic conduction. Tachydysrhythmias associated with orthodromic conduction are more common than antidromic conduction.

ECG findings for WPW depend on whether antidromic or orthodromic conduction mechanism is present. Orthodromic conduction usually manifests as a tachydysrhythmia with a **narrow** QRS complex (duration of <120 milliseconds). It may be impossible to distinguish the ECG of a patient with WPW syndrome and orthodromic conduction from a patient with supraventricular tachycardia from other etiologies. Antidromic conduction usually manifests as a tachydysrhythmia with a **wide** QRS complex (duration >120 milliseconds). The ECG may resemble ventricular tachycardia or supraventricular tachycardia with aberrancy.

Patients with WPW syndrome may present with rapid atrial fibrillation and wide QRS complexes. This usually occurs only in the context of antidromic conduction. The presence AF in association with WPW is significant; extremely rapid ventricular response, deterioration into ventricular fibrillation (VF), and cardiac arrest are well described in the literature.

Safe ED management of WPW depends on whether the QRS complex is narrow or wide (indicating orthodromic or antidromic conduction, respectively), and whether the patient is stable or unstable. Unstable patients should receive synchronized electrocardioversion. Stable patients with known WPW complicated by tachydysrhythmias with narrow QRS complexes may be treated with adenosine, procainamide, or amiodarone. Stable patients with known WPW complicated by tachydysrhythmias with wide QRS complexes may be treated with procainamide or amiodarone.

Medications with AV nodal blocking properties (eg, diltiazem, verapamil, digoxin, β-adrenergic antagonists, adenosine) promote antidromic conduction through the accessory pathway, and can produce extremely rapid tachydysrhythmias which may deteriorate into VF.

77. Answer: B[59,61]. A junctional rhythm occurs when the site of origin for cardiac depolarization is located within the AV junction. The junctional rhythm is differentiated from other dysrhythmias based on the rate, the absence of normal P wave positioning/morphology, and narrow QRS morphology. Most junctional rhythms produce a heart rate of 40 to 60 beats per minute. Junctional tachycardia may present as a narrow-complex tachycardia (QRS duration is <0.10 seconds) with a rate ranging from 120 to 200 beats per minute (usually not >130 beats per minute in most patients).

The presence and morphology of P waves is dependent upon the location within the AV junction where depolarization occurs. P waves are not visible ("buried" within the QRS complex) when atrial depolarization and ventricular depolarization occur contemporaneously, which happens when the site of depolarization is centrally located between the atria and the ventricles. When the site of depolarization within the AV junction is asymmetrically positioned between the atria and the ventricles, depolarization of the atria and the ventricles does not occur simultaneously, and P waves are more likely to be visible. The morphology and positioning of the P waves is variable: they may be normal or inverted (representing retrograde depolarization). P waves also may be found either before or after QRS complexes.

Causes for junctional rhythms include sick sinus syndrome, myocardial ischemia/infarction, inflammatory cardiac processes, increased vagal tone, therapeutic drug effect (eg, β-adrenergic antagonists), drug toxicity (eg, digoxin toxicity), and structural cardiac disease. Diagnosis is usually made on the basis of electrophysiologic testing. Treatment depends on the degree of instability (and rate), the severity of coexistent symptoms, and underlying cause for the dysrhythmia, and includes observation and expectant management, pharmacotherapy, cardioversion (for refractory tachycardias), or permanent pacemaker placement.

78. Answer: A[61,62]. Long QT syndrome (LQTS) is a hereditary disorder. Mutations of the genes coding for cardiac sodium, calcium, and/or potassium channels result in prolongation of ventricular depolarization. Prolongation of ventricular depolarization results in prolongation of the QT interval, and is associated with a high risk of ventricular dysrhythmia (R-on-T phenomenon) and sudden cardiac death.

Hereditary conditions causing LQTS are Romano-Ward syndrome and Jervell and Lang-Nielsen syndrome. Romano-Ward syndrome is the most common (90% of all cases) and is an autosomal dominant condition. Jervell and Lang-Nielsen syndrome is an autosomal recessive condition; in addition to causing QT prolongation, this syndrome causes congenital deafness.

LQTS manifests in otherwise healthy individuals, especially children and young adults. Although people with LQTS may be asymptomatic, most have a history of at least one episode of syncope or other symptoms (eg, dizziness, lightheadedness, palpitations) during their childhood. Symptoms are classically precipitated by exercise, swimming (sudden exposure to cold water), or psychological stress, although events have been reported during sleep. Many people with LQTS have a family history of the disorder or of sudden cardiac death. Diagnosis is most commonly made on the basis of ECG findings (QT prolongation >0.46 seconds), clinical presentation, and family history. Management includes administration of β-adrenergic antagonists and placement of an implantable cardioverter-defibrillator in high-risk patients.

Acquired causes of QT prolongation, which should be considered among the differential diagnoses include electrolyte disturbances (hypokalemia, hypomagnesemia, hypocalcemia), hypothyroidism, hypothermia, drugs/toxins (Ia/Ic antidysrhythmics, phenothiazines, antihistmines, cyclic antidepressants, organophosphates), starvation (suspect anorexia in cachetic adolescents), MI, and cerebrovascular events.

79. Answers: D, C[63,64]. The ECG is consistent with pericarditis. Pericarditis results from inflammation of the pericardium. The causes of pericarditis include idiopathic (most common), infection (viral, bacterial, and tuberculosis), inflammatory and autoimmune disorders (rheumatoid arthritis, SLE, sarcoidosis), neoplasm, post-MI pericarditis (Dressler syndrome), uremia, trauma, and postradiation therapy.

The most common presenting symptom of pericarditis is chest pain, retrosternal in location, and often described as sharp, stabbing, pleuritic, movement related, and positional (most severe with supine positioning, and relieved with upright positioning). Other signs and symptoms include fever, tachypnea, dyspnea, and a pericardial friction rub (often transient). If a pericardial effusion develops, signs and symptoms of cardiac tamponade may be evident (eg, anxiety, shortness of breath, chest pain, hypotension, muffled heart sounds, jugular venous distention, pulseless electrical activity, cardiac arrest).

Diagnosis is made on the basis of the history, physical examination, and ECG. The findings on ECG are described in stages. In the first stage, diffuse ST segment elevations with concave-upward ST segments are seen throughout all leads, and may persist for several days. PR segment depression may precede or accompany ST segment elevation. ST segments then return to the baseline as T waves initially flatten, then invert. Resolution is evident by normalization of the ECG. An echocardiogram is useful to determine whether a coexistent pericardial effusion is present, and whether it is causing a tamponade effect.

Management includes supportive care with NSAIDs and analgesics; corticosteroids, colchicine, antibiotics (when an infectious etiology is likely), and dialysis (for patients with uremic pericarditis). Other conditions in the differential diagnosis of ST segment elevation include acute MI, LBBB, left ventricular aneurysm, and early repolarization.

80. **Answers: D, B**[65,66]. The echocardiogram shows a pericardial effusion. The major complication of a pericardial effusion is cardiac tamponade. Cardiac tamponade results when the external pressure exerted by the pericardial fluid on the heart is greater than the internal intraventricular pressure. Because the right side of the heart has lower filling pressures than the left, when tamponade develops, the right ventricle collapses, left ventricular filling is diminished, and hypotension and cardiovascular collapse develop. Impending tamponade should be suspected when a pericardial effusion, and right ventricular diastolic collapse are visualized on echocardiography.

Causes of pericardial effusions and tamponade include trauma, infarction (secondary to postinfarct pericarditis or ventricular rupture), infection, autoimmune/inflammatory illness (eg, rheumatoid arthritis, SLE, sarcoidosis), neoplasm, uremia, and iatrogenic (after placement of inferior vena cava [IVC] filters).

Physical examination findings of a pericardial effusion (and pericardial tamponade) are variable, depending on the rate of pericardial fluid accumulation and the degree of hemodynamic compromise. Acutely, the pericardial sac is unable to accommodate even modest fluid accumulations (50 to 150 cc); however, much larger volumes of pericardial fluid are tolerable if fluid accumulation is slower. Pulsus paradoxus (an exaggeration of the normal decrease in systemic blood pressure with inspiration of >20 mm Hg), friction rubs, and narrowed pulse pressures are described. However, these findings are not universally present and may be difficult to appreciate. Kussmaul sign, the paradoxical increase in jugular venous distention and central venous pressure with inspiration, is a classic physical examination finding. The presence of all three components of Beck triad (hypotension, muffled heart sounds, and jugular venous distension) in a patient with cardiac tamponade is the exception, not the rule.

ECG findings include electrical alternans (beat-to-beat variability of the QRS complex amplitude caused by swaying of the heart within the fluid-filled pericardium), tachycardia, and right heart strain. ECG shows low voltage when there is a sizeable effusion. Chest radiographs show an enlarged "water bottle" heart. Patients with large pericardial effusions causing significant tamponade may present in cardiac arrest, with pulseless electrical activity or asystole as the predominant finding on ECG.

In dyspneic patients with pericardial effusions and cardiac tamponade, chest radiographs reveal clear lungs, whereas the chest radiographs of patients with CHF have findings consistent with fluid overload. Echocardiography may reveal a pericardial effusion and swaying of the heart within the fluid-filled pericardium. The classic sign of cardiac tamponade on echocardiography is diastolic right ventricular collapse. Increased caliber of the IVC during inspiration ("IVC plethora") is another ultrasonographic finding consistent with tamponade.

Management of the patient with cardiac tamponade includes intravenous fluid administration (to maintain preload) and pericardiocentesis (blind or ultrasonographically guided). A pericardial drain (single lumen catheter) or pericardial window represents definitive therapy to prevent tamponade from recurring. Nonsteroidal antiinflammatory medications and corticosteroids may have a role in management of inflammatory conditions that cause pericardial effusions. Intensification of dialysis is indicated in those patients with uremic pericardial effusions.

81. Answer: E[67]. Torsade de pointes ("twisting of the points") is a paroxysmal variant of ventricular tachycardia. ECG findings include

Ventricular rate >200 beats per minute
QRS structure has an undulating axis; the polarity of the complexes rotates around the baseline
Occurs in short episodes (usually <90 seconds, although sustained runs can be seen)

Torsade is associated with conditions that result in QT interval prolongation. When the QT is prolonged, the likelihood of the "R-on-T phenomenon" increases. The R-on-T phenomenon describes the effect of a premature ventricular impulse that interrupts the relative refractory period of ventricular repolarization. Depolarization of the ventricles during this vulnerable period can induce ventricular tachycardia, torsade de pointes, or ventricular fibrillation. Conditions and drugs which prolong the QT interval include cocaine, carbamazepine, cyclic antidepressants, phenothiazines, antihistamines, and Ia and Ic antiarrhythmics; hypomagnesemia, hypokalemia, and hypocalcemia; hypothyroidism; hypothermia; starvation; MI; and cerebrovascular events. **Unstable** torsade (without a pulse or blood pressure) requires immediate defibrillation. **Stable** torsade is classically treated with magnesium sulfate. Overdrive pacing, β-adrenergic antagonists, lidocaine, phenytoin, amiodarone, and isoproterenol have all been described as appropriate interventions (depending on the etiology of the torsade). Ia and Ic antidysrhythmics (eg, procainamide) are contraindicated because they prolong the QT interval, and may worsen the patient's clinical condition.

82. Answer: A[68,69]. The ultrasound image shows an AAA. The presence of an AAA on ultrasonography in the context of this patient's symptoms makes aneurismal leak a likely etiology for the patient's symptoms. The best test to assess whether there is a leak from an AAA is CT of the abdomen so long as the patient is stable enough to undergo CT scanning. In patients with other more likely diagnoses (eg, elderly patients with hematuria and symptoms of "renal colic"), ultrasonography or CT can be used to exclude an AAA. Because urolithiasis (renal colic) is the most common misdiagnosis made in the patient with a leaking AAA, it is important to consider imaging in patients with risk factors for development of an AAA (eg, hypertension) and with a clinical presentation that suggests "renal colic."

In the unstable patient with symptoms that indicate a ruptured AAA, bedside ultrasonography (if accessible quickly) to demonstrate the presence of an AAA is the best test in the ED. The patient should then be brought to the operating room for emergent repair. The normal aortic diameter is ≤2 cm. AAAs >4 cm in diameter are at risk of rupture; the larger the aneurysm is, the more likely it is to rupture.

Definitive management of leaking AAAs involves either emergency surgical repair via laparotomy using a synthetic graft or percutaneous endovascular stent-graft insertion. ED management involves early diagnosis, rapid surgical consultation, and fluid resuscitation. Patients with asymptomatic, nonleaking AAAs should be referred for elective surgical or endovascular repair if the AAA is ≥5 cm or if the aneurysm is saccular. Elective repairs on nonleaking AAAs, regardless of the method chosen, have significantly reduced mortality in comparison with with emergent repairs.

83. Answer: B[70]. The structure shown in this ultrasound is a gallbladder. The findings seen on this ultrasound (pericholecystic fluid, thickened gallbladder wall, gallstone within the neck of the gallbladder) in a patient with RUQ abdominal pain, fever, nausea, and vomiting are consistent with the diagnosis of acute cholecystitis.

The diagnostic imaging modalities used to establish the diagnosis of cholelithiasis and acute cholecystitis include ultrasonography, contrast-enhanced CT, and cholescintigraphy. Ultrasonography is the fastest, least invasive, and most readily available. It has almost 100% sensitivity for detecting gallstones when properly performed. The sensitivity of ultrasonography for acute cholecystitis ranges from ~75% to 90%. Findings of acute cholecystitis include gallbladder wall thickening (normal wall thickness is normally <3 mm), a sonographic Murphy sign (inspiratory arrest and tenderness of the gallbladder using the ultrasound transducer both to palpate and to visualize the gallbladder), and pericholecystic fluid. Of these, the sonographic Murphy sign is the most sensitive (~90%), but the specificity for acute cholecystitis is variable.

Cholescintigraphy involves the intravenous administration of a radioactive tracer. This tracer is taken up by the liver and excreted into the biliary tree. Visualization of tracer within the hepatic ducts, the cystic duct, the gallbladder, the common bile duct, and the small intestine is evidence of a patent biliary system. Nonvisualization of tracer within the gallbladder is consistent with cystic duct obstruction that results from cholelithiasis or cholecystitis. Nonvisualization of tracer within the small intestine is consistent with choledocholithiasis ("high-grade" obstruction of the biliary collecting system).

Contrast-enhanced CT is indicated in the ED workup of these patients when ultrasound is equivocal or when the clinical presentation suggests a different diagnosis. Contrast-enhanced CT may visualize gallstones, gallbladder wall thickening, and pericholecystic fluid; and it has the added benefit of allowing visualization of the pancreas, intestine, colon, liver, and other structures of the abdomen.

The management of acute cholecystitis includes antibiotics, analgesics, and cholecystectomy. Usually the cholecystectomy is deferred until several doses of antibiotics have been administered, unless the patient's initial presentation indicates peritonitis or if the patient deteriorates. The most serious complication of cholecystitis is gangrene of the gallbladder; this may be seen on ultrasound (although sensitivity is poor), but is usually well visualized on CT.

84. Answer: D[71]. This ultrasound image demonstrates hydronephrosis—a dilated renal pelvis with distortion of the renal pelvis (especially the calyces). The severity of the hydronephrosis is graded from 1 to 5 (most severe). In patients with renal colic, ultrasonography reveals hydronephrosis in 85% to 94% of patients. Ultrasonography, however, is not as good at detecting ureteral calculi (sensitivity of 64%). Ultrasonography is useful as an adjunct in the evaluation of a patient with new flank or back pain when the patient has a well-described history of urolithiasis, or has symptoms suggesting an alternative diagnosis (eg, appendicitis), assisting the emergency physician in deciding between a contrast-enhanced and noncontrast-enhanced CT.

Noncontrast-enhanced CT is the modality of choice in patients with flank and back pain from presumed renal colic. The sensitivity and specificity of noncontrast-enhanced CT for detecting ureteral calculi and ureteral obstruction are 97% and 98%, respectively. Noncontrast-enhanced CT is able to visualize other pathologies that mimic renal colic (eg, appendicitis, AAA).

This patient has hydronephrosis presumably from an obstructing ureteral calculus. Most renal stones are composed of calcium oxalate alone or in combination with calcium phosphate. Stones may also be comprised of oxalate, uric acid, cysteine, and magnesium-ammonium-phosphate (struvite). Struvite stones form almost exclusively in patients with urinary tract infections caused by urea-splitting

organisms such as *Proteus*, *Pseudomonas*, and *Staphylococcus*. The most important factor that relates to passage of a calculus though the genitourinary tract is its size; the critical size is 5 mm. Stones <5 mm are usually passed spontaneously. <5% of stones >8 mm will pass spontaneously; surgical intervention or extracorporeal shock-wave lithotripsy (ESWL) is required in these patients. Patients who require surgical intervention or ESWL, and patients with complicated urolithiasis (coexistent pyelonephritis, pregnancy, a solitary kidney, intractable pain, inability to tolerate oral intake) require admission.

85. Answer: E[72]. The finding on this ultrasound is significant for an intrauterine pregnancy. Visualizing an intrauterine pregnancy on transvaginal ultrasound is possible when the quantitative β-hCG is between 1000 and 1200 IU/L. In most patients, however, the serum β-hCG has to reach levels >1800 to 2000 IU/L before definitive evidence of intrauterine pregnancy is evident. An intrauterine pregnancy can, on average, be visualized ~1 or 2 weeks earlier using a transvaginal in comparison with a transabdominal approach.

The earliest sonographic sign of pregnancy is the gestational sac. Visualization of a yolk sac, however, is a more dependable sign of intrauterine pregnancy. Pseudosacs, collections of fluid within the uterine cavity surrounded by symmetrically thickened endometrium, may be interpreted as gestational and yolk sacs by inexperienced ultrasonographers (the pseudosac is a classic finding associated with an ectopic pregnancy). As pregnancy progresses, a fetal pole and, eventually, fetal heart motion can be detected. Fetal heart motion is visualized on or after the sixth-to-seventh week of gestation. Mean HCG levels at 7 to 10 weeks of gestation are 50,000 IU/L, with a range from 20,000 to 200,000 IU/L.

Ultrasound of a patient with an ectopic pregnancy will demonstrate an empty uterus despite a quantitative β-hCG that suggests a pregnancy of appropriate maturity for ultrasonographic visualization. As mentioned above, a pseudosac within the uterus may be visualized. In addition, an adnexal "mass," an adnexal gestational sac, or free fluid within the pelvis (with ruptured ectopic pregnancy) may also be seen.

The management of a pregnant patient within the early first trimester with ambiguous signs and symptoms for ectopic pregnancy at presentation and without sonographic evidence of either an intrauterine or ectopic pregnancy is challenging. If the patient presents early in pregnancy (β-hCG <1800 IU/L), and if the clinical presentation reveals no obvious cause for concern (eg, intractable pain, hemodynamic instability) the patient must be carefully followed in the outpatient setting; serial examinations by an obstetrician, in addition to serial β-hCG determinations, should be recommended. The rationale for serial β-hCG determinations is to determine if an early pregnancy is progressing normally (spontaneous abortion is also among the differential diagnoses). In the first trimester, the serum HCG level doubles every 48 to 72 hours) until ~8 to 11 weeks of gestation, when the levels begin to decline (usually with drops at 12 and at 16 weeks).

If the β-hCG level is >1800 IU/L, and ultrasound does not detect an intrauterine pregnancy, then ectopic pregnancy must be considered. The patient with a clinical presentation that reveals no obvious cause for concern (eg, intractable pain, hemodynamic instability) must be carefully followed if discharged. Frequent serial examinations by an obstetrician, as well as serial β-hCGs determinations, should be recommended. As mentioned, this patient could have had an unrecognized completed spontaneous abortion. Following serial β-hCGs is an appropriate management pathway if the clinical presentation makes spontaneous abortion more likely. The patient with β-hGC levels >1800 IU/L, without evidence of intrauterine pregnancy on ultrasound, but with a concerning clinical presentation requires, at a minimum, close inpatient observation and monitoring.

The management of confirmed ectopic pregnancy is based on the patient's hemodynamic stability, the size of the developing ectopic pregnancy, the location of implantation, and the length of gestation. Methotrexate can be administered to treat early, uncomplicated ectopic pregnancies in the hemodynamically stable patient. Other patients usually require surgical resection.

Determining whether anti-D immunoglobulin administration is indicated is a management consideration which should not be overlooked in the pregnant woman with vaginal bleeding. Current recommendations are to administer 50 mcg IM within 72 hours after termination of pregnancy ≥12 weeks. For termination that occurs >12 weeks, one 300 mcg dose is usually sufficient to prevent future complications.

86. **Answer: D**[73]. These ultrasonographic images demonstrate free fluid in the peritoneum. The FAST (focused acute sonography in trauma) examination has, in many centers, replaced the DPL as the initial procedure of choice to assess the hemodynamically unstable patient with blunt abdominal trauma in whom intraperitoneal hemorrhage is suspected. The advantages of FAST versus DPL are that FAST is less invasive, readily available, and easier to perform. In stable patients, FAST is often employed initially as the primary and secondary surveys are performed. FAST includes examination of the subxiphoid areas (heart and pericardium), the hepatorenal recess (Morison pouch), the splenorenal recess, and the bladder.

The presence of intraperitoneal hemorrhage in the context of blunt trauma is most frequently the result of injury to the spleen. The liver is the second most commonly injured organ. The small intestine is the most commonly injured hollow viscus. Hemodynamically unstable patients with free fluid on FAST examination require rapid ED stabilization. These patients should be moved expeditiously from the ED to a site where definitive care can be provided (usually, the operating room). In hemodynamically patients, the FAST examination is usually followed by contrast-enhanced CT, which is better at assessing the solid organs (kidneys, liver, spleen), diaphragm, and retroperitoneum.

87. **Answer: B**[74-76]. This ECG demonstrates an inferior **and** posterior wall MI. Patients who present with chest pain of <12 hours duration and with ECG evidence of acute MI are candidates for emergent fibrinolytic therapy, as long as no absolute contraindications exist. The currently accepted ECG criteria for fibrinolytic therapy includes: ST segment elevation of >1 mm in two or more contiguous precordial or adjacent limb leads, and new (or presumably new) LBBB.

The only MI which is not associated with ST segment elevations with conventional ECG lead placement is the posterior wall MI (PWMI). Using conventional lead placement, the ECG findings indicating PWMI include horizontal ST segment depressions in V1 and V2 in association with prominent R waves and an R/S-wave ratio of >1 in V2. By extending the precordial leads around the left lateral chest wall (leads V7 through V9) in patients with PWMIs can one visualize ST segment elevations ≥1 mm using conventional ECG.

Patients with acute PWMIs are eligible for and should receive fibrinolytic therapy or PCI even though, when using conventional leads, they do not seem to demonstrate the criteria necessary for these interventions. Fortunately, as in the ECG pictured, most PWMIs occur in conjunction with more-obvious ST-segment elevation IWMIs.

88. Answer: A[77]. Cyclic antidepressant toxicity classically produces prolongation of the QT interval and increased QRS duration. By blocking fast sodium channels, cyclic antidepressants prolong phase 0 of the cardiac myocyte action potential (depolarization). This quinidine-like effect results in an increased QRS duration >100 milliseconds. Increased QRS duration is associated with increased risk for seizures (30% of patients with QRS duration >100 milliseconds) and ventricular dysrhythmias (50% of patients with QRS duration >160 milliseconds). Additionally, cyclic antidepressants block potassium efflux during phase 3 of the cardiac myocyte action potential (repolarization); this blockade creates prolongation of the QT interval. Prolongation of the QT interval increases the chances of torsade de pointes, and ventricular dysrhythmias. Other ECG changes (include a right axis deviation of the terminal 40 milliseconds of the QRS (an R wave of >3 mm in aVR), PR interval prolongation, and Brugada syndrome-like waveforms (RBBB with ST segment elevations in V1 through V3).

Administration of intravenous sodium bicarbonate is indicated in the management of intraventricular conduction delays, other ECG changes, and dysrhythmias resulting from cyclic antidepressant poisoning. The sodium load provided with the administration of sodium bicarbonate corrects arrhythmias that result from sodium channel blockade in the context of cyclic antidepressant toxicity.

89. Answer: B[78-80]. Type 1 second-degree AV block (Mobitz I; Wenckebach) is a conduction disturbance which is often asymptomatic, transient, and occurs at the level of the AV node. Second-degree AV block is distinguished by its characteristic grouping of beats. With Mobitz I (Wenkebach), there is progressive lengthening of the PR interval until a sinus impulse is not conducted ("dropped"). In addition, the distance between the preceding R wave and the next P wave becomes shorter with consecutive beats until a sinus impulse is dropped. This gives the appearance of shortening of each consecutive R-R interval. This is known as "RP/PR reciprocity."

Type 1 second-degree AV block usually requires no immediate treatment if the heart rate and blood pressure are normal. However, a patient with syncope still requires admission, continuous telemetric monitoring, and further evaluation by a cardiologist to determine if the conduction abnormality found (the type I second-degree AV block) is an etiology for dysrhythmia resulting in syncope. Patients with dysrhythmias as the underlying etiologies for their episodes of syncope usually have the following risk factors: age >65 years; previous history of MI or CHF; structural cardiac disease, and abnormal ECG. Young patients (<45 years) with explainable mechanisms for syncope, without histories of CHF, MI, or structural heart disease, and without ECG changes, are candidates for discharge from the ED with outpatient referral and follow-up.

90. Answer: E[81]. Third-degree AV block represents a high-grade block of cardiac conduction, and indicates pathology at the level of the AV node, bundle of His, or bundle branches. No impulses are conducted between the atria and the ventricles. The initial treatment of a patient with bradycardia should focus on support of airway, breathing, and circulation while obtaining an ECG to define the rhythm. Identification of signs and symptoms that are associated with instability, and determination if unstable signs and symptoms are caused by the bradycardia are an important part of patient management. Unstable signs and symptoms include hypotension, chest pain, shortness of breath, acute altered mental status, CHF, seizures, syncope, or signs of shock. Patients with a symptomatic or unstable bradycardia that results from high-grade AV block require immediate cardiac pacing. Pacing may be performed transcutaneously or transvenously.

Patients with high-grade AV block often do not respond to atropine, although they may respond to dopamine or epinephrine infusions that are started as bridges to pacing. Atropine use for symptomatic bradycardia in the context of acute coronary syndromes may worsen ischemia. Patients with symptomatic bradycardia that results from calcium channel blocker or β-adrenergic antagonist overdose may show improvement with calcium or glucagon administration. Patients with symptomatic bradycardia resulting from cardiac glycoside toxicity (eg, digoxin) may require treatment with digoxin-antibody fragments; calcium administration in this setting should be avoided.

91. Answer: B[82]. Patients with symptomatic bradycardias resulting from cardiac glycoside toxicity (eg, digoxin) require treatment with digoxin-antibody fragments. The primary indication for treatment with digoxin-antibody fragments is hyperkalemia (serum potassium level >5.5 mEq L or ECG changes consistent with hyperkalemia), which is associated with an increased mortality risk. Elevated potassium may be treated with temporizing measures (eg, sodium bicarbonate, glucose/insulin, nebulized albuterol, sodium polystyrene sulfonate) until the digoxin-antibody fragments are available. Calcium administration in the setting of digoxin toxicity should be avoided based on reports in animal models showing potentiation of cardiac tetany and asystole ("stone heart").

Patients with digoxin toxicity and symptomatic bradycardia may not respond to other routinely used interventions, including atropine and pacing. Transcutaneous pacing should be avoided in the setting of digoxin toxicity, because lead insertion into the myocardium may provoke dysrhythmias in the more irritable, easily inducible myocardium (unless digoxin-antibody fragments have been given). The antiarrhythmics of choice for digoxin toxicity-associated ventricular dysrhythmias are phenytoin and lidocaine. There is no role for magnesium sulfate or procainamide in the management of digoxin toxicity.

92. Answer: A[83]. The image pictured demonstrates free fluid adjacent to the uterus (along the right side of the image). This finding, in a woman of childbearing age who presents to the ED with acute lower quadrant abdominal pain and unstable vital signs, is consistent with a ruptured ectopic pregnancy. Ruptured ectopic pregnancy must be presumed until it is definitively excluded. In a patient with a positive pregnancy test, the presence of an empty uterus, free fluid, a pseudosac, adnexal mass/gestational sac, or combinations of the above on transabdominal or transvaginal sonography are indicative of a ruptured ectopic pregnancy.

In the ED, aggressive resuscitative measures should be initiated, including isotonic crystalloid fluid boluses and blood transfusion. Emergent gynecologic consultation should be obtained, and the patient should undergo laparoscopy or laparotomy.

93. Answer: C[5,84]. The ECG pictured shows a RBBB. The criteria for RBBB are as follows:

QRS complex duration exceeds 120 milliseconds. Right precordial leads show prominent and notched R waves with rsr', rsR', or rSR' patterns. Leads I, aVL, and the left precordial leads demonstrate wide S waves that are longer in duration than the preceding R wave.

ST-T waves are discordant with the QRS complex, meaning that the T waves are opposite the major vector of the QRS complex. T waves are, therefore, inverted in the right precordial leads and upright in the left precordial leads and in leads I and aVL.

Blocks involving the anterior or posterior fascicles of the left bundle may coexist with RBBBs. These are termed fascicular blocks (or hemiblocks). Fascicular blocks involve either the left anterior or posterior fascicles. A left anterior fascicular block (LAFB) results in a small Q wave in leads I and one or more S waves in the inferior leads (S wave in lead III is most common). A left posterior fascicular block (LPFB) results in a small Q wave in lead III and S waves in lead I, avL, or both. A fascicular block in conjunction with a RBBB is called a bifascicular block. A LAFB with a RBBB is the most commonly seen bifascicular block. Bifascicular and trifascicular (AV nodal) blocks indicate significant cardiac conduction system disease.

RBBBs are common. Their appearance does not always represent acute structural or ischemic heart disease; in patients without overt heart disease, its presence does not have prognostic significance. However, when RBBBs are new, or when they are found in patients with a history of ischemic heart disease, their presence may suggest advanced conduction system disease. In these situations, RBBBs are often associated with complicated coronary artery disease and increased cardiovascular mortality.

Although not applicable to this question, the Brugada syndrome is well-described in the literature and is appropriate to mention here. The Brugada syndrome is a genetic disorder leading to cardiac ion channel dysfunction. The abnormalities in depolarization and repolarization result in an ECG with ST segment elevations in leads V1 through V3 and in aVR, associated with complete or incomplete RBBB and T wave inversions. The significance of these ECG changes is that they are associated with ventricular dysrhythmias, cardiac arrest, and sudden cardiac death.

REFERENCES

1. Aujesky, D, Auble, TE, Yealy, DM, et al: Prospective comparison of three validated prediction rules for prognosis in community-acquired pneumonia. *Am J Med.* 2005;118,384.

2. Fine MJ, Auble TE, Yealy DM, et al. A prediction rule to identify low-risk patients with community-acquired pneumonia, *N Engl J Med.* 1997;336:243.

3. Mandell LA, Wunderink RG, Anzueto A, et al: Infectious Diseases Society of America/American Thoracic Society Consensus Guidelines on the Management of Community-Acquired Pneumonia in Adults. *Clin Infect Dis.* 2007 Mar 1;44 Suppl 2:S27.

4. Marx JA, Hockberger RS, Walls RM, eds: *Rosen's Emergency Medicine: Concepts and Clinical Practice.* 6th ed. Philadephia: Mosby; 2006.

5. Paller, Mancini, Hurwitz : *Clinical Pediatric Dermatology.* 3rd ed. Philadelphia: WB Saunders; 2005.

6. Tintinalli JE, Kelen GD, Stapczynski JS: *Emergency Medicine: A Comprehensive Study Guide.* 6th ed. New York: McGraw-Hill; 2003.

7. Roberts JR, Hedges JR, eds: *Clinical Procedures in Emergency Medicine.* 4th ed. St. Louis, MO: Saunders; 2004.

8. Maisel A, Krishnaswamy P, Nowak RM, et al: Rapid measurement of B-type natriuretic peptide in the emergency diagnosis of heart failure. *N Engl J Med.* 2002;347:161.

9. Maisel A, Hollander JE, Guss D, et al: Primary results of the Rapid Emergency Department Heart Failure Outpatient Trial (REDHOT): a multicenter study of B-type natriuretic peptide levels, emergency department decision making, and outcomes in patients presenting with shortness of breath. *J Am Coll Cardiol.* 2004;44:1328.

10. Mueller C, Scholer A, Laule-Kilian K, et al: Use of B-type natriuretic peptide in the evaluation and management of acute dyspnea. *N Engl J Med.* 2004;350:647.

11. Sackner-Bernstein JD, Kowalski M, Fox M, Aaronson K: Short-term risk of death after treatment with nesiritide for decompensated heart failure: a pooled analysis of randomized controlled trials. *JAMA.* 2005;293:1900.

12. Flomenbaum NE, Goldfrank LR, Hoffman RS et al, eds: *Goldfrank's Toxicologic Emergencies.* 8th ed. New York: McGraw-Hill; 2006.

13. Mohsen AH, McKendrick M: Varicella pneumonia in adults. *Eur Respir J.* 2003 May;21(5):886.

14. Rodrigo GJ, Rodrigo C, Hall JB: Acute asthma in adults: a review. *Chest.* 2004;125(3):1081.

15. Taylor Z, Nolan CM, Blumberg HM: American Thoracic Society; Centers for Disease Control and Prevention; Infectious Diseases Society of America. Controlling tuberculosis in the United States. Recommendations from the American Thoracic Society, CDC, and the Infectious Diseases Society of America. *MMWR.* 2005;54:1.

16. Griffin XL, Pullinger R: Are diagnostic peritoneal lavage or focused abdominal sonography for trauma safe screening investigations for hemodynamically stable patients after blunt abdominal trauma? A review of the literature. *J Trauma.* 2007;62:779.

17. Rogers RL, McCormack R: Aortic disasters. *Emerg Med Clin North Am.* 2004;22:887.

18. Sanchez-Ross M, Anis A, Walia J, et al: Aortic rupture: comparison of three imaging modalities. *Emerg Radiol.* 2006; 13:31.

19. Scaglione M, Pinto A, Pinto F, et al: Role of contrast-enhanced helical CT in the evaluation of acute thoracic aortic injuries after blunt chest trauma. *Eur Radiol.* 2001; 11:2444.

20. Lappas JC, Reyes BL, Maglinte DD: Abdominal radiography findings in small-bowel obstruction: relevance to triage for additional diagnostic imaging. *AJR Am J Roentgenol.* 2001;176:167.

21. Miller G, Boman J, Shrier I, Gordon PH: Etiology of small bowel obstruction. *Am J Surg.* 2000;180:33.

22. Barkun A, Bardou M, Marshall JK, et al: Consensus recommendations for managing patients with nonvariceal upper gastrointestinal bleeding. *Ann Intern Med.* 2003;139:843-57.

23. Chen K, Varon J, Wenker OC, et al: Acute thoracic aortic dissection: the basics. *J Emerg Med.* 1997;15:859.

24. Donovan AJ, Berne TV, Donovan JA: Perforated duodenal ulcer: an alternative therapeutic plan. *Arch Surg.* 1998; 133:1166.

25. Hogg K, Brown G, Dunning J, et al: Diagnosis of pulmonary embolism with CT pulmonary angiography: a systematic review. *Emerg Med J.* 2006;23:172.

26. Practice Parameters Committee of the American College of Gastroenterology. Medical treatment of peptic ulcer disease. Practice guidelines. *JAMA.* 1996;275:622.

27. Bouyer J, et al: Risk factors for ectopic pregnancy: A comprehensive analysis based on a large case-control, population-based study in France. *Am J Epidemiol.* 2003; 157:185.

28. Gan SI, Beck PL: A new look at toxic megacolon: an update and review of incidence, etiology, pathogenesis, and management. *Am J Gastroenterol.* 2003; 98: 2363.

29. Cervenakov I, Fillo J, Mardiak J, et al: Speedy elimination of ureterolithiasis in lower part of ureters with the alpha 1-blocker tamsulosin. *Int Urol Nephrol.* 2002;34:25.

30. Dellabella M, Milanese G, Muzzonigro G: Efficacy of tamsulosin in the medical management of juxtavesical ureteral stones. *J Urol.* 2003;170:2202.

31. Dellabella M, Milanese G, Muzzonigro G: Randomized trial of the efficacy of tamsulosin, nifedipine and phloroglucinol in medical expulsive therapy for distal ureteral calculi. *J Urol.* 2005;174:167.

32. Ege G, Akman H, Kuzucu K, Yildiz S: Acute ureterolithiasis: incidence of secondary signs on unenhanced helical CT and influence on patient management. *Clin Radiol.* 2003;58:990.

33. Erturhan S, Erbagci A, Yagci F, et al: Comparative evaluation of efficacy of use of tamsulosin and/or tolterodine for medical treatment of distal ureteral stones. *Urology.* 2007; 69:633.

34. Healy KA, Ogan K: Nonsurgical management of urolithiasis: an overview of expulsive therapy. *J Endourol.* 2005; 19:759-67.

35. Labrecque M, Dostaler LP, Rousselle R, et al: Efficacy of nonsteroidal anti-inflammatory drugs in the treatment of acute renal colic. A meta-analysis. *Arch Intern Med.* 1994;154:1381.

36. Porpiglia F, Ghignone G, Fiori C, et al: Nifedipine versus tamsulosin for the management of lower ureteral stones. *J Urol.* 2004;172:568.

37. Segura JW, Preminger GM, Assimos DG, et al: Ureteral Stones Clinical Guidelines Panel summary report on the management of ureteral calculi. The American Urological Association. *J Urol.* 1997;158:1915.

38. Sowter SJ, Tolley DA: The management of ureteric colic. *Curr Opin Urol.* 2006;16:71.

39. Bhalla S, Menias CO, Heiken JP: CT of acute abdominal aortic disorders. *Radiol Clin N Am.* 2003;41:1153.

40. Ernst CB: Abdominal aortic aneurysm. *N Engl J Med.* 1993;328:1167.

41. Lederle FA, Simel DL: The rational clinical examination. Does this patient have abdominal aortic aneurysm? *JAMA.* 1999;281:77.

42. Canele ST, ed: *Campbell's Operative Orthopaedics.* 10th ed. St. Louis, MO: Mosby; 2003.

43. Neviaser RJ, Neviaser TJ, Neviaser JS: Anterior dislocation of the shoulder and rotator cuff rupture. *Clin Orthop.* 1993;291:103.

44. Zahiri CA, Zahiri H, Tehrany F: Anterior shoulder dislocation reduction technique—revisited. *Orthopedics.* 1997; 20:515.

45. Neviaser RJ, Neviaser TJ, Neviaser JS: Anterior dislocation of the shoulder and rotator cuff rupture. *Clin Orthop.* 1993; 291:103.

46. Zahiri CA, Zahiri H, Tehrany F: Anterior shoulder dislocation reduction technique—revisited. *Orthopedics.* 1997; 20:515.

47. Goldfarb CA, Yin Y, Gilula LA, et al: Wrist fractures: what the clinician wants to know. *Radiology.* 2001;219:11.

48. Seitz WH, Papandrea RF: Fractures and dislocations of the wrist. In: *Rockwood and Green's Fractures in Adults.* 5th ed. Phliadelphia: Lippincott, Williams & Wilkins; 2001:749.

49. Yealy DM, Delbridge TR: Dysrhythmias. In: Marx JA (editor): *Rosen's Emergency Medicine: Concepts and Clinical Practice,* 6th ed. Philadelphia: Mosby, 2006.

50. Yealy DM, Delbridge TR: Dysrhythmias. In: Marx JA: *Rosen's Emergency Medicine: Concepts and Clinical Practice,* 6th ed. Philadelphia: Mosby, 2006; 1218.

51. *Circulation.* 2005;112:IV-136-IV138.

52. Brady WJ, et al: Acute Coronary Syndromes. In: Marx JH: *Rosen's Emergency Medicine: Concepts and Clinical Practice,* 6th ed. Philadelphia: Mosby, 2006; 1167.

53. Sgarbossa EB, et al: ECG diagnosis of evolving acute myocardial infarction in the presence of left bundle branch block. *N Engl J Med.*1996;334:481. *Circulation.* 2005;112:IV97.

54. *Circulation.* 2005;112:IV126.

55. *Circulation.* 2005;112:IV-93-IV-103,IV-126-IV-131.

56. *Circulation.* 2005;112:IV-100.

57. Hemingway TJ, et al: *Wolff-Parkinson-White syndrome.* eMedicine Available at http://www.emedicine.com/ emerg/topic664.htm

58. *Circulation.* 2005;112:IV69.

59. Beinart SC: *Junctional rhythm.* eMedicine Available at http://www.emedicine.com/med/topic1212.htm

60. Yealy DM, Delbridge TR: Dysrhythmias. In: Marx JA: *Rosen's Emergency Medicine: Concepts and Clinical Practice,* 6th ed. Philadelphia: Mosby, 2006;1213.

61. Sovari AA: Long QT syndrome. eMedicine Available at http://www.emedicine.com/med/topic1983.htm

62. Yealy DM, Delbridge TR: Dysrhythmias. In: Marx JA: *Rosen's Emergency Medicine: Concepts and Clinical Practice,* 6th ed. Philadelphia: Mosby, 2006; 1237.

63. Jouriles N: Pericardial and myocardial disease. In: Marx JA:, *Rosen's Emergency Medicine: Concepts and Clinical Practice,* 6th ed. Philadelphia: Mosby, 2006; 1280.

64. Inaba AS: Cardiac disorders. In: Marx JA: *Rosen's Emergency Medicine: Concepts and Clinical Practice,* 6th ed. Philadelphia: Mosby, 2006; 2592.

65. Jouriles N: Pericardial and myocardial disease. In: Marx JA: *Rosen's Emergency Medicine: Concepts and Clinical Practice,* 6th ed. Philadelphia: Mosby, 2006; 1280.

66. Inaba AS. Cardiac disorders. In: Marx JA: *Rosen's Emergency Medicine: Concepts and Clinical Practice,* 6th ed. Philadelphia: Mosby, 2006; 2592.

67. Yealy DM, Delbridge TR: Dysrhythmias. In: Marx, JA: *Rosen's Emergency Medicine: Concepts and Clinical Practice,* 6th ed. Philadelphia: Mosby, 2006; 1242.

68. Bessen HA: Abdominal aortic aneurysm. In: Marx DA: *Rosen's Emergency Medicine: Concepts and Clinical Practice,* 6th ed. Philadelphia: Mosby, 2006; 1330.

69. Dillon M, Cardwell C, Blair PH, et al: Endovascular treatment for ruptured abdominal aortic aneurysm. Cochrane Collaboration Review. No. CD005261. DOI: 10.1002/14651858.CD005261.pub2.

70. Guss DA: Liver and biliary tract. In: Marx DA: *Rosen's Emergency Medicine: Concepts and Clinical Practice,* 6th ed. Philadelphia: Mosby, 2006; 1418.

71. Kahler J, Harwood-Nuss A: Selected urologic problems. In: Marx JA: *Rosen's Emergency Medicine: Concepts and Clinical Practice,* 6th ed. Philadelphia: Mosby, 2006; 1586.

72. Houry DE, Abbott, JT: Acute complications of pregnancy. In: Marx JA: *Rosen's Emergency Medicine: Concepts and Clinical Practice,* 6th ed. Philadelphia: Mosby, 2006; 2739.

73. Isenhour J: Abdominal trauma. In: Marx JA: *Rosen's Emergency Medicine: Concepts and Clinical Practice,* 6th ed. Philadelphia: Mosby, 2006; 489.

74. *Circulation.* 2005;112:IV89.

75. Brady W, Erling B, Pollack M, et al: Electrocardiographic manifestations: acute posterior wall myocardial infarction. *J Emerg Med.* 2001;20:391.

76. Van Gorselen EOF, et al: Posterior myocardial infarction: the dark side of the moon. *Neth Heart J.* 2007;15(1):16.

77. Bilden EF, Walter FG: Antidepressants. In: Marx JA: *Rosen's Emergency Medicine: Concepts and Clinical Practice,* 6th ed. Philadelphia: Mosby, 2006; 2352.

78. Yealy DM, Delbridge TR: Dysrhythmias. In: Marx DA: *Rosen's Emergency Medicine: Concepts and Clinical Practice,* 6th ed. Philadelphia: Mosby, 2006; 1219.

79. *Circulation.* 2005;112:IV67.

80. Sarasin FP, et al: A risk score to predict arrhythmias in patients with unexplained syncope. *Acad Emerg Med.* 2003; 10:1312.

81. *Circulation.* 2005;112:IV67.

82. Roberts DJ: Cardiovascular drugs. In: Marx DA, *Rosen's Emergency Medicine: Concepts and Clinical Practice,* 6th ed. Philadelphia: Mosby, 2006; 2368.

83. Houry DE, Abbott, JT: Acute complications of pregnancy. In: Marx JA, *Rosen's Emergency Medicine: Concepts and Clinical Practice,* 6th ed. Philadelphia: Mosby, 2006; 2739.

84. Mirvis DM, Goldberger AL: Electrocardiography. In: *Braunwald's Heart Disease: A Textbook of Cardiovascular Mediicne,* 7th ed. Philadelphia: Saunders, 2005.

INDEX

Note: Page numbers followed by *f* or *t* indicate figures or tables, respectively.